Contents

Companion website

A companion website is available at:

www.lecturenoteseries.com/emergencymed

featuring a selection of MCQs on common pitfalls in emergency medicine.

Emergency Medicine
Lecture Notes

Chris Moulton

Consultant in Emergency Medicine
Emergency Department
Royal Bolton Hospital
Bolton, UK

David Yates

Emeritus Professor of Emergency Medicine
University of Manchester
Salford Royal Hospital
Salford, UK

Fourth edition

WILEY-BLACKWELL

A John Wiley & Sons, Ltd., Publication

This edition first published 2012 © 2012 by Blackwell Publishing Ltd

Blackwell Publishing was acquired by John Wiley & Sons in February 2007. Blackwell's publishing program has been merged with Wiley's global Scientific, Technical and Medical business to form Wiley-Blackwell.

Registered office: John Wiley & Sons, Ltd, The Atrium, Southern Gate, Chichester, West Sussex, PO19 8SQ, UK

Editorial offices: 9600 Garsington Road, Oxford, OX4 2DQ, UK
The Atrium, Southern Gate, Chichester, West Sussex, PO19 8SQ, UK
111 River Street, Hoboken, NJ 07030-5774, USA

For details of our global editorial offices, for customer services and for information about how to apply for permission to reuse the copyright material in this book please see our website at www.wiley.com/wiley-blackwell.

The right of the author to be identified as the author of this work has been asserted in accordance with the UK Copyright, Designs and Patents Act 1988.

First published 1985
Second edition 1999
Third edition 2006.

Library of Congress Cataloging-in-Publication Data
Moulton, Chris.
   Lecture notes. Emergency medicine / Chris Moulton, David Yates. – 4th ed.
      p. ; cm.
   Emergency medicine
   Includes bibliographical references and index.
   ISBN 978-1-4443-3666-5 (pbk. : alk. paper)
   I. Yates, David W.   II. Title.   III. Title: Emergency medicine.
   [DNLM: 1. Emergencies.   2. Emergency Medicine–methods.   3. Emergency Treatment.   WB 105]
   616.02'5–dc23
                                    2012007481

Cover design by Grounded Design

A catalogue record for this book is available from the British Library.

Wiley also publishes its books in a variety of electronic formats. Some content that appears in print may not be available in electronic books.

Set in 8/10.5 pt Utopia by Toppan Best-set Premedia Limited
Printed and bound in Malaysia by Vivar Printing Sdn Bhd

1   2012

Preface to the fourth edition

The intervals between editions of this text are getting shorter, perhaps reflecting the increasing speed of change in medicine in general and emergency medicine in particular. We have introduced new material on emerging topics and updated information on established topics and now support this with a bank of multiple-choice questions (MCQs) available online. The MCQs are supplemented by short explanations to reinforce your understanding.

The original layout has been retained – providing immediately accessible didactic advice supported by evidence-based rationale. The latter is now firmly established in the practice of the specialty, vindicating the aspiration in our first preface that 'future developments must ensure that the scientific method is woven into the fabric of the department'.

There is an increasing tendency for more professionals to be exposed to the emergency department for shorter periods of time and, to many, the sometimes deceptive lure of the internet as a source of immediate knowledge seems to be all-satisfying. We hope that you will agree that, although search engines can reinforce a book, they can never replace it. Using both, you will gain knowledge and understanding. Your patients will then be treated by the experienced rather than be used by you to gain experience.

We are very grateful to Anne Bassett whose help improved the quality of this book.

Chris Moulton and David Yates, 2012

Preface to the second edition

Emergency physicians work in an environment where measured interrogation is a luxury, where life-saving skills can be required urgently and where the art of rapid and effective communication is essential. Add to this list the expectation that the doctor will have an encyclopaedic knowledge of the emergency aspects of every medical condition -and not a few social crises – and it is not surprising that most medical students and young doctors approach the emergency department with an excitement that is tinged with anxiety.

This book is designed, in its approach, layout and content, to address these fears. Information is presented in an order that is relevant to the enquirer. It is demand led. Pathophysiology and relevant explanations follow. The reader learns how to deal with the emergency and then reads the background to the crisis and how, perhaps, it could have been avoided. This link with prevention is an increasingly emphasised part of emergency medicine, together with its concern to blur the boundaries between hospital and community care. Our primary aim has been to equip the reader with the knowledge to deal with crises, but we hope that we have shared, in these pages, our concern to ensure that doctors are also trained to try to avoid them.

Professor AD Redmond was the co-author of the first edition of this work, with Professor Yates. Although the book has been completely rewritten we have retained all the innovations that were so successfully introduced in *Lecture Notes on Accident and Emergency Medicine* in 1985. Professor Redmond has provided valuable advice on the development of this new edition and it is a pleasure to record our appreciation of this support and encouragement.

The authors are very grateful for the support of their families, whose accidents and emergencies were neglected during the writing of this book.

Chris Moulton and David Yates
Manchester, UK, 1999

Preface to the first edition

Our aim has been to cover all aspects of the work of a doctor in a busy accident and emergency department. Much of the text should be of interest to medical students during their clinical studies, but we hope that the book will be of special value to doctors studying for postgraduate diplomas.

Clearly some restriction must be placed on our definition of accident and emergency work unless we are to be overwhelmed, both here as authors and in our departments as casualty officers. These lecture notes have not been conceived as comprehensive treatises on the management of the many topics discussed – for only some aspects of most diseases and injuries are germane to the accident and emergency department. But it is precisely these aspects that are often inadequately covered in the standard texts. This book is based on our daily experience of the plethora of conditions presenting to what is inevitably an unstructured environment.

Sections devoted to 'Urgent action' are designed to facilitate the book's use during emergencies. The remaining text continues this rather didactic format but is supported by background material, which attempts to justify our dogma. It is, however, not always enough to state that the advice given here has worked in practice (but it has!). Emergency medicine, like all other branches of medicine, must be based on sound scientific principles. A significant recent development has been the acceptance that emergencies are better treated by the experienced than used to gain experience. Future developments must ensure that the scientific method is woven into the fabric of the department.

The academic base for accident and emergency medicine in Manchester has been created by the foresight and hard work of three men. We wish to record our thanks to Professor MH Irving, Dr GS Laing and Professor HB Stoner who have given so much to the specialty in its early days and who have supported us during the preparation of this book. The doctors, nurses, clerical staff and patients of Salford and Stockport have also given us invaluable help. Their encouragement has been greatly appreciated. Jackie Fortin typed some of the preparatory work and Julie Rostron exercised great skill and patience in compiling the manuscript.

Veronica Yates responded to our vague requests for pictures with precise illustrations, and our publishers displayed remarkable tolerance during a long gestation.

DW Yates and AD Redmond,
August 1984

What every emergency physician must know

People from many different backgrounds, with an enormous variety of problems, present to an emergency department (ED) both by day and by night. Fortunately, certain basic principles are applicable to the care of them all.

WHAT TO DO IN AN EMERGENCY

In all cases, swift and accurate assessment must immediately lead to appropriate action:

Cardiac arrest → p. 150.
Children → p. 329.

A – Airway

The airway may be:

- patent, partially obstructed or completely obstructed (this results from physical obstruction or loss of muscle tone)
- adequately protected or at risk (this depends on the protective reflexes of the airway).

Check for responsiveness

Is the patient alert and responsive to questions? A verbal reply confirms that there is:

- a maintained and protected airway
- temporarily adequate breathing and circulation
- cerebral functioning.

If responsive, then the patient will usually be able to elaborate on the cause of the sudden deterioration that has brought him or her to an ED.

Failure to respond indicates a significantly lowered level of consciousness and therefore an airway that may be obstructed and is definitely at risk. There may be a need for airway-opening manoeuvres and action to protect the airway.

Look, listen and feel for breathing

The absence of breath sounds indicates the need to attempt airway-opening manoeuvres (see below) and if unsuccessful to consider the possibility of a foreign body obstruction.

> Foreign body obstruction may initially present as a distressed, very agitated, cyanosed patient – 'choking'.

Cardiorespiratory arrest → p. 150.
Choking → p. 196.
Respiratory arrest → p. 199.

If breathing is present then do the following.

Look for the signs of partial upper airway obstruction

- *Snoring*: the familiar sound of obstruction caused by the soft tissues of the mouth and pharynx. Often it accompanies the reduced muscle tone of a lowered level of consciousness.
- *Rattling or gurgling*: the sound of fluids in the upper airway.
- *Stridor*: a harsh, 'crowing' noise, which is heard best in inspiration. It is thus different from

Emergency Medicine Lecture Notes, Fourth Edition. Chris Moulton and David Yates.
© 2012 Blackwell Publishing Ltd. Published 2012 by Blackwell Publishing Ltd.

wheezing, which is usually loudest in expiration. Stridor suggests obstruction at the level of the larynx and upper trachea. General illness and temperature usually indicate an infection causing swelling. Obstruction by a foreign body is the other main cause.

> In cases of suspected supraglottic swelling, examination or instrumentation of the throat should not be carried out for fear of causing complete obstruction.

- *Drooling*: the inability to swallow saliva. It suggests blockage at the back of the throat.
- *Hoarseness*: gross voice change. This suggests obstruction at the level of the larynx.

> Cyanosis and reduced haemoglobin saturation readings on a pulse oximeter are very late signs of airway obstruction.

Allergic reactions → p. 299.
Laryngotracheal obstruction → p. 196.
Surgical airways → p. 22.

> Assess the need for cervical spine protection before any airway intervention.

Clearance and maintenance of the airway

A patent airway is a prerequisite for life; a blocked airway is a common harbinger of death in emergency situations. There are two main ways in which the airway becomes blocked.

1 **Depressed level of consciousness:** most common cause. The tone of the muscles controlling the patency of the mouth and the pharynx is under neural control, in much the same way as the activity of the other striated muscles of the body. When this control is lost, the soft tissues around the airway prolapse and fail to maintain patency (simplistically, the tongue falls back).

This is overcome by:

- tightening these tissues (chin-lift manoeuvre)
- pushing the jaw and the hyoid bone and their attached soft tissues forward (jaw-thrust manoeuvre)
- putting an artificial airway down the anatomical airway (oro- or nasopharyngeal airways, endotracheal tubes, laryngeal masks, etc. → *Figure 1.1*).

2 **Physical obstruction:** many things can do this (direct trauma, external or intramural mass, etc.)

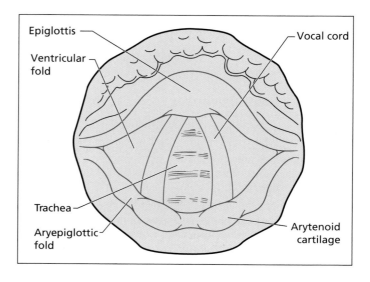

Figure 1.1 Visualisation of the larynx.

Epiglottis — Vocal cord
Ventricular fold
Trachea
Aryepiglottic fold — Arytenoid cartilage

However, in emergency practice, there is usually either something in the airway (vomitus, blood or foreign body) or there is swelling in the wall of the airway (oedema, haematoma, etc.).

This is overcome by:

- removing the cause of the obstruction (suction, manual removal or choking manoeuvres)
- passing an artificial airway (as detailed above) past the obstruction
- reducing the swelling with vasoconstrictor drugs (adrenaline)
- bypassing the obstruction with a surgical airway.

Protection of the airway

The airway is normally kept clear of foreign matter by the gag, cough and laryngeal reflexes. These may be attenuated by specific palsies, the effects of drugs or a generalised depression of conscious level. They may also be impaired at the extremes of age and in states of general debilitation. Special vigilance is required in all such situations; the recovery position should be used whenever possible.

Paradoxically, these same reflexes may make advanced airway care extremely difficult in situations where they are not completely absent. At such times, the airway should be managed by a person skilled in both its assessment and the use of sedating and paralysing drugs.

> Over 10% of normal individuals have no gag reflex.

Laryngospasm, bleeding, vomiting and consequent hypoxia can result from ill-judged attempts at intubation. It should be noted that the absence of the gag reflex is not a good predictor of the need for (or the ease of) endotracheal intubation.

> In a patient with a reduced level of consciousness, the airway must be assumed to be at risk until proved otherwise.

On-going protection of the airway requires continual vigilance. The following are also essential:

- The recovery position uses gravity, both to drain fluid matter away from the airway and to allow the soft tissues to be positioned in such a way that they do not cause obstruction. Once the airway is clear, this position can be used to both maintain and protect the airway.
- A high-flow suction catheter must always be near the patient's head.
- The patient's trolley must be capable of tilting 'head down' so as to drain vomitus out of the airway.
- If endotracheal intubation is attempted, the airway must be protected by the manoeuvre known as cricoid pressure throughout the period of instrumentation. Pressure is applied to the front of the patient's cricoid cartilage by an assistant using the thumb and two fingers. This compresses the oesophagus against the cervical spine and thus prevents the passive regurgitation of gastric contents. The airway is vulnerable from the start of induced paralysis until the cuff is inflated on a correctly positioned endotracheal tube.

Protection of the cervical spine

If the patient has an injury to the cervical spine, there is a risk of damage to the spinal cord during the procedures needed to maintain the airway. Because of the terrible outcome of such damage, it is mandatory to protect the neck immediately in patients who are:

1 unresponsive with a history of trauma or no clear history
2 suffering from multiple trauma
3 difficult to assess
4 showing any symptoms or signs that might be attributable to the cervical spine.

Adequate protection of the potentially unstable cervical spine consists of a rigid collar and either a purpose-made cervical immobiliser or sandbags and tape.

Exclusion of cervical spine injury → p. 55.

B – Breathing

Breathing is the means by which oxygen is delivered to the alveoli and thus made available to the circulating red cells. At the same time carbon dioxide (CO_2) is eliminated.

Look for

- *Difficulty in talking*
- *Abnormal respiratory rate*: usually fast, laboured breathing. Very slow respiratory rates may occur just before respiratory arrest or as a consequence of poisoning with narcotic drugs, e.g. methadone
- *Nasal flaring and use of shoulder and neck muscles.*

- *Paradoxical respiration*: a see-sawing movement of the chest and abdomen, which indicates obstruction of either the upper or lower airways or fatigue of the diaphragm.
- *In children, recession of the chest wall*: indrawing of the elastic tissues caused by increased respiratory effort.

All the above suggest that the patient is struggling to achieve normal respiration. Failure to oxygenate the blood adequately and hence the tissues is shown by:

- *Tachycardia* – the nervous system has detected hypoxia and is stimulating the heart
- *Pallor and sweating* – caused by sympathetic stimulation
- *Cyanosis* – a late sign
- *Irritability, confusion or reduced responsiveness* – the brain is short of oxygen. This is an extremely worrying sign
- *A low SaO_2 (<94%)* – pulse oximetry should be established as soon as possible
- *Unequal, diminished or abnormal breath sounds*
- *Hyperresonance or dullness to percussion*
- *Displacement of the trachea or apex beat*
- *A flail segment*

Allergic reactions → p. 299.
Chest decompression and drainage → p. 74.
Chest injuries → p. 72.
Respiratory distress → p. 196.

Oxygen therapy

The common denominator of all life-threatening illness, regardless of cause, is a failure to deliver adequate amounts of oxygen to the tissues. In normal circumstances, the oxygen content of atmospheric air (21%) is perfectly adequate but when the mechanisms for breathing are diseased or traumatised supplemental oxygen should be given. The physiological compensatory mechanisms for hypoxia and hypovolaemia all consume oxygen themselves; the immediate administration of supplemental oxygen may maintain these reflexes while more definitive measures are put in place. There are really only two main types of oxygen therapy:

1 High-concentration oxygen (40–100%)
2 Low-concentration oxygen (24–30%).

The dangers of high-concentration therapy are known to every medical student. The patient with a chronically raised blood CO_2 level may depend on a hypoxic drive to stimulate breathing – give him or her oxygen and the breathing slows, CO_2 levels rise even

higher and the patient becomes comatose with CO_2 narcosis. In practice, these patients are a small group in whom the speed of onset of symptoms can be used to determine treatment (→ *pp. 199 and 205*).

> Oxygen therapy should be prescribed and used carefully, like any other therapeutic intervention. Effectiveness of treatment should be guided by pulse oximetry → *Box 1.1*.

Hypoxia is a swift killer and so patients in the resuscitation room invariably require a high concentration of oxygen. The use of a mask that has a reservoir bag improves the effectiveness of oxygen delivery (to perhaps 60–80%) and should be standard. (The reservoir bag is needed because a patient's inspiratory flow is always greater than the 15 L/min maximum flow from the oxygen supply.) Blood gases must be obtained at an early stage to monitor the effect of supplemental oxygen. If improvement is not satisfactory, then ventilation may be needed. Continuous positive airway pressure (CPAP) is another method of increasing oxygenation.

Mechanical ventilation

This should always be considered when:

- the patient cannot maintain a clear airway
- oxygen enrichment of the inspired gases fails to prevent the signs of cerebral hypoxia
- CO_2 narcosis is present
- there has been a successful but prolonged resuscitation from cardiac arrest
- the patient is multiply injured
- the patient has a severe chest injury (particularly multiple rib fractures and/or flail segments)
- the patient is to be transferred and there is a risk of severe deterioration en route.

The emergency induction of anaesthesia for the purpose of intubation and ventilation in a hypoxic patient is a difficult and demanding task. It requires considerable anaesthetic skills.

> A pneumothorax is more likely to tension in a ventilated patient. Chest drains must be inserted before ventilating patients with chest injuries.

Box 1.1 Summary of the BTS Guideline for Emergency Oxygen Use in Adult Patients (British Thoracic Society Emergency Oxygen Guideline Group 2008)

Oxygen is a treatment for hypoxaemia, not breathlessness. Oxygen has not been shown to have any effect on the sensation of breathlessness in non-hypoxaemic patients. The essence of this guideline can be summarised simply as a requirement for oxygen to be prescribed according to a target saturation range and for those who administer oxygen therapy to monitor the patient and keep within that target saturation range.

The guideline recommends aiming to achieve normal or near-normal oxygen saturation for all acutely ill patients apart from those at risk of hypercapnic respiratory failure or those receiving terminal palliative care. The recommended target saturation range for acutely ill patients not at risk of hypercapnic respiratory failure is 94–98%. However, some normal individuals, especially people aged over 70 years, may have oxygen saturation measurements below 94% and still do not require oxygen therapy when clinically stable. For most patients with known chronic obstructive pulmonary disease (COPD) or other known risk factors for hypercapnic respiratory failure (e.g. morbid obesity, chest wall deformities or neuromuscular disorders), a target saturation range of 88–92% is recommended pending the availability of blood gas results.

Supplementary oxygen therapy is required for all acutely hypoxaemic patients and for many other patients who are at risk of hypoxaemia, including patients with major trauma and shock. Most acutely breathless patients will require supplementary oxygen therapy, but there are some conditions such as acute hyperventilation or diabetic ketoacidosis in which an apparently breathless patient will not benefit from oxygen therapy. Conversely, there are some other clinical situations such as carbon monoxide poisoning where a patient may benefit from oxygen therapy despite a lack of hypoxaemia or breathlessness because carbon monoxide binds more avidly than oxygen to the haemoglobin molecule. Similarly, high-concentration inhaled oxygen can increase the rate of reabsorption of gas from a pneumothorax by up to fourfold. For this reason, the British Thoracic Society (BTS) guideline on the management of pneumothorax recommends the use of high-concentration oxygen (by reservoir mask) in all non-COPD patients who require hospital admission for observation due to a moderate-sized pneumothorax that does not require drainage.

C – Circulation

Check for a central pulse (over 5 seconds)

The absence of a central pulse (*or a rate of <60 beats/ min in infants*) indicates the need to follow procedures for cardiorespiratory arrest:

Arrest rhythms:
Asystole → p. 150.
Pulseless electrical activity (PEA) or electromechanical dissociation (EMD) → p. 151.
Ventricular fibrillation (VF) → p. 150.

Look for

- *Pallor and coolness of the skin* – the body diverts blood away from the skin when there are circulatory problems and these signs are thus very useful indicators of shock.

- *Pallor and sweating* – signs of gross sympathetic disturbance.
- *Active bleeding or melaena*
- *A fast or slow heart rate* – fast heart rates usually mean that either there is a cardiac arrhythmia or more commonly the sympathetic nervous system has detected a problem with the body (such as hypoxia, hypoglycaemia, pain or fear) and is 'instructing' the heart to beat faster. A slow heart rate usually means that something is wrong with the heart itself. The worst cause of this is severe hypoxia (or hypovolaemia) and, in this case, it means that terminal bradycardia and asystole are only seconds away.
- *Abnormal systolic blood pressure*
- *A raised capillary refill time* – it should be less than 2 s if the circulation is satisfactory. However, peripheral shutdown in a cold, wet patient can easily produce a prolonged refill time.
- *Absent or quiet heart sounds and raised jugular venous pulse (JVP)* – suggestive of tamponade if

accompanied by hypotension and tachycardia; JVP will not be raised if there is also hypovolaemia.

- *A precordial wound*
- *An abnormal electrocardiogram (ECG) trace on the monitor*
- *Signs of left ventricular failure* (dyspnoea, gallop rhythm and crepitations)
- *Signs of abdominal, pelvic or occult bleeding* (may need per rectum examination and a nasogastric tube or ultrasound scan)
- *Signs of dehydration* (especially in children)
- *Purpura* (meningococcal septicaemia)

Inadequate circulation will reduce tissue oxygenation and thus may also cause:

- a raised respiratory rate
- altered mental status.

Bolus fluid therapy should be calculated at 20 mL/kg and repeated as necessary after further assessment. (Reduced to 10 mL/kg for patients with bleeding after trauma in hospital and no more than 5 mL/kg for patients with trauma in the prehospital setting → *p. 7*.)

Abdominal bleeding → *pp. 81 and 308.*
Allergic reactions → *p. 299.*
Anaphylaxis → *p. 299.*
Blood transfusion → *p. 25.*
Cardiac arrhythmias → *p. 164.*
Cardiac failure → *pp. 208 and 238.*
Cardiac tamponade → *pp. 78 and 238.*
Emergency thoracotomy → *p. 80.*
Pelvic bleeding → *p. 84.*
Renal effects of shock → *p. 247.*
Shock → *p. 24.*

Cardiac function

The stroke volume is the amount of blood ejected from the heart with each beat. It is determined by the left ventricular filling pressure, myocardial contractility and systemic vascular resistance. The product of heart rate and stroke volume is the cardiac output – the most important parameter of cardiac function. (Cardiac index is cardiac output divided by body surface area.) An increase in heart rate will directly increase the cardiac output and is the earliest cardiac response to hypoxia. However, the faster the heart beats the less time there is for it to fill and, eventually, a rise in heart rate will no longer be matched by a rise in cardiac output.

Myocardial function is compromised at high pulse rates because coronary blood flow occurs chiefly in diastole. When the heart rate rises above about 130 in an adult, the filling time is so reduced that cardiac output will actually fall.

Pulse and blood pressure

The autonomic response to hypovolaemia is complex. Rapid blood loss produces a reflex bradycardia, but, when associated with tissue damage, it produces the more familiar tachycardia. Systolic blood pressure is the product of the cardiac output and the systemic vascular resistance. A high catecholamine response to hypoxia and hypovolaemia will produce a high systemic vascular resistance. This will maintain a 'normal' blood pressure in the presence of a falling cardiac output.

Knowledge of the systemic blood pressure provides only very limited information about cardiac function and is a very late indicator of haemodynamic instability.

Blood pressure when measured by a cuff depends on the production of Korotkoff's sounds by turbulent flow in the artery. When systemic vascular resistance is high and flow through the artery is relatively low (e.g. in the immediate aftermath of cardiac arrest), these sounds may not be heard easily, even when the mean arterial pressure is good. Great care must be taken when deciding if such patients are beyond salvage or have pulseless electrical activity.

Maintenance of systemic vascular resistance is a vital response to hypovolaemia and hypoxia. (Skin pallor reflects this early on but is an imprecise clinical sign.) Similar to other compensatory mechanisms to hypoxia, this vasomotor response consumes oxygen and will eventually fail.

Measurements of pulse and blood pressure are very poor indicators of haemodynamic function in critically ill patients. Central venous pressure may not reflect the functioning of the left side of the heart and is thus of limited use in the assessment of overall cardiac performance. Indwelling pulmonary artery flotation and systemic arterial catheters will provide much more useful information and allow measurement of the cardiac output. Critically ill patients should be moved to an intensive care unit where such monitoring facilities are available as soon as possible.

Direct ultrasound measurement of cardiac output may soon become routine in EDs, but this facility must not delay consultation with intensivists.

Fluid replacement

Left ventricular filling pressure (and hence cardiac output) is a function of the circulating blood volume. Increases in heart rate, systemic vascular resistance and myocardial contractility can maintain cardiac output and blood pressure in the early stages of hypovolaemia. However, this will be at the expense of increased oxygen demands by the cardiovascular system and reduced tissue perfusion in many other areas. The rapid restoration of circulating volume will prevent a sudden failure of these mechanisms and an often irreversible fall in cardiac output.

> Early restoration of blood pressure by transfusion does not necessarily indicate correction of the circulatory deficit.

The delivery of oxygen to the tissues depends not only on the pumping mechanism of the heart but also on the red cells in the circulating blood. A modest fall in haematocrit can reduce viscosity and increase blood flow while maintaining oxygen delivery, but will still require an increase in cardiac output to be effective. Maintenance of haemoglobin levels by blood transfusion reduces the impact of hypoxia by increasing the effectiveness of each cardiac cycle and reducing the need for an increase in cardiac output. Transfused blood will also maintain the oncotic pressure of the circulating fluid, thereby increasing the filling pressure. However, adequate levels of 2,3-diphosphoglycerate (2,3-DPG) are also necessary for satisfactory oxygen delivery → *p. 26*.

Maintenance of adequate tissue perfusion is not synonymous with the return of a normal blood pressure. Indeed, the latter may be contraindicated in the ED in an actively bleeding patient (e.g. with an aortic aneurysm). Resuscitation can be achieved while keeping the blood pressure relatively low. This has been shown to improve survival until definitive surgery can be undertaken. A similar approach is recommended in the prehospital management of injured adults and older children with presumed blood loss. Intravenous (IV) fluids should not be administered if a radial pulse can be felt (or, in the case of penetrating torso injuries, if a central pulse can be felt). In the absence of these pulses, IV crystalloids should be administered, en route to hospital, in boluses of no more than 250 mL until the relevant pulse becomes palpable. The same advice is probably applicable for young children and infants also, in which case boluses of 5 mL/kg should be used.

When rapid fluid replacement is required, warmed IV fluids (40°C) should be used. A ratio of crystalloids to colloids of at least 50 : 50 has been shown to be safe. Many doctors believe that Hartmann's solution is preferable to 0.9% saline if large volumes are to be given. The role of hypertonic saline in resuscitation looks promising but has yet to be fully established.

The management of massive blood loss is summarised in *Figures 1.2* (adults) and *1.3* (children).

D – Disability

After A, B and C (airway, breathing and circulation) have been attended to, it is necessary to look at the state of the brain. In this context, the term *disability* is now widely used to describe a brief assessment of neurological functioning.

Look for

1 A reduced level of consciousness – this is the most important sign of any problem affecting the brain. AVPU scoring is useful initially:
   A Alert
   V Voice elicits a response
   P Pain elicits a response. (Attending relatives are usually in a highly distressed state so be careful how you elicit this sign. Pressure on a fingernail [with a pencil] is probably the most subtle way.)
   U Unresponsive
   Later, the Glasgow Coma Scale (GCS) should be used (→ *p. 34 for adults and* → *p. 332 for children*).

> Always consider hypoglycaemia as a cause for a reduced level of consciousness.

2 Abnormal pupils – look for size, equalness and reactivity. These features can be affected by both drugs and brain disease.
3 Abnormal posture and limb movements.

Severe intracerebral problems may also cause:

- airway obstruction
- respiratory depression (respiration, unlike the heart beat, requires an intact brain stem)
- bradycardia and hypertension (Cushing's response)
- neurogenic pulmonary oedema (caused by massive sympathetic vasoconstriction).

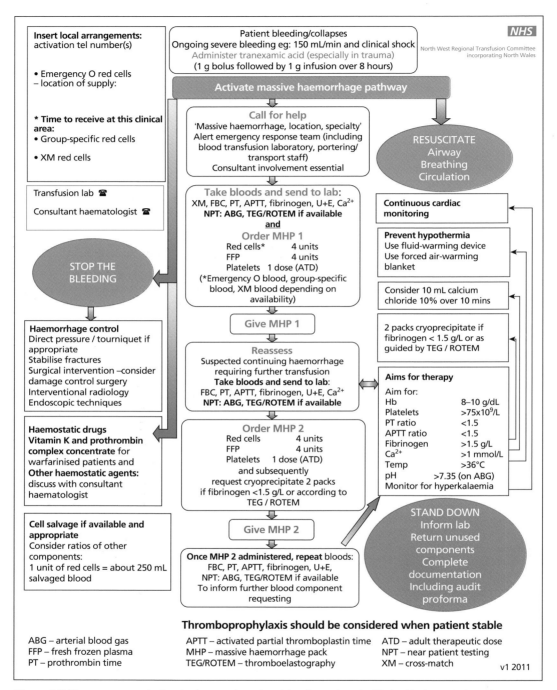

Insert local arrangements: activation tel number(s)

• Emergency O red cells – location of supply:

* Time to receive at this clinical area:
• Group-specific red cells
• XM red cells

Transfusion lab ☎
Consultant haematologist ☎

STOP THE BLEEDING

Haemorrhage control
Direct pressure / tourniquet if appropriate
Stabilise fractures
Surgical intervention –consider damage control surgery
Interventional radiology
Endoscopic techniques

Haemostatic drugs
Vitamin K and prothrombin complex concentrate for warfarinised patients and **Other haemostatic agents:** discuss with consultant haematologist

Cell salvage if available and appropriate
Consider ratios of other components:
1 unit of red cells = about 250 mL salvaged blood

Patient bleeding/collapses
Ongoing severe bleeding eg: 150 mL/min and clinical shock
Administer tranexamic acid (especially in trauma)
(1 g bolus followed by 1 g infusion over 8 hours)

North West Regional Transfusion Committee incorporating North Wales

Activate massive haemorrhage pathway

Call for help
'Massive haemorrhage, location, specialty'
Alert emergency response team (including blood transfusion laboratory, portering/ transport staff)
Consultant involvement essential

RESUSCITATE
Airway
Breathing
Circulation

Take bloods and send to lab:
XM, FBC, PT, APTT, fibrinogen, U+E, Ca^{2+}
NPT: ABG, TEG/ROTEM if available
and
Order MHP 1
Red cells*   4 units
FFP   4 units
Platelets   1 dose (ATD)
(*Emergency O blood, group-specific blood, XM blood depending on availability)

Give MHP 1

Reassess
Suspected continuing haemorrhage requiring further transfusion
Take bloods and send to lab:
FBC, PT, APTT, fibrinogen, U+E, Ca^{2+}
NPT: ABG, TEG/ROTEM if available

Order MHP 2
Red cells   4 units
FFP   4 units
Platelets   1 dose (ATD)
and subsequently
request cryoprecipitate 2 packs if fibrinogen <1.5 g/L or according to TEG / ROTEM

Give MHP 2

Once MHP 2 administered, repeat bloods:
FBC, PT, APTT, U+E,
NPT: ABG, TEG/ROTEM if available
To inform further blood component requesting

Continuous cardiac monitoring

Prevent hypothermia
Use fluid-warming device
Use forced air-warming blanket

Consider 10 mL calcium chloride 10% over 10 mins

2 packs cryoprecipitate if fibrinogen < 1.5 g/L or as guided by TEG / ROTEM

Aims for therapy
Aim for:
Hb   8–10 g/dL
Platelets   >75x10⁹/L
PT ratio   <1.5
APTT ratio   <1.5
Fibrinogen   >1.5 g/L
Ca^{2+} >1 mmol/L
Temp   >36°C
pH   >7.35 (on ABG)
Monitor for hyperkalaemia

STAND DOWN
Inform lab
Return unused components
Complete documentation
Including audit proforma

Thromboprophylaxis should be considered when patient stable

ABG – arterial blood gas
FFP – fresh frozen plasma
PT – prothrombin time

APTT – activated partial thromboplastin time
MHP – massive haemorrhage pack
TEG/ROTEM – thromboelastography

ATD – adult therapeutic dose
NPT – near patient testing
XM – cross-match

v1 2011

Figure 1.2 The management of major haemorrhage in adults. Reproduced with the kind permission of Dr Kate Pendry, Consultant Haematologist, on behalf of the North West Regional Transfusion Committee.

Figure 1.3 The management of major haemorrhage in children (→ *also Tables 1.1 and 1.2*). Reproduced with the kind permission of Dr Kate Pendry, Consultant Haematologist, on behalf of the North West Regional Transfusion Committee.

Table 1.1 Major haemorrhage pack 1 (MHP 1) **order** these volumes, which are also the maximum volumes to be administered from this pack in each weight category

Weight (kg)	Red cells: group O, group specific, cross-matched depending on availability	FFP	Platelets
<5	2 paediatric units (80–100 mL)	2 'neonatal' units of MB-treated FFP (100 mL)	1 paediatric pack of platelets (50 mL)
5–10	1 adult unit (250 mL)	1 paediatric unit MB-treated FFP (225 mL)	2 paediatric packs of platelets (100 mL)
10–20	2 adult units (500 mL)	2 paediatric units MB-treated FFP (450 mL)	1 adult apheresis pack (200 mL)
>20	4 adult units (1000 mL)	4 paediatric units MB-treated FFP (900 mL)	1 adult apheresis pack (200 mL)

FFP, fresh frozen plasma; MB, methylene blue.
Calculate volumes to be administered as detailed in Figure 1.3, but do not exceed these maxima (see example below Table 1.2).

Table 1.2 Major haemorrhage pack 2 (MHP 2) **order** these volumes, which are also the maximum volumes to be administered from this pack in each weight category

Weight (kg)	Red cells	FFP	Cryoprecipitate – request if fibrinogen <1 g/L or according to TEG/ROTEM	Platelets
<5	2 paediatric units (80–100 mL)	2 'neonatal' units of MB-treated FFP (100 mL)	1 single donor unit MB treated (40 mL)	1 paediatric pack of platelets (50 mL)
5–10	1 adult unit (250 mL)	1 paediatric unit MB-treated FFP (225 mL)	2 single donor units (80 mL)	2 paediatric packs of platelets (100 mL)
10–20	2 adult units (500 mL)	2 paediatric units MB-treated FFP (450 mL)	1 pool (5 units) (200 mL)	1 adult apheresis pack (200 mL)
>20	4 adult units (1000 mL)	4 paediatric units MB-treated FFP (900 mL)	2 pools (10 units) (400 mL)	1 adult apheresis pack (200 mL)

FFP, fresh frozen plasma; MB, methylene blue; TEG/ROTEM, thromboelastography.
Calculate volumes to be administered as detailed in Figure 1.3, but do not exceed these maxima (see example).
An example: in a 5-kg child, you may administer up to 200 mL red blood cells (RBCs: 40 mL/kg) and 50 mL platelets (10 mL/kg); however, in a 30-kg child do not administer more than 4 adult units of RBCs (33 ml/kg) or 1 adult therapeutic dose of platelets (6 mL/kg).

Brain-stem death → p. 386.
Head injury → p. 33.
Hypoglycaemia → p. 240.
Intracranial pathology → p. 223.
Poisoning → p. 268.

Depression of consciousness

A decreased level of consciousness indicates that something is wrong with the brain or its fuel supply → Box 1.2. There is a continuum of consciousness that ranges from an alert and oriented patient to one with brain-stem death.

Unconsciousness is an imprecise term usually describing a condition of an unaware patient with whom verbal communication is not possible; unresponsive is thus a better description. Such patients will usually be amnesic for the duration of the unresponsiveness.

The ability to maintain the airway decreases as the coma score falls and finally the ability to protect the airway is also lost. Breathing indicates a functioning

Box 1.2 Causes of impaired consciousness

- Hypoxia, hypovolaemia or cerebral ischaemia
- Hypoglycaemia
- Hypothermia
- Poisoning or gross metabolic disturbance (including CO_2 narcosis)
- Injury to the brain
- Intracranial pathology (bleeding, thrombosis, embolism, infection, swelling, tumour, fits, etc.)

If prolonged, many of the above problems (including hypoxia, ischaemia, hypoglycaemia and status epilepticus) will lead to a remarkably similar outcome – selective neuronal necrosis and permanent brain damage.

brain stem; in an arrested patient it often returns quickly after cerebral circulation is restored. Sudden cerebral trauma may cause transitory apnoea and all of the causes of impaired consciousness listed in Box 1.2 may lead to terminal apnoea. The heart beat is less immediately dependent on an intact brain but asystole is inevitable within hours of brain-stem death.

> Coma is defined as a Glasgow Coma Scale score of ≤8.

E – Environment and exposure

In cases of trauma, collapse and depressed conscious level, the whole body must be exposed – including the back – so that nothing important is missed. However, control of body temperature is important to successful resuscitation. So remove wet clothes and, if high volumes of IV fluids are to be given, they should be warmed. Even at this early stage avoid extrinsic factors that may harm the patient.

Look for

- Cold extremities
- Shivering
- Wet clothing
- Pyrexia and clamminess
- The position in which the patient is most comfortable
- Uncomfortable splints (including collars and spinal boards)

- Loss of the protective reflexes of the eyes
- Areas where pressure sores might form (→ *p. 222*)
- The proximity of the next of kin.

Attention to these details early on can radically change the wellbeing (and demeanour) of a patient.

> If a patient cannot blink, then the eyes should be covered to protect them.

Hyperpyrexia → p. 245.
Hyperthermia → pp. 245 and 271.
Hypothermia → p. 243.

F – Fits

Fits deprive the brain of oxygen and make assessment almost impossible. Stopping them is as important as the ABCs.

Look for

- Frank tonic or clonic activity
- Spasmodic twitching
- Post-ictal drowsiness
- Gurgling, rattling or other signs of post-ictal airway obstruction
- Cyanosis: there is increased demand for oxygen and also respiratory distress
- Signs of head injury
- Signs of other injury caused by a convulsion (e.g. a bitten tongue and intraoral bleeding)
- Reasons to consider hypoglycaemia
- Pyrexia or other signs of infection (especially in children).

Convulsions must be terminated before any further action can be effective. Meanwhile, the patient must be prevented from harming him- or herself.

Convulsions in adults → p. 231 and in children → p. 343
Hypoglycaemia → pp. 240 and 333.

Fitting indicates that something is wrong with the brain or its fuel supply. The list of possibilities is almost the same as that for causes of reduced consciousness → *Box 1.3*. Convulsive activity causes a dramatic increase in cerebral and muscle oxygen demand; a post-ictal acidosis is inevitable. The unco-ordinated muscle action that occurs during the tonic or clonic stages of a fit makes control of the airway extremely difficult; some regurgitation may also occur. Ventilation of the lungs is usually reduced for the same reason. Alveolar oxygenation is thus poor

> Box 1.3 **Causes of fits**
>
> - Hypoxia
> - Shock
> - Hypoglycaemia
> - Poisoning
> - Metabolic disturbance
> - Intracranial pathology:
>   - bleeding
>   - trauma
>   - thrombosis
>   - embolism
>   - infection
>   - swelling
>   - tumour
>   - epilepsy

at a time of high oxygen demand. This combination explains why prolonged fitting is associated with permanent neurological damage.

G – Glucose

The human body can be compared to an engine that needs an oxygen supply (airway and breathing) delivered in the bloodstream (circulation). However, we should not forget that the oxygen is required to burn fuel (glucose). Fat and protein are, of course, also important but the brain uses glucose almost exclusively.

Look for

- Restlessness, agitation or other mental change ('jitteriness' in a neonate)
- Inappropriate lack of cooperation or aggression
- A reduced level of consciousness
- Convulsions
- Signs of insulin usage
- A low blood sugar level on testing with a reagent strip.

A reagent-strip measurement of blood glucose should be performed in all patients who have depression of consciousness. If hypoglycaemia is found it should be immediately treated with IV glucose solution (50 mL of 50% glucose for a normal adult, 0.2 g/kg for a child). If no venous access can be found, then glucagon 1 mg by intramuscular injection is a useful standby.

Hypoglycaemia → pp. 240 and 333.

> Hypoglycaemia is always waiting to catch you out. A comatose patient with profuse sweating should always make you think of a low blood sugar.

H – History

At this juncture a brief history becomes a necessity and brief is AMPLE:

A	Allergies
M	Medication
P	Past and present illnesses of significance
L	Last food and drink
E	Events leading up to the patient's presentation

The people who accompany the patient to the department are a vital source of this information, hence the need to collect facts before the paramedical staff leave the ED.

> **Adrenocortical suppression**
>
> Patients who are undergoing prolonged treatment with steroids (i.e. for more than 3 weeks) may develop adrenocortical suppression. This can also occur for up to a year after stopping long-term steroid therapy. During a medical crisis, such patients should be given supplementary corticosteroids (e.g. IV hydrocortisone 200 mg) in the ED.

I – Immediate analgesia and investigations

> This is the point (if you have not already done it) to call for help. There should be no hesitation in seeking another pair of hands or a more experienced opinion.

In many patients who are not in extremis, the above will take only a matter of seconds. Once life-threatening problems have been identified and treated, it is necessary to perform the tasks that are at the very heart of emergency medicine – to ensure the immediate relief of suffering. This will include the following:

Box 1.4 Assessment of pain

Pain is a subjective experience. Clinical assessment of a patient's level of pain depends on:

- the patient's description of the pain
- the patient's behaviour
- the known injuries or condition
- any observed signs of pain (sweating, etc.)
- the use of visual pain scales – analogue or image type (pain ladders and faces, etc.)

 Box 1.5 Summary of immediate assessment and management

Airway
  Establish and maintain a clear airway
  Ensure airway protection
  Consider the need for cervical protection
Breathing
  Give high-concentration oxygen
  Ensure adequate ventilation of the lungs
  Decompress pneumothoraces
  Begin to correct severe respiratory problems
Circulation
  Restore the circulating blood volume
  Ensure adequate cardiac function
  Commence monitoring
Disability
  Assess cerebral functioning
  Consider causes of depression of consciousness
Environment/exposure of the whole body
  Check the body temperature and positioning
  Ensure protection from further harm
  Expose the whole body for examination
Fits
  Control convulsive activity
Glucose
  Correct hypoglycaemia
History
  Take brief but AMPLE details
Immediate analgesia and investigations
  Provide analgesia and splintage
  Relieve remaining dyspnoea
  Give reassurance
  Request major investigations

- Administration of analgesia: *assessment of pain →
  Box 1.4*
- Provision of splintage and support for injuries: *lower limb → p. 94; upper limb → p. 112*
- Further relief of dyspnoea
- Reassurance.

This is not just a matter of humanity. The trust of the patient (and the relatives and friends) is more easily gained by staff who are seen to 'do something'. This trust leads to the provision of more information and better compliance with treatment. Conversely, nothing agitates relatives more than the sight of a doctor or nurse asking endless questions while the patient continues to suffer. It is always better to over-estimate pain rather than to underestimate it.

Major radiographs can now be requested. In patients who have suffered multiple trauma, these are views of the chest, lateral cervical spine and pelvis. In other instances a CXR is usually sufficient. Twelve-lead ECG and blood gas analysis are also helpful early on.

Analgesia

The administration of analgesia does not mask significant clinical signs. Conscious level is not greatly depressed by the judicious administration of small doses of IV opioids; abdominal signs remain unchanged. Tenderness can still be located and guarding is an involuntary mechanism, which is unaffected. The biggest change will be in the ease of examining a trusting, cooperative patient who was previously distressed and agitated.

The immediate relief of suffering, in all its forms, is the most important function of an ED.

The needs of relatives and friends

The needs of the carers cannot be ignored. These may vary from simple reassurance to medical treatment. As soon as practicable, the relatives must be informed of the patient's current situation and what is going to happen next.

*For a summary of this section on immediate assessment and management of emergency patients →
Box 1.5.*

FURTHER MANAGEMENT IN THE ED

How much history, how much examination?

History-taking in emergencies should be guided by the presenting complaint. The familial medical history will rarely be relevant in a patient with a dog bite; it might be vital in someone with haemophilia and a swollen joint. The art of adjusting the acquisition of information is a difficult one.

Most new ED staff take an over-long history for the first few days; they then record less than a bare minimum for the next few months. Mechanism of injury is particularly important in trauma; events that lead to the patient's presentation, the timing and speed of onset are essential in medical cases.

The examination must also be tailored to the patient. At times it can be limited, but often it must be thorough. Experience teaches the relative uselessness of some physical signs and the enormous value of others. The examination in trauma patients is usually performed from top to toe rather than in systems and is called the secondary survey. The back of the patient and the perineum are the parts that are often missed.

Investigations

Investigations should be requested only if the results could have an impact on immediate care or disposal. Major radiographs are initially requested. In patients who have suffered multiple trauma, these are views of the chest, lateral cervical spine and pelvis. In other patients a chest radiograph (CXR) is usually sufficient. Twelve-lead ECG and blood gas analysis are also helpful early on.

Other tests should be performed for precise indications rather than as a general screen. The exception to this is in elderly patients who present with non-specific events such as collapse. They can be very difficult to evaluate clinically. Consequently, before considering sending them home, it is best to carry out a brief screen including CXR, ECG, haemoglobin, white cell count and blood urea level – and a pelvic radiograph if concerned about mobility.

Definitive care

This may involve:

- accurate liaison with other specialists in the hospital or community
- safe transport to another facility
- careful follow-up arrangements
- rehabilitation

Homelessness

> The standardised mortality rate for homeless people is three times higher than that of the UK population as a whole.

Many patients who come to an ED have nowhere to sleep or to shelter. People with psychiatric disease often become homeless, and there are many other illnesses (such as tuberculosis and alcohol abuse) that are associated with homelessness.

> The average life expectancy for someone on the streets is just 47 years.

Efforts should always be made to find temporary accommodation for these patients. The most likely sources of help are:

- the Social Services
- the Salvation Army
- Shelter Nightline (in London).

> Health inequalities in the UK are increasing. The differences in life expectancy between rich and poor areas of the country are at their greatest since the Victorian era.

Prehospital care

Outside the hospital situation, there is a clear organisational hierarchy:

- The police are in overall control of the scene.
- The fire service is in charge of rescue and extrication, and of scene safety for the other personnel.
- The ambulance service is responsible for the evacuation of casualties.
- The medical team is present at the request of the ambulance service.

Entrapment of casualties is now the most common reason for paramedics to request the assistance of a hospital team – either prolonged entrapment (more than 20 min) or situations where release requires analgesia.

An on-site medical team must be formed from experienced, regularly trained staff who have:

- high-visibility protective clothing
- adequate equipment
- insurance cover for this type of work.

Furthermore, the parent department must be left adequately staffed.

The only measures that have been shown conclusively to save lives in the prehospital situation are ABC:

Airway	Clearance, maintenance and protection
Breathing	Oxygen and ventilation
Circulation	Chest compression and defibrillation

> In cardiac arrest, the time taken to initiate the above interventions is crucial to survival → p. 151.

Extensive clinical examination and the establishment of IV infusions are of no proven benefit. Nevertheless, other prehospital treatments may contribute greatly to the relief of pain and suffering.

> Time at the scene must not be extended by anything other than essential treatment. The priority is to get the patient to a major ED as soon as possible.

The basic principles of prehospital care are the same as those for in-hospital care. Specific resuscitation courses are now available where the applied skills may be mastered.

Major incidents

The management of major incidents is outside the scope of this book, but in essence the following should be implemented:

- All departments should have a written policy for dealing with events that have the potential to overwhelm the standard facilities of the hospital.
- Action cards for all personnel should be available together with a special supply of equipment and drugs.
- Regular practice sessions are essential.

(Note that the last is a legal obligation in the UK under the Civil Contingencies Act 2004. The Act is divided into two parts – Civil Protection (Part I) and Emergency Powers (Part II). For the purposes of Civil Protection, local responders are divided into two categories. Category 1 responders (which include hospitals, primary care trusts and ambulance services) have a duty to make and execute effective plans for major incidents. Category 2 organisations (such as utility and transport companies) are obliged to cooperate with other responders.)

Contamination and irradiation → p. 145.

SEDATION AND GENERAL ANAESTHESIA

Most ED patients are self-referred and many will return to their homes or workplaces within a matter of hours. Some patients arrive in a coma and others will require sedation. All are, by definition, unexpected. This combination of circumstances leads to special problems with the safe administration of sedative drugs:

- Most patients are not fasted.
- Painful conditions delay gastric emptying.
- Many patients will have ingested alcohol.
- There is no opportunity for preplanned assessment of fitness or review of case notes.
- The need for sedation is invariably immediate.
- The fitness of patients for discharge and the circumstances to which they depart require very careful consideration.

The techniques used for assessment and monitoring of pathological coma are applicable to the depression of consciousness that occurs during sedation. The safety of the patient is paramount; emergency situations do not obviate the need for standard precautions. Consideration must be given to the medical preparedness and fasting state of all patients. If in doubt, senior staff should be consulted.

Preparation for sedation and selection of patients

The immediacy of the situation does not obviate the need for a concise but adequate work-up of the patient. Most patients will not require investigations to assess their fitness for the procedure; those who do are generally not suitable for sedation in the ED. Pulse oximetry (while breathing air) is a useful screening test – a fit patient will invariably have an SaO_2 of >94%.

Patients with the following problems are unsuitable for sedation in the ED:

- Severely intoxicated
- Full stomach
- Previous problems with sedation
- Chronic illnesses – may complicate sedation or aftercare
- Other severe injuries
- Coexistent significant head injury
- At the extremes of age
- Inadequate circumstances for discharge.

Patients who are deemed unsuitable for sedation but whose condition does not allow delay (e.g. vascular compromise distal to a dislocation) must be discussed with a senior colleague immediately.

The urgency of most of the conditions that present to an ED does not allow for the conventional period of preoperative fasting. However, in all but the most pressing circumstances, a period of 2 h should separate sedation from the last ingestion of food or drink to allow for gastric emptying. No further food or drink must be allowed from the moment of entering the department.

Painful conditions, such as dislocations, must be alleviated with parenteral analgesia (before the radiograph) and the subsequent doses of sedative drugs then adjusted accordingly.

> Sedation is not the same as analgesia. Pain relief is still needed.

Facilities for the administration of sedation or general anaesthesia

The minimum requirements include the following:

- Medical and nursing staff trained in the management of patients with a depressed level of consciousness
- Areas suitable for high-dependency observation
- A full range of resuscitation and monitoring equipment
- All necessary drugs for resuscitation, including the specific benzodiazepine antagonist flumazenil and the opioid antagonist naloxone.

> When a doctor is performing a procedure on a sedated patient, a separate member of staff must be responsible for the overall care of that patient. The operator should never try to monitor the patient at the same time.

Conditions during the period of sedation

During sedation, and until recovery is complete, all patients should:

- be accompanied by a responsible member of staff
- be on a trolley with side rails, which can be tipped head-down
- have an IV cannula *in situ*
- be given a high concentration of oxygen by mask
- be monitored by pulse oximetry as a minimum standard – respiratory rate, ECG and BP recording are also highly desirable
- have a high-volume suction catheter in place under their pillow.

The protective reflexes of the airway are depressed by all sedative and opioid/narcotic drugs to an unpredictable degree. Even at a high GCS there may be enough impairment of airway protection to allow aspiration of gastric contents. Therefore, all sedated patients must be placed in the recovery position as soon as is practically possible.

Effective sedation is greatly facilitated by pleasant, quiet surroundings and the presence of attentive, reassuring and obviously competent staff.

Assessment of the level of sedation

> The scores for measuring coma (AVPU and GCS) must be understood and practised by all ED staff. They are ideal for use in assessing the level of sedation.

General anaesthesia and sedation are both induced states of depression of consciousness. Sedation is characterised by an ability to maintain verbal contact at all times. This does not mean that the patient either speaks sensibly or remembers the conversation afterwards. It is equivalent to 'V' on the AVPU scale and 10 or above on the GCS. It is certainly not the same as a GCS of 8 (coma). Full general anaesthesia is characterised by a GCS of 3. Gentle stroking of the upper eyelashes usually causes blinking (the eyelash reflex) and the loss of this reflex (at a GCS of around 8) is a good guide as to the imminent onset of general anaesthesia.

Drugs for sedation in the ED

All drugs that are used for sedation are capable of inducing general anaesthesia and vice versa. The main difference between the two groups of agents is the speed of onset of action and thus the ability to control the level of consciousness. (Thiopental acts in 20 seconds whereas diazepam takes several minutes to work.)

Sedation should always be accompanied by adequate analgesia, before, during and after the procedure. Antiemetics may be given as required but there is little evidence that their routine use reduces the risk of aspiration.

Sedation and analgesia for children → p. 352.
Sedation of the disturbed patient → p. 358.

Intravenous benzodiazepines

Intravenous benzodiazepines such as midazolam or diazepam emulsion are the standard drugs for ED sedation:

- Initial adult dose of IV midazolam = 1–2 mg
- Initial adult dose of IV diazepam = 2.5–5.0 mg.

The correct initial dose can be estimated from the age, weight and general health of the patient. Elderly people may need only very small amounts. Subsequent doses, given after a delay of a few minutes, should be titrated against apparent effect. The muscle relaxation that is a feature of sedation with benzodiazepines makes these drugs ideal for use in the reduction of dislocations.

Short-acting opioids

Short-acting opioids such as fentanyl can provide an excellent combination of sedation and analgesia:

- IV dose of fentanyl = 1–3 mcg/kg.

This should be titrated slowly at a rate of no more than 1 mcg/kg per min up to a maximum dose of 5 mcg/kg in 1 h. The onset of action is within 3 min and the effects of a single dose wear off in less than 1 h. Opioids may cause some muscular rigidity.

Low-dose inhaled nitrous oxide

Low-dose inhaled nitrous oxide is useful as a supplement to other drugs or to give background sedation. It is often administered, for the purpose of analgesia rather than sedation, in a fixed concentration (50%) from a cylinder premixed with oxygen (e.g. Entonox) via a demand valve. Such valves require a negative pressure to open them (which varies greatly with the make of the demand apparatus). The generation of this pressure may be beyond the ability of younger children and some adults.

Proper sedation with nitrous oxide requires a constant flow of gas and this is best achieved with a purpose-built system such as the Quantiflex machine. Using this apparatus, nitrous oxide may be administered in subanaesthetic concentrations of 30–70% via a non-re-breathing circuit with a guaranteed minimum of 30% oxygen.

Ketamine

Ketamine is a derivative of phencyclidine and is often recommended as an anaesthetic for prehospital use. This is because it has both sedative and analgesic effects and does not compromise the airway or the circulation as much as other comparable drugs. In a lower range of doses, it is also an excellent and safe sedative for use in the ED with a success rate of more than 90%. Contraindications to sedation with ketamine include:

- Age <12 months due to an increased risk of laryngospasm and airway complications (children aged between 12 and 24 months should receive ketamine sedation only from expert staff)
- High risk of laryngospasm (active respiratory infection, active asthma)
- Unstable or abnormal airway
- Active upper or lower respiratory tract infection
- Proposed procedure within the mouth or pharynx
- Significant cardiac disease
- Recent significant head injury or reduced level of consciousness
- Intracranial hypertension with cerebrospinal fluid (CSF) obstruction
- Intraocular pathology (glaucoma, penetrating injury)
- Uncontrolled epilepsy
- Hyperthyroidism or thyroid medication
- Porphyria
- Previous psychotic illness
- Severe psychological problems such as cognitive or motor delay or severe behavioural problems
- Prior adverse reaction to ketamine.

The recommended doses are as follows:

- IV dose of ketamine for sedation = 1 mg/kg. The sedation starts within 60 s and lasts for 5–10 min.
- Intramuscular (IM) dose of ketamine for sedation = 2.5 mg/kg. The onset of sedation is around 5 min with an effective duration of up to 35 min. A top-up dose of a further 1 mg/kg can be given if either the first dose proves to be inadequate or there is a requirement to prolong the duration of the sedation. The effects of ketamine are surprisingly predictable and reliable when it is administered by the IM route.

In these low doses, laryngospasm and dysphoria are uncommon and excess salivation is not a problem. Consequently, emergence from sedation is usually uneventful and prior administration of atropine is unnecessary. However, around 5% of children will have transient clonic movements and the same number will vomit during the recovery phase.

Discharge of patients who have received sedative drugs in the ED

The patient who is fit for discharge after sedation must fulfil all of the following criteria:

- Alert and oriented
- Able to walk steadily and unaided
- Able to drink liquids
- Not suffering from any disabling condition such as
  - vomiting
  - dizziness
  - shortness of breath
  - severe pain
- Accompanied by a responsible adult
- Suitable for the available transport
- Returning to adequate home circumstances.

Aftercare advice for patients who have received sedative or opioid (narcotic) drugs in the ED → p. 390.

Major trauma and multiple injuries

Epidemiology

There is a pandemic of trauma throughout the world. In the developed countries, trauma is the leading cause of death in the first four decades of life and is surpassed only by cancer and atherosclerosis throughout life. Moreover, because it affects young people, trauma wastes more years of life than any other cause – an average of 36 years per trauma death. It is responsible for 8.3% of all 'life-years' lost in people under the age of 75 years in the UK. In addition, for every death from trauma, there are more than two survivors with serious or permanent disabilities.

> In the UK, accidents cause almost 2% of all deaths and account for 7% of total NHS expenditure.

The absolute number of accidental deaths is greatest in people aged 65 years and over. In this age group, more than half of all fatal trauma results from falls. However, for most of the population, road traffic is the greatest danger, being responsible for about 40% of trauma deaths and seriously injuring somebody every 20 minutes in the UK. Falls from a height and motor vehicle accidents commonly lead to multiple injuries ('polytrauma').

> People from deprived backgrounds are more likely to be injured than those from higher social classes.

Alcohol is a significant factor in about one in seven of all fatal car crashes and in over 40% of deaths from falls. (*For further information on alcohol and injury → p. 374.*)

Speed also kills. A car hitting 100 pedestrians:

at 20 mph	†††††††††††††††††††††††	kills 5
at 30 mph	†††††††††††††††††††††††	kills 45
at 50 mph	†††††††††††††††††††††††	kills 85

Deaths from trauma were commonly said to occur in a triphasic distribution:

1 Immediate death, within minutes of injury: damage to the brain, brain stem, proximal spinal cord, heart, aorta or other large vessels
2 Delayed deaths, within hours of injury: intracranial bleeding or blood loss into the chest, abdomen or pelvis
3 Late deaths, days or weeks after injury: sepsis and organ failure.

However, in the UK, most fatalities (around 80%) actually occur at the scene of the injury and later deaths do not neatly fit into this classification. Prevention is thus the best way to reduce the effect of injury, next is protection to mitigate its impact and finally there must be timely and effective treatment.

TRAUMA CARE

The Advanced Trauma Life Support (ATLS) system, developed by the American College of Surgeons in the late 1970s, has become the standard method for initial assessment and management of trauma victims. There are three main phases:

Emergency Medicine Lecture Notes, Fourth Edition. Chris Moulton and David Yates.
© 2012 Blackwell Publishing Ltd. Published 2012 by Blackwell Publishing Ltd.

1 Primary survey and resuscitation
2 Secondary survey
3 Definitive care.

> This chapter adopts the ATLS approach but is no replacement for attendance on a 3-day ATLS course. The practical skills and team approach to trauma care cannot be learned from a book.

Preparation for reception of trauma victims

If warned of the imminent arrival of patients who are multiply injured:

- Assemble a team in the resuscitation area
- Warn appropriate in-patient specialties
- Allocate tasks: doctor/nurse to airway and breathing, doctor/nurse to circulation, nurse to record findings and interventions, nurse to support relatives, senior doctor as team leader
- Check equipment and put on protective clothing
- Meet the ambulance with doctor/nurse to ensure continuous care of the airway
- Detain the ambulance crew for a subsequent report on the biomechanics of impact (*Box 2.1*), initial clinical state and prehospital care

> **Box 2.1 Factors associated with severe injury**
>
> Fall from a height of 5 m or more or a road traffic accident involving:
>
> - impact at high speed
> - fatality of other passenger(s)
> - ejection from vehicle
> - pedestrian struck by vehicle
> - motorcyclist with no crash helmet
> - steering wheel or windscreen damage
> - significant intrusion into passenger compartment

The primary survey and resuscitation phase (initial assessment and management)

Also → Chapter 1.

- Assess and secure the airway while guarding the neck. Manual in-line stabilisation may be needed.
- Give high-flow 100% oxygen.
- Protect the neck with a rigid cervical collar and a head holder (or sandbags and tape).

- Assess the breathing; exclude/treat tension pneumothorax and other critical chest injuries. Cover 'sucking' chest wounds with a flap dressing:
    - stop external bleeding by direct pressure and establish venous access at two sites – large cannulae in large veins
    - take 20 mL blood for cross-matching, a coagulation screen and baseline glucose, electrolytes and haemoglobin
    - commence infusions of 0.9% saline and then colloid (a 50:50 ratio of the two is probably a good start).
- Take and record the pulse, BP and respiratory rate. Attach the patient to a pulse oximeter and a cardiac monitor.
- Determine the level of consciousness (*AVPU →* *p. 7*) and the size and reactivity of the pupils.
- Assess limb movements to confirm spinal cord integrity.
- Remove remaining clothing and expose the patient to allow further assessment.
- Measure the blood glucose with a reagent stick in all unresponsive patients.
- Obtain brief details of the patient and the trauma that he or she has suffered (*AMPLE → p. 12*).
- Consider early analgesia.
- Request the three major radiographs of trauma: chest, lateral cervical spine and pelvis.

> An understanding of the biomechanics of the trauma will suggest the likely extent of the injuries – many of which may not be obvious at this stage.

The secondary survey (further assessment)

- When resuscitation is successfully under way, begin a head-to-toe examination. If any features in the primary survey are still giving cause for concern, return to the assessment of oxygenation and circulation.
- When the front of the trunk and the limbs have been assessed, call for help to log-roll the patient. Four people are required, one controlling the head alone and taking charge of the timing of the turn.
- When rolled, examine the thoracolumbar spine, listen to lung fields, examine the perineum and do a rectal examination. The last will reveal the anal tone, presence of perineal injuries, position of the prostate and any blood.
- Document the injuries discovered.
- Consider the priorities for investigation and treatment. Discuss the patient with doctors from other

specialties who should, by now, have arrived in the resuscitation room.
- Maintain contemporary notes and repeat the ABCs and baseline observations frequently.

The chain of care

Patients appear deceptively stable even after significant injury – particularly blunt trauma. Inadequate assessment and treatment are commonplace, yet the consequences are not immediately evident. Complications on the intensive care unit (ICU) may be a result of inadequate resuscitation in the emergency department (ED) and deterioration in an ED may be caused by inadequate treatment at scene.

Prehospital

In urban areas, with short transfer times to a definitive care centre and no delay involved in releasing the injured patient, a 'scoop and run' prehospital policy is best. Pause only to secure the airway and protect the neck. In other situations (e.g. entrapment or prolonged transfer time) field resuscitation may be helpful (*Box 2.2*). Try to treat in transit; don't delay and play!

In the prehospital management of untrapped injured adults and older children with presumed blood loss, IV fluids should not be administered if a radial pulse can be felt (or, in the case of penetrating torso injuries, if a central pulse can be felt). In the absence of these pulses, IV crystalloids should be administered, en route to hospital, in boluses of no more than 250 mL until the relevant pulse becomes palpable. The same advice is probably applicable for young children and infants – use boluses of 5 mL/kg.

Emergency department

The primary concerns here are:

1 adequate oxygen delivery to vital tissues
2 treatment of critical problems as soon as they are identified
3 prevention of further deterioration.

This can be achieved by a well-rehearsed team working to agreed protocols and integrated into a comprehensive trauma care system.

 Box 2.2 Prehospital management

- Secure the airway – jaw thrust, oropharyngeal or nasopharyngeal airway. Consider intubation
- Protect the cervical spine – collar and head holder
- Ensure adequate ventilation and oxygenation (this may necessitate decompression of the chest: → *p. 74*)
- Cover open chest wounds
- Control external haemorrhage by direct pressure
- Start intravenous (IV) infusions only if this does not delay transfer
- Protect thoracic and lumbar spine – backboard or 'scoop' stretcher
- Provide analgesia
- Record initial assessment of cardiorespiratory and neurological status
- Communicate with the hospital – assessment, management and expected time of arrival

PRIMARY SURVEY AND RESUSCITATION

This must be carried out in a strict order of priority. Problems are corrected as they are identified. The ATLS formula for the primary survey is:

A Airway
B Breathing
C Circulation
D Disability
E Exposure

Airway

Check for responsiveness.

In an unresponsive patient the airway is always at risk.

Then look for the following:

- No movement of air (complete airway obstruction or apnoea)

Box 2.3 Causes of upper airway obstruction in trauma

Oropharyngeal – tongue, teeth, dental plates, foreign bodies, blood and vomit
Facial – fractures of the maxilla or mandible
Cervical – laryngeal injury
Intracerebral – altered level of consciousness after head injury, alcohol or drugs

 Box 2.4 Artificial airways in trauma

Standard orotracheal intubation: this is the route of choice in the apnoeic patient or where cervical spine injury has been excluded by good quality radiographs.
Nasotracheal intubation: this may be useful in patients in whom cervical spine injury has not been excluded because it involves less extension of the neck. It is also a valuable technique in some special situations, such as for the non-paralysed patient. It should not be performed in the presence of a possible fracture of the base of the skull. The traditionally advocated method of 'blind' nasal intubation requires considerable skill and must not be attempted by inexperienced staff.
Surgical cricothyroidotomy: this is the method of choice in adults. It is contraindicated in children aged <12 years because of the importance of the cricoid cartilage in tracheal support and the long-term problems that result if it is damaged ($\rightarrow$ *Box 2.5*).
Needle cricothyroidotomy: this procedure is performed using a large cannula. Bag-and-mask ventilation is ineffective via such a small opening. The patient must be ventilated with high-flow oxygen from either a flow meter or the wall supply (at 50 lbf/in² [psi], or 4000 cmH₂O pressure). Intermittent flow is achieved using a Y-piece, a three-way tap or a hole in the side of the tubing. Exhalation takes place through the upper airway and not through the cannula. CO₂ retention occurs and thus this technique should not be used for more than 20 min if a more effective airway can be obtained ($\rightarrow$ *Box 2.6*).

- Noises from the upper airway (partial airway obstruction); there may be snoring, rattles, stridor or other sounds

Causes of upper airway obstruction in trauma → Box 2.3.

Any injury severe enough to compromise the airway may also have damaged the cervical spine.

Tx All severely injured patients require a high inspired oxygen concentration. The airway must be:

- *cleared* of foreign material with suction, Magill's forceps and fingers, if necessary
- *maintained* using a jaw-thrust manoeuvre, a Guedel oropharyngeal airway, a nasopharyngeal airway or by endotracheal intubation (the nasopharyngeal airway is safe and well tolerated in the conscious patient and is much less likely to stimulate gagging than the Guedel airway)
- *protected* by vigilance, suctioning and positioning.

When traumatic disruption of the facial or laryngeal structures prevents intubation, surgical access to the airway must be obtained. Emergency tracheostomy is difficult and dangerous and has been superseded by the technique of cricothyroidotomy. Needle puncture of the cricothyroid membrane is preferable in children aged <12 years ($\rightarrow$ *Box 2.4*).

The cervical spine

Neck injury must be assumed to have occurred in all patients who have sustained polytrauma until excluded by clinical examination and good quality imaging. Patients at particular risk include those who have sustained:

- any injury above the clavicle
- head injury associated with depressed consciousness
- a high-speed injury
- a fall from a height.

A normal neurological examination does not exclude cervical spine injury. Moreover, conscious patients with other painful injuries may not always complain of neck discomfort.

Tx The neck must be splinted to prevent damage to the spinal cord from the movement of an unstable injured spine. This should be achieved with a well-fitting hard collar and a purpose-built head holder. However, if the patient is struggling violently, attempts to control the head may inadvertently lead to further injury. In these circumstances, it is better to use a collar alone. The cause of the agitation should be sought. It is often hypoxia, pain or both. In a patient with a depressed level of consciousness, a full bladder may be responsible.

Box 2.5 **Cricothyroidotomy**

- Extend the patient's neck while controlling the head
- Mark the skin over the centre of the cricothyroid membrane (which lies between the thyroid and cricoid cartilages → *Figure 2.1*)
- Support the larynx and tighten the overlying skin with the non-dominant hand
- Make a small transverse incision through the skin and spread the edges outwards
- Make a transverse incision through the cricothyroid membrane and open the wound with the handle of the scalpel
- Insert an appropriate size of endotracheal or tracheostomy tube
- Start ventilation and check for air entry
- Secure the tube

 Box 2.6 **Needle cricothyroid puncture**

- Extend the patient's neck while controlling the head
- Mark the skin over the centre of the cricothyroid membrane (which lies between the thyroid and cricoid cartilages → *Figure 2.1*)
- Attach a cannula and needle of an appropriate size (at least 12 G for an adult) to a small syringe
- Support the larynx and tighten the overlying skin with the non-dominant hand
- Puncture the skin and cricothyroid membrane with the needle, aiming for the small of the back, aspirating as the needle is advanced
- When air is easily aspirated, advance the cannula and withdraw the needle
- Recheck the ease of aspiration of air (it is surprisingly easy to miss the trachea with a needle, especially in children)
- Attach the cannula to either the wall or the flow-meter oxygen supply via an in-line Y-connector. In a child, start with a flow meter set at a delivery rate in litres equal to the child's age in years
- Adjust the flow rate and inspiratory time until adequate chest movement is achieved. Expiration may take several seconds
- Secure the cannula

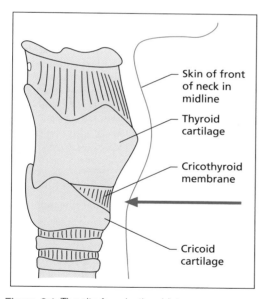

Figure 2.1 The site for cricothyroidotomy.

Labels in figure:
- Skin of front of neck in midline
- Thyroid cartilage
- Cricothyroid membrane
- Cricoid cartilage

Breathing

Look for

- External signs of injury
- Abnormal respiratory rate or pattern
- Unequal chest movement
- Tracheal shift and displacement of the apex beat

- Decreased breath sounds
- Increased or decreased resonance
- Low SaO_2 (arterial O_2 saturation)
- Signs of hypoxia (tachycardia, agitation or confusion and cyanosis).

Five major chest injuries require immediate recognition and treatment during the primary survey:

1 Tension pneumothorax
2 Open pneumothorax (sucking chest wound)
3 Massive haemothorax
4 Flail segment of the chest
5 Cardiac tamponade.

Other injuries, which may cause dyspnoea or shock, may become apparent in the secondary survey:

- Pulmonary contusion
- Myocardial contusion
- Aortic disruption
- Traumatic diaphragmatic hernia

- Tracheobronchial disruption
- Oesophageal disruption.

Tx

*Diagnosis and treatment of major chest injuries →
Chapter 6.*

Upper airway patency does not ensure adequate ventilation. Assisted breathing using a bag, mask and airway or tracheal intubation may be required. Before attempted intubation, the patient must be preoxygenated using a bag, mask and airway technique, and intubation should be performed quickly by an experienced operator. Prolonged, unsuccessful attempts at intubation must be avoided.

> Attempted intubation in a patient who is not paralysed may cause a dramatic rise in intracranial pressure.

Even the apparently 'flat' apnoeic trauma patient must be assessed by a doctor with anaesthetic training before intubation. (These cases are not analogous to the cardiac arrest patient, where intubation without paralysis is acceptable.)

A small, uncomplicated, and possibly undiagnosed, simple pneumothorax may rapidly develop into a life-threatening tension pneumothorax if the patient is mechanically ventilated, in either the operating theatre or ICU. Prophylactic chest drains should be considered in any patient with chest injury requiring ventilation.

Circulation

In the primary survey the state of the circulation is quickly assessed by observation of:

- skin colour and temperature
- pulse rate and volume
- capillary refill time at a finger pulp or nail bed (usually 2 seconds or less)
- BP (blood pressure)
- JVP (jugular venous pressure) and heart sounds
- level of consciousness (in the patient who has not sustained a brain injury).

> Hypotension with a raised JVP and absent heart sounds suggests cardiac tamponade: → *p. 78.*

The assessment of hypovolaemia in the trauma patient is difficult because of the following:

- The interaction of autonomic reflexes, head injury, pain, drugs and blood loss is complex.
- Compensatory mechanisms may prevent a fall in systolic blood pressure until 30% of the blood volume has been lost.
- Rapid blood loss may produce a reflex bradycardia.
- In elderly people, tachycardia may not be present as a result of a limited cardiac response to catecholamines or treatment with β blockers.
- Haematocrit is an unreliable index of shock; a nearly normal value does not rule out significant blood loss.

> All abnormalities of colour, pulse, BP and consciousness should be regarded with suspicion.

*Methods of assessing organ perfusion → Box 2.8.
Signs of shock → Box 2.7.*

The blood loss potential of evident injuries should be considered (→ *Table 2.1*); the mechanism of injury may suggest occult blood loss. Hypovolaemia is seldom caused by head injury alone, except occasionally in infants. Open fractures will cause greater blood loss than similar closed injuries.

Tx

*General management of major haemorrhage → Figure
1.2 on p. 8.*

- Control external blood loss by direct pressure at the bleeding site.
- Insert at least two large-calibre (14 G) cannulae into large veins. If percutaneous venous access is difficult, use the interosseous route. Alternatively, cut down to the antecubital veins or the long saphenous vein or insert a long line into the femoral vein. Central veins should not be used as routes for fluid

> **Box 2.7 Signs of shock**
>
> - Altered mental state
> - Delayed capillary refill (>2 s)
> - Tachycardia
> - Pale, cool skin

Box 2.8 **Guides to organ perfusion**

- Mental state
- Urinary output: adequate volume replacement produces a urine output in the adult of about 50 mL/h
- Arterial blood gases: metabolic acidosis implies inadequate tissue oxygenation requiring increased oxygen and fluids (not bicarbonate)
- Shock index: calculated by dividing the pulse rate in beats/min by the systolic BP in mmHg. The normal range is 0.5–0.7. Values >0.9 suggest significant haemorrhage
- Core/periphery temperature gradient
- Aortic flow (measured by Doppler ultrasound probe)
- Serum lactate: high lactate is increasingly recognised as a good indicator of tissue hypoxia and a poor prognosis
- ICU determination of oxygen demand and supply

Table 2.1 **Estimation of traumatic blood loss in an adult (closed injuries)**

Site	Volume (L)
Pelvis	0.5–3
Shaft of femur	1–2
Tibia	0.5–1
Chest	>2
Abdomen	>2
Arm	0.5–1
Forearm	0.5–1

replacement in the initial stages of resuscitation, but should be preserved for use in the ICU.
- Take a sample of blood (20 mL in an adult) for group and cross-match, and coagulation screen.
- Commence rapid fluid replacement with a bolus of 10 mL/kg. After reassessment of the patient, this can be repeated. A ratio of crystalloids to colloids of 50:50 is safe. Some prefer Hartmann's solution to 0.9% saline if large volumes are to be given. The role of hypertonic saline in resuscitation looks promising but has yet to be fully established. Ideally, IV fluids should be warmed to 40°C.

- In prehospital management of patients with presumed blood loss, IV fluids should not be administered if a radial pulse can be felt or, in the case of penetrating torso injuries, if a central pulse can be felt. In the absence of these pulses, IV crystalloids should be administered, *en route* to hospital, in boluses of not more than 250 mL (5 mL/kg for infants and young children) until the relevant pulse becomes palpable.
- Consider the possibility of intra-abdominal bleeding and the need for surgical advice.
- Consider the possibility of blood loss from a major pelvic fracture. Do not try to 'spring' the pelvis to demonstrate its instability – this may increase bleeding. Vessel damage is difficult to identify surgically, instability is best treated with an external fixation device, which can be applied rapidly in the ED by the orthopaedic team. This should be thought of as a resuscitation manoeuvre to help control the circulation in the primary survey.

Military anti-shock trousers (MASTs) or pneumatic anti-shock garments (PASGs) are no longer recommended. Controlled trials have not shown them to be of benefit and their sudden removal causes significant volume loss into the lower limbs.

The return of a normal BP after the infusion of, for example, 1000 mL does not mean that only a litre has been lost – the true amount is likely to be much higher. When blood pressure can be maintained only by continuing infusion, cardiovascular collapse is imminent; the cause of the hidden blood loss must be sought.

Failure to respond to fluids usually means inadequate transfusion or unrecognised fluid loss. However, it may also be caused by:

- tension pneumothorax → *p. 74*
- cardiac tamponade → *p. 78*
- myocardial infarction
- acute gastric distension
- neurogenic shock → *p. 51*.

Blood transfusion

Indications for blood components→ Box 14.29 on p. 258.
Overview of the management of major haemorrhage → Figure 1.2 on p. 8.

Military surgeons avoid 'old blood' and crystalloids and use large volumes of whole blood with fresh frozen plasma (FFP).

Modest haemodilution and a fall in haematocrit to 30% improve erythrocyte passage through the microcirculation. This allows optimal oxygen delivery to the tissues – until the haematocrit falls below 25%. However, when estimated blood loss exceeds 1.5 L in an adult, blood should be transfused to maintain the haematocrit >25% or a haemoglobin concentration >8 g/dL.

SAG-M blood (which consists of plasma-poor red blood cells in saline, adenine, glucose and mannitol) is frequently supplied by the National Blood Service in the UK. (The adenine maintains 2,3-diphosphoglycerate or 2,3-DPG activity in stored blood to allow more normal uncoupling of oxygen from oxyhaemoglobin and thus improved tissue oxygenation.) This red cell concentrate is presented in units of 300 mL, each with a packed cell volume (haematocrit) of 0.55–0.65.

If a blood sample is taken when the initial intravenous lines are established, grouped blood (type specific) should be available within 20 min. Cross-matched blood (whether by urgent or full cross-match) is seldom available within 1 h and is therefore not normally appropriate for unstable hypovolaemic patients. These patients should receive blood that is matched only for the recipient's ABO and rhesus group. This will, of course, increase the incidence of transfusion reactions.

In situations of such urgency that delay – even for grouped blood – is unacceptable, O-negative (universal donor) blood should be given. However, the risks of a transfusion reaction must be outweighed by the benefits of immediate blood replacement; such occasions are rare.

Rapid blood transfusion may produce the following:

- *Coagulopathy*: requiring platelets and/or FFP
- *Hypocalcaemia*: as a result of calcium binding by anticoagulants in stored blood (at infusion rates of <50 mL/min this should not be a problem); plasma calcium must not be allowed to fall <1 mmol/L
- *Hypothermia* (which may itself cause a significant reduction in coagulation).

Thus, if a large volume of blood is transfused rapidly, it should be filtered and warmed.

Immunocompromised and pregnant patients should always receive CMV-negative blood (i.e. blood that is free of cytomegalovirus).

Control of severe bleeding

The 'coagulopathy of trauma' is due to many factors: consumption of fibrinogen and clotting factors, dilution of plasma proteins, hypothermia, acidosis, inflammation and shock. If present on admission, it is associated with a mortality rate of almost 50%.

In the presence of intractable bleeding, deficiency of clotting factors should be considered and haematological advice sought. In particular, in the absence of any known disease, acquired haemophilia may be a possibility ($\rightarrow$ p. 257). If a site for bleeding is identified, further investigation should never delay surgical attempts to 'turn off the tap'.

Tranexamic acid: tranexamic acid inhibits fibrinolysis. It has been shown to safely reduce mortality in bleeding trauma patients without increasing the risk of adverse events, provided that it is given within 3 h of the time of injury. It is particularly useful when other treatments directed at coagulopathy (e.g. FFP, platelets and cryoprecipitate) are unavailable. A loading dose of 1 g is given intravenously over 10 min, followed by an infusion of 1 g over the next 8 h.

Recombinant factor VIIa: recombinant factor VIIa (rFVIIa or activated eptacog alfa) is licensed for the treatment of bleeding in patients with inhibitors such as congenital and acquired haemophilia, inherited factor VII deficiency and Glanzmann's thrombasthenia ($\rightarrow$ p. 258). It may also be a useful treatment in patients with continuing severe haemorrhage despite optimal surgical management and on-going attempts to correct coagulopathy. It is more effective if used early in the course of bleeding and, for maximum benefit, it should be given before the onset of the complications associated with a massive blood transfusion. Every effort should be made to correct deficiencies in platelets and coagulation factors by administering appropriate platelet, plasma and cryoprecipitate, or fibrinogen concentrate transfusions, before considering treatment with rFVIIa. Treatment with factor VII is expensive and may not be suitable for all patients, especially those with risk factors for thromboembolic disease or disseminated intravascular coagulation. It is not derived from human blood and is therefore acceptable for use in Jehovah's Witness patients. The dose is 90 mcg/kg (4.5 kIU/kg) by slow IV bolus injection and this can be repeated after 2 h if there is still significant blood loss. If there is no response after two doses, further amounts should not be given. Full blood count (FBC), prothrombin time (PT), activated partial thromboplastin time (APTT) and fibrinogen should be measured before treatment and 20 min after factor VII has been given. The PT will shorten dramatically and the APTT may also be reduced. However, these effects do not last long and further monitoring is required according to the clinical situation. It may be appropriate to consider bilateral lower limb ultrasonography to check for deep venous thrombosis (DVT) 3–5 days after rFVIIa administration.

Haemostatic substances for local application: severe bleeding from damaged tissue, blood vessels or even organs may sometimes be controlled by the local application of haemostatic substances. The most effective of these is MPH (Microporous Polysaccharide Hemospheres), a patented powder synthesised from raw materials derived from potatoes! The MPH particles dehydrate the blood and concentrate blood solids on their surfaces, thus creating a high concentration of gelled, compacted. clotting material.

Emergency thoracotomy

Emergency thoracotomy may be life saving for some patients with penetrating injuries to the chest ($\rightarrow$ p. 79). A left anterolateral thoracotomy in the fourth intercostal space allows cardiac tamponade to be relieved; cross-clamping of the thoracic aorta optimises cerebral circulation during the critical period. Thoracotomy is of no value if the patient is already lifeless on arrival at the department or has sustained blunt trauma.

Disability

A rapid assessment of the patient's neurological status completes the primary survey:

- Level of consciousness
- Pupil size and reaction
- Posture and spontaneous movements.

A simple classification of level of consciousness is the AVPU system:

A Alert
V Responds to voice
P Responds to pain
U Unresponsive

Alternatively, if time allows, the Glasgow Coma Scale (GCS) can be used.

Exposure

All parts of the patient should be exposed and examined. The spine must be well controlled when clothing is disturbed. Some clothes can only be safely removed during log-rolling. The areas most often missed are the back and the perineum.

> Beware of hypothermia.

At the end of the primary survey, attention must be given to the following:

- *Glucose*: check for hypoglycaemia with a reagent stick. Some degree of hyperglycaemia is inevitable in most trauma patients; hypoglycaemia can precipitate trauma ($\rightarrow$ pp. 240 and 333)
- *History*: the AMPLE format ($\rightarrow$ p. 12)
- *Immediate analgesia*: small aliquots of IV morphine carefully titrated against response
- *Investigations*: the three initial radiographs of multiple trauma (chest, lateral cervical spine and pelvis).

> Do not forget to communicate as frequently as possible with the patient's relatives ($\rightarrow$ pp. 13 and 334)

FURTHER CARE OF THE TRAUMA PATIENT
The secondary survey

On completion of the primary survey – when resuscitation is well under way and appropriate inpatient team members have been called – remove all the patient's remaining clothing while controlling the entire spine. The detailed secondary survey can now begin. It should be carried out in a top-to-toe rather than a systems-oriented order.

> Much of the information of the secondary (and primary) survey is best recorded on a purpose-designed trauma form.

The following features must be included in the examination.

Head and neck

- GCS score
- Pupillary size and reactions
- Posture, movement and cranial nerve function – lateralising signs
- Scalp – haematomas, lacerations, depressed fractures; insert gloved finger into lacerations to detect fractures
- Ears and nose for cerebrospinal fluid and/or bleeding. Look with an auroscope for haemotympani
- Facial skeleton
- Mouth and teeth
- Neck – swelling, wounds and tenderness.

Chest

- Respiratory rate, pattern and depth; watch and feel for the abnormal movement of a flail segment
- Clothing imprints or bruising
- Wounds – especially small penetrating injuries
- Surgical emphysema
- Rib tenderness
- Tracheal displacement
- Air entry, percussion note and breath sounds
- Heart sounds and position of the apex beat
- Trends in SaO_2
- Arterial blood gases
- ECG.

Abdomen

- Clothing imprints or bruising – which usually indicate severe compression
- Wounds
- Localised or generalised tenderness and guarding
- Bowel sounds – an unreliable guide to injury
- Buttocks, anus, genitalia and perineum
- Consider rectal and vaginal examination ($\rightarrow$ p. 303).

Back (will need log-roll)

- Bruising, swelling and wounds
- Gaps and swellings in the line of the spinous processes
- Tenderness – especially ribs, spine and loins
- Perineum and anus ($\rightarrow$ p. 84).

Limbs

- Swelling and bruising
- Tenderness
- Wounds
- Deformity and compound fractures

- Circulation, nerve and tendon function distal to injuries
- General peripheral neurological function.

At the end of the secondary survey, re-examine the ABCs.

Tx

- Summon further appropriate specialist help
- Reduce any fracture or dislocation that is threatening distal circulation or overlying skin; a mixture of IV morphine and inhaled nitrous oxide will be the minimum analgesia required for this in a conscious patient ($\rightarrow$ p. 15)
- Splint other fractures
- Clean and dress wounds
- Catheterise the bladder and measure the urine output
- Obtain further information from the patient, paramedics, bystanders, relatives or the GP
- Consider further investigations ($\rightarrow$ below).

Prophylactic antibiotics: These are indicated for:

- severe contaminated wounds with tissue destruction
- compound limb fractures
- penetrating intestinal injuries.

> Antibiotics are not indicated for simple contaminated wounds but thorough surgical toilet is always required. Delayed primary suture may be appropriate.

Tetanus prophylaxis: Tetanus immune status should be confirmed as soon as possible and antitetanus toxoid and immunoglobulin given as appropriate ($\rightarrow$ p. 394). If no history is available, the patient should be treated as unimmunised.

Investigations in trauma

Blood tests

Blood should be taken for FBC, blood group and cross-match, coagulation screen and biochemistry (including glucose). Arterial blood gases should be checked as soon as possible. When the cause of coma is in doubt, plasma osmolality can be useful ($\rightarrow$ p. 221).

Radiological priorities

Radiological priorities are chest, lateral cervical spine and pelvis. Portable or overhead machines should be used so that the patient does not have to be moved out of the resuscitation area. CT of the brain and radiographs of the dorsal and lumbar spine or extremities should be delayed until resuscitation is under way and the patient stable.

Assessment of cervical spine injury → p. 54.
Assessment of chest injury → p. 73.
Assessment of pelvic injury → p. 84.

Trauma radiograph of the chest: The ideal view of the chest is the erect posteroanterior (PA) film, which will demonstrate:

- pneumothorax
- haemothorax
- mediastinal widening
- subphrenic air
- rib fractures.

However, positioning the patient upright is potentially hazardous if spinal injury has not been excluded or the patient is unresponsive. Diagnosis of intrathoracic injury on an anteroposterior (AP) (supine) film is difficult. A lateral decubitus film, i.e. taken with a patient lying on his or her side (literally 'elbow down'), may be helpful in diagnosing pneumothorax, free intraperitoneal air or fluid levels, but to achieve the correct position requires careful in-line log-rolling.

Trauma radiograph of the cervical spine: A good cross-table lateral view of the cervical spine will exclude many significant injuries. Often, the body of C7 and the C7–T1 junction are not adequately visualised on the initial film, and a coned view of this area with gentle shoulder traction is needed.

If the lateral radiograph of the neck is normal and the patient is fully conscious without significant neck pain, then the cervical collar may be removed to allow clinical assessment of the cervical spine. In the patient with depressed consciousness, the cervical spine must remain immobilised while awaiting AP and odontoid peg views, discussion with an orthopaedic surgeon and, if necessary, a CT scan.

Clearance of the cervical spine → p. 55.

Trauma radiograph of the pelvis: Clinical assessment of pelvic injury by pressure on the anterosuperior iliac spines is unreliable and may restart or exacerbate pelvic bleeding. An AP radiograph of the pelvis is taken to assess the potential for blood loss rather than to obtain detailed information about the nature of any fractures.

CT scan: CT provides excellent assessment of intracranial injuries and their sequelae. It is also essential for:

- clearance of the cervical spine where there remains clinical doubt after plain films
- further assessment of spinal injuries seen on plain films
- detailed examination of thoracic injuries, especially those involving the mediastinum
- assessment of abdominal injuries in relatively stable patients before laparotomy
- detailed assessment of pelvic fractures.

If CT is to be performed, all necessary images should be obtained at the same time. Routine use of 'top-to-toe' scanning is now recommended in the adult trauma patient if no indication for immediate intervention exists. A CT scan with contrast is often required.

Ultrasound scan: In experienced hands, ultrasonography can be a highly sensitive diagnostic technique. It is particularly useful for the detection of free fluid and the identification of solid organ injury. It is less valuable in the assessment of bowel damage. The ultrasound machine can be brought to the patient rather than moving an unstable patient to the CT room.

Further assessment of the abdomen in multiple trauma

Abdominal injuries have special significance because of the following:

1 They can cause profound haemorrhage.
2 They can be difficult to diagnose clinically – especially in unresponsive patients. Signs may be poorly localised or equivocal.

Exclusion of intra-abdominal damage is particularly important in any patient who:

- is shocked or unstable
- has signs attributable to the abdomen
- has a reduced level of consciousness or is otherwise difficult to assess clinically
- is about to be anaesthetised or transferred to another department for the management of other injuries.

Methods of abdominal assessment include:

- immediate laparotomy
- diagnostic peritoneal lavage
- ultrasound examination
- CT scan.

More on assessment of abdominal injuries → p. 81.

Definitive care of the trauma patient

The trauma patient should be moved to an area for definitive care as soon as possible. This may be an operating theatre, a specialised surgical unit, an ICU or a bed in a ward. Rapid disposal of a properly assessed and stabilised patient is associated with a decreased risk of complications and is (obviously) a reassurance for both patients and relatives.

> Do not forget the continuing need for analgesia.

Refer to appropriate chapters for specific injuries.

SPECIAL SITUATIONS

Choking → p. 196.
Electrocution → p. 144.
Exposure to radiation and contamination by radioactive substances → p. 145.
Gunshot wounds → pp. 371 and 398.
Major burns → Chapter 10 on p. 136.

Blast injuries

Explosions have the potential to cause complex and varied polytrauma to large numbers of people. These injuries are compounded when the explosion occurs in a confined space. Blast injuries are divided into four classes – primary, secondary, tertiary and quaternary:

1 Primary injuries are caused by the effect of blast overpressure waves (shock waves) on human tissue. The degree of injury depends on the level of pressure and its duration. These type of injuries are especially likely when a person is close to exploding munitions, such as a landmine. Unlike water, air is easily compressible and so a primary blast injury almost always affects air-filled structures. The ears are most often injured, followed by the lungs and the hollow organs of the gastrointestinal (GI) tract. GI injuries may present after a delay of hours or even days and are very hard to diagnose.

2 Secondary injuries are caused by flying shrapnel, glass, debris and other objects propelled by the explosion. These injuries may affect any part of the body and often result in penetrating trauma and bleeding.

3 Tertiary injuries are a feature of high-energy explosions. Displacement of air by the explosion creates a blast wind that can throw victims against solid objects. There may be both blunt and penetrating injuries. Fractures are common. Children are particularly vulnerable because of their low body weight.

4 Quaternary (or miscellaneous) injuries include all other injuries not included in the first three classes such as burns, crush injuries, toxic inhalations and radiation exposure.

All patients exposed to a significant explosion must be carefully examined with special attention paid to their tympanic membranes, lungs and abdomen. The urine should be screened for blood. A chest radiograph (CXR) is indicated in the presence of dyspnoea or ruptured tympanic membranes. Blunt injuries, fractures, crush injuries, burns and superficial injuries from flying glass should all receive standard investigation and treatment. Penetrating injuries from shrapnel and other debris are best regarded as low-velocity gunshot wounds.

Burns → Chapter 10 on p. 136.
Burns from white phosphorus in incendiary munitions → p. 143.
Exposure to radiation and contamination by radioactive substances → p. 145.
Gunshot wounds → pp. 371 and 398.

Drowning

Drowning is suffocation resulting from submersion or immersion in a liquid and as such causes injury by the effects of fluid in the airway and lungs and by generalised hypoxia. There may also be:

- precipitating causes, e.g. alcohol or drug intoxication, myocardial infarction, hypoglycaemia, fit
- coincidental injury, e.g. from a fall or dive into water (especially injury to the cervical spine)
- other consequences, e.g. hypothermia.

Toddlers and teenagers are the most common victims of drowning – which is the leading cause of accidental death in children worldwide.

The difference between the effects of sea water (hypertonic) and fresh water (hypotonic) drowning is probably less important than once believed. In many cases, there is immediate laryngospasm and thus little inhalation into the lungs (dry drowning). The patient is likely to be unresponsive and hypotensive with signs of cerebral hypoxia and perhaps also pulmonary oedema. Beware the danger of an 'after-drop' in exhausted patients pulled out of very cold water; the core temperature may fall further as resuscitation progresses.

Tx

Cardiac arrest → p. 150.

- Clear the airway of debris and then secure it. Consider the need for cervical spine protection.
- Give high-flow oxygen with a continuous positive airway pressure (CPAP) circuit if possible. Patients in whom breathing is inadequate should be ventilated immediately – with the help of an anaesthetist if possible. These patients will usually need decompression of the stomach with a wide-bore tube.
- Establish IV access and fluid infusion.
- Monitor SaO_2, respiratory rate, pulse, BP, ECG and core temperature.
- Send blood for FBC, blood chemistry, glucose and blood gases.
- Obtain a 12-lead ECG and CXR.
- Treat hypotension, wheezing or pulmonary oedema. Severe acidosis can be corrected with bicarbonate.
- Treat hypothermia ($→ p. 243$).

All patients must be admitted – most to an ICU. Delayed exacerbations may occur up to 24 h after injury. Patients with signs of cerebral hypoxia (usually unresponsive) should be ventilated even in the presence of satisfactory oxygenation because they are likely to have cerebral oedema.

Suffocation and asphyxiation

Suffocation is a state in which there is inadequate availability of air for inhalation – usually as a result of external obstruction of the mouth and nose. Asphyxiation describes oxygen deficit from a wider range of causes such as gassing and strangulation. The signs of both are those of prolonged hypoxia and developing cerebral oedema. The treatment is similar to that detailed above for drowning.

Paediatric trauma

The principles of the management of trauma are the same for both adults and children. Differences in anatomy, physiological parameters and equipment are dealt with in *Chapter 18*. The most important aspects of a child when compared with an adult in trauma care are as follows:

- The airway is narrower, floppier and more difficult to maintain.
- The lungs have a very limited oxygen reserve but the body has a higher metabolic rate.

- The circulation may suddenly decompensate and thus shock appears with very little warning.
- The vertebrae are relatively elastic and so there may be spinal cord injury without radiological abnormality (abbreviated to the acronym SCIWORA).
- The ribs are also elastic and so underlying viscera may be injured without evidence of rib trauma.
- A child becomes hypoglycaemic and hypothermic very easily.

> A child's lungs, liver and spleen are like fresh eggs in an AMBU bag. Hit the bag with a hammer and the eggs are smashed but the bag (the ribs) returns to its former shape. An adult's organs are like hard-boiled eggs in a tin can. Hit the can and it is damaged (there are rib fractures) but the eggs may survive intact.

Trauma in pregnancy

The relevant anatomical and physiological changes of pregnancy must be considered during assessment:

- The tidal volume is increased, respiratory rate is stable and so $PaCO_2$ (arterial CO_2 partial pressure) is slightly reduced.
- The BP is normally slightly reduced and the pulse is increased.
- Compression of the inferior vena cava in the supine patient in the last trimester of pregnancy is very significant and reduces cardiac output. The risk of sudden collapse is reduced by turning the patient partially on to the left side.
- Gastric emptying is delayed.

Systemic (maternal) hypovolaemia results in a selective reduction in placental blood flow. The fetus is very vulnerable to hypoxia but the maternal circulation is partially protected by a physiological hypervolaemia. Deterioration in oxygen supply to the fetus can occur very rapidly after a period of apparent normality.

XR Consider early ultrasound scan of the abdomen, uterus and fetus.

Tx There are, of course, two patients:

1 **The mother:** for the most part, the care of a pregnant woman is identical to that of a non-pregnant patient. Important additions are the following:

- Hypoxia and hypovolaemia must be treated particularly quickly and vigorously. If blood is to be given, it must be CMV negative.
- Patients in the last trimester of pregnancy should be nursed wedged on to the left side. This is to prevent compression of the inferior vena cava by the pregnant uterus with consequent reduction in cardiac filling and circulatory collapse.
- There is an increased risk of aspiration pneumonia (Mendelson's syndrome), especially if the mother has a reduced level of consciousness or needs sedation or anaesthesia. Prophylaxis is aimed at reducing the acidity of the gastric contents as quickly as possible – give at-risk patients IV ranitidine (50 mg diluted to 20 mL over 2 min) or IV omeprazole (40 mg diluted to 100 mL over 20 min).
- Rhesus D-negative women with abdominal injury are at risk of developing antibodies against a rhesus-positive fetus. Any pregnant woman who may have had abdominal trauma should be blood grouped and, if found to be rhesus D negative, given anti-D immunoglobulin.

2 **The fetus:** the wellbeing of the fetus depends almost entirely on the state of the mother.

> The initial management of the fetus is the support of the maternal airway, breathing and circulation.

Once the mother is stabilised, then obstetric advice should be sought. Methods of assessing the fetus include:

- auscultation with a Pinnard's stethoscope or Doppler fetoscope
- fetocardiotocography (FCTG)
- abdominal ultrasonography.

In some cases, in late pregnancy, caesarean section will be required for the health of both parties.

Postmortem caesarean section may occasionally save the life of the baby when the mother is recently deceased. For this purpose, the modern operation of lower uterine segment caesarean section is too slow. A 'classic' section is usually performed through the muscle of the upper uterine segment, leading to a rapid delivery.

Abdominal trauma in pregnancy → p. 83.

OTHER ASPECTS OF TRAUMA CARE

Bereaved relatives

As with cardiac arrest, a fatality from trauma will leave relatives in a state of sudden and unexpected bereavement. The care of these people is part of the complete spectrum of trauma management.

Outline of bereavement care → p. 163.

Trauma scores

Trauma scoring systems are useful for audit, research and planning purposes but should not be used to determine in-hospital care. They have a limited use in prehospital triage. There are four main types:

1 Scores used at the site of an incident, which are based on direct observation of evident abnormalities
2 Scores that are based retrospectively on the anatomical injuries, e.g. the Injury Severity Score (ISS)
3 Scores that are calculated from the currently observed physiology, e.g. the Revised Trauma Score (RTS)
4 More complex scores – usually derived on the ICU – which take account of both the current status and the pre-existing health of the victim, e.g. the Acute Physiology and Chronic Health Evaluation (APACHE score).

Head injuries

Around 10% of patients who attend UK emergency departments (EDs) have head injuries; half of them are children.

> Over 5000 people die from traumatic brain injuries in England and Wales every year and over 1500 patients survive with severe brain damage. Most will have a severely reduced employment potential and many will require long-term nursing care. The majority are men, with a mean age of 30 years.

Primary damage to the brain occurs at the time of injury. Secondary damage is the result of extracranial factors such as hypoxia or hypovolaemia, which lead to impaired cerebral oxygen delivery. Reperfusion of damaged brain (with the release of oxygen free radicals and lipid peroxidation) is now recognised as an additional secondary factor that can complicate recovery from traumatic brain injury. The problems that cause secondary damage can be minimised by systemic resuscitation. In the future, intracranial factors may be amenable to pharmacological interventions.

A decreased level of consciousness indicates that something is wrong with the brain or its fuel supply. It may be injury or:

- hypoxia or shock
- hypoglycaemia
- hypothermia
- poisoning or gross metabolic disturbance (including CO_2 narcosis)

- intracranial pathology (bleeding, thrombosis, embolism, infection, swelling, tumour, fitting).

> Over half of all patients who are in a traumatic coma for more than 6 h will die; only a fifth will recover without significant disability.

Biomechanics and brain injury

Direct trauma may cause:

1 Focal scalp injury
2 Depressed vault fracture
3 Extradural haemorrhage
4 Focal brain injury
5 Contre-coupe injury
6 Brain laceration and intracerebral haemorrhage
7 Subdural haemorrhage.

1–5 may not be associated with loss of consciousness. **Sudden acceleration/deceleration** causes shearing injury to the brain and diffuse axonal injury (DAI). This is associated with loss of consciousness but external evidence of head injury may be lacking. DAI is more common with the longer deceleration time characteristic of restrained passengers in traffic crashes. Extradural haemorrhage is more common in falls.

Cervical spine injury is more likely to be associated with a brain injury if the mobile head hits a fixed object (deceleration/acceleration), than if a mobile object hits the fixed head (assault).

Emergency Medicine Lecture Notes, Fourth Edition. Chris Moulton and David Yates.
© 2012 Blackwell Publishing Ltd. Published 2012 by Blackwell Publishing Ltd.

THE PATIENT WITH A DEPRESSED LEVEL OF CONSCIOUSNESS

This section deals with the management of those patients who when first seen have a Glasgow Coma Scale (GCS) score <15 (→ *Table 3.1*). Serious brain injury must be suspected. The principal objective of emergency management is to limit the effects of this primary insult by preventing deleterious secondary events, which could impair cerebral oxygen supply. A detailed neurological examination to determine the extent of the primary injury must be deferred until treatable secondary events have been controlled.

Immediate assessment and management

The ABC approach is vital:

- Clear and maintain the airway and give high-concentration oxygen. Have suction available.
- Ensure that the cervical spine is protected.

Table 3.1 The Glasgow Coma Scale (GCS)

Response elicited	Score
Response of eyes	
Open spontaneously	4
Open to speech	3
Open to pain	2
No response	1
Best motor response	
Obeys commands	6
Localises pain	5 (supraorbital ridge pressure)
Withdraws from pain	4 (normal flexion)
Abnormal flexion	3 (decorticate response)
Extension to pain	2 (decerebrate response)
None	1
Best verbal response	
Oriented	5
Confused	4
Inappropriate words	3
Incomprehensible sounds	2
None	1

- Obtain anaesthetic assistance as soon as possible. Emergency induction of anaesthesia, intubation and ventilation are likely to be required.

> Ensure that cardiorespiratory resuscitation is initiated and the neck is protected before assessing brain injury.

- Obtain intravenous (IV) access.
- Monitor and record pulse, BP, SaO_2, respiratory rate and ECG.
- Assess neurological status by AVPU criteria:
  A Alert
  V Responds to voice
  P Responds to pain
  U Unresponsive
  and assess the pupils for size, equality and reaction.
- Check blood glucose with a reagent strip.
- Treat reversible conditions (and reassess after therapy):
  Hypoglycaemia: take blood for glucose estimation before giving IV dextrose (0.2– 0.5 mg/kg); avoid hyperglycaemia
  Fits: give IV lorazepam 4 mg (0.1 mg/kg) or IV diazepam 10 mg (0.25 mg/kg) slowly
  Narcosis: give IV naloxone 0.4 mg
  Aggression and restlessness: give 100% oxygen; check the airway and the SaO_2; catheterise the bladder; sedation should be given only after consideration of the causes.
- Ask witnesses/paramedics if the level of consciousness has changed since the impact. Did the patient briefly recover and speak and then deteriorate? Obtain a brief history (*AMPLE* → *p. 12*). Try to establish the mechanism of the injury.
- Obtain radiographs of the cervical spine. Measure the blood gases.

> Steroids are of no benefit in the treatment of head injuries.

Further assessment and management

- Carry out a detailed secondary survey
- Seek surgical/neurosurgical advice
- Consider catheterising the bladder.

The secondary survey searches for other injuries and establishes the neurological status. It must include examination of the following:

- The scalp
- The auditory canals and tympanic membranes (caution → p. 44)
- The pupils and limbs
- The face
- The neck.

Neurological assessment

There are three groups of observations:

1 *Global*: the level of consciousness should be assessed using the GCS (→ Box 3.1). This is a sensitive and reproducible indication of early neurological deterioration.
2 *Focal*: neurological signs (e.g. variation in muscle tone, asymmetrical limb movement and reflexes, disconjugate eye movements) help to identify the site and severity of brain damage.
3 *Physiological*: the components of 'Cushing's response' (slow pulse, raised BP and dilated, sluggish pupils) are easily measured but are very late indicators of high intracranial pressure.

All of the above observations should be repeated at appropriate intervals and plotted on a chart.

> GCS maximum score = 15 (not necessarily equivalent to alert and oriented)
> GCS minimum score = 3 (even if dead!)
> GCS of 8 or less = coma

Children's Coma Score → p. 332.

Other injuries

About 50% of patients with major brain injury have serious injuries elsewhere. The more injuries there are, the greater the risk of missing some of them.

Multiple injuries → Chapter 2 on p. 19.

Imaging

As soon as the patient with a depressed level of consciousness is stabilised, a CT scan of the brain should be obtained (→ Boxes 3.1 for adults and 3.8 for children). Most patients will be intubated and ventilated before scanning. If a patient who is aged over 65 presents 'out of hours' and the only positive CT indicator from Box 3.1 is amnesia of events for more than

 Box 3.1 Indications for CT of the brain in adults with head injuries

Children aged < 16 years → Box 3.8

(Incorporating the UK National Institute for Health and Clinical Excellence's [NICE's] head injury guideline, 2007)

1 The threshold for CT examination should be lowered if there are other life-threatening injuries, particularly if these will require surgery under general anaesthetic
2 The CT brain scan should extend down to the second cervical vertebra with 3-mm cuts from the level of the foramen magnum to C2. If the lower cervical spine has not been well visualised on plain radiographs, this should also be scanned
3 Patients who return to the ED after discharge with persistent complaints that could be attributed to their head injury should be discussed with a senior clinician and considered for CT

Immediate CT scan (= *imaging performed and results analysed within 1 h of the request*)

- GCS <13 when first assessed in the ED
- GCS <15 when assessed in the ED 2h after injury
- Suspected open or depressed skull fracture
- Sign of fracture of skull base (→ p. 43)
- Focal neurological signs
- Post-traumatic seizure
- More than one episode of vomiting
- Coagulopathy with a history of loss of consciousness or amnesia (history of bleeding or clotting disorder or current anticoagulant treatment)

Delayed CT scan (= *imaging performed and results analysed within 8 h of the time of injury*)

- Dangerous mechanism of injury with a history of loss of consciousness or amnesia (pedestrian or cyclist hit by motor vehicle; occupant ejected from motor vehicle; fall from a height of >1 m or five stairs; lower heights are applicable for infants and young children)
- Amnesia >30 min for events before the impact
- Age 65 years with a history of loss of consciousness or amnesia

...ry or a dangerous mechanism ...eptable to admit them for over-... CT the next morning.

...al and resource reasons, MRI is ...cated as a primary investigation in patients with head injuries. Moreover, it is contraindicated in both head and cervical investigations unless there is absolute certainty that the patient is not harbouring an incompatible device, implant or metallic foreign body.

Skull radiographs do not contribute to initial management. Therapy is concerned with brain injury rather than bone injury and this is detected initially by the neurological signs.

The indications for imaging of the cervical spine in patients with head injuries are summarised in *Box 3.2*. In most circumstances, plain radiographs are the initial investigation of choice – three views in adults, two in children under 10 years.

Management of specific problems

Airway and breathing

Inadequate respiration leads to hypoxia, hypercapnia and acidosis. This results in cerebral vasodilatation and a rise in intracranial pressure (ICP). Although simple manoeuvres to clear and maintain the airway may be initially successful, intubation and ventilation are required for most patients with impaired respiration (→ *Box 3.3*).

Intubation should not be attempted without sedation, analgesia and muscle paralysis (even in apparently 'flat' head-injured patients) because this would cause a sudden rise in intracranial pressure.

> In ventilated patients with a head injury, aim for a PaO_2 >100 mmHg (13 kPa) and a $PaCO_2$ of 35–38 mmHg (4.5–5.0 kPa).

Box 3.2 Indications for imaging of the cervical spine in adults and children with head injuries

(Incorporating NICE's head injury guideline, 2007)

Assessment of the injured neck → p. 55.

Immediate plain radiographs:
- Cannot actively rotate neck to 45° (left and right)
- Not safe to move neck (→ *p. 54*)
- Focal neurological signs (including paraesthesia in the extremities)
- Neck pain or midline tenderness with:
  - dangerous mechanism of injury (fall >1 m or five stairs; axial load to head: diving injury, ejection from a motor vehicle, high-speed motor vehicle collision or roll-over, bicycle collision, crash involving motorised recreational vehicles; use lower threshold for falls for infants and children <5 years)
  - aged >65 years
- Definitive diagnosis required urgently, e.g. before surgery

Immediate CT scan:
- GCS <13 on initial assessment
- Has been intubated
- Plain films technically inadequate, suspicious or definitely abnormal
- Continued clinical suspicion despite normal plain films
- Patient is being scanned for multi-region trauma

Note that CT is now recommended more often than previously but the risks from irradiation to children <10 years limits CT in this group to those with severe head injury (GCS <8) and where there is a strong clinical suspicion of injury despite normal plain films.

Even patients with no apparent respiratory disturbance may benefit from controlled ventilation. (→ *Box 3.4*). Hyperventilation to a $PaCO_2$ <40 mmHg (5.3 kPa) causes cerebral vasoconstriction and a consequent fall in intracranial pressure (ICP). Excessive hyperventilation can, however, be dangerous. Only the undamaged brain responds to changes in blood gas tension, and vasoconstriction in normal areas may result in redistribution of blood flow to the injured tissue. This increases the penumbra around the damaged area. Brain ischaemia leads to lactic acidosis and reflex vasodilatation.

Circulation

In a healthy person, changes in arterial BP between 80 and 200 mmHg do not influence cerebral blood flow. Brain injury impairs this autoregulatory function and hence cerebral blood supply in damaged

Box 3.3 Indications for immediate intubation and ventilation after head injuries

Aiming for PaO$_2$ >100 mmHg (13 kPa) and PaCO$_2$ of 35–38 mmHg (4.5–5.0 kPa)

- Coma or deteriorating conscious level
- Apparent loss of protective airway reflexes
- Ventilatory insufficiency as judged by oximetry/blood gas measurement:
  - *PaO$_2$* <75 mmHg (10 kPa) on air or <100 mmHg (13 kPa) on oxygen
  - *PaCO$_2$* >45 mmHg (6 kPa)
- Spontaneous hyperventilation causing a *PaCO$_2$* <30 mmHg (4 kPa)
- Irregular respiration
- Multiple fits
- Significant facial injuries
- Bleeding into the airway
- Extreme agitation

Box 3.4 Reasons for intubating and ventilating patients with brain injuries

1 To clear, maintain and protect the airway
2 To maintain adequate gas exchange
3 To reduce ICP and *PaCO$_2$*
4 To facilitate CT
5 To allow safe patient transport

areas is less well protected from changes in the systemic circulation.

Hypotension is only very rarely caused by brain injury. Trauma to the trunk and neck must be considered together with the biomechanics of the impact.

Cushing's response (bradycardia and hypertension) is a late sign and indicates rising ICP.

Neurogenic pulmonary oedema is occasionally seen. It is thought to be caused by vasoconstriction resulting from sympathetic overactivity (an alpha effect). It should be treated aggressively with standard drugs and always necessitates ventilation ($\rightarrow$ p. 208).

Raised intracranial pressure

Hyperglycaemia increases brain swelling and must be avoided. IV mannitol 1 g/kg is used as a short-term agent to reduce brain swelling before clot evacuation; IV furosemide 0.5 mg/kg is an alternative. Mannitol actually causes a transient ICP rise and leaks into the extracellular space, exerting an osmotic effect.

Furosemide does not have these deleterious effects and causes a reduction in cerebrospinal fluid production. Neither drug should be used for the long-term management of cerebral oedema.

Fits

Both ICP and metabolic demand for oxygen rise dramatically during a fit and this may increase the extent of the brain damage. Intravenous lorazepam or diazepam is usually effective, but be aware of the possibility of respiratory arrest.

Suspected alcohol intoxication

Drunkenness increases the risk of sustaining a head injury and of that injury causing brain damage. Nevertheless, changes in conscious level must not be attributed to alcohol or other drugs except after exclusion of all other possible causes – and in retrospect. The plasma osmolality may be a useful investigation in this circumstance ($\rightarrow$ p. 221) if direct measurement of plasma alcohol is unavailable.

Patients with a diagnosis of alcohol intoxication who have not regained full consciousness within 6–8 h of arrival should have a CT scan of the brain.

Urine output

Catheterisation of the bladder is mandatory in an unresponsive, brain-injured patient. A full bladder leads to increasing restlessness. In addition, the urine output is a good indicator of adequate tissue perfusion – it should be at least 1 mL/kg per h.

Pain

Analgesia may be needed if the patient is not deeply unconscious and has other painful injuries. Initially, it can be achieved by fracture splintage. Once baseline observations are established, give small doses of opiates intravenously.

Bleeding from the scalp

Examination of the scalp must be meticulous; the hair must be shaved off to a distance of at least 1 cm around the wound edges. Lacerations should be palpated with a gloved finger to detect fracture lines and foreign bodies. Severe bleeding can be controlled with a single layer of deep sutures, using 2/0 silk on a hand-held needle. A pressure dressing should then be applied. The application of Raney clips to the wound edges can be a useful holding measure.

Deterioration

Early, rapid, neurological deterioration is very rarely caused by a remedial intracranial lesion but more often is due to:

- severe primary brain injury
- hypoxaemia
- hypovolaemia.

Guidelines for neurosurgical consultation

> Before telephoning a neurosurgeon, ensure that resuscitation has been initiated and that extracranial injuries have been addressed.

Regional neuroscience centres should collaborate with their linked EDs and ambulance service to provide clear written guidance on consultation and referral practices. In particular, the definition of 'surgically significant' must be agreed by both parties. There is increasing evidence that all seriously brain-injured patients will benefit from care at a neuroscience centre, whether or not neurosurgical intervention is required, but clearly it is imperative that all those requiring surgery should be transferred as soon as possible. Seek neurosurgical/neurointensive care advice in any of the following instances:

- Positive intracranial findings on CT scan including cerebral oedema
- Penetrating injury
- Depressed skull fracture
- Basal skull fracture
- Skull fracture with any depression of consciousness, repeated fits, severe headache, persistent vomiting or acute focal neurology
- CSF leak
- GCS <13 after resuscitation
- Unexplained confusion persisting after >4 h
- Deterioration of GCS (especially motor score)
- Progressive focal neurological signs.

Transfer from an ED to a neuroscience centre should be well planned, well resourced, speedy and documented. In all circumstances complete initial resuscitation and patient stabilisation, and establish comprehensive monitoring, before transfer, to avoid complications during the journey. If the patient is persistently hypotensive despite resuscitation, do not transport until the cause has been identified and the patient stabilised.

A doctor with appropriate training should accompany the patient. Child or infant transfer requires relevant paediatric critical care expertise. A communication system capable of being used en route is essential; it must not interfere with on-board equipment function.

THE AMBULANT PATIENT WITH A HEAD INJURY

These patients will mostly have a GCS score of 15. This score does not necessarily imply normal mental functioning because the GCS score is not sensitive to changes in alertness or higher intellectual function. Some ambulant patients may be confused (GCS score = 14).

The diagnosis of a minor head injury can be made only in retrospect. The following points should help to distinguish between those with no significant brain injury and those at risk of serious complications.

History

The history of the incident is important because it often influences management. When the history is unknown or unreliable the patient must be considered for admission to hospital.

- Establish the speed of impact and the nature of the object struck by the head. The part of the head involved and the area of contact are also important (e.g. occiput hitting a carpeted floor is less serious than temple hitting the corner of a radiator).
- Establish the pattern of subsequent behaviour and ask about any period of unconsciousness, confusion, amnesia or fitting. Ask about the occurrence of headache and vomiting. Changes to hearing and vision, including diplopia, must also be noted.

Post-traumatic amnesia

The duration of post-traumatic amnesia (PTA) correlates fairly well with the degree of primary brain injury. Under 1 h usually denotes mild injury, whereas over 24 h is associated with severe injury. PTA is often underestimated. It should be measured up to the time when memory of consecutive events returns. This usually corresponds with the duration of spatial disorientation and is much longer than the period during which the patient did not speak.

> PTA is often longer than initially estimated.

Retrograde amnesia

Retrograde amnesia (for events before the accident) can be very unreliable and extremely variable, especially in patients who have been drinking alcohol. However, in others, it is a useful indicator of injury severity.

Drugs and alcohol

These are often implicated in the aetiology of head injury, but deterioration in a patient should not be attributed to their effects. Very high blood alcohol levels (>6000 mg/L) have been recorded in ambulant patients. Put alcohol at the bottom of the list of causes of altered consciousness.

Medical history

A medical history is usually obtained from relatives, neighbours, a phone call to the GP or by searching clothing. It is valuable in two respects:

1 Factors relevant to present management (e.g. diabetes, steroid treatment)
2 Factors relevant to the prevention of a further incident (e.g. transient ischaemic attack, alcohol abuse).

> Always enquire about any bleeding diathesis or anticoagulant therapy – especially warfarin or clopidogrel.

Assessment

- Behaviour: it is common for a patient to appear normal on casual assessment whereas enquiry a few days later reveals no recollection of the first interview.
- Cognition: pupil changes and the other classic signs of raised ICP are very late indicators of deterioration. Eighty per cent of the rise in pressure required to cause brain-stem coning occurs without any change in these indicators.
- Movement: look especially for loss of coordination and ataxia. Examine limb movement, sensation and reflexes.
- GCS ($\rightarrow$ Table 3.1).
- Pupil size and reactivity.
- BP, pulse, respiratory rate, SaO_2, temperature.

- Examine the head, noting any wounds, swellings or depressions. Palpate, as well as inspect, with gloved hand. Interpretation of imaging is facilitated by being able to link common areas of radiological and clinical abnormality.
- Examine the neck.
- Exclude injuries elsewhere.
- Imaging.

Imaging

CT allows visualisation of the brain and almost all pathology that may require operative treatment. Fractures of the base and vault of the skull may be seen on 'bony windows'. Depressed fractures may be identified and the depth of depressions calculated.

Indications for CT of the brain in patients with head injuries $\rightarrow$ Boxes 3.1 and 3.8.

Skull radiographs have been largely replaced by CT and observation on short-stay wards. However, they still have a place in the management of physical child abuse and the assessment of some complicated patients. Moreover, 24-hour CT is not universally available – hence a section on skull radiography is provided on p. 46.

Patients at risk of developing complications after a head injury

Patients with one or more of the following features have a significant risk of developing intracranial complications:

- Impaired level of consciousness at time of presentation (including those who are showing GCS = 15 but not fully alert)
- Post-traumatic amnesia of over 15 min duration
- Abnormal neurological signs
- Fits
- Symptoms of raised ICP (severe headache, persistent vomiting)
- Vault fracture on radiograph ($\rightarrow$ Tables 3.2 and 3.3)
- Clinical evidence of basal skull fracture ($\rightarrow$ p. 43).

Table 3.2 Risk of intracranial haematoma in adults with head injuries

	No skull fracture	Skull fracture
Fully conscious	1 in 8000	1 in 45
Impaired consciousness	1 in 180	1 in 5
Comatose	1 in 27	1 in 4

Table 3.3 Risk of intracranial haematoma in children with head injuries

	No skull fracture	Skull fracture
Fully conscious	1 in 13000	1 in 157
Impaired consciousness	1 in 580	1 in 25
Comatose	1 in 65	1 in 12

Box 3.5 Indications for observation in hospital after head injuries

(Adapted from NICE's head injury guideline, 2007)
Patients with head injuries who have any of the following features should be admitted to hospital for observation:

- New clinically significant abnormalities on imaging
- Failure to return to GCS of 15 regardless of any imaging results
- Fulfil the criteria for CT imaging (→ *Boxes 3.1 and 3.8*) but cannot be scanned because of patient state or equipment failure
- Continuing symptoms or signs for concern (e.g. persistent vomiting, severe headache)
- Other coexisting problems (e.g. drug or alcohol intoxication, other injuries, CSF fluid leak, suspected non-accidental injury, meningism)

In patients who are fully alert on examination, a history of an altered level of consciousness before arrival at hospital increases the risk of intracranial haematoma by a factor of 4

Indications for observation in hospital following a head injury → Box 3.5.

Xʀ CT scans are of great value in this group of patients.

Tx All patients with a significant risk of developing complications must be admitted and observed carefully by nurses who understand the GCS and are trained in the early detection of changes in neurological status. The following observations should be made:

- Best eye-opening response
- Best motor response (noting lateralising signs)

Box 3.6 Changes requiring urgent review in patients admitted to hospital with head injuries

(Adapted from NICE's head injury guideline, 2007)
Consider immediate CT scan if:

- Development of agitation or abnormal behaviour
- Drop of 1 point in GCS score for 30 min or more (especially in motor score)
- Drop of ≥2 points in GCS score regardless of duration or of GCS component affected
- Development of persistent severe headache
- Persistent vomiting
- New or evolving focal neurological symptoms or signs (e.g. pupil inequality or asymmetry of limb or facial movements)

- Best verbal response
- Pupil size and reaction to light
- Respiratory rate
- Pulse and BP
- Temperature.

Perform and record these observations at 30-min intervals until the GCS=15. Thereafter, continue at 30 min for 2 h, then hourly for 4 h and then 2-hourly.

Changes requiring urgent review in patients admitted to hospital with head injuries → Box 3.6.

Ambulant patients with head injuries who are not obviously at risk

There is a remote possibility that intracranial complications will occur after the most trivial head injury. A council of perfection might suggest that all patients should be admitted. This would result in a vast number of people being admitted to make an uneventful recovery. Quite apart from economic and social implications, this would be counterproductive. Staff would have an increased threshold for the recognition of abnormalities when their everyday experience was of large numbers of relatively well patients. Thus only those patients who have histories, symptoms or signs that put them at risk should be detained. However, if the home conditions appear inadequate or the relatives are unhappy about looking after the patient, admission is essential.

Advice to discharged patients ('head injury instructions')

*Discharge criteria for patients with head injuries →
Box 3.7.*

1 Insist on the presence of a relative or a friend and
never discharge a head-injured patient unless a
third party is aware of the injury and will accompany the patient home.
2 Ensure that there is a telephone in or near the
patient's home and encourage the relatives to
phone the hospital if they have any anxieties.
3 Provide verbal and written advice. The following
points should be made:
- Nausea and mild headache are common but the
ED should be contacted if these symptoms
persist or increase. Any vomiting must be taken
seriously.
- Alterations in the level of consciousness are an
important early sign of the development of complications and necessitate urgent referral back to
hospital. Changes should not be attributed to
drugs or alcohol.
- Any other unusual change in vision, hearing or
movement should prompt a discussion with the
hospital.
- Recovery from a mild traumatic brain injury
often takes much longer than commonly
expected. A period of rest and time off work
is usually appropriate. Alcohol may delay
recovery.

4 Every patient who has had a CT brain scan and/or
been admitted to hospital should be referred
to their GP for follow-up within 1 week of discharge. If problems persist the GP should arrange
referral back to an outpatient clinic for specialist
assessment.

Head injuries in children

In a school-age child the most common cause of
death is a brain injury from a road traffic incident.
Minor head injuries are also important, even if they
do not produce immediate major complications;
repeated minor head trauma in children has been
linked to lowered IQ. Young children are less likely
to lose consciousness than adults. Significant
brain injury may thus occur without a history of
unconsciousness.

*Risk of intracranial haematoma in children after head
injuries → Table 3.3.*

Assessment can be difficult. The Children's Coma
Scale (a modified GCS) should be used for children aged <5 years (→ p. 332). In the evening, children
may be sleepy but, nevertheless, a normal child is
easily woken. Parents are in the best position to
judge minor alterations in their children's level of
consciousness.

Children are more prone to head injury when frac-
tious, feverish or in the prodromal stage of an acute
illness. A cause for unsteadiness should always be
sought and the temperature recorded.

Child abuse: Unexplained or atypical head injuries
may be a result of physical abuse, especially if bilateral. Non-accidental head injury (NAHI) is most frequently seen in infants aged <6 months. It has a
mortality rate of around 30% and is the most common
cause of death after abuse. The triad of injuries sometimes called the 'shaken baby syndrome' is subdural
haematoma, hypoxic cerebral injury and retinal
haemorrhage, usually without skull fracture. It is
thought to be caused by either violent shaking alone
or shaking with head impact. The presentation of
NAHI may be very variable – fits, coma, drowsiness,
irritability, apnoeic attacks, poor feeding or general
malaise.

Child abuse → p. 353.

Box 3.7 Discharge criteria for patients with head injuries

*Patients who fulfil **all** of the following criteria
may be discharged home to a caring relative
or friend:*

- Fully conscious on presentation
- No abnormal neurological signs
- Loss of consciousness or post-traumatic
amnesia of <5 min
- No severe headache or vomiting
- No suspicion of skull fracture
- No bleeding disorder
- Good home conditions, supervision by carer
arranged
- Reliable relative or friend available to take
patient home from the ED (in appropriate
transport)

Most serious head injuries in the first year of life
result from physical abuse.

> **Box 3.8 Selection of children (aged < 16) for CT of the head**
>
> *(Adapted from NICE's head injury guideline, 2007)*
>
> - Witnessed loss of consciousness lasting >5 min
> - Amnesia (anterograde or retrograde) lasting >5 min
> - Abnormal drowsiness
> - Three or more episodes of vomiting
> - Clinical suspicion of non-accidental injury
> - Post-traumatic fit but no history of epilepsy
> - Age >1 year: GCS <14 on assessment in ED
> - Age <1 year: GCS (paediatric) <15 on assessment in ED
> - Suspicion of open/depressed skull injury or tense fontanelle
> - Any sign of basal skull fracture (→ *p. 43*)
> - Focal neurological deficit
> - Age <1 year: bruise/swelling/laceration >5 cm on the head
> - Dangerous mechanism of injury (→ *Box 3.1*)

X**R**

Imaging of the cervical spine is summarised in Box 3.2.
Indications for CT of the head in children aged <16 years are summarised in Box 3.8.
Radiology of the skull in both adults and children → p. 46.

- Skull radiographs still have a valuable part to play in the assessment of children aged <12 years with suspected abusive injuries. The most common cause of skull fractures in children aged <18 months is NAHI. There may be multiple, branching fractures that involve more than one skull bone. Occipital fracture is characteristic and underlying brain injury is relatively common.
- Early cerebral oedema may not be visible on the CT scan of a child's brain.
- Separation of the suture lines of the skull (diastasis) may sometimes be seen after injury. This can fail to close, resulting in a 'growing fracture'.

T**x** Most aspects of the management of a child's head injury are identical to that in the adult. Children are unique in invariably having a carer with them. This means that most can go home with their parents and written head injury instructions. They often sleep after trauma and should not be kept awake. Instead, they should be examined by their parents two or three times during the night. All that is required is for the parents to be confident that their child has a normal response to a mild stimulation (verbal or tactile). It is not necessary to wake the child completely or to examine the pupils. Parents are much better judges of their children's night-time behaviour than hospital doctors or nurses.

Some injuries, especially those to the occiput, may cause severe and prolonged vomiting. Children in this situation require observation in hospital and a CT scan is usually indicated (→ *Box 3.8*).

> Pituitary damage occurs in around 25% of moderate-to-severe head injuries. It may lead to endocrine failure (e.g. short stature or delayed puberty) that is only discovered several years after the injury.

Delayed presentations

Occasionally, young children are brought to the ED by their parents with a large fluctuant swelling over the parietal area (cephalohaematoma). There is a history of an injury a few days before but the child is otherwise well. CT scan (or skull radiograph) usually shows a long, linear fracture that may extend over most of the side of the skull. It is normal for the swelling to be delayed and for a relatively late presentation. Although unlikely, child abuse must still be considered and excluded. Most of these children will need observation over a period of 24 h and assessment by paediatricians.

SPECIFIC INJURIES
Fracture of the vault of the skull

Fracture of the skull vault most commonly results from a fall on to a hard surface. The lateral parts of the skull are the most vulnerable; intoxication is a predisposing factor.

X**R** A CT scan of the cranium will detect most fractures of the vault of the skull.

Radiology of the skull → p. 46.

X**R** A skull radiograph is indicated only when CT is not available (except in suspected child abuse – see above).

Indications for skull radiographs → Box 3.9

Box 3.9 Indications for skull radiographs

In the absence of facilities for CT or other problems in adhering to the NICE guidelines, skull radiographs are indicated if any of the following is present:

- Altered consciousness or amnesia at any time
- History unknown or unreliable
- Significant mechanism of injury (e.g. high-speed incident, injuring agent heavy/sharp, fall on hard surface)
- Abnormal neurological signs
- Swelling or bruising to temporal or parietal areas
- Extreme headache
- Vomiting (even once)
- Clinical suspicion of depressed vault fracture (e.g. trauma with hammer, golf club, etc.)
- Clinical suspicion of penetrating injury
- Clinical suspicion of basal skull fracture
- 'Drunk' patient with uncertain history of any event

Skull radiographs are unnecessary if all of the following apply:

- No loss of consciousness
- Occipital or frontal injury
- Low-speed impact or injuring agent flat/soft
- Normal neurological status at time of examination
- No scalp damage (or, if laceration, no associated swelling)

Child abuse is the most common cause of a skull fracture in an infant (→ *p. 41*).

Tx All patients with a new skull fracture should be admitted for observation. In the same way that a broken egg box may contain smashed eggs, a fractured skull may contain traumatised brain. Expressed more scientifically, the presence of a skull fracture greatly increases the risk of a patient developing an intracranial haematoma (→ *Tables 3.2 and 3.3*).

Around 70% of intracranial haematomas occur in the presence of a skull fracture.

Compound fracture of the skull

Antibiotics are not routinely indicated for compound linear fractures of the skull. Lacerations over fractures that are not depressed can be closed in the normal way and the injury then treated in the same way as a simple vault fracture.

Depressed fracture of the skull

Depressed fractures are often missed. The history is the key to diagnosis – direct force will have been applied over a small area of the head, e.g. a blow from a hammer or a golf club. The injury is usually compound. Cerebral irritation may manifest itself as fitting.

XR A CT scan is required when there is a suspicion of a depressed skull fracture (→ *Boxes 3.1 and 3.8*). Fractures can be easily overlooked on plain skull films. It appears as an area of whiteness rather than as the usual black line because of the increased density of the compressed and overlapping bone. The fracture may be stellate in appearance. In the absence of a CT scan, a plain film tangential view can be used to assess the amount of depression, but will give no indication as to the extent of any underlying damage.

Tx Treat the brain injury first. Discuss management of all depressed fractures with a neurosurgeon. Surgical elevation of the fragments is usually indicated.

Fracture of the base of the skull

This is usually the result of indirect violence. It often occurs in a drunken patient and may follow uncontrolled 'rag doll'-type falls.

The patient may sometimes feel unwell and vomit. A complaint of reduced hearing in one ear points to a haemotympanum. There will be one or more signs:

- Bleeding from the ear canal
- Haemotympanum (causes reduced hearing)
- Bleeding from the nose in the absence of direct injury
- Nasopharyngeal bleeding (may be torrential and compromise the airway)
- Cerebrospinal fluid leakage from the nose or ear
- Subconjunctival haemorrhage without a posterior edge
- Retro-orbital haematoma (*for emergency treatment → p. 66*)
- Bilateral periorbital haematomas ('raccoon' or 'panda eyes')
- Bruising around the mastoid area (Battle's sign) (occurs late).

Blood in the external auditory meatus after trauma is usually caused by basal fracture but is occasionally secondary to temporomandibular joint injury.

> Deep auroscopic examination of the canal should be avoided because it may introduce infection via torn meninges.

X𝗥 A CT scan of the cranium will detect most fractures of the base of the skull. High-resolution sections may be required.

There is usually no evidence of a basal skull fracture on plain radiographs. However, there may be:

1 Blood in the sphenoid sinus (look for a fluid level)
2 A vault fracture line that appears to continue towards the base of the skull.

T𝗑
- Admission for observation for 48 h or until any discharge has ceased for at least 24 h
- Discussion with a neurosurgeon, ophthalmologist or ENT surgeon as appropriate
- Antibiotics (e.g. phenoxymethylpenicillin or ampicillin) are not of proven value.

Aerocele

A fracture involving a bony sinus may result in intracranial air. The presence of this aerocele is suggested by periorbital surgical emphysema.

X𝗥 An aerocele is usually an incidental finding on a CT scan of the brain or a plain skull radiograph. Look for a fluid level (under the vault or in the sphenoid fossa) but be aware of the orientation of the head when the film/scan was taken – it could appear as a 'vertical' line if the patient was supine.

T𝗑 The aerocele may expand if the pressure in the sinuses is increased, so the patient should be warned not to blow his or her nose. Discuss with a neurosurgeon; early decompression is sometimes necessary.

Extradural haematoma

A blood clot in the extradural space results from direct trauma and, in adults, is usually associated with a skull fracture (of the squamous temporal bone). A lucid interval between initial trauma and the onset or return of depressed consciousness is said to be characteristic but is by no means inevitable.

The signs are those of increasing ICP. An impaired level of consciousness is the first feature. The classic,

unilateral, fixed, dilated pupil is a very late sign; it occurs as the result of an ipsilateral third nerve palsy that is caused by cerebral herniation through the foramen magnum. Limb weakness, from direct pressure on the motor cortex, is usually found on the contralateral side. Lateralising signs may be preterminal.

X𝗥 CT will detect almost all extradural bleeds. In the very early stages, the blood may have the same density as the brain tissue and thus be difficult to identify. Extradural collections usually appear biconvex on CT scan, whereas subdural collections have inner concave borders (→ *Figure 3.1*). On plain skull radiographs, a fracture that overlies the vascular markings of the middle meningeal artery may be associated with an extradural bleed.

T𝗑 Resuscitation and stabilisation (→ p. 34) should precede transfer to a neurosurgical centre. Major coincidental extracranial injuries must always be identified before transport is initiated.

> Outcome in a patient with an extradural haematoma is compromised if the time to decompression is more than 2 h from the point of deterioration.

Acute subdural haematoma

Bleeding from the veins that traverse the subdural space results in a more insidious clinical picture than extradural haemorrhage. Alteration in conscious level is the cardinal feature; lateralising signs may be absent or minimal. A unilateral increase in limb tone is sometimes apparent.

Acute subdural haematomas are most commonly seen in those:

1 Who are intoxicated with alcohol. There may be no apparent injury. The first sign may be a failure to wake up after an episode of heavy drinking. A CT scan should be obtained in all patients with head injuries who do not recover to GCS score of 15 within 2 h of injury (→ *Box 3.1*). Intoxication may make this difficult. In such cases, consider general anaesthesia. Even in patients with a diagnosis of alcohol intoxication, a CT scan is indicated if they do not reach a GCS score of 15 within 6–8 h of arrival.
2 Who are on anticoagulant or anti-platelet therapy (e.g. warfarin or clopidogrel). The trauma may be minimal.
3 Who have coexisting extensive brain injury from major trauma (lacerations and contusions).

Figure 3.1 Comparison of (a) extradural and (b) subdural haemorrhages. **Extradural:** There is injury to the middle meningeal artery or to one of its branches. The expanding haematoma strips the strongly-attached dura from the skull to form a characteristic biconvex shape with a well-defined inner margin. **Subdural:** There are often ruptured veins in the subural space. The bleeding spreads between the dura and the arachnoid to make a crescentic appearance with an irregular inner margin.

Xʀ A CT scan is diagnostic, showing a collection with an irregular, inner concave border (compare extradural → *Figure 3.1*).

Tx Patients with subdural haematomas must be discussed with a neurosurgeon immediately.

> Outcome in a patient with an acute subdural haematoma is compromised if the time to decompression is more than 4 h from the accident.

Chronic subdural haematoma

This is usually seen in elderly patients with a history of a trivial head injury, or no injury at all. The symptoms and signs develop after a latent period of days or even months and, characteristically, fluctuate in severity as a result of alternating bleeding and resorption of clot. There is headache, memory loss, confusion and drowsiness. Localising signs are rare.

A CT scan should be performed if the diagnosis is suspected. Neurosurgical intervention has a very good outcome.

Subarachnoid haemorrhage

A subarachnoid haemorrhage (SAH) may sometimes occur after trauma. In a conscious patient there may be severe headache, neck stiffness and photophobia (→ *p. 224*). Diagnosis is confirmed by CT scan and then neurosurgical advice must be sought. IV nimodipine is not indicated in the treatment of traumatic SAH.

Cerebral contusions

Bruising to the brain may result in a similar clinical picture to subdural haematoma, with a delayed recovery from trauma or alcohol intoxication. Frontal contusions cause disinhibition.

Xʀ CT scan is diagnostic.

Tx All patients with contusions should be discussed with a neurosurgeon. Spontaneous resolution may take several weeks.

Transient complications after minor head injury

Cortical blindness

Sudden visual loss after a head injury is uncommon but very frightening. The loss of vision can be confirmed by testing for the absence of the blink reflex (i.e. an object rapidly approaching the eye will not cause blinking). A CT scan of the brain is required to exclude serious pathology. The patient should be admitted and examined by an ophthalmologist. Vision usually returns spontaneously within a few hours.

Transient apnoea

A brief (but totally unexpected!) period of apnoea may sometimes follow an otherwise relatively minor head injury. Irregular respirations may also occur independently. A CT scan should be obtained to exclude significant intracranial pathology. Total recovery is to be expected. The mechanism is presumably similar to that of cortical blindness and temporary abducens palsy.

Abducens palsy

Unilateral sixth nerve palsy is occasionally seen after an otherwise uncomplicated minor head injury. CT scan should be obtained to exclude significant intracranial pathology. The condition resolves spontaneously.

Prolonged symptoms after apparently minor traumatic brain injury

Many patients with a minor traumatic brain injury, who do not have demonstrable intracranial lesions or abnormal signs, will have persisting symptoms for a surprisingly long period of time. These complaints include the following:

- Minor lapses in concentration and memory
- Inability to undertake complex tasks
- Fatigue
- Occipitofrontal headache.

Symptoms may progress to a more chronic post-concussional stress disorder. It is probable that some patients will have structural brain damage – a minor form of diffuse axonal injury. This is unlikely to be seen on CT scan but has been demonstrated on MRI.

XR A CT scan may be undertaken (as a delayed procedure) to exclude treatable causes and to give a more reliable prognosis.

TX The patient should be reassured that recovery will occur but may take several weeks. Advise against alcohol and propose a gradual resumption of normal activities. Follow-up by the GP or specific care by a psychologist or neurologist may be valuable.

RADIOLOGY OF THE SKULL

This section is included in the recognition that CT is not universally available.

Skull radiographs must be taken with suitable equipment (not portable) and should include an AP, Townes' and a lateral view. Basal views should not be requested because they require extreme extension of the cervical spine. Occipitomental and special tangential views may be required after the first set of films has been viewed.

Indications for skull radiographs in the absence of CT facilities→ Box 3.9 on p. 43.

To gain the maximum information from skull radiographs:

- Insist on good-quality films.
- Look at them carefully on a good viewing box with a rear spotlight.
- Use specific films for specific purposes:
  1 AP view for frontal bone, orbits and upper occiput. If the pineal gland is calcified (above the shadow of the ear lobe on the lateral film) it should appear in the midline on the AP view.
  2 Townes' view for occipital injury.
  3 Left lateral (plate next to the left side of the head) shows lesions on the left clearly but those on the right will be slightly out of focus ($\rightarrow$ *Figure 3.2*).
  4 Laterals taken from both sides, together with a careful examination of the head for bruising and haematoma, will help to indicate the significance of linear markings in the temporal regions.

- A fracture classically produces a finite, crisp, linear mark ($\rightarrow$ *Figure 3.2*). Fractures of the skull may persist on a radiograph for many years. However, if there is any doubt about the age of a fracture, it should be presumed to be new.
- A vascular marking is usually of indefinite length, wide and curvilinear. Vessels in the temporal region tend to radiate upwards from the base of the skull, predominantly posteriorly. Any markings at right angles to these should be considered to represent fractures.
- A shift of the calcified pineal gland from the midline is evidence of movement of the falx, usually by an expanding haematoma. If only the choroid plexus

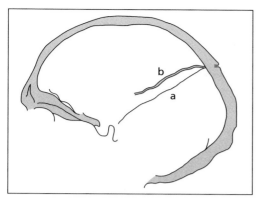

Figure 3.2 Characteristics of an extensive linear vault fracture. This shows as a crisp thin line (a) on the side of the skull adjacent to the film, but as a wide hazy line (b) on the opposite side of the skull.

are calcified, they cannot be used reliably to indicate brain shift because of their variable positions in the normal brain.

- The small linear fracture, which is classically overlooked and overlies an extradural haematoma, is often near the soft-tissue marking of the pinna as seen on the lateral film.

It is essential to be aware of the characteristics of the normal suture lines and vascular markings of the skull in both adults and children (→ *Figures 3.3–3.5*). The common anatomical variants should also be recognised (→ *Figures 3.6–3.8 and the accompanying legend in Box 3.10*).

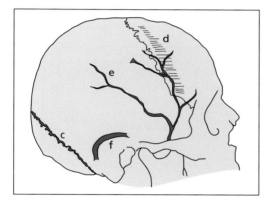

Figure 3.3 Lateral view of adult's skull. The coronal (d) and lambdoid (c) sutures are fused but persist as wide irregular structures in contrast to the curvilinear branching radiolucencies produced by the meningeal vessels (e). Note the superoposterior radiation of the vessels. Darker lines at right angles in the region of the pterion (just in front of and above the pinna (f)) usually represent undisplaced vault fractures.

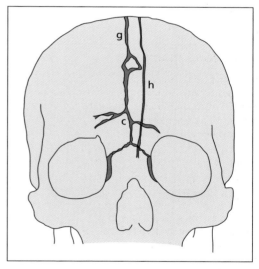

Figure 3.4 AP view of child's skull. Note the persisting metopic suture (h) in the frontal bone. This does not overlie the sagittal suture (g) because the radiograph has not been correctly centred. The division of the sagittal suture into the two lambdoid sutures (c), at the lambda, is an imprecise feature in this particular skull.

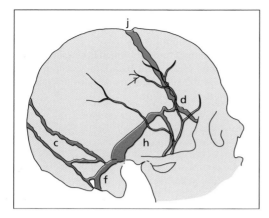

Figure 3.5 Lateral view of child's skull. Note that sutures on both sides of the skull are seen on this projection. Although the bregma is often very thin, the lambda is thick and irregular. (c) Lambdoid suture, (j) bregma (position of anterior fontanelle in infant), (d) coronal suture, (h) squamosal suture and (f) pinna.

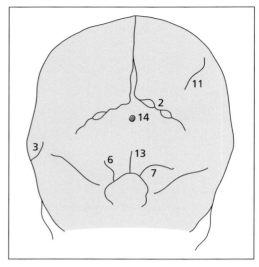

Figure 3.7 Normal anatomical variants – Townes' view (key in *Box 3.10*).

Figure 3.6 Normal anatomical variants – AP view (key in *Box 3.10*).

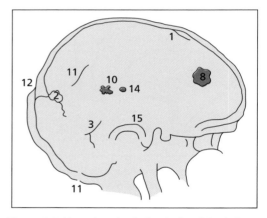

Figure 3.8 Normal anatomical variants – lateral view (key in *Box 3.10*).

Box 3.10 **Normal anatomical variants (numbers correspond to those in Figures 3.6–3.8)**

Neonate

- Vault disproportionately larger in neonate than in adult (vault:face ratio in neonate 4:1 but in adult 3:2)
- Overlapping sutures may be seen in neonate secondary to moulding occurring during labour
- Scalp folds may mimic fracture line (e.g. wrinkle in occiput)

Child

Suture spreading is very common between the ages of 4 and 8 years.

1 Anterior fontanelle: fusion may mimic depressed fracture on lateral projection but is clearly outlined on Townes' view
2 Wormian (accessory) bones: normal variant in both children and adults
3 Posterior part of squamosal suture: may simulate a fracture
4 Metopic suture: may persist throughout life
5 Prominent nasofrontal suture: may persist into adult life
6 Persistent membranous fissure: may simulate a fracture. Most common in infancy but may persist into adult life

7 Normal synchrondrosis between two parts of occipital bone in infant

Adult

8 Localised focal dural calcification
9 Focal calcification of falx cerebri
10 Calcification in the glomus of the choroid plexus of the lateral ventricle
11 Subsagittal suture of parietal bone
12 Overlapping of occipital bone (bathrocephaly): may be confused with a fracture
13 Midline occipital suture: also a common site for a fracture!
14 Calcified pineal structure: visible on lateral view in 50% of adults. Less frequently seen on AP view

All ages

15 Upper part of the pinna: often seen on the lateral projection

Matted hair, lacerations, clothing, hair buns and pillows may all simulate a fracture. However, the line may be seen to extend out past the bone into the soft-tissue shadow.

4

The neck and the back

The possibility of spinal injury should always be considered in:

- major trauma
- multiple injuries
- high-speed injuries
- falls
- sports injuries (especially in diving, trampolining, riding and rugby accidents)
- head injuries
- all unresponsive patients.

Immediate assessment and management

- Ensure an adequate airway and give high-concentration oxygen. The jaw-thrust manoeuvre is safer than the chin-lift technique in this situation. The neck must be protected by manual in-line stabilisation if more extensive airway intervention is needed. As soon as possible, immobilise the neck with a hard collar fitted with a chin piece and prevent head movement with a purpose-made head holder (or sandbags and tape).
- Assess respiratory function and rate, and measure oxygen saturation with a pulse oximeter.
- Set up an intravenous (IV) infusion and monitor BP (blood pressure) and pulse.
- Record the Glasgow Coma Scale (GCS) score. Check if the patient can move and feel his or her fingers and toes. *For spinal cord injury → later.*
- Protect the thoracolumbar spine with a long spinal board wherever the signs or mechanism of injury suggest thoracolumbar injury or when there are evident injuries both above and below the spine.
- Log-rolling will be necessary to examine the back of the patient. Look for bruising, swelling, tenderness and palpable steps in the vertebral column.

- Pay special attention to pressure points (sores develop rapidly) and core temperature (the patient may be thermolabile).
- Consider the need for early analgesia.
- Complete the primary survey and continue resuscitation.
- Call for senior advice and then start the secondary survey.

Radiographs in spinal trauma → p. 54.

> Whenever spinal protection is removed to aid examination, the neck and spine must be held still by one staff member who has no other responsibilities.

INJURY TO THE SPINAL CORD

Few injuries produce the devastating disability of damage to the spinal cord. In the fully conscious adult, the presence of paralysis and anaesthesia after trauma immediately points to spinal cord injury. However, in the obtunded patient the diagnosis may be difficult. Similarly, incomplete cord damage is often misdiagnosed. *For cord syndromes → p. 53.*

Initial management of spinal cord injury

Initial assessment and management → before.

- Keep the patient calm, warm, splinted and immobile.
- Request orthopaedic advice.

Emergency Medicine Lecture Notes, Fourth Edition. Chris Moulton and David Yates.
© 2012 Blackwell Publishing Ltd. Published 2012 by Blackwell Publishing Ltd.

- Record respiration and SaO_2 (arterial O_2 saturation). The onset of respiratory failure may be insidious.
- Monitor pulse, BP and ECG. Watch carefully for peripheral vasodilatation and the onset of neurogenic shock. Copious IV fluids may be required, but there is a potential for volume overload if too much is given.
- Catheterise the patient.

Anaesthetic help will be required for both respiratory failure and neurogenic shock.

> Paralysis may mask multiple injuries. Pain may be absent as may the signs of intra-abdominal trauma.

Steroid therapy

High-dose steroid therapy in patients with spinal cord injuries remains controversial. However, as the negative effects of steroids in acute head injury are now established, it would seem inadvisable to give steroids routinely to patients with spinal cord damage on current evidence.

Special problems that may accompany injury to the spinal cord

Respiratory failure

Intercostal muscle paralysis occurs with most cervical cord lesions. High lesions transect the phrenic nerve nucleus (C3–5) and are usually fatal. Even when the diaphragm is spared, vital capacity is greatly reduced and a compensatory tachypnoea occurs. The tidal volume and vital capacity should be measured if possible.

Paradoxical respiration is an important sign. As the diaphragm descends during inspiration to create a negative intrathoracic pressure, intercostal muscle paralysis allows rib retraction rather than the normal expansion. Deteriorating respiratory function (rate >35 breaths/min) is an indication for senior anaesthetic advice to consider the need for ventilation.

Neurogenic shock

Impairment of descending sympathetic pathways in the spinal cord (i.e. cord damage at T6 or above) leads to relative hypovolaemia and bradycardia. Paralytic ileus often occurs in addition with a risk of vomiting and aspiration. Other injuries may have been sustained and can cause true hypovolaemia and either a bradycardia or a tachycardia. Any reduction of blood supply to the damaged cord will further impair its function. Hypotension from loss of sympathetic tone is one of the very few indications for therapy with vasopressor agents (e.g. ephedrine). Bradycardia usually responds to atropine. Symptoms last from several hours to several weeks depending on the level and the severity of the cord damage.

Retention of urine

Bladder tone is lost immediately after spinal transection. Distension leads to ureteric reflux and renal damage. Intermittent catheterisation may be the treatment of choice in the spinal unit, but it is preferable to insert and retain a fairly thin catheter during the initial period of resuscitation and interhospital transfer. Catheterisation must be performed by an experienced member of staff using an aseptic technique.

Impaired thermoregulation

The patient is unable to sweat and thereby lose heat at high ambient temperatures. More commonly, too much heat is lost at low temperatures because of a failure of cutaneous vasoconstriction. The environmental temperature should be near to normal body temperature if the patient has to be exposed for long periods (e.g. for the diagnosis and treatment of other injuries). At other times, insulation is used to prevent heat loss to a cooler environment. Core temperature must be measured regularly.

Associated injuries

The signs of abdominal, pelvic and major limb injury may be masked by the motor and sensory loss. CT scan or ultrasound examination should be performed if there are external signs of abdominal trauma or if the patient is haemodynamically unstable. Abdominal swelling may occur with a full bladder or from a paralytic ileus. Severe swelling from any cause may splint the diaphragm. Multiple fractures are present in around 5% of patients with spinal injuries.

Localisation of spinal cord damage

Twisting forces are most likely to cause fractures at the junction of mobile and fixed parts of the column, i.e. at C7–T1 and T12–L1. Upper thoracic spine injury may be associated with sternal fractures – massive forces attempting to buckle the thoracic cage. Direct blows are commonly associated with injuries elsewhere.

Partial transection of the cord may be inflicted by a knife or a bullet but complete separation is unusual. A twisting or bending movement resulting from indirect blunt violence is more common. This causes a combination of crushing and tearing which produces a mixed picture of neuronal damage. There is often total loss of neural continuity with complete distal motor and sensory loss.

Distal reflex activity may not be clearly related to the extent of cord section in the immediate post-injury phase. Complete section usually causes immediate flaccid paralysis with later return of reflex activity. Rarely, some reflexes are preserved throughout.

The level of cord injury may be difficult to determine because of the following:

1 Most muscles receive efferent fibres from more than one level.
2 Dermatomes have imprecise boundaries.
3 Closed cord lesions usually extend over several centimetres, involving more than one level.

It is important to detect change in neurological status over time. Identify and document the lowest functional muscle groups and the extent of skin anaesthesia (→ *Table 4.1 and Figure 4.1*).

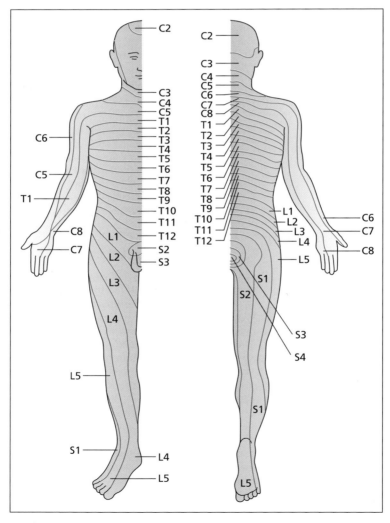

Figure 4.1 Sensory dermatomes of the body.

Table 4.1 Nerve roots supplying tendon and superficial reflexes			
Tendon reflexes		**Superficial reflexes**	
Biceps	C5	Abdominal	T8–12
Supinator	C5–6	Cremasteric	L1–2
Triceps	C7	Plantar	S1
Knee	L3–4	Anal	S3–4
Ankle	S1–2		

Delayed improvement or deterioration after spinal cord injury

Spinal shock

This is rare. After a cord injury, spinal concussion causes a generalised flaccidity below the level of the lesion. Reflex activity may initially be present but later disappears. Neurological signs begin to improve spontaneously within 8 h and the effects of the concussion are variably reversed within 48 h.

This diagnosis can be made only in retrospect. An initial finding of proximal paralysis with sparing of distal neurological function (e.g. sphincter tone) is likely to be associated with cord concussion and carries a more favourable prognosis. Concussion and permanent cord damage may coexist.

Late-onset paralysis

Secondary deterioration can occur after spinal injuries in a similar way to the much more common complications of brain injury. Paralysis that develops hours after the incident is rare and is usually a result of cord ischaemia or oedema (causing infarction or vascular occlusion, respectively). An extradural haemorrhage may cause cord compression. Delayed signs are very unlikely to result from direct injury. Gentle handling, as described above, will not further damage a spine that has been subjected to forces sufficient to render it unstable. The doctor would be expected to be less violent than the injuring agent.

Cord syndromes

Incomplete cord damage produces a number of discrete syndromes. Some degree of recovery is more likely than in complete lesions where there is no sign of any spinal cord function below the level of the injury. The mixed nature of the signs leads to misdiagnosis.

Lesser degrees of damage produce spinal cord contusions. There may be non-specific weakness, poor mobility and myoclonus. The diagnosis is usually only made on an MR scan. Recovery is usually slow but complete.

Central cord syndrome

This usually occurs in older patients with spondylitic spines following a relatively minor hyperextension injury. The spinal cord is compressed between the osteophytic vertebral body anteriorly and the stiff ligamentum flavum posteriorly. The more centrally situated parts of the corticospinal and spinothalamic tracts are the worst injured. These fibres supply the arms where the damage results in a flaccid (lower motor neuron) paresis. The legs are less affected with a spastic (upper motor neuron) type of weakness. The sacral fibres are often spared, so perineal sensation and bladder and bowel function may be normal.

> Central cord syndrome should be suspected in the elderly patient with a forehead injury who can walk but complains of altered function in the upper limbs. These symptoms are often mistakenly diagnosed as hysterical.

Anterior cord syndrome

The anterior part of the spinal cord is usually injured by a mixture of bony encroachment and ischaemia. Typically, a flexion–rotation force causes a dislocation or a compression fracture of the vertebral body with accompanying anterior spinal artery compression. There is loss of power as well as reduced pain and temperature sensation below the lesion.

Traumatic herniation of a cervical vertebral disc

This may occur during an acute flexion injury and cause extensive injury to the anterior part of the spinal cord. There is impaired motor function with reduced pain and temperature sensation. The posterior horns and posterior columns are usually undamaged so that touch and proprioception remain intact. *Also → p. 58.*

Posterior cord syndrome

Hyperextension injuries with fractures of the posterior elements of the vertebrae may injure the posterior columns. Loss of proprioception may cause profound ataxia in the presence of normal power and pain and temperature sensation.

Brown–Séquard syndrome

This lateral cord syndrome can be precisely produced only by a knife or gun, although closed injuries (lateral mass fractures) may also give rise to some of its classic features. These are the signs of a hemisection of the cord. On the injured side there is reduced power, but relatively normal pain and temperature sensation because the spinothalamic tract crosses over to the opposite side. The uninjured side has normal power, but reduced sensation for pain and temperature.

IMAGING AND CLEARANCE OF THE SPINE IN TRAUMA

Radiographs taken to confirm a clinically proven injury to the spine are less important initially than those requested for patients who are asymptomatic but at risk. Splints should be radiolucent and retained during radiography.

CT and MRI in spinal trauma → Box 4.1.

Radiographs of the cervical spine

These should be obtained for all patients with:

• multiple injuries
• injuries caused by the mobile head striking a fixed object.

Clearance of the spine → p. 55.

There are three standard views of the cervical spine in UK practice:

1 Lateral
2 Upper anteroposterior (AP) ('open-mouth' or 'peg')
3 Lower AP.

Supplemental oblique views are used to visualise the apophyseal joints, looking for facet joint dislocation. Radiographs in flexion and extension are used to reveal instability. They should be taken only in the presence of a senior clinician.

Lateral view

Adequacy: This is the view that causes the most trouble. The first film is adequate (C7–T1 disc space shown) in only about two-thirds of cases. Often, only the first five vertebrae are demonstrated.

Suggested sequence to follow, if lateral radiograph of cervical spine is inadequate, → Box 4.2.

> The lateral view of the cervical spine must include the C7–T1 junction.

Alignment: Confirm the continuity of the curve along the following four lines:

1 Anterior borders of the vertebral bodies
2 Posterior borders of the vertebral bodies (the anterior edge of the vertebral canal)

Box 4.1 Indications for CT and MRI in spinal trauma

CT scan
• Areas of the spine poorly visualised on plain films
• Fracture not excluded by plain films
• Significant or possibly significant fracture on plain films (requiring further visualisation)
• Unexplained neurology after trauma

MR scan
• Fracture on plain films or CT scan with unknown associated soft-tissue injuries
• Suspected ligament or disc injury
• Neurological symptoms and signs referable to the spine
• Suspicion of vascular injury to the spinal cord

Box 4.2 Suggested sequence to be followed if the lateral radiograph of the cervical spine is inadequate

If the patient is thought to be at high risk of cervical injury, proceed immediately to CT scan of the neck. In low-risk cases:

1 Request a coned view of the lower cervical spine with the shoulders pulled down OR
2 Request a swimmer's view of the lower cervical spine (the swimmer's view is better at demonstrating the previously obscured vertebrae but is much harder to interpret)

If one of the above views does not allow visualisation of the C7–T1 junction, proceed to a CT scan of the neck.

3 Posterior edge of the vertebral canal
4 Tips of the spinous processes.

Look for steps. Normal slight lordosis is lost when there is painful muscle spasm.

C2 may appear to be subluxed forward on C3 in young children; the same appearance is less frequently seen of C3 on C4. These are normal variants that occur in up to 10% of children aged <7 years and disappear on extension of the neck.

Bones: Compare the height and shape of each vertebral body, looking for wedging and fractures.

Examine each apophyseal joint and spinous process for malalignment and fractures.

Look at the integrity of the odontoid peg and for increased space between the peg and the anterior arch of C1. Look for fracture of the posterior arch of C1 and for 'hangman's fracture' of the pedicles of C2.

Cartilages: Examine each intervertebral joint looking for osteophytes and narrow disc spaces.

Soft tissue: The soft-tissue shadow, anterior to the vertebral bodies, is increased if there is a fracture, haematoma or anterior ligament injury. Air is trapped in this area if there is damage to the posterior pharyngeal wall. Above the larynx, the width of the prevertebral soft-tissue space should be less than a third of the diameter of the vertebral body. Below this level, the space is accepted as normal if it is no wider than a whole vertebral body.

Look for widening of the space between the spinous processes (torn interspinous ligaments).

Upper AP (odontoid peg) view

Adequacy: The upper AP view is adequate in only about two-thirds of first films. The odontoid peg may be superimposed on the base of the skull or on the upper incisors. Simple repositioning is usually sufficient.

Alignment: Look at the lateral masses of C1, on either side of the odontoid peg. They should line up with the equivalent parts of C2. Spread suggests a burst (Jefferson's) fracture.

Bones: Look at the integrity of the odontoid peg.

Anteroposterior view

Adequacy: The first attempt at this view is invariably adequate.

Alignment: Look for symmetry of the apophyseal joints.

Bones: Examine the transverse processes for fracture, or buttressing of C7 or a cervical rib. Thyroid cartilage wings are often misinterpreted as calcified vertebral arteries.

Cartilages: Confirm that the disc spaces are equal. Spaces above and below the centre of the X-ray beam appear narrower but should be bilaterally symmetrical.

Soft tissue: Confirm the central shadow of tracheal air.

> A CT or MR scan may be necessary for absolute clearance of the cervical spine → *Box 4.1.*

Radiographs of the thoracolumbar spine

These are indicated when:

- the history suggests violent impact
- there are significant injuries above and below the diaphragm
- there are positive clinical findings on log-rolling (such as bony tenderness, swelling or a palpable step).

Thoracolumbar films must include good views of the T12–L1 junction. Transverse process fractures, although not associated with spinal cord damage, are often overlooked and are important indicators of retroperitoneal injury. They may also cause severe pain.

Clearance of the spine

Patients with circumstantial evidence of multiple injuries, e.g. those involved in high-speed incidents or falls, are assumed to have neck injuries until proven otherwise. Appropriate splintage will have been applied by the resuscitation team or paramedics. To remove this cervical protection, the examiner must be satisfied of the following points:

1 The patient is able to cooperate fully with the assessment, i.e.:
  - fully conscious, cooperative and mentally normal
  - an adult or older child
  - free from severe pain in other regions of the body.
2 The patient has no neck pain.
3 The patient has no neurological deficit (normal peripheral movements and no paraesthesia).

Also, when the splintage is gently removed:

4 The patient has no bony tenderness of the cervical spine.

5 The patient has a good range of movements without pain or paraesthesia (specifically lateral rotation to 45° bilaterally).

Patients who fulfil the above criteria will not generally need radiographs of the cervical spine unless the mechanism of injury indicates the possibility of significant forces applied to the neck (→ *p. 50*).

In patients who require imaging, clearance of the cervical spine can be surprisingly difficult because there is no perfect modality:

- A single, plain, lateral film will reveal about 80% of the fractures.
- The addition of the two standard AP views will increase the detection rate to about 90% of fractures.
- A CT scan of the neck will pick up about 98% of bony injuries.

The removal of splintage from the thoracolumbar spine should follow the same principles as outlined above.

> Patients who have sustained injuries more than 24–48 hours ago (and have been mobile since) should not have immediate splintage applied in the ED.

CERVICAL INJURY AND NECK PAIN

Patients with neck pain who can be safely moved and examined → Box 4.3.

Cervical spine fractures and dislocations

Bony injury is suggested by the following:

- A likely mechanism of injury (→ *p. 50*)
- Severe pain of immediate onset
- Marked paraesthesia
- Other neurological signs.

XR
Interpretation of plain cervical films → p. 54.

Fractures may be difficult to see. The most common cause of a step on the lateral view is a unilateral facet joint dislocation with or without an accompanying fracture.

> **Box 4.3 Patients with neck pain who can be safely moved and examined**
>
> Even in the presence of neck pain, a patient who is fully conscious with no paraesthesia or neurological deficit, and no significant midline cervical tenderness, can be safely moved and examined if any of the following apply:
>
> - No history of trauma
> - Simple rear-end motor vehicle collision (excludes rollover, hit by bus or large truck or high-speed vehicle, or pushed into oncoming traffic)
> - Ambulatory at any time since the injury
> - Sitting position when seen
> - Delayed onset of neck pain

Tx
Immediate assessment and management of potentially serious spinal injuries → p. 50.

The patient must be kept splinted and immobile. Orthopaedic advice must be sought immediately.

> The atlantoaxial joint of the cervical spine in a patient with Down's syndrome can be unstable. Subluxation and subsequent cord compression may occur after comparatively minimal force or even vigorous exercise. Similar problems are sometimes seen in rheumatoid arthritis.

Whiplash injury (strain injury to the neck)

Whiplash strain injury to the neck is poorly understood and is usually the result of a motor vehicle accident. It is much more common than similar injuries to other spinal regions for all vehicle occupants in all crash configurations. Drivers, females and younger people seem to be most at risk. The strain injury appears to be caused by sudden hyperextension and -flexion of the cervical spine. The circumstances of the incident will help assessment of the forces applied to the neck and so aid prognosis. The most common story is of a stationary vehicle being hit from behind. Whiplash-type injuries are often the cause for legal claims and so notes should, as usual, be of a high standard.

Mobility may be good initially, with little pain, and then symptoms typically increase over the first 24 h. There may be an associated headache, and pain may radiate to the shoulders. Sometimes there is slight paraesthesia in one or both hands, but there are no long tract signs. Occasionally, the patient complains of difficulty in swallowing as a result of inflammation of the adjacent muscles.

> The patient may arrive in the ED wearing a cervical collar. *For safe removal of splintage →* *Clearance of the spine on p. 55.*

On examination, there is usually tenderness of the paravertebral areas. Movements are restricted, particularly lateral flexion (in the direction of tenderness), and flexion and extension of the lower cervical spine. Movement at the atlanto-occipital joint is normal and will allow the head to flex forward without movement of the rest of the cervical spine. Rotation is variably restricted; forward flexion against resistance is always painful.

Xʀ Radiographs of the cervical spine should be taken only if any of the following apply:

- The patient is aged >50 years.
- The mechanism of injury suggests a violent application of force (e.g. the vehicle rolled over or the patient's head hit the windscreen).
- The pain occurred immediately after the accident or is unusually severe.
- There is bony tenderness.
- There are abnormal physical signs additional to those described above (including severe paraesthesia).

Radiographic findings include the following:

- *Evident recent bony injury:* a cervical collar should be applied and no further radiographs taken without orthopaedic advice.
- *Loss of the normal lordosis with no bony injury:* this is caused by muscle spasm and usually indicates a more severe injury. Recovery may take longer than average but treatment remains as described below.
- *Pre-existing osteoarthritis:* the patient may have been asymptomatic previously. Some clinicians believe that spondylosis is associated with prolonged symptoms.
- *No radiographic abnormality:* this is the most common finding but does not equate to nothing wrong. There is a problem and it will get worse over the next 24 h.

> The prognosis is difficult to determine on initial presentation to the ED. Symptoms are usually worse and more protracted than most clinicians anticipate.

Tx

- Reassure the patient that symptoms will gradually settle over the next few weeks but warn him or her that they may increase over the first 24 h.
- Prescribe an oral non-steroidal anti-inflammatory drug (NSAID). Consider a parenteral NSAID for patients in severe pain.
- Do not prescribe a soft cervical collar. The use of these devices has been shown to prolong symptoms without short-term benefit.
- Consider physiotherapy (heat lamp and massage at home may suffice). Early treatment probably reduces the incidence of chronic symptoms.

Clay shoveller's shoulder

The muscular effort associated with strenuous digging – classically in clay – may avulse the spinous process of C7. There is localised pain over this vertebra prominens, which worsens on attempted flexion and extension.

Xʀ Lateral radiographs clearly demonstrate the lesion.

Tx Fracture clinic referral is indicated for all spinous process fractures, although they heal spontaneously with conservative treatment.

Torticollis

Pain and spasm of one of the sternomastoid muscles may occur spontaneously (wry neck) or reflect local or generalised pathology. Most commonly, the symptoms occur on waking or after a sudden neck movement. The head is turned to the opposite side and cannot be rotated, but slight flexion and extension are usually possible. The muscle may be locally tender.

Local causes include throat infection, direct trauma, overuse or strain of neck muscles and spinal pathology. In small children, a submandibular or retropharyngeal abscess may cause painful torticollis (→ p. 423). Athetoid movements as a result of extrapyramidal excitation may present as atypical torticollis (*For acute dystonias → p. 300*).

XR When there are no other positive findings and there is no history of trauma, radiographs are unnecessary.

TX Idiopathic torticollis may be extremely painful but usually responds to reassurance, oral analgesia and the local application of NSAID cream. The neck should be manipulated gently with slight longitudinal traction into the neutral position and a soft collar applied. Consider referral for physiotherapy. If symptoms persist for more than 2 or 3 days, review with radiographs is indicated.
Atlantoaxial rotary subluxation is one of the most common structural neck injuries of childhood. It may present with torticollis after trauma and is very difficult to identify on plain radiographs. If suspected, a CT scan of the neck is indicated.

Cervical spondylosis

Degenerative disease of the cervical spine is very common and often asymptomatic. The condition is usually diagnosed incidentally in the ED, on radiographs taken to exclude bony injury after trauma. Neurological function should be assessed and recorded.

If symptoms are longstanding and attributable to the cervical spondylosis, referral to the orthopaedic department or the patient's GP is appropriate.

Diffuse neck pain

The history is important:

- Mode of onset
- Site and character of pain and any radiation
- Associated headache and systemic symptoms.

The temperature must be taken and the mouth, ears and neck examined. A brief neurological examination should also be performed. Consider:

- Meningeal irritation (meningitis or subarachnoid haemorrhage)
- Spinal disease (infection, degenerative disease or rheumatoid arthritis)
- Intervertebral disc herniation
- Herpes zoster
- Pathology in the chest (e.g. myocardial infarction or pneumomediastinum → p. 194).

Standard cervical spine radiographs should be taken in most cases. The direction of further investigation and treatment is dictated by the clinical findings.

Cervical nerve root pain

Cervical nerve entrapment can be caused by degenerative disease, prolapsed intervertebral disc or in a relatively normal neck for reasons that are unclear.
Cervical spondylosis: degeneration often affects the C7 distribution and causes pain and paraesthesia in the upper arm, dorsal forearm and dorsum of the hand, extending to the index and middle fingers. There may be weakness of triceps and the extensors of the wrist and fingers. The triceps reflex may be absent. Despite the acute nature of the presentation (and a lack of previous symptoms), most patients will have established degenerative changes on plain cervical radiographs. Treatment is difficult. Adequate analgesia is essential and physiotherapy may be helpful. Specialist review may be indicated for patients whose symptoms or signs fail to resolve.
Cervical intervertebral disc prolapse: this may arise spontaneously or after a sudden lifting or twisting movement. There is acute pain and spasm of the neck muscles with pain and paraesthesia radiating down the arm. In severe cases, there is anaesthesia, weakness and loss of reflexes in the arm. An MR scan is diagnostic. Treatment consists of a soft collar, analgesia and physiotherapy. Patients with prolonged symptoms (more than 2 weeks) or any neurological signs require specialist referral (Also → p. 53).

BACK INJURY AND BACK PAIN

Fractures of the thoracolumbar spine

> Injuries to the thoracolumbar spine are easily overlooked in patients with polytrauma.

Knowledge of the mechanism of the injury will help in the assessment of the forces involved. The spine should be assumed to be unstable until cleared by a radiograph and a senior clinician.

- Log-roll the patient carefully. Look for swelling, bruising, tenderness and steps in the vertebral column. Examine the bony spines, paravertebral structures and perineum.
- Perform a neurological examination. This should include the anus (tone) and rectum (blood and swelling).

- Consider the possibility of renal injury; test the urine for blood.
- Chest injuries may coexist and include:
  - aortic rupture
  - haemopneumothorax
  - fractures of the sternum and ribs.

XR Obtain radiographs of the thoracic and/or lumbar spine (→ p. 55). Visualisation of the thoracolumbar junction is important because there is a high incidence of fractures at this site. Look carefully for separation of the transverse processes.

Tx

Immediate assessment and management of potentially serious spinal injuries → p. 50.

The patient must be kept splinted and immobile. Orthopaedic advice should be sought immediately. Urinary catheterisation is required.

Suspected renal injury → p. 83.

Severe soft-tissue injury to the back

Patients with severe bruising to the back are often unable to walk. Many such patients require admission for analgesia and mobilisation. The possibility of renal injury must always be considered; the urine should be tested for blood.

Fractures of the transverse processes

These fractures, which are often multiple, are caused by either direct trauma – usually a fall from a height – or psoas muscle avulsion. Significant force is required and so other concomitant injuries are common. The retroperitoneal structures are particularly vulnerable; the urine must always be tested for the presence of blood. Over 10% of patients with a fractured transverse process also have a further lumbar spine fracture.

XR The bisected transverse process is often missed on a plain AP radiograph. A CT scan is usually indicated to detect both retroperitoneal and more severe spinal injuries.

Tx Admission is required for observation, bed rest and especially for analgesia.

Suspected renal injury → p. 83.

Acute back pain

Back pain of sudden onset is a common presentation in young or middle-aged patients and affects 60% of the population to a significant degree at some point in their lives. It usually occurs while lifting. The clinician should enquire about the following:

- Onset of the pain/relation to lifting or injury
- Site and character of the pain
- Aggravating and relieving factors
- Radiation and referral of the pain, especially sciatica
- Neurological symptoms, including bladder and bowel function
- Previous episodes
- Coexisting diseases and drug therapy (especially steroids).

The clinician should then do the following:

- Observe the patient's degree of mobility.
- Examine the spine and paravertebral areas for tenderness.
- Check the mobility of the lumbar spine with the patient erect and supine.
- Determine the extent of sciatic nerve sheath tethering by measuring straight-leg raising bilaterally.
- Record subjective or objective sensory loss in the lower limbs.
- Look for muscle weakness (commonly at ankle or toe) and reflex loss.
- In severe cases, examine the perineum for sensory loss and sphincter laxity.

Atypical (and thus worrying) features in a patient with back pain of sudden onset are listed in *Box 4.4.*

> **Box 4.4 Atypical ('red flag') features in a patient with back pain**
>
> - Age <20 years or >55 years
> - Recent onset of pain without trauma or lifting
> - Severe pain at rest or progressively worsening pain
> - Bilateral sciatic pain
> - Thoracic pain
> - Obvious structural deformity
> - Neurological symptoms or signs
> - Urinary or bowel symptoms
> - Malaise or weight loss
> - History of carcinoma, HIV infection, drug abuse or recent steroid therapy

> **Box 4.5 Indications for radiography of the lumbar spine in patients with back pain**
>
> - History of significant trauma → *p. 50*
> - History suggestive of non-mechanical back pain (i.e. the pain is constant, progressive, worse at night and unrelated to activity)
> - History of coexisting condition that may give rise to non-mechanical back pain (i.e. malignancy or inflammation)
> - Patient at risk of spontaneous vertebral collapse (on steroids, elderly)
> - Neurological symptoms or signs
> - Pain persisting for more than 4–6 weeks

> Mechanical low back pain is usually exacerbated by movement in specific directions. Global pain (with all movements) is either more sinister or associated with psychological overlay.

XR Urgent plain radiography is unhelpful in most younger patients (→ *Box 4.5*). Older men (>55 years) and postmenopausal women should have a radiograph taken to exclude osteoporotic collapse of the vertebrae or other diseases. The differentiation between new and old collapse of the bone can be very difficult on plain films.

Tx Negative neurological findings in the presence of low back pain suggest minor ligamentous injury in the young or degeneration in the older patient. Most patients will be helped by the following:

- An immediate injection of an NSAID (e.g. diclofenac 75 mg intramuscularly)
- Analgesia to take home (to be taken on a regular basis). The muscle relaxant baclofen (or even diazepam) may occasionally be helpful, especially where muscle spasm is a prominent feature.
- Written instructions on the care of the injured back
- Review by the GP after this time if there is no improvement. A letter should accompany the patient.

Physiotherapy should also be considered. Regular exercise is important and patients should be advised to return to work as soon as possible. Some patients may be confined to bed as a consequence of their pain but this should be limited to 2 days as a maximum and should not be considered as a primary treatment.

> Over 95% of patients with simple mechanical low back pain will recover spontaneously within 6 weeks. However, there is an 85% chance of recurrence, with around 8% of affected patients becoming chronically disabled. Psychosocial factors are the only known predictors of long-term problems.

Collapsed vertebral bodies are an indication for an orthopaedic opinion. Nursing care and analgesia are usually required before mobilisation. Female patients with osteoporotic collapse who are referred back to their GP should be considered for hormone replacement therapy or for treatment with calcium and vitamin D tablets.

Bladder, bowel and perineal symptoms and signs suggest central prolapse of an intervertebral disc (→ *p. 62*). Immediate orthopaedic referral is essential. Positive findings in the limbs suggest lateral intervertebral disc protrusion (→ *p. 61*).

Atypical back pain

> No one would be satisfied with a diagnosis of front pain so why accept back pain? A more specific diagnosis should be sought.

If back pain is not related to direct trauma and did not come on while the patient was lifting or twisting, the insidious onset of a more sinister disease should be considered. (*For atypical or warning features* → *Box 4.4*.) This could include the following:

- Secondary deposit (breast, bronchus, prostate, thyroid, kidney)
- Myeloma
- Pelvic neoplasm or infection
- Epidural abscess or other spinal infection (→ *p. 61*)
- Aortic aneurysm
- Renal or pancreatic disease or peptic ulceration
- Ankylosing spondylitis
- Paget's disease
- Herpes zoster.

> A leaking aortic aneurysm commonly presents with pain experienced in the back and myocardial infarction may cause isolated back pain.

The examination should be tailored to the history but may need to include:

- abdominal palpation and rectal examination
- urinalysis
- breast examination
- a search for causes of weight loss.

Investigations: Full blood count (FBC), blood chemistry, C-reactive protein (CRP) and erythrocyte sedimentation rate (ESR) may be helpful as screening tests. To obtain radiographs of the lumbar spine requires the highest doses of radiation of any plain films and thus these views should be requested only in specific circumstances ($\rightarrow$ *Box 4.5*). CT and MR scans are often of more diagnostic value than plain films. The advice of a radiologist should be sought.

Tx Assess the patient and ask for advice. Older people with backache tend to be under-investigated.

Spinal epidural abscess

Infection of the spinal epidural space is easily overlooked; the diagnosis is delayed in around half of all cases. During this time, damage to the spinal cord by direct infection, compression or vascular compromise may occur. Epidural abscess may be found at all ages but is more common in males and in high-risk groups such as intravenous drug abusers. Haematogenous spread from almost any site can infect the epidural space but, often, no source is identified. The most common pathogen is *Staphylococcus aureus.*

Back pain – often of disproportionate severity – is the main symptom, although irritation of nerve roots may cause the patient to complain of chest or abdominal pain. Unlike mechanical and sciatic back pain, symptoms get progressively worse rather than better. Only a third of patients have a raised temperature; some have neck stiffness. Neurological features may initially be absent and, when present, can be very variable and atypical. There may be motor and sensory deficits in isolation or findings suggestive of incomplete cord syndromes. Reflexes may be absent or increased and sphincter disturbance can occur.

Investigations: Only half of patients with an epidural abscess have a raised white cell count. ESR and CRP are more sensitive. Lumbar puncture is relatively contraindicated. An MR scan (or CT myelography) is diagnostic. Oedema of the paraspinal muscles may be seen in addition to the epidural infection.

Tx The patient should be discussed with a spinal surgeon. Antibiotics are required for 3–4 weeks ± surgical decompression. Anti-staphylococcal therapy (such as IV flucloxacillin and vancomycin) may be given initially until cultures are available (following CT-guided aspiration of the abscess).

Other spinal infections: subdural abscess, vertebral osteomyelitis and paraspinal infections may all occur. Diagnosis and treatment is similar to that for epidural abscess. Tuberculosis of the spine may also cause severe, intractable back pain.

Sciatica

Pain in the distribution of the sciatic nerve is most commonly caused by the lateral prolapse of an intervertebral disc (PID). The pain, which may be severe, radiates across the buttock, down the back of the thigh and along the medial aspect of the leg to the foot. Backache may be absent, especially when the sciatic pain is of more gradual onset. Bilateral buttock and thigh pain, which does not cross the knee joint, is not usually associated with PID.

The examination should be the same as that detailed above for low back pain. Consider alternative, particularly vascular, causes of the pain.

XR Plain films are not helpful. An MR scan will demonstrate the prolapsed disc(s), the degree of protrusion and any impingement on the cauda equina.

Tx The initial management of sciatica is similar to that for back pain. In severe cases, strong analgesics may be needed. A short course of prednisolone can sometimes speed resolution (especially where there is a marked inflammatory element to the nerve entrapment) but should generally be avoided. The patient should be warned that sciatica can be slow to settle. Fortunately, the majority of sufferers will be better in 6 weeks and many of the remainder will have resolved before 6 months have elapsed.

Cauda equina syndrome

Central prolapse of the L4–5 or L5–S1 intervertebral disc may cause compression of the terminal branches of the spinal cord. In the absence of prompt treatment, cauda equina syndrome results in severe and permanent neurological damage. Consequently, the presenting symptoms and signs must not be missed:

- Acute low back pain (which may be superimposed upon a chronic history of recurrent pain)
- Radiation of pain to the legs – usually but not always bilateral
- Weakness or sensory disturbance in the legs – often present but not invariable; this may cause an abnormal gait
- Alteration of perineal sensation ('saddle anaesthesia') – usually but not exclusively bilateral
- Sphincter dysfunction presenting as urgency, frequency or incontinence
- Alteration of bladder and bowel habit (leading to retention and constipation).

XR Plain films are not helpful. An MR scan will demonstrate the prolapsed disc(s), the degree of protrusion and compression of the cauda equina.

TX Immediate admission and referral for urgent decompression is essential. Surgery undertaken more than 48 h after presentation is rarely successful.

Injury to the coccyx and coccygodynia

The coccyx may be injured by a fall on to the buttocks. There is local pain and extreme tenderness. Dyschezia (pain on defecation) may also occur. A haematoma can sometimes be felt between the coccyx and rectum, but pain usually prevents a rectal examination. Prolonged symptoms are inevitable; sitting is likely to be uncomfortable for months.

Pain in this region (coccygodynia) can also be caused by prolapse of an intervertebral disc, pelvic inflammatory disease, and tumours of the spine and sacrum.

XR Films of the sacrum and coccyx are often of poor quality, especially in obese patients. Moreover, management is rarely changed by an initial radiograph. If imaged, a fractured coccyx is often seen to be anteverted or displaced. Anterior subluxation of the entire coccyx can also occur, with or without an accompanying fracture of the distal sacrum.

TX Analgesia is the mainstay of treatment and the patient should be advised to sit on an inflatable rubber ring cushion. A swimming ring is a cheap and easily available alternative. Constipation must be avoided. The patient should be warned that pain will persist for several months. Physiotherapy (ultrasound treatment) can sometimes be helpful. For severe, prolonged coccygodynia, excision of the coccyx may be necessary.

WOUNDS TO THE NECK AND THE BACK

Major wounds to the neck

A major neck wound is defined as any injury in which the platysma muscle is thought to be divided. Look for further wounds if the patient has been stabbed. Neck wounds are often deeper than a casual examination might suggest, and wounds near the base of the skull and the root of the neck are particularly dangerous.

- Major vascular injury may remain occult for many hours or even days. A normal carotid pulse does not exclude arterial damage.
- Air embolisation may follow venous injury.
- Surgical emphysema will follow division of the trachea or oesophagus.
- Hoarseness and stridor are associated with laryngeal trauma.

XR A lateral soft-tissue view of the neck may show surgical emphysema or air tracks.

TX Position the patient with a slight head-down tilt to lessen the risk of air embolism. Gain venous access and ensure antitetanus cover.

Major neck wounds should not be explored under local anaesthesia in the ED. Patients with such wounds must be referred for specialist assessment, observation and surgical exploration.

Stab wounds to the back

Stab wounds to the back are common.

XR A chest radiograph should be taken to exclude pneumothorax.

TX The wound should be cleaned, dressed and antitetanus cover given. Suturing usually creates a large haematoma under the stitches. The injury will need to be inspected and the dressing changed on the following day.

Leakage of cerebrospinal fluid: Midline wounds to the back may occasionally puncture the dura and cause leakage of cerebrospinal fluid (CSF). Wet dressings are often the first clue. Patients with a suspected CSF leak need admission for bed rest and antibiotics (e.g. oral phemoxymethylpenicillin and flucloxacillin). The inevitable 'spinal' headache will be slow to settle and need prolonged analgesia.

Injuries to the trunk → Chapter 6 on p. 72.

5

Facial injuries

Facial injuries are commonly seen following assaults in adults and falls in children. They need special consideration because:

- the airway may be compromised
- the eyes, nose, mouth and ears are functionally and cosmetically important
- the skin is closely bound to underlying tissue, which complicates wound care and local anaesthesia
- deep tissue injuries may be masked; delay in their treatment can lead to major disability.

FRACTURES OF THE FACIAL BONES

Management of fractures in the emergency department (ED) is confined to:

- airway care (may be difficult)
- control of profuse bleeding
- pain relief
- initial clinical and radiographic assessment
- administration of antibiotics for compound fractures
- tetanus prophylaxis
- consideration of other injuries.

The airway

Airway patency may be threatened by profuse bleeding and distortion of the skeleton and soft tissues. The airway may be maintainable in a fully conscious patient, but in the unresponsive patient endotracheal intubation becomes essential. Rarely, very extensive facial injuries may make this technically difficult or impossible and warrant urgent cricothyroidotomy or tracheostomy (→ pp. 22 and 23).

Neck injuries

These must be considered when facial injury is sustained by the moving head striking a fixed object (e.g. in a car). Although neck damage is less likely if the immobile head is struck by a mobile object (e.g. in an assault), it is essential to examine the cervical spine of all patients with facial injuries.

> An elderly patient with a bruise on the forehead and weak arms should be assumed to have sustained a central cord injury (→ p. 53).

The facial skeleton is designed to withstand the vertical forces associated with mastication but it collapses readily when struck from the front. Injuries can be divided into lower third (mandible), middle third and upper third (frontal). The last type is considered in Chapter 3.

Facial fractures are not always obvious. Examination begins with an assessment of facial contours often best achieved by looking at the face from above and behind. Bony tenderness may be difficult to detect if soft-tissue bruising and swelling are already present. However, pressure for a few seconds over bony points (e.g. the infraorbital margin) will usually displace sufficient interstitial fluid to allow assessment of bony contours and orbital contents.

Facial radiography

The head position required to obtain basal skull and occipitomental views can be dangerous in the presence of cervical spine injuries. These can never be excluded immediately in the severely injured patient and so it is unwise to request these views in such

Emergency Medicine Lecture Notes, Fourth Edition. Chris Moulton and David Yates.
© 2012 Blackwell Publishing Ltd. Published 2012 by Blackwell Publishing Ltd.

patients. The usual brow-up, lateral view has two advantages: (1) minimal patient movement and (2) easier demonstration of paranasal sinuses. A CT scan overcomes these problems but should not be undertaken at the expense of treating more immediately important injuries.

Antibiotics for compound fractures

Flucloxacillin is appropriate prophylaxis for fractures associated with skin wounds. When there is a fracture into a sinus, then phenoxymethylpenicillin or equivalent is probably a better choice.

Special features associated with facial fractures

Surgical emphysema of the face

This indicates the presence of a fracture into an air-containing sinus. Antibiotics and referral are required.

Facial sensory loss

Anaesthesia in the area of distribution of the infraorbital nerve (terminal branches of Vb) is often associated with:

- fractures of the malar complex
- fractures of the floor of the orbit
- Le Fort II and III fractures
- severe soft-tissue injuries to the cheek.

The area of numbness may include the ipsilateral upper lip and also the anterior gums and teeth (anterior superior alveolar nerve). Oedema in the infraorbital canal is the usual cause. This is where the dental nerve separates off, leaving the terminal part of the maxillary nerve to exit from the infraorbital foramen as the infraorbital nerve. Oral surgical follow-up is indicated.

Intraoral damage

Examination inside the mouth is very important. Malocclusion of teeth, or displacement of dentures in the absence of primary dental damage, is always associated with injury to bone or to the temporomandibular joint (TMJ). Palatal irregularities suggest a Le Fort fracture. Inability to open the mouth fully should provoke a careful look at the mandible.

Injuries affecting the eye

Assessment of visual acuity, conjunctival sac, cornea, anterior chamber and fundus is an essential part of facial assessment. Displacement of the eye, inwards

or downwards, is associated with injury to the infraorbital plate. Extraocular muscle damage or distortion may complicate any damage to the bony wall of the orbit and is clearly demonstrated on testing the full range of eye movements. The presence of a subconjunctival haemorrhage without evidence of direct trauma to the eye is a strong indication of the presence of a facial fracture, usually in the infraorbital region.

Other causes of subconjunctival haemorrhage →
  pp. 43 and 414.

Wounds associated with major fractures

Closure of major wounds associated with displaced facial fractures must await reduction of the fractures. The wounds may offer surgical access to bone and facilitate reduction. Until this has been carried out it may not be possible to achieve cosmetically acceptable reconstruction of the soft tissues.

Mandibular fractures

The most common mandibular fracture, through the extracapsular part of the neck of the condyle, is usually sustained by a blow on the chin. It can be unilateral or bilateral. Examination reveals dental malocclusion, often a lateral cross-bite and absence of forward movement of the condylar head on opening the mouth. The force may have been sufficient to drive the head of the condyle backwards and cause a fracture of the squamous temporal bone. This produces bleeding and a cerebrospinal fluid (CSF) leak into the external auditory meatus.

Fractures of the ramus, angle and body will be revealed by local tenderness of the cheek and difficulty in opening the mouth. There may be surprisingly little swelling. The presence of mucosal lacerations and irregular dentition helps confirmation. Displacement is determined by the configuration of the fracture line in relation to the pull of the masticatory muscles. Mental anaesthesia may reflect damage to the inferior dental nerve.

> The ability to open the mouth fully and to clench the teeth normally makes the presence of a fracture of the jaw very unlikely.

XR An orthopantomogram (OPT or OPG), a rotational tomogram that gives a circumferential view of the face, is especially helpful and easy to interpret.

The best plain radiographs are lateral oblique, posteroanterior (PA) and Townes' views (for the condyles).

Tx No immediate treatment is required in the ED for any of these fractures themselves. Unstable and painful fractures will require early repair; the remainder – the majority – can be referred for specialist management later. Some displaced condylar fractures can be managed conservatively with good functional results, but there is an increasing trend towards internal fixation. All patients will need analgesia and a light diet.

> **Mumps** is often unilateral in its early stages and unwell children are more likely to fall. Swelling at the angle of the jaw may reflect parotid engorgement and not a mandibular fracture. Take the temperature.

Temporomandibular joint dislocation

This may occur spontaneously (as inability to close the mouth after yawning) or result from a blow to the open mouth. It is often recurrent and is particularly common in elderly people.

XR An OPT of the jaw is usually diagnostic. TMJ views may be requested but can be difficult to interpret. Fractures of the condyles must be excluded.

Tx Reduction can usually be achieved without general anaesthetic, but must be carried out by an experienced clinician using appropriate analgesia or sedation. The jaw is held by putting both thumbs inside the mouth along the line of the lower teeth on each side while the forefingers grasp the bone from outside. Pressure is then applied downwards and backwards by the thumbs intraorally pressing bilaterally against the angle of the jaw. Post-reduction radiographs are taken to confirm relocation although the patient is usually in no doubt. Specialist follow-up on an outpatient basis is appropriate.

Malar fractures

The malar complex provides the bony prominence on the cheek and is commonly fractured in isolation by a blow to that area. The strong central part of the bone usually remains intact, the force being transmitted to the three buttresses. These bones then fracture or dislocate either individually or, more frequently, simultaneously (a 'tripod fracture'):

1 **Infraorbital fracture:** fracture in the infraorbital region usually causes neuropraxia of the infraorbital nerve. Subconjunctival haemorrhage may occur.

> Sensory loss after a facial injury merits specialist follow-up. It may involve the upper lip, gum and front teeth on the affected side (→ p. 65).

2 **Displacement of the zygomaticofrontal suture:** this may be associated with injury to the suspensory ligament of the eye.
3 **Fracture of the zygomatic arch (zygoma):** this may be sufficiently displaced to impinge on the coronoid process of the mandible and prevent normal jaw movement. Even if this does not occur at the time of injury, exuberant callus formation may cause problems later.

Examination will reveal tenderness over one or more malar processes. Bony irregularity is assessed by intraoral examination behind and above the upper molars, and by careful palpation along the inferior and lateral borders of the orbit and along the line of the zygomatic arch. Diplopia may occur because of injury to the suspensory ligament or displacement and damage to the extraocular muscles. The latter is usually transient.

> Surgical emphysema in the area of a malar injury indicates a (compound) fracture into an air sinus. Antibiotics and follow-up are indicated.

XR Facial radiographs confirm the diagnosis. The most common pair of views are occipitomental projections at 10° and 30°.

Tx Once the diagnosis has been made, the patient should be referred for specialist care. If reduction and elevation of the displaced malar are required, this can be achieved relatively simply, under a short general anaesthetic on a day-case basis within the following week.

Retrobulbar haemorrhage

This may occasionally occur after a fracture of the zygomatic complex. It causes:

- retrobulbar pain
- very marked proptosis
- diminished vision (which may quickly become permanent)
- massive facial swelling.

> Severe retrobulbar bleeding with orbital displacement is a surgical emergency. The area must be decompressed by lateral canthotomy. This entails division of the lateral check ligament, which extends between the edge of the globe and the lateral bony margin of the orbit. Seek urgent ophthalmic advice.

Middle third fractures

When the face is struck directly from the front, the delicate bony skeleton formed by the maxilla, palatine, nasal and ethmoid bones may be crushed and forced backwards and downwards. The nasal bones may be broken in isolation (→ *below*) but the other bones tend to collapse en masse. Le Fort first described the three fracture complexes that are commonly seen (→ *Box 5.1*).

Examination may reveal a dished-in face if the middle third has moved backwards and downwards. The nose appears flattened and widened. This appearance is best confirmed from the side and from above. Swelling and bruising are usually marked. Holding the vault of the skull with one hand and the maxilla complex with the other (between gloved index finger on the hard palate and thumb over the upper incisors), instability may be elicited with surprising ease and without too much pain.

There may be diplopia on upward gaze and damage to the lacrimal system. Damage to the cribriform plate may produce anosmia, but this can be difficult to

> **Box 5.1 Le Fort fractures**
> **(see *Figure 5.1*)**
>
> *Le Fort I* fracture runs across the lower face, including the hard palate and alveolus.
> *Le Fort II* is pyramidal, extending variably upwards in the midline to involve the ethmoids. An associated leak of CSF may occur.
> *Le Fort III* is more transverse but at a uniformly higher level than Le Fort I. Essentially, it separates the face from the skull and has been described as craniofacial disjunction.

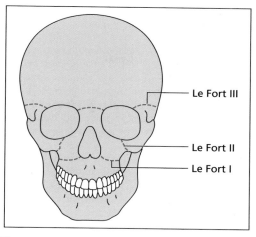

Figure 5.1 Le Fort classification of fractures of the middle third of the face.

confirm in the ED because blood is usually present in the nasal cavity and will seriously impair the sense of smell even in the absence of damage to the olfactory apparatus. Any minor occlusion deformity is readily appreciated by the patient and is a reliable indicator of bony injury. The backward displacement of the middle third of the face will produce a reverse overbite (upper incisors behind lower incisors). The associated tilting results in an anterior open bite.

XR Le Fort fractures can be difficult to spot on facial views. A CT scan may be required.

Tx Immediate specialist inpatient care is required. Significant bleeding and airway compromise may occur, and in this case an anaesthetist should be called.

Nasal fractures

The nasal bones may be dislocated from their normal relationship with the maxilla or fractured. The nasal cartilages usually deform to accommodate violence and do not break. The nasal septum may be deformed, deviated laterally and fractured.

> Trauma to the nose may produce a large septal haematoma that can obstruct the nostril and damage the nutrient vessels to the septum. This can result in avascular necrosis of the bone and septal collapse.

The nose has a good blood supply and all these injuries are associated with epistaxis.

Examination should first exclude more serious facial injuries. Local tenderness over the nasal bones will be present but the appearance of swelling may be delayed. The tip of the nose may be upturned. Lateral deviation may not be obvious to the examiner. The patient should be given a mirror and asked to compare present and previous facial appearance. An obvious deformity may relate to a previous injury.

More extensive fractures involving the ethmoids are associated with widening of the intracanthal distance, a transverse cleft across the glabella and CSF rhinorrhoea. Intranasal examination should be carried out with a speculum and good light; it is essential to exclude a septal haematoma.

XR Radiological confirmation of nasal fractures is of no immediate value. Indeed, an undisplaced fracture may be difficult to distinguish from a vascular marking.

TX Bleeding usually settles with alar pressure (→ p. 419). Septal haematoma or uncontrolled bleeding is an indication for immediate referral. Patients with clearly deformed noses should be seen at the next ENT clinic. However, there is a large group of patients who have marked swellings but an uncertain amount of deformity. They should be told to let the swelling settle over 5–7 days and then return to the ED for reassessment if they are unhappy with their appearance.

FACIAL WOUNDS

Minor wounds to the face → Chapter 21 on p. 391.

Facial skin is unusual. It is an integral part of the deep structures, bound to them by the facial muscles that arise from and insert into the subcutaneous tissues. Consequently, it is difficult to undermine and close quite small defects without causing deformity. Wounds near the circular muscle around the eyes or mouth may influence their function.

Initial assessment should include the following:

- Mechanism and direction of injury
- Wounding agent (especially glass)
- Contamination
- Delay to presentation
- Sensation and function (before anaesthetising the wound)
- Involvement of specialised areas.

Record details of wound site, size and configuration. A drawing on a rubber-stamped facial outline is best. Many such injuries are the result of assaults and you may be called to describe the wound in court.

> Wounds to the chin may be associated with fractures of the condyles of the jaw.

Prerequisites for definitive care in the ED are:

- patience (and time)
- good operating conditions
- adequate anaesthesia
- an immobile patient
- a knowledge of facial anatomy
- a knowledge of the general principles of plastic surgery
- technical skill.

Standard suture sets, provided in EDs, often contain large and unreliable instruments. A special set of fine, good-quality instruments for face and hand use should be available.

Anaesthesia

This is essential to permit adequate exploration and cleaning. In children, a general anaesthetic may be required for a relatively small wound; this may warrant admission.

> Do not use local anaesthetics containing adrenaline near the extremities of the nose and ears.

Exploration

Deep wounds may damage the facial or infraorbital nerves, or the parotid, submandibular or tear ducts. The suspicion of damage to any of these structures requires expert assessment by the appropriate specialist. Early referral is essential.

Cleaning

This must be very thorough. Dirt and foreign bodies such as windscreen glass may be driven deep into facial wounds. An appreciation of the direction and force of the injuring agent will facilitate exploration. Remove dirt from grazes as soon as possible because, otherwise, some of it is taken up by inflammatory cells, producing a tattoo effect. It may be necessary to use a scrubbing brush or toothbrush to remove ingrained dirt. A second operation to retrieve a foreign body is always more difficult and produces a more pronounced scar.

Special areas

Wounds involving the eyelid margins should always be referred to an ophthalmic surgeon. Incorrect apposition of the various layers may produce entropion or ectropion. Extreme care is also required when repairing wounds that involve the red margin of the mouth and nose. A slight malalignment will produce a major cosmetic defect.

Similarly, the line of the eyebrows must be carefully preserved. Adequate local anaesthesia can be difficult to achieve around the nose and ears.

Tissue loss

Undermining facial wound edges is technically difficult and can increase rather than decrease the deformity associated with tissue loss. Large defects are best closed by swinging whole flaps of facial tissue. An experienced plastic surgeon should be involved in the management of such wounds from the outset. The excellent blood supply of the face allows even the most tenuous flap to survive. Trimming of wound edges should be left to a senior doctor with plastic surgery experience.

Closure with sutures

Two layers are usually adequate. Troublesome bleeding may require the occasional ligature, but haemostasis is usually achieved on wound closure. Haematoma formation is rarely a problem. Subcutaneous closure with interrupted, plain catgut (about 4/0) is advisable in larger wounds. The skin is then apposed with interrupted sutures. Tension must be avoided. Correct alignment is best achieved by initial insertion of a few sutures at intervals along the wound.

Fine-diameter sutures are generally recommended for use on the face, but the contused wounds often seen in an ED do not lend themselves to very fine sutures. Placing adhesive tapes on top of a sutured wound may reduce the tension on the sutures and improve the final result.

Suture removal

Facial wounds heal rapidly. Those not subject to undue stress (e.g. on the forehead or cheek) will be sufficiently strong to allow suture removal at 4–5 days. Wounds over convex surfaces may open up at this stage and can be protected by adhesive tapes. The early replacement of sutures by tapes has the advantages of reducing scarring around the needle puncture marks. This is not recommended under the chin and other areas where saliva or excessive movement may impair their adhesion.

Closure with adhesive tapes

Some facial wounds can be closed with adhesive tapes. Cleaning before the application of these tapes must be just as thorough as cleaning before the insertion of sutures. This often requires local anaesthesia. Wounds on convex surfaces will tend to open up in the early stages of healing, as a result of a combination of reduced tissue strength and oedema. Tapes should not be used if the wounds cannot be kept dry and immobile (e.g. the chin or eyebrows of children), but are ideal for small wounds of the forehead and cheek.

Closure with tissue glue

This can also be considered for some small wounds. The same precautions apply as for adhesive tapes.

Bites

This type of wound is considered in detail on p. 399.

The practice of leaving bites open, to heal by secondary intention, should not be applied to the face. Primary closure usually gives good cosmetic results. The wounds must be cleaned meticulously and then a broad-spectrum antibiotic (e.g. co-amoxiclav) prescribed. Follow-up in the ED is advisable.

INJURIES INSIDE THE MOUTH

> Wounds associated with dental damage should be explored for tooth fragments, which may lead to a severe infection if not removed. The possibility of tooth aspiration should also be considered.

Injuries to the tongue

Isolated lacerations rarely require any specific treatment. Healing is rapid and the cosmetic result good, despite initial deformity caused by the pull of the intrinsic muscles. An antiseptic, analgesic, oral rinse (e.g. benzydamine HCl 0.15% solution) may be valuable. This is particularly important in patients who are reluctant to drink and in whom a dry mouth may predispose to secondary infection.

Injuries to the buccal mucosa and gingiva

Simple lacerations are treated in the same way as injuries to the tongue; if more extensive then look for a fracture.

> The patient (or the parents) should be warned that a yellow exudate will form over the wound. This is caused by the normal commensal bacteria of the mouth. It will last a few days and may give rise to slight halitosis.

Injuries to permanent teeth

Teeth may be chipped, displaced or avulsed. The site of injury should be described using the dental formula shown in *Box 5.2*.

Tx
Conditions that require immediate dental advice → *Box 5.3*.

- A chip confined to enamel or dentine (→ *Figure 5.2*) will be very sensitive but does not pose any immediate threat to the viability of the tooth. Varnish may be applied to reduce thermal pain and the patient referred to his or her own dentist the next day.
- If the pulp is exposed (→ *Figure 5.2*) there is a risk of infection and immediate dental referral is necessary. The pulp is recognised by its red colour.

> **Box 5.2 Dental formula**
>
> **1** Determine the quadrant (as if you are looking into the mouth):
>
> | upper right | upper left |
> | lower right | lower left |
>
> **2** Count out from the midline:
>
> 1, 2 incisors   3 canines
> 4, 5 premolars   6, 7, 8 molars
>
> e.g. outer upper right incisor 2|
>   lower left canine |3

> **Box 5.3 Dental injuries for which immediate specialist advice is needed**
>
> - Exposed pulp of any tooth
> - Avulsed permanent tooth
> - Subluxed permanent tooth
> - Mobile segment of alveolar bone
> - Severe soft-tissue injury with dental damage

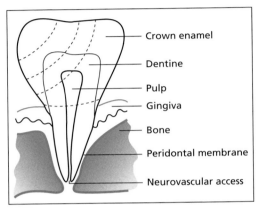

Figure 5.2 Types of dental injury in relation to the dental anatomy.

- Incisor teeth may be displaced (subluxed) but otherwise apparently undamaged. Immediate specialist advice should be obtained in the case of permanent teeth because there is only a 4-h window of opportunity for easy repositioning. Manipulation of the tooth in the ED may loosen it further, with subsequent risk of inhalation.
- Sometimes, several incisor teeth are loosened together with a segment of the underlying alveolar bone (alveolar plate fracture). Again, this needs immediate specialist treatment including splintage and antibiotics.
- Avulsed (permanent) teeth should immediately be:
  - washed very gently with saline
  - kept in saline
  - handled as little as possible
  - reimplanted and splinted in place by a dental surgeon.

Reimplantation is often successful but the chances of a good outcome are directly related to the speed of reimplantation – within 30 min is ideal. If definitive care is delayed, the socket can be cleaned with saline, local anaesthetic gel instilled and the tooth replaced. Temporary stabilisation is obtained by the patient biting on damp gauze. Aftercare includes tetanus prophylaxis and antibiotics.

Injuries to deciduous (milk) teeth

For the purposes of treatment, it is important to differentiate the permanent dentition from the deciduous teeth. Permanent teeth are bigger and have a different shape from milk teeth. They usually appear after age 6 years in the lower jaw and after age 7 years in the upper jaw. The 32 permanent teeth replace 20 deciduous teeth. The first milk tooth erupts at about 6 months of age and thereafter one or more appears every month. They are all shed by the age of 13. For children, the dental formula is written in the usual way (→ *Box 5.2*) but the letters A–E are used to designate the deciduous teeth.

Avulsed milk teeth are common and require no immediate treatment. However, there are two possible long-term effects on the permanent teeth:

1 The gap may affect their positioning.
2 The trauma may impair their development. This risk is increased by attempts at reimplantation.

The child should see his or her own dentist on the following day.

Deciduous teeth that are subluxed or intruded (pushed into the jaw) should also be seen by the dentist on the following day.

Very loose deciduous teeth should be removed but other loose milk teeth can be safely left to the patient's dentist. We all have 20 loose milk teeth at some time in our lives and survive without aspiration.

Chipped deciduous teeth are dealt with in the same way as the permanent dentition.

INJURIES TO THE EAR

Injuries involving the cartilage of the ear

The elastic cartilage of the ear receives its blood supply from the overlying skin. If the cartilage is exposed on both sides by skin avulsion or is separated from the skin by haematoma, it will necrose and collapse, resulting in a 'cauliflower' ear.

Tx Most lacerations of the pinna involving cartilage require specialist care. Small pieces of cartilage exposed at the edge of the pinna may be trimmed, before skin closure, without causing significant cosmetic problems.

Bites to the ear

Bites to the ear may result in extensive mixed flora infection and cartilage destruction. They are usually caused by humans.

Tx Most such injuries should not be closed. Clean the area thoroughly, give antibiotics (e.g. co-amoxiclav) and ensure protection against tetanus. The advice of an ENT or plastic surgeon will usually be required.

Bites (general considerations) → *p. 399.*

INJURIES AROUND THE EYE

Assessment of the eye → *p. 411.*
Corneal and other ocular injuries → *p. 411.*

Blow-out fractures of the orbit

These injuries result because the eyeball is stronger than the floor of the orbit. A direct blow on the eye by a fairly large object (e.g. a squash ball) may cause little damage to the eye – acuity may not be impaired – but push it backward and downward through the infraorbital plate. Surprisingly, the condition may go unrecognised. Suspicion is aroused by the mechanism of injury and sometimes by restriction of the extraocular muscles, resulting in double vision.

Xʀ There may be a fluid level in the maxillary antrum on the AP radiograph and sometimes a 'teardrop' soft-tissue shadow at the top of the antrum. An associated fracture of the malar may occur but the infraorbital plate fracture is often difficult to identify. A CT scan shows the 'tear drop' to be orbital contents herniating into the antrum through the fracture.

Tx Elevation and reconstruction of the orbital floor may be necessary; early referral is essential.

Eyelid lacerations

These wounds require expert assessment and repair and so must be referred to an ophthalmic surgeon immediately. Injuries below the medial canthus may involve the lacrimal apparatus; this damage is easily overlooked.

6

Injuries to the trunk

Injuries to the trunk can be difficult to diagnose and are easily overlooked, especially when associated with:

- a depressed level of consciousness
- painful skeletal injuries.

They may be immediately life threatening but can also cause delayed deterioration. *Primary survey and resuscitation are described on p. 1; details specifically concerned with injury to the trunk are dealt with in this chapter.* A careful and repeated systematic review of the chest, abdomen, pelvis and thoracolumbar spine should be undertaken in all patients who may have sustained multiple injuries.

> If blunt trauma results in injuries both above and below the trunk (e.g. to the head and femur), then the trunk itself is also likely to be injured.

Bruises, clothing imprints and friction burns, together with any history available from the patient or witnesses, can help to determine the direction and severity of the injuring agent.

> Stab wounds must be assumed to involve vital organs until proven otherwise.

Repeated physical examination is essential.

> Always examine the back and the perineum – they are often forgotten.

CHEST INJURIES

Chest injuries are commonly caused by major trauma such as assaults, road traffic accidents and falls. They vary in severity from minor bruising or an isolated rib fracture to severe chest wall, pulmonary and cardiac injuries that may:

- disrupt the mechanism of respiration
- impair gas exchange
- produce hypovolaemia
- cause cardiogenic shock.

Immediate assessment and management

- Attend to ABCs as described in *Chapter 1*.
- Give a high-concentration of oxygen.
- Consider tension pneumothorax ($\rightarrow$ *p. 74*).
- Cover open (sucking) wounds of the chest wall with firm, waterproof dressings. Note that this may allow a tension pneumothorax to develop.
- Obtain intravenous (IV) access. *For a discussion of the rate and type of fluid infusion $\rightarrow$ pp. 7 and 331.*
- Connect the patient to appropriate monitors (arterial O_2 saturation [SaO_2], ECG and blood pressure [BP]) and measure the respiratory rate.
- Request an urgent chest radiograph (CXR).
- Obtain an urgent 12-lead ECG.
- Consider early analgesia.
- Consider blood gas analysis.

Further assessment and management

Ask about

- Site and character of pain
- Dyspnoea

Emergency Medicine Lecture Notes, Fourth Edition. Chris Moulton and David Yates.
© 2012 Blackwell Publishing Ltd. Published 2012 by Blackwell Publishing Ltd.

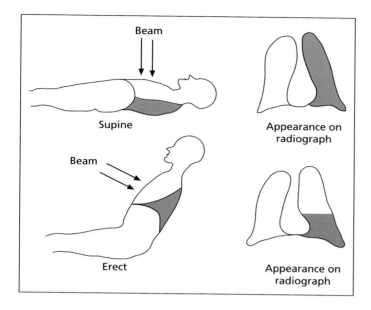

Figure 6.1 The appearance of fluid on erect and supine CXRs.

- Mechanism of injury
- Past medical history.

Look for

- Sweating, pallor, cyanosis
- Increased respiratory rate, work of breathing
- Uneven or abnormal chest movements
- Areas of tenderness, bruising, abrasions or crepitus
- Dullness or hyperresonance on percussion
- Reduced air entry, abnormal breath sounds
- Abnormal position of apex beat or trachea
- Increased pulse rate or paradoxical pulse
- Inaudible heart sounds (tamponade)
- Distended neck veins
- Abdominal tenderness
- SaO_2, BP and ECG abnormalities.

> The chest has a back as well as a front: log-roll the patient.

Radiographs of the chest

Ideally, the CXR should be performed with the patient erect to permit fluid level detection (→ *Figure 6.1*). With the patient supine, fluid present in the pleural cavity will lie behind the lung and produce a diffusely opaque lung field. A lateral decubitus film ('sick side down') may also reveal a fluid level, even in a supine patient.

> Radiography must not precede or prevent careful initial clinical assessment.

Wounds to the chest wall

Sucking wounds, although unusual, attract immediate attention. In contrast, small stab wounds may be underestimated. They must be assumed to penetrate the parietal pleura until proved otherwise. This entails confirmation of the mechanism of wounding, observation of progress (if necessary, with repeated CXRs or CT scan) and occasionally careful examination of the anaesthetised wound by an experienced surgeon in an operating theatre (but not in the ED). A long, incised wound at right angles to the line of the ribs is usually superficial.

XR All patients with stab wounds to the trunk should have a CXR. A CT scan of the thorax may be required.

Tx The presence of surgical emphysema, pneumothorax or haemothorax confirms pleural penetration.

A chest drain will usually be required but should not be inserted through the wound (→ *later*). Most cases settle without surgical management; thoracotomy is indicated only if bleeding is severe or if a large air leak persists.

Antitetanus cover must be established and the wound covered with an antiseptic dressing. Be aware that an open wound may effectively prevent the development of a tension pneumothorax. Stab wounds are best left unsutured to allow drainage of any intramuscular bleeding.

Pneumothorax and haemothorax

Traumatic pneumothorax may follow rib injury, stab wounds or barotrauma. The degree of pleuritic pain and dyspnoea is very variable. Clinical suspicion should be followed by radiographic confirmation except in the case of tension pneumothorax (→ *later*).

> A simple pneumothorax may develop into a tension pneumothorax – particularly when the patient receives intermittent positive-pressure ventilation (IPPV).

Management of spontaneous pneumothorax → *p. 192.*

Haemothorax may also follow multiple rib fractures as a result of intercostal vessel damage. The bleeding is often brisk and continuous from the high systolic pressure of the intercostal arteries. In contrast, bleeding from the low-pressure pulmonary vessels usually stops with the collapse of the lung. A stab wound may cause profound bleeding from the internal thoracic artery or other intrathoracic structures. Symptoms and signs usually reflect the initial injury.

XR Look carefully for small pneumothoraces – especially apically, laterally and medially (close to the heart border). Haemothorax may appear as blunting of the costophrenic angles. A large quantity of blood lying parallel to the diaphragm is often missed (a sub-pulmonary haemothorax). If this area looks slightly abnormal consider requesting a lateral decubitus film (→ *p. 73*) that may reveal the problem. A CT scan of the thorax may be required.

Tx
- Give high-concentration oxygen by mask
- Monitor SaO_2, BP and ECG
- Consider early analgesia
- Insert a chest drain (→ *Box 6.1 and Figure 6.2*).

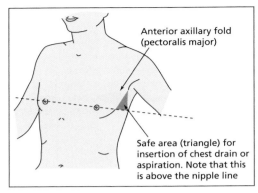

Figure 6.2 The triangle of safety for insertion of a chest drain.

The 'open' technique is described but new equipment is now available on the market that makes 'closed' techniques much safer than was previously the case. In particular, catheters that are small diameter and wire guided (Seldinger type) are quick and easy to insert and relatively comfortable for the patient.

Some small haemopneumothoraces can be managed conservatively if the patient is stable and there are no plans to institute IPPV. Such patients should be discussed with senior staff and must be observed closely for signs of deterioration. A repeat radiograph will be needed after 4 h to check for radiological enlargement of the pneumothorax.

> Do not use nitrous oxide mixtures for pain relief if there is a possibility of pneumothorax or pneumomediastinum. It may result in expansion of a gas-filled space.

Tension pneumothorax

This is a life-threatening emergency; the rapid increase in intrapleural pressure moves the mediastinum, compressing the opposite lung and impairing venous return. The patient has:

- dyspnoea
- unilaterally reduced breath sounds
- distended neck veins
- tracheal deviation
- impaired cardiac output
- cyanosis (a late sign).

The patient may look and feel as if they are 'about to die'. (They are!) The clinical picture may be mistaken for that of a cardiac tamponade (→ *p. 78*). However,

Box 6.1 **Insertion of a chest drain**

In a dire emergency, the need for a chest drain should be determined clinically, without waiting for radiographic confirmation. However, this is the exception rather than the rule. Bilateral drains may sometimes be needed. The preferred site in emergency practice is the fifth intercostal space in the midaxillary line (*Correct area →* *Figure 6.2*). There are three equally important phases to the procedure:

1 Analgesia and preparation
- Position the patient in a semi-recumbent position with the affected side uppermost
- Administer oxygen, attach a pulse oximeter and obtain venous access
- Consider IV morphine if there is adequate respiratory effort. Sedation with a small dose of midazolam is also an option in some patients
- Perform intercostal blocks posterior to the anticipated site of drain insertion. This is done by injecting 2 mL of 1% lidocaine around the neurovascular bundle (just below the inferior border of the rib). About three intercostal nerves should be blocked to include a space above and a space below
- Infiltrate local anaesthetic down to the parietal pleura at the site of insertion. Aspiration of air bubbles into a syringe containing residual local anaesthetic is a useful confirmatory sign

2 Insertion technique
- Clean the skin and use surgical gloves and drapes
- Make a small incision down to parietal pleura. Aim for the upper border of the lower rib, to avoid the neurovascular bundle

- Open the incision with forceps. Some blunt dissection over the superior border of the rib may be required with the tips of scissors
- Consider inserting a gloved finger and sweeping the cavity to establish lung collapse
- Insert a chest drain (up to 28 G in an adult) using either a pair of curved artery forceps or a blunt trocar. Better still, use a modern drainage tube that includes a flexible introducer within its lumen
- Attach the drain to an underwater seal or a double Heimlich ('flutter') valve. In the case of the former, check for movements with respiration
- Advance the drain up to 15–20 cm in an upward, posterior direction

3 Fixation of the tube
- Close the wound with large sutures on either side of the drain
- Cover the site with a waterproof dressing
- Cover the dressing completely with strips of tape
- Secure the drain with a 'mesentery' of adhesive tape
- Confirm the position of the chest drain on CXR

Remember that the patient will have to live with the tube for several days and that some other poor doctor will have to remove it!

tension pneumothorax is more common and there is hyperresonance to percussion over the affected side.

XR This delays treatment and so is inappropriate in the case of a clinically obvious tension. If taken, it would show a hyperexpanded lung field that is displacing the mediastinum, depressing the diaphragm and compressing the opposite lung.

Tx Immediate needle decompression (→ *Box 6.2*). This is part of the initial assessment or primary survey and resuscitation phase of management.

Insertion of a needle does not always decompress a tension pneumothorax because the underlying pleura and lung can be 'sucked' into the needle and occlude it. If this happens, a second attempt should be made. Failure to achieve decompression at this point indicates the need to proceed immediately to rapid insertion of a chest drain.

> **Box 6.2 Treatment of tension pneumothorax (needle thoracocentesis)**
>
> - On the affected side, identify the second intercostal space in the midclavicular line
> - Insert a cannula with a syringe attached just above the rib, until air is aspirated (a cannula of at least 4.5 cm in length will be required)
> - Remove the syringe and needle. There should be a hissing decompression followed by an immediate clinical improvement
> - Tape the cannula in place
> - Proceed to chest tube drainage (→ *Box 6.1* and *Figure 6.2*)
> - Once the chest drain is working, remove the cannula and dress the site
> - Obtain a CXR
>
> Note that a syringe with the plunger removed can be attached to the needle instead of a normal syringe. If it is filled with saline and the needle inserted with the patient supine, air bubbles will reveal the presence of a pneumothorax.

Surgical emphysema

Gas under the skin can be caused in three main ways:

1 As a complication of injury to gas-containing structures (usually lung or oesophagus – rib fracture is the most common cause)
2 After assault with a high-pressure hose
3 As a result of infection with gas-forming organisms.

Subcutaneous gas in the chest or neck can usually be felt as crepitus. Other symptoms and signs result from the original insult.

Surgical emphysema after blunt trauma is usually a direct result of damage to the lung, but clinical and radiological examination may not initially confirm this. Stab and gunshot wounds may injure the pharynx or oesophagus. Infection spreading from such wounds into the mediastinum is a major, life-threatening complication.

X<small>R</small> Subcutaneous or mediastinal gas may easily be seen on a plain CXR (or CT scan) as streaking in the soft tissues.

T<small>x</small> Look for the injury that has caused the air leak. Observe in hospital.

Pneumomediastinum and pneumopericardium → *p. 194*

Pneumothorax → *p. 192.*
Rib fractures → *below.*

In the case of suspected oesophageal or pharyngeal injury, prophylactic antibiotics should be started and surgical advice sought.

Rib fractures

Fractured ribs are common and result from direct blows or falls. There is local tenderness, pain on inspiration and coughing, and difficulty with trunk movements. The patient must be asked about shortness of breath and previous cardiorespiratory problems. Careful observation should reveal any significant dyspnoea. The chest should be examined thoroughly to exclude underlying pneumohaemothorax and contusion.

X<small>R</small> A CXR is mandatory in the presence of dyspnoea or past history of respiratory problems. There are usually more ribs fractured than can be seen on a plain film.

> Multiple old rib fractures on an adult's CXR usually indicate past episodes of alcohol abuse; non-accidental injury must be considered in a child.

T<small>x</small>
Simple pneumothorax/haemothorax → *p. 74.*

Multiple rib fractures

- Give high-concentration oxygen by mask
- Monitor SaO_2, BP and ECG and measure the respiratory rate
- Consider early analgesia
- Measure the blood gases.

Request an urgent anaesthetic opinion; the patient often requires intensive care. The inevitable underlying contusion will cause severe hypoxaemia. Pain may require a thoracic epidural infusion.

Fewer than three fractured ribs

- Exclude underlying problems and respiratory difficulty
- Assess mobility in the light of home circumstances
- Assess the level of pain.

The patient may go home if the above considerations do not contraindicate it. Adequate analgesia and GP follow-up will be required. For patients with a past history of cardiorespiratory problems, also consider the following:

- Prophylactic antibiotics
- Prophylactic steroids
- Community physiotherapy.

The patient must take analgesics and cough rather than refuse to do both. Winding a scarf around the chest and pulling on the crossed-over ends while coughing provides a surprising amount of pain relief. Strapping of the ribs, however, is contraindicated.

Patients with clinical signs of chest injury who do not have fractures on radiograph should be treated in exactly the same way as those with radiographic signs.

Flail segment

When a rib is broken at two points, the middle section is not mechanically linked to the rest of the rib cage and tends to move in the opposite direction during breathing.

A flail chest occurs when a part of the thoracic cage moves independently from the rest of the chest wall. There is paradoxical movement of this free segment – it is drawn inwards on inspiration and moves outwards on expiration – and thus impedes ventilation. Flail chest has been defined in a variety of ways, but at least two fractures per rib in at least two ribs are needed to produce a flail segment. Large flail segments may extend bilaterally or even involve the sternum. This injury is best detected clinically but is often overlooked. A large area of crepitus is usually apparent on palpation. Respiratory movements are best observed from the bottom of the trolley, looking for an area of the chest wall that moves out in expiration. Even apparently minor degrees of 'paradoxical respiration' are associated with significant hypoxaemia, because there is usually a large underlying pulmonary contusion.

XR Radiographs may initially look normal, because rib fractures and costochondral junction separation may not be visible; later, a pulmonary contusion becomes apparent. An erect chest film is helpful before intubation to exclude other major intrathoracic injuries.

Tx
- Give a high concentration of oxygen by mask
- Monitor SaO_2, BP and ECG

- Give sufficient analgesia as soon as possible
- Consider local direct pressure to stop gross flailing
- Request an urgent anaesthetic opinion; intubation and ventilation are usually required
- Measure the blood gases.

Surgical stabilisation with metal rib reinforcements may be considered to allow earlier weaning from ventilatory support, to reduce acute complications and to avoid the chronic pain that is sometimes associated with permanent deformity of the chest wall.

Tracheobronchial tree injuries

Larynx

There is localised pain, hoarseness, subcutaneous emphysema and local crepitus. An urgent ENT opinion is indicated and a surgical airway may be required ($\rightarrow$ *p. 22*).

Trachea

The signs may be subtle and overlooked. If suspected, obtain anaesthetic and surgical advice. Plain radiographs may be followed by CT scan and bronchoscopy.

Bronchus

This is rare, difficult to detect (without a CT scan) and often fatal. A large air leak after a thoracotomy is suspicious. Bronchoscopy is diagnostic. Ventilation of patients with tracheobronchial injuries may be difficult and indeed hazardous.

Fracture of the sternum

Sternal fractures are not usually associated with instability of the rib cage and may be overlooked in patients with multiple injuries. Local examination reveals tenderness and sometimes swelling. Respiratory movements may not be affected. Consider associated injury to the heart and great vessels. The ECG should be checked. There may also be associated crush injuries to the upper thoracic spine.

XR CXRs do not show sternal injuries clearly. Specific lateral views are required.

Tx This consists of observation, exclusion of associated injuries to thoracic contents and symptomatic pain relief. Reduction or internal fixation is not usually indicated, although fractures with a large amount of depression of the inner table should be discussed with a cardiothoracic surgeon.

Traumatic asphyxia syndrome

Diffuse crushing of the chest (e.g. by a trench collapse) will cause transient venous engorgement and petechial haemorrhages over the upper chest and face. There may also be subconjunctival haemorrhages. Maximal barotrauma occurs in the presence of airway obstruction.

The prognosis is good if the patient is rescued promptly. If crushing is not quickly relieved, hypoxia is severe with lung contusion and alveolar collapse. Some patients may initially appear deceptively well. Pulmonary oedema gradually develops and gas exchange is impaired – a form of adult respiratory distress syndrome.

Tx Oxygen is given in high concentration and the patient admitted for intensive care. Steroids are of no benefit. If there is associated bronchospasm in the early stages nebulised salbutamol will be useful.

Injury to the heart

Damage may be inflicted by a gunshot, a stabbing or blunt decelerating forces. Contrary to popular belief, these injuries may not be instantly fatal and may remain undetected in the patient who is slowly dying from 'multiple injuries'. The paucity of specific signs may frustrate early and precise diagnosis.

Stab wounds anywhere between the midclavicular lines, from the lower third of the neck to the epigastrium, have the potential to involve mediastinal structures. Beware of small entry wounds, especially in the back.

Laceration of the thick left ventricular wall may not be as catastrophic as damage to less muscular structures. Pump failure may occur because of valve damage, hypovolaemia or tamponade.

Haemopericardium may produce a life-threatening cardiac tamponade at any time, with high venous pressure, muffled heart sounds and falling BP (Beck's triad). There may be distended neck veins. Classically, the systolic BP is lower during inspiration (pulsus paradoxus). Tamponade may also cause a paradoxical rise in venous pressure during inspiration (Kussmaul's sign). Profound shock and IPPV may invalidate these signs.

Blunt injuries are more common. Most minor contusions probably resolve without detection. At the other extreme, fatal dysrhythmias may not be associated with structural damage *post mortem*. A few patients, in between, present with symptoms and signs typical of myocardial ischaemia, including ECG changes.

Box 6.3 Needle aspiration of the pericardium (pericardiocentesis)

The subxiphisternal approach is recommended (→ *Figure 6.3*) although parasternal and apical approaches have also been described. Ideally, the procedure should be performed under ultrasonic (e.g. echocardiographic) guidance.

- Consider the need for sedation or general anaesthesia
- Position the patient with a 30° head-up tilt
- Monitor the patient's SaO_2 and ECG
- Clean and anaesthetise the subxiphoid area with 2% lidocaine, if time allows
- Make a 5-mm incision through the skin, just below a point midway between the tip of the xiphoid process and the left costal margin (→ *Figure 6.3*)
- Attach a 20-mL syringe to a three-way tap and a long 16 G over-the-needle catheter (or use a central venous Seldinger-type set)
- Enter the skin through the 5-mm incision (→ *Figure 6.3*), just below and to the left of the xiphochondral junction, at a 30–45° angle to the skin
- Carefully advance the needle, aiming for the tip of the left scapula. Contact with the pericardium will occur at about 6–8 cm. Watch the ECG – ventricular ectopics suggest myocardial irritation whereas QRS or ST changes may indicate actual entry into the ventricular muscle. If these ECG changes are seen, the needle should be withdrawn and repositioned
- Once fluid is reached (i.e. the needle has entered the pericardial sac), remove the needle and aspirate blood or straw-coloured fluid down the cannula. Removal of as little as 15 mL blood may result in a dramatic clinical improvement. Large amounts of blood suggest that the ventricle has been entered
- After aspiration remove the syringe, leaving the cannula *in situ* with a closed three-way tap attached
- Secure the cannula to the skin. If the symptoms recur, aspiration can then be repeated
- Obtain an ECG and CXR and arrange definitive care

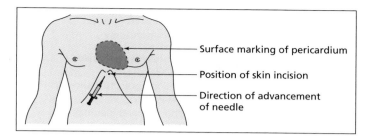

- Surface marking of pericardium
- Position of skin incision
- Direction of advancement of needle

Figure 6.3 The site of entry for percutaneous pericardiocentesis.

Figure 6.4 ECG of a 16-year-old driver involved in a road traffic accident. The CT scan showed a mediastinal haematoma and a small aortic tear.

Direct damage to coronary arteries is rare but septal rupture, damage to papillary muscle and chordae tendineae, and tears of the atria or right ventricle do occur. Rupture of the sturdy left ventricle is rare.

It is useful to distinguish between cardiac contusion and concussion. The latter is defined as the occurrence of a dysrhythmia without ECG or biochemical evidence of muscle necrosis. Most of these dysrhythmias are transient, but sudden death has been reported after relatively minor blows to the sternum.

Tx
- Give a high concentration of oxygen
- Obtain IV access
- Consider aspiration of the pericardium (→ *Box 6.3 and Figure 6.3*)
- In dire cases of penetrating injury consider emergency thoracotomy (→ *below*)
- Seek cardiothoracic advice
- Perform routine blood tests and cross-match blood
- Obtain an ECG (→ *Figure 6.4*).

In less urgent cases the problem is always the initial paucity of physical signs. Admit the patient to a high-dependency area and monitor carefully.

Emergency thoracotomy may be life saving after stab wounds, but is rarely helpful after gunshot wounds, and never after blunt trauma. The criteria for this operation are defined in *Box 6.4* and the

Box 6.4 **Criteria for thoracotomy in the emergency department**

- History of penetrating trauma
- Signs of life in the field
- Short transport time to hospital (up to 15 min)
- Agonal vital signs or electromechanical dissociation (EMD; for <5 min)
- Cardiopulmonary resuscitation in progress if pulseless (for <5 min)

Patients with asystole or ventricular fibrillation will not benefit from thoracotomy

 Box 6.5 **Technique of thoracotomy in the emergency department**

1 Intubate and ventilate the patient
2 Start the incision in the fourth left intercostal space, 2 cm to the left of the sternum (the internal mammary artery runs within 2 cm of the sternal border)
3 Extend the incision along the upper border of the rib as far as the anterior axillary or even the midaxillary line (the intercostal vessels and nerve run behind lower rib border)
4 Incise the pleura and sweep the area with a gloved finger
5 Insert a rib spreader and crank it open to allow visualisation of the thoracic cavity
6 Open the pericardium transversely parallel to and above the phrenic nerve, without damaging surface vessels on the heart

 Box 6.6 **Procedures after an emergency thoracotomy**

- Pericardotomy to relieve tamponade
- Open cardiac massage
- Internal defibrillation (up to 10 J energy)
- Cardiac haemostasis
  (An 18 G French Foley catheter may be inserted through a wound in the heart and the balloon inflated inside. Gentle traction on the distal catheter then achieves temporary haemostasis. If the catheter is connected to an IV infusion, fluids and drugs can be given by the intracardiac route.)
- Clamping of major lacerations of the lung
- Cross-clamping of the descending aorta to optimise cerebral circulation and reduce major abdominal blood loss

technique is described in *Box 6.5*. Some possible intrathoracic procedures are listed in *Box 6.6*.

Injuries to the great vessels

Immediate survival depends on the formation of an acute false aneurysm. Stab wounds may inflict injury at any site, but the more common deceleration injury usually produces a lesion at the level of the aortic isthmus. The intima and media rupture, but the adventitia and adjacent mediastinal structures may provide a sufficiently strong sheath to contain the arterial pressure for a few hours, or indeed many years.

The expanding haematoma may occlude the origin of one or more of the vessels arising from the aortic arch. Blood pressure and pulse may differ in the two arms. Pain radiating to the back is more common than precordial pain.

These injuries can be overlooked, even at thoracotomy. The history is important. Most are associated with injuries elsewhere after high-speed road traffic accidents or falls.

Investigations: A plain CXR may show haemorrhage into the mediastinum and other indirect signs of blood vessel injury:

- Widened mediastinum (mediastinum/chest width >25%; may be obscured by lung injury and not present in 10% of cases)
- Trachea (or nasogastric tube) displaced to the right
- Left main-stem bronchus depressed
- Aortic knuckle absent
- Left apical pleural cap (the left paraspinal line is displaced laterally and extends up and over the apex of the left lung)
- Broad right paratracheal stripe
- Separation of calcium deposits in the aortic wall
- Other signs of severe chest trauma (rib fractures, pulmonary contusion, haemopneumothorax, ruptured diaphragm).

On an AP (portable) film the mediastinum always appears to be widened. Other benign causes of a widened mediastinum are as follows:

- Supine as opposed to upright film
- Rotated positioning of the patient
- X-ray beam directed cranially (lordotic view)
- Short distance between the film and the X-ray source
- Poor inspiratory effort.

High-resolution CT (HRCT) provides much more information, especially with contrast angiography, and is the definitive investigation once the diagnosis is suspected. Transoesophageal ultrasonography and arch aortography may also be useful in some circumstances.

ECGs in thoracic trauma are usually unremarkable although they may sometimes show dramatic changes ($\rightarrow$ *Figure 6.4*).

Tx The role of the ED is to:

- have a high index of suspicion
- begin fluid replacement (but beware of overload)
- refer urgently for specialist care.

Oesophageal injury

This may be caused by penetrating trauma. Blunt rupture may follow vomiting or a direct blow to the epigastrium; it may also complicate endoscopy. Consider oesophageal injury if there is:

- gas in the mediastinum on radiograph
- inexplicable shock after trunk injury
- left pneumothorax without rib fracture
- gastric contents in a chest drain.

Mediastinitis develops insidiously and is often fatal.

XR There is mediastinal gas on plain radiographs and CT scan.

Tx Early diagnosis, antibiotics and surgery are essential.

Diaphragmatic injuries $\rightarrow$ p. 83.

ABDOMINAL INJURIES

Immediate action

- Repeat ABCs as described in *Chapter 1*.
- Cover eviscerated gut with warm saline packs – do not try to push it back. Manipulating mesentery potentiates shock.
- Obtain IV access and commence an IV infusion.

> Fluid loss into the abdomen is usually underestimated.

- Examine the abdomen, noting areas of tenderness, guarding and lacerations, clothing imprints and grazes. Listen for bowel sounds.
- Consider early analgesia.

> Intravenous analgesia is unlikely to mask significant signs in the abdomen. On the contrary, it usually makes the following procedures much easier to perform.

- Log-roll the patient and examine the back and perineum.
- Consider performing a rectal examination (noting injuries, sphincter tone, presence of blood, the wall and contents, and prostate gland).
- Obtain details of the incident, past medical history, medication and time of last food and drink.
- Insert a urinary catheter if there is no urethral injury ($\rightarrow$ p. 84).
- Consider passing a large-bore nasogastric tube if there is no basal skull fracture ($\rightarrow$ p. 43).

> Closed abdominal injuries may easily be overlooked especially when they are less painful than injuries elsewhere and not immediately associated with signs of hypovolaemic shock.

- Give antibiotics if gut perforation suspected.
- Obtain surgical advice early on. There are three possible courses of action:

1 Obvious injury $\rightarrow$ immediate operation
2 Apparently stable $\rightarrow$ admission and observation
3 Equivocal signs or impaired level of consciousness $\rightarrow$ repeated / further assessment in ED.

Methods of assessment $\rightarrow$ below.

Methods of assessment of intra-abdominal damage

Diagnostic peritoneal lavage: DPL is decreasingly used where sophisticated imaging is available. It tends to change the clinical signs in the abdomen and introduces air into the peritoneum, thus complicating CT scan interpretation. It does not rule out hollow visceral perforation (bladder and bowel), diaphragmatic tears or retroperitoneal injuries (i.e. to pancreas or duodenum). It is unsuitable for young children and is contraindicated in patients with bleeding diatheses, morbid obesity and advanced pregnancy.

However, there are some circumstances where the technique may be useful and so it is described in *Box 6.7*. DPL is carried out in the resuscitation area of the ED but normally only after discussion with the admitting general surgeons. Iatrogenic damage to intraperitoneal structures and false-positive taps are unusual (2% of cases) and may be reduced by using the mini-laparotomy technique described. False negatives may also occur (again in 2% of cases) especially with diaphragmatic and pelvic injuries.

Computed tomography: CT is the imaging modality of choice. Any delay that it may cause must be balanced against a corresponding delay in definitive care. It should be performed only in relatively stable patients with continuous monitoring. It is good for retroperitoneal examination but may miss gastrointestinal injury.

Ultrasonography: this is widely used in the ED. In experienced hands, it is good for solid organ assessment and detection of free fluid.

Stab wounds to the abdomen

Small lacerations should be assumed to be deep until proved otherwise. Injury to the intestine and mesentery may not be accompanied by the rapid clinical deterioration usually associated with stab wounds to the liver, spleen and major vessels.

X$_R$ An erect CXR is the most important plain film. Free gas is a strong, but not absolute, indication for laparotomy. Ultrasonography and CT have better diagnostic accuracy.

T$_X$ Obtain surgical advice. Laparotomy has an associated morbidity. This can be reduced if a selective approach is used.

Patients with immediate evidence of an intra-abdominal catastrophe must be taken straight to theatre. Resuscitation with oxygen and IV fluids is started in the ED; 4–8 units of blood should be cross-matched.

The remaining patients (the majority) can be treated by admission and careful observation. This must include serial examination of the abdomen

 Box 6.7 Peritoneal lavage

- Catheterise the bladder to decompress it
- Insert a nasogastric tube if the stomach is distended
- Clean and drape the abdomen
- Inject local anaesthetic in the midline, a third of the distance from the umbilicus to the symphysis pubis. The use of lidocaine with adrenaline helps to limit bleeding from the wound into the abdomen
- Make a small longitudinal skin incision
- Identify and open the peritoneum under direct vision
- Introduce a dialysis catheter, directing it towards the pelvis
- Connect the catheter to a syringe and attempt to aspirate blood

If gross blood is not obtained:

- Flush in 500 mL (10 mL/kg) of warm isotonic saline
- Leave the fluid in the peritoneum for 5–10 min, then lower the infusion bag to the floor to allow drainage
- Send a sample of the lavage fluid to the laboratory

A positive result is shown by:

- Immediate aspiration of heavily blood-stained, non-clotting fluid
- Lavage fluid containing >100 000 erythrocytes/mm^3
- Lavage fluid containing >500 leukocytes/mm^3
- Lavage fluid leaking from other sites (e.g. bladder catheter or chest drain)
- Lavage fluid containing bile, food, faecal matter or bacteria

(initially every 1–2 h) and frequent recordings of pulse and BP.

Early administration of antibiotics (e.g. metronidazole and cefotaxime) reduces the risk of intraperitoneal infection and septic shock. Patients with perineal injuries may develop gas gangrene and so should also receive benzylpenicillin.

The wound should be covered with an antiseptic dressing. Antitetanus prophylaxis is required. Stab wounds are best left unsutured when first seen, to allow drainage of any deep bleeding or infection.

Blunt abdominal trauma

Blunt abdominal injury should be considered if any of the following apply:

- Localising symptoms or signs
- Marks on the abdominal wall
- Suspicious mechanism of injury
- Injuries both above and below the abdomen
- Unexplained hypovolaemia
- Abnormally pale patient
- Reduced conscious level, so patient difficult to assess.

In the conscious patient, the site and character of abdominal pain will help to determine the need for laparotomy. It may be possible to determine the direction and severity of the injuring agent from details of the incident, an examination of clothing and distribution of skin injuries and clothing imprints.

Most bleeding is caused by damage to the liver or spleen. As in the case of stab wounds, damage in the absence of bleeding is much slower to present and more difficult to diagnose.

XR An erect CXR can be difficult to obtain. Ultrasonography and CT are the investigations of choice.

Methods of assessment of intra-abdominal damage → p. 81.

Tx Resuscitation should be started and blood cross-matched. Patients need close observation and laparotomy at the first indication of significant problems.

Abdominal pain may be caused by acute gastric dilatation or paralytic ileus associated with an injury elsewhere. Gastric dilatation is a well-recognised complication of head injury, particularly in children. Insertion of a nasogastric tube may resolve distension and pain. If the tube is wide-bore it will also remove partially digested food and thus reduce the risk of aspiration into the lungs.

Splenic injuries are common. They may occur with very little in the way of external signs. Very careful monitoring, with repeat ultrasound or CT scan is essential. Conservative management or repair of a bleeding spleen is preferable to splenectomy. In children, especially, surgeons will attempt to preserve the spleen because of the risk of sudden, overwhelming sepsis that can occur at any time of life after splenectomy.

Rupture of the diaphragm

This injury is often overlooked. It is more common on the left side. Blunt injury usually causes a large defect in the diaphragm whereas stab wounds may cause a small defect with delayed presentation.

XR Rupture of the diaphragm may be missed on a CXR. If suspected, the insertion of a nasogastric tube will aid interpretation of both plain radiographs and CT scans.

Tx The stomach should be decompressed with a nasogastric tube and the patient kept sitting up if possible. Surgical repair will be necessary.

Retroperitoneal injuries

These are associated with back pain, significant blood loss and paralytic ileus. Consider the involvement of:

- paravertebral muscles with avulsion of lumbar transverse processes (→ p. 59)
- kidneys and ureters
- pancreas and duodenum.

XR A plain film may show associated bony damage as above. A CT scan is diagnostic. Investigate renal injury as below.

Tx Resuscitation should be followed by surgical referral. Blood should be cross-matched. A raised serum amylase may point to pancreatic injury.

Renal injury

Injuries to the loins are common after falls and assaults. Many soft-tissue injuries in this area cause severe pain. The urine should always be tested for blood.

XR In a stable patient, with only microscopic haematuria, ultrasonography can be performed during the next 24 h. A CT scan (with contrast) or intravenous urography (IVU) is indicated for macroscopic haematuria and before exploratory laparotomy in an unstable patient.

Tx All patients with suspected renal injury should be admitted for observation and analgesia.

Abdominal trauma in pregnancy

General principles of management of major trauma in pregnancy → p. 31.

Signs of intra-abdominal bleeding tend to be reduced or modified in pregnancy. Gastric emptying is delayed.

XR Consider early ultrasound scan of the abdomen, uterus and fetus.

Tx The treatment of an injured pregnant patient follows the usual ABCs, but in addition there should be the following:

- Left lateral positioning to avoid inferior vena cava compression
- Extra vigilance in treating early hypovolaemia. Signs of shock are delayed because of maternal hyperaemia
- Confirmation of the normal fetal heart beat (usually for maternal reassurance, because the fetus is well protected inside the amniotic sac). A Doppler ultrasound probe is better for this purpose than a fetal stethoscope. Consider early monitoring of the fetal heart rate by fetocardiotocograph (FCTG) in seriously injured patients ($\rightarrow$ p. 32)
- Prophylaxis against aspiration pneumonia with an IV gastric acid suppressant ($\rightarrow$ p. 32)
- Administration of anti-RhD immunoglobulin to rhesus D-negative women.

PELVIC INJURIES

Bony injury to the pelvis

There are two distinct types of pelvic fracture:

1 After violent injury, the fracture is:
   - unstable
   - crushed or displaced at more than one point
   - associated with major blood loss and visceral injury.
2 After a fall in an osteoporotic patient, the injury is:
   - stable
   - anterior and minimally displaced
   - associated with pre-existing general medical problems.

Tenderness is usually apparent. Testing stability by attempting to move the iliac wings is unreliable and contraindicated – it provokes bleeding. Straight-leg raising is usually reduced or impossible.

XR An AP radiograph is essential initially. Oblique views and CT scan are useful later. A cone view of the pubic rami may sometimes be helpful.

Tx Initial management of major pelvic fractures includes:

- fluid resuscitation
- assessment of visceral injury
- pain control
- external fixation.

External fixation can be used as an emergency intervention in the management of an unstable pelvic fracture. Modern fixators are quick to apply and are suitable for use in the ED. They may help to control haemorrhage.

Single fractures of the pubic rami are rarely associated with visceral injury or significant blood loss ($\rightarrow$ p. 90). They are, however, painful and restrict the mobility of the elderly patients in whom they most commonly occur. Hospital admission is usually required for a few days before gentle mobilisation. No specific treatment is necessary in the ED. Look for the cause of the fall. Also consider fracture of the neck of the femur ($\rightarrow$ p. 89). This presents itself in a similar way in the same group of patients.

Injury to the pelvic viscera

Injury within the pelvis may cause profound blood loss.

XR A CT scan is essential if visceral injury is suspected.

Tx Transfuse and refer. External fixation may be helpful with pelvic instability ($\rightarrow$ *above*).

Urogenital injuries

Perineal injury is easily missed. There may be:

- a painful desire to micturate
- local swelling or bruising
- blood at the external meatus.

In a male patient, there may be cranial migration of the prostate (the 'missing prostate' sign). This is associated with rupture of the membranous urethra and is diagnosed by rectal examination. The corresponding sign in a female patient is bogginess of the anterior vaginal wall on pelvic examination.

Extravasation of urine into the perineal tissues is unusual immediately after injury, more commonly developing after 1 or 2h. It suggests injury to the extraperitoneal part of the bladder or urethra. Intraperitoneal rupture of the bladder produces the earlier abdominal signs of pain and shock.

XR Retrograde urethrography is easy to perform and must precede catheter placement. Alternatively, a suprapubic catheter may be inserted directly into the bladder.

Tx The majority of urethral injuries are incomplete transections. The maintenance of urothelial continuity will reduce the severity of late stricture formation. It is therefore important that these injuries are diagnosed early and treated gently by an experienced surgeon.

Other perineal injuries

Lacerations of the perineal body or the anal or vaginal margins should be assumed to penetrate deeply until proven otherwise. This will entail careful and skilled examination under good operating conditions. If there is any suggestion of intraperitoneal extension, laparotomy will be required – possibly with faecal diversion. Early referral is essential. Antibiotics should be started in the ED.

7

The lower limb

GENERAL APPROACH TO LIMB PROBLEMS

This section should be read before turning to the relevant anatomical site.

Crush injuries and myoglobinuria → p. 265.
Hand → p. 128.
Small wounds and localised infections → p. 391.
Upper limb → p. 111.

> **Do not consider the limb in isolation as:**
> - Injuries around the shoulder and thigh may cause hypovolaemia
> - Painful limb injuries may be associated with life-threatening, but less painful, trunk trauma
> - Limb infection may have systemic effects
> - Limb pain may be symptomatic of trunk pathology (e.g. cardiac pain, sciatica and herpes zoster infection)

> Four four-letter words describe a structured approach to examination of the limbs: LOOK, FEEL, MOVE, X-RAY.

Immediate assessment and management

- Start with the ABCs as discussed in *Chapter 1*.
- Apply direct pressure to stop any bleeding.
- Expose the affected part; cut off clothes as necessary.
- Take a brief but comprehensive history.
- Confirm that the presenting problem is confined to the limb.
- Confirm the presence of distal pulses and the integrity of the nerve supply.
- Splint fractures.
- Give analgesia early on; this may be systemic or local.
- Finally undertake a detailed local examination including a comparison with the opposite limb.

If there is a clear history of trauma, it is useful to reconstruct the incident to appreciate the forces applied and to consider the biomechanics of the injury:

- Healthy young bones will undergo considerable elastic deformation (e.g. the femoral shaft will bend over 10° before breaking). At breaking point, stored energy is released and the limb suddenly deforms further, inflicting secondary soft-tissue injury. Often, this is more important than the underlying fracture.

Emergency Medicine Lecture Notes, Fourth Edition. Chris Moulton and David Yates.
© 2012 Blackwell Publishing Ltd. Published 2012 by Blackwell Publishing Ltd.

- Twisting tends to produce spiral fractures.
- Direct blows cause transverse fractures, which may be compound.
- Sheering forces raise contused skin flaps.
- Forces applied to the heel of the falling body and causing a fracture of the os calcis will be transmitted cranially and may produce a fracture of the lumbar spine or the base of the skull.
- An evident knee injury, sustained by a front-seat car passenger, may draw attention away from an occult hip dislocation.

Wounds

Wounds should not be explored at this stage. Sterile dressings or iodine soaks are the only necessary treatment. An instant photograph of the injury will prevent the need for frequent re-examination by attending doctors. Foreign bodies must be left alone, even if they are grossly protruding, until resuscitation has begun and the environment and staff are prepared for a careful, controlled assessment. Patients with grossly contaminated wounds and compound fractures should receive intravenous (IV) antibiotics (e.g. flucloxacillin) and antitetanus prophylaxis as soon as possible.

Pain

Splintage and reassurance are very important. Pain may be controlled by nitrous oxide while a splint is applied. Intravenous injection of opiates should be given as soon as contraindications have been excluded. In some situations a local anaesthetic block may be preferable.

Radiographs

Radiographs complement but do not replace a full clinical examination. Good radiographs demand good viewing facilities. The doctor should have a high-quality screen and charts showing the times of appearance and fusion of primary and secondary ossification centres.

> Do not attempt to interpret a colleague's radiographs without first examining the patient.

Vascular problems related to injury

Specific vascular problems → p. 107.

> All urgent limb problems are related to blood supply.

Occlusion

Fractures around the elbow and the knee are commonly associated with vascular occlusion. Do not assume that distal ischaemia has been caused by transient vascular spasm. Urgent specialist referral is necessary. Limb viability is threatened if a major occlusion persists for 4 h or more.

> Healthy young limbs are more at risk from vascular occlusion of main vessels than are old ischaemic limbs because the latter have had time to develop a collateral circulation.

Bleeding

Elevation is an effective first-aid measure for major venous haemorrhage but is often impossible to achieve because of associated bony injury. Applying artery clips to spurting vessels in the emergency department (ED) will usually inflict further injury, especially as most major limb vessels run alongside peripheral nerves. Instead, local pressure should be applied. Bleeding into damaged muscle is a much more common problem.

Compartment syndrome

The closed fascial compartments of the limbs prevent contused muscles and haematomas from expanding indefinitely. Interstitial pressure rises causing pain and ischaemia (→ *p. 110*).

Plaster casts

Application of a cast is the most common way of immobilising an injured area of a limb, be it an injury to the bone or to the soft tissue. However, acute injuries may swell considerably in the first 48 h and restriction of that expansion by a cast can cause severe ischaemia. The inelasticity of fascial compartments, particularly in the lower leg, can have a similar effect.

Splitting a cast (a single, longitudinal split is the best) or prescribing an incomplete slab-type plaster does not necessarily protect the limb from the underlying ischaemia. All ED plasters must be well padded, especially over bony protuberances, and the patient must have:

- instructions to elevate the limb and crutches or a sling if needed
- advice on the care of the cast and a written list of the signs of ischaemia (plaster instructions)
- early review.

All staff who deal with patients in casts must be aware of the need to look out for the signs of compartment syndrome (→ p. 110) as well as the more widely appreciated changes to the warmth, colour and capillary refill of the digits.

The National Institute for Health and Clinical Excellence (NICE) recommends that all patients who are being treated with a plaster cast on the lower limb should be risk assessed for venous thromboembolism (VTE). If they are found to be at significant risk of VTE, they should be offered thromboprophylaxis for the duration of the treatment.

Diagnosis and management of suspected deep vein thrombosis (DVT) → p. 108.
Prophylaxis against VTE → p. 222.
Risk factors for VTE → Box 13.13 on p. 215.

Physiotherapy

The help of the physiotherapist can be invaluable in treating a wide range of soft-tissue injuries and other conditions. Particular benefits are seen with early physiotherapy and include the following:

- Reduction in pain, bruising and swelling
- Maintenance of muscle fibre length and range of movements
- Early mobilisation and restoration of function.

The physiotherapist also offers:

- Re-examination of the injury and the level of function
- Assessment for and training with walking aids
- Restoration of the patient's confidence
- Skilled follow-up.

Crutches

Crutches are required for emergency patients with a large variety of differing problems. They may be designed to enable a limb to be:

- non-weight-bearing (axillary crutches)
- partial weight-bearing (elbow crutches).

All patients given crutches must be instructed about their safe care and usage and should also be observed in action.

Local injection of steroids

The injection of a long-acting steroid-type drug into a joint, tendon sheath, bursa or other suitable area can bring long-lasting relief to a large number of inflammatory soft-tissue conditions. The steroid is often premixed with local anaesthetic to:

- minimise the discomfort of the injection
- give some immediate relief of the underlying condition
- act as a marker of successful localisation of an injection.

> The patient must be warned that symptoms may increase over the first 24 h before gradual resolution.

Complications of depot steroid injection include the following:

- Local damage
- Introduction of infection
- Rupture of a tendon
- Fat necrosis and atrophy and disfigurement of overlying skin.

As such, it is a technique that requires the following knowledge:

- The local anatomy
- The best approaches to the target area
- The correct drug dosage for each site (→ *Table 7.1*).

Table 7.1 Dose of methylprednisolone for local injection

Joint	Dose	
	(mg)	**(mL)**
Large joint (knee, ankle, shoulder)	20–80	0.5–2
Medium joint (elbow, wrist)	10–40	0.25–1
Small joint (MCPJ, IPJ, ACJ)	4–10	0.1–0.25
Bursa	4–30	0.1–0.75
Periarticular (for epicondylitis)	4–30	0.1–0.75
Tendon sheath (never into a tendon)	4–30	0.1–0.75

ACJ, acromioclavicular joint; IPJ, interphalangeal joint; MCPJ, metacarpophalangeal joint.

Local injections of steroid should not be given by inexperienced staff or in circumstances where there are no facilities for review of the patient.

Sports injuries

Soft-tissue and bony injuries, secondary to trauma sustained during sport, are common presentations. Many such injuries can also occur during non-sporting activities. There are three specific needs of the sportsperson:

1 A quick return to normal training and activity
2 Maintenance of muscle fibre length
3 Protection from re-injury when the activity is resumed.

Accurate diagnosis is essential. A good general recipe for treating sports injuries is:

- 3 days' complete rest (crutches/sling if required)
- appropriate analgesia
- early physiotherapy.

Ice, compression and elevation are useful in the early stages to reduce discomfort and swelling. There should be a return to about 50% training levels as soon as possible and then a gradual build-up to full activity.

See also the appropriate anatomical sections of this chapter and Chapters 8 and 9.

THE HIP AND THIGH

> The hip joint capsule is innervated from the L2–4 level. These dermatomes extend to the knee, hence the common complaint of hip pathology apparently arising in the knee. The hip must be examined whenever a patient complains of a knee problem.

Dislocation of the hip

This is caused by axial violence such as a force applied to the knee. The dislocation is usually posterior with a fracture of the acetabular rim. Sometimes the sciatic nerve is injured – most frequently that part destined to be the common peroneal nerve. Pain is usually severe and the hip is held partially flexed and adducted. Central dislocation into the pelvis is associated with major (concealed) blood loss. Dislocation of an arthroplasty of the hip is often seen after relatively minor trauma.

XR When resuscitation has been established and analgesia given, radiographs are obtained. Later a CT scan will aid identification of complex acetabular rim fractures.

Tx Resuscitate and provide analgesia; support the limb but do not attempt reduction in the ED. The distal neurovascular function must be assessed and the secondary survey completed, looking for other injuries. The patient needs an urgent referral to the orthopaedic department.

Both types of traumatic dislocation can be difficult to reduce by closed manipulation. Posterior dislocation may be treated more appropriately by open reduction and internal fixation of the bone fragments.

Fracture of the hip (fracture of the proximal femur)

There are three circumstances in which this may occur:

1 At any age – associated with major violence and multiple injuries
2 In elderly people – after a simple fall
3 Spontaneously – as a result of osteoporosis or bony secondary deposits.

> Hip fracture is a major public health issue in countries with an ever-increasing ageing population. In the UK, these fractures account for 90% of the enormous cost of osteoporosis to the NHS. The human cost is equally high – around 10% of people with a hip fracture die within 1 month and almost a third within 12 months of the injury. Most of these deaths are due to associated co-morbidities.

A detailed history must be taken and other injuries excluded. Consider the reason for an unexplained fall (medication, domestic disorganisation) and assess general health. The following notes assume that systemic examination has been undertaken and relate to the care of the typical elderly patient with an isolated injury.

The patient (usually female) presents as unable to weight-bear after a relatively minor fall. Some patients may be able to walk, albeit with a painful limp. There is pain in the hip, thigh or knee but usually no visible swelling, bruising or deformity. The affected leg may be shortened and externally rotated but this classic appearance is dependent on the grade of the fracture.

A more valuable sign is pain on gentle passive rotation of the extended leg. If the fracture has impacted, other movements may be good with minimal pain including even straight-leg raising. Tenderness is most marked posteriorly. Significant blood loss is unusual and associated vascular and tendon damage is rare.

Examination of the hip joint → Box 7.1.

XR Radiological examination must include an anteroposterior (AP) view of the hips and pelvis, and a lateral radiograph of the affected hip. In the AP view, look for a break in the normal apparent continuity of trabeculae across the joint.

Osteoarthrosis is associated with intertrochanteric rather than subcapital fractures, so it is very unlikely that an undisplaced subcapital fracture will be hidden in the disorganised radiological pattern around an arthritic joint.

> The lateral view may be difficult to obtain and interpret but is nevertheless the best film on which to see a minimally displaced fracture.

Up to 5% of fractures in osteoporotic bone are not immediately visible on plain radiographs. An MR scan should be performed if a hip fracture is suspected but initial radiographs are normal. A CT scan is an alternative if MRI is not available within 24 h of admission. *For different types of proximal femoral fractures → Box 7.2.*

Tx A box splint may be used to control leg movements and analgesia should be given immediately (and the effect of these measures assessed after 30 min). Long waits on hard trolleys must be avoided because these patients acquire pressure sores very quickly. (*For risk factors for pressure sores → p. 222.*) Internal fixation, hemiarthroplasty or total arthroplasty is usually performed on the day of admission or at least within 24 h of injury.

Fracture of the pubic rami

The anterior pelvis should be carefully examined in all cases. Fracture of the pubic rami occurs in the same group of patients as those with fracture of the hip and gives a very similar clinical picture. The pain may be felt in the buttock or groin but otherwise symptoms are localised to one leg and may divert attention away from the pelvis. Patients with this injury need initial bed rest and analgesia and then gradual mobilisation (*also → p. 84*).

 Box 7.1 How to examine the hip joint

- Assess gait and continue inspection of mobility and pain as clothes are removed and the patient gets on to the couch
- Look for shortening or rotation of the leg. True shortening is caused by collapse or angulation of bone (distance between anterosuperior iliac spine and medial joint line of knee – both legs in the same position). Apparent shortening is the difference between the two sides when the patient is lying supine (distance from umbilicus to medial malleoli). It is usually caused by pelvic tilt or fixed deformity at the hip joint
- Look at the groin, perineum, buttock and lateral bony prominences, and feel for tenderness in these areas. A sinus or old scar may point to established disease but there are usually no surface signs of acute inflammation or of joint effusion
- Assess flexion, abduction, adduction and rotation in each leg (active before passive). Keep one hand under the lumbar spine when testing flexion and one hand on the opposite iliac crest when testing abduction and adduction. Rotation is most accurately measured with the knee at right angles (lower leg over the end of the couch or patient prone). With the patient lying on his or her side attempt to extend the hip joint backwards; 5–10° is often possible
- Examine the relationship between hip movement and lumbar spine and pelvic movement. Fixed flexion of the hip can be camouflaged by excessive lumbar lordosis. Fixed adduction is usually compensated for by pelvic tilt. The easiest way to abolish the lordosis is to fully flex the leg that is not being measured. Any passive movement off the bed of the leg under assessment is fixed flexion. Similarly, setting the pelvis square may cause fixed adduction of one leg
- Finally, ask the patient to stand on one leg. The pelvis should rise on the non-weight-bearing side. Failure to do this is a positive Trendelenburg sign and indicates disease in the weight-bearing hip or its associated abductor muscles

Box 7.2 **Hip fractures (or proximal femoral fractures)**

Fractures occurring between the edge of the femoral head and 5 cm below the lesser trochanter.

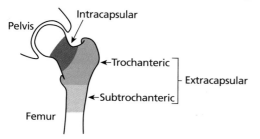

Extracapsular fractures

Fractures between the insertion of the capsule of the hip joint and a line 5 cm below the lesser trochanter. There are two subgroups:

1 Trochanteric fractures: including intertrochanteric (pertrochanteric) and reverse oblique trochanteric fractures
2 Subtrochanteric fractures: fractures up to 5 cm below the lesser trochanter

Intracapsular fractures

Fractures between the edge of the femoral head and the insertion of the capsule of the hip joint. Also known as femoral neck fractures. There are three types:

1 Subcapital
2 Transcervical
3 Basal cervical

Garden classification of subcapital (intracapsular) hip fractures

The classification relies only on the appearance of the hip on an AP radiograph:

Grade 1: incomplete (impacted) fracture
Grade 2: complete fracture without displacement
Grade 3: complete fracture with partial displacement
Grade 4: complete fracture with full displacement

The elderly patient with failure to weight-bear after a fall

All such patients must be admitted for reassessment and mobilisation. A considerable number prove to have a fracture that was not evident on the initial radiograph. An MR scan should be performed if a hip fracture is thought to be a possibility (i.e. in most elderly patients) but initial radiographs are normal. A CT scan is an alternative if MRI is not available within 24 h of admission. Patients with soft-tissue injuries may require prolonged rehabilitation before they are ready for discharge. Local policy dictates whether care for these patients is provided by the geriatric or orthopaedic department.

Degenerative disease of the hip

The patient presents with pain and stiffness and may relate this to a recent injury. The hip joint has a restricted range of movement. Fixed flexion may be obscured by compensatory lumbar lordosis. Fixed adduction causes pelvic tilt and an apparently short leg. Pain is usually most marked at the extremes of the range and there is little muscle spasm. A general examination is always indicated to exclude systemic disease and injury.

XR Radiographs show reduced joint space, irregular articular surface, osteophytes, sclerosis and bone cysts. Such changes, however, are common and may not be related to the patient's symptoms.

Tx In the absence of other pathology, symptomatic treatment with analgesia and a walking aid should be offered. The patient should be advised to consult his or her GP. Physiotherapy may help with initial mobilisation.

Irritable hip

This is a common condition in children. The child, usually under the age of 5 years, presents with a limp that is unrelated to trauma. Occasionally, the sore hip gives way and creates the illusion of a traumatic injury. Pain in the hip region may not be immediately evident and passive movements are usually normal. Sometimes mild protective spasm may limit abduction. There may be a history of a prodromal upper respiratory infection.

The condition is thought to be caused by a transient synovitis, possibly of viral origin, and is invariably unilateral. It is important to exclude a septic arthritis

Management of a young child with a limp → Box 7.3.

Box 7.3 The management of a young child who is limping or not weight-bearing

- Ask about duration and severity of limp
- Ask about a history of trauma, viral infection or previous episodes
- Take the temperature
- Observe the gait
- Ask the child to stand on alternate legs
- Examine the whole limb, feeling carefully, especially for tibial tenderness and hip spasm in abduction
- Consider the need to obtain radiographs of the whole limb
- If there are no specific clinical or radiological findings, reassure the parents and recommend rest and paracetamol elixir for the child. Arrange for review within 72 h

XR Radiographs of the affected limb from hip to ankle are usually required. The foot may need to be included if there is any tenderness in this area. The main differential diagnosis is a toddler's fracture or other tibial injury (→ p. 100).

Ultrasound examination can demonstrate an effusion in the hip joint but cannot differentiate synovial fluid, blood and pus. A difference of >3 mm of effusion between the normal and the affected hip is considered to be pathological. A positive ultrasound scan obviates the need for radiographs.

Tx If there is an unexplained pyrexia and/or hip muscle spasm refer the child to the orthopaedic department for admission. A child who is apyrexial with no hip spasm and no evidence of bony injury can be discharged with analgesia and instructions to rest but must be reviewed in the ED review clinic within 72 h.

The age of a limping child will help with diagnosis:

Irritable hip – usually seen in children who are <5 years old
Perthes' disease – most common in children aged 5–10 years
Slipped femoral epiphysis – occurs at the age of 10–15 years

Perthes' disease

Perthes' disease is an idiopathic avascular necrosis of the proximal femoral epiphysis. It is often called an 'osteochondritis' and belongs to a group of similar diseases of epiphyseal growth (→ p. 350). In the UK, it affects 1 in 10 000 children and is four times more common in boys than in girls. In 10% of cases it is bilateral. Children aged between 3 and 15 years may be affected, although it is most common in children between 5 and 8 years of age. It presents with a painful or painless limp or sometimes with hip or knee pain after exercise. Pain may be mild and is often of several months' duration. There is restriction of hip movements with muscle spasm, especially internal rotation and abduction. Flexion is usually unaffected.

XR Radiographs may be normal in very early disease. However, they often show remarkably advanced changes in contrast to the short clinical history. The femoral neck may be widened, bone density reduced, joint space increased and the femoral head fragmented (→ Figure 7.1). An ultrasound scan reveals an effusion and bone scanning shows reduced uptake in the affected epiphysis. Blood tests are all normal.

Tx The child should be referred to the orthopaedic department for admission. Bed rest until the muscle spasm has resolved is now the mainstay of treatment for this condition.

Slipped upper femoral epiphysis

The capital (or proximal femoral) epiphysis may slip suddenly or gradually, usually in a teenager who is having a pubertal growth spurt. The onset may be linked to minor trauma. There is limping and pain, which may be localised to the distal thigh or knee. Hip abduction is restricted but adduction is often increased. Flexion and internal rotation may increase the pain because these movements stretch the joint capsule. An acute slip is more likely to lead to ischaemia and avascular necrosis of the epiphysis than the more common chronic slip.

XR Radiographs may be difficult to interpret and should include AP and lateral views of both hips. Posterior movement of the epiphysis is sometimes the first radiographic sign and is best seen on the lateral view. Slight medial displacement of the epiphysis is usually the initial change and is sometimes likened to 'an ice-cream sliding off its cone' (→ Figure 7.2). More specifically, a line drawn parallel to the femoral neck (Klein's line) will normally intersect with

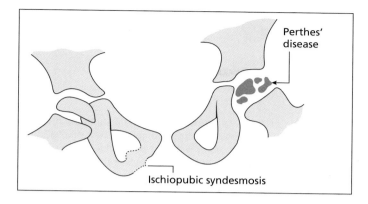

Figure 7.1 Perthes' disease, with incidental normal enlargement of the ischiopubic syndesmosis.

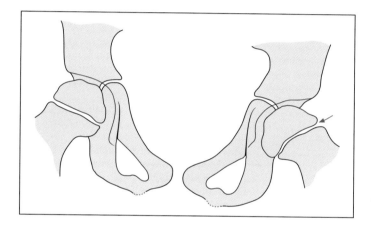

Figure 7.2 Slipped left proximal femoral epiphysis (arrowed) (anteroposterior view).

the lateral portion of the femoral epiphysis (Trethowan's sign).

Tx Immediate referral to the orthopaedic department is essential. Surgical reduction of an acute slip followed by prophylactic pinning is usually recommended.

Extra-articular problems around the hip

Spinal and abdominal lesions may present with hip symptoms:

- Infection of the lumbar spine may produce a psoas abscess, which points just below the inguinal ligament. This may be tuberculous or as a result of a variety of agents in drug addicts.
- A femoral hernia may be overlooked, especially in an obese, elderly woman.

- A high lumbar disc lesion may present with anterior thigh pain and limitation of hip extension (the femoral stretch test).
- Constriction of the lateral cutaneous nerve of the thigh as it passes through the inguinal ligament may cause persistent pain over the thigh (meralgia paraesthetica).
- A child with haemophilia may present with hip joint spasm caused by haemorrhage into the psoas muscle.

Fracture of the femoral shaft

This is associated with extensive soft-tissue injury and internal bleeding but is not usually compound. The level of trauma required to fracture the femur should suggest the possibility of serious injuries elsewhere.

XR The diagnosis should be clinically evident without immediate resort to radiographs, which are mainly used to exclude other injuries and to check the position of the bone after the application of a splint.

Tx Priorities are as follows:

- Complete ABCs
- Give effective analgesia, initially nitrous oxide mixture and then IV opiates and/or a femoral nerve block (→ Box 7.4)
- Apply Thomas' or other traction splint (→ Box 7.5)
- Check distal pulses; vascular damage can occur with supracondylar fractures
- Withdraw blood for baseline values and cross-match
- Complete the secondary survey
- Take radiographs as appropriate
- Involve the orthopaedic team early in management.

 Box 7.4 Femoral nerve block

Indications: fractures at any level of the femur.
Contraindications: hypersensitivity to local anaesthetics; neurovascular complications of the injury.
Method: clean and drape the skin. Insert a short needle lateral to the femoral artery just below the inguinal ligament. Advance it perpendicularly to the skin. Feel for loss of resistance when the fascia is penetrated. Inject up to 10 mL 0.5% bupivacaine. The patient may experience paraesthesia during the injection.
Onset: within 15 min.
Duration: variable, but often over 5 h.

THE KNEE
Assessment of the knee joint

The knee can be very difficult to assess acutely. A detailed history will help to distinguish between the many types of injury and symptoms that may occur:

- Ask about the relationship between the onset of symptoms (especially pain and swelling) and the time of injury.
- Ask about and observe the ability to weight-bear.
- Look, feel and move the joint (→ Box 7.6).
- Confirm the presence of distal pulses.

 Box 7.5 Splinting a femoral shaft fracture

Traction splints and Thomas' splints are commonly available. Apply the splint before the radiograph. It will give immediate pain relief and reduce blood loss.

- If Thomas' splint is to be used, obtain the appropriate size and cover it with tubular bandage or webbing slings. If a traction splint is to be used much of the following can be omitted, but ensure that you know how it works before trying to apply it
- Apply the strapping from the skin traction kit to the leg. Adhesive strapping must not be used on elderly or fragile skin because its removal later may damage the skin. Instead, use a non-adhesive traction kit
- Protect the malleoli by padding
- Secure the strapping with crepe bandages
- Ensure adequate analgesia. Intravenous analgesia can be supplemented with nitrous oxide while applying the splint
- Grip the heel and forefoot of the injured leg and apply firm continuous traction. Muscle spasm will gradually disappear and angulation of the thigh will decrease. Transient increase in pain is usually reduced by continuous traction
- Instruct an assistant to manoeuvre the splint over the foot and ankle
- Maintain constant traction while the assistant pushes the splint towards the pelvis
- Protect the genitalia
- Fasten the strapping by its ropes to the end of the splint
- Tighten the traction by inserting a wooden spatula between the two ropes and twisting it until the required tension is achieved (Chinese windlass method)
- Check the foot pulses and toe movements
- Request a radiograph to check the position of the splint

- Exclude referred pain, especially from the hip and spine.

Vascular problems are relatively common in fractures around the knee. They are of two types:

1 Direct trauma to a major vessel by a bone fragment or by the interosseous ligament at the trifurcation of the popliteal artery

2 Raised interstitial pressure within a closed fascial compartment of the lower leg (→ *p. 110*).

Damage to the distal part of the popliteal artery is particularly serious in young people, because here it is an 'end'-artery. Elderly patients may have developed a collateral circulation around the knee in response to the main vessel disease.

Examination of the knee joint → Box 7.6.
Indications for radiography of the knee after injury →
Box 7.7.

Wounds around the knee

Even apparently trivial wounds around the knee may involve the joint capsule and synovium.

XR Intra-articular air may be seen on the radiograph as a radiolucent area.

Tx Suspicion of joint involvement warrants orthopaedic referral, thorough assessment, usually under general anaesthesia. and prophylactic antibiotics (flucloxacillin, started before surgery).

Soft-tissue injuries to the knee

Ligamentous and meniscal injuries to the knee are often difficult to diagnose precisely on first presentation. The patient generally has variable degrees of:

- pain
- difficulty weight-bearing
- swelling
- reduction of the range of movements – due to restriction by fluid, pain and sometimes by mechanical blocks.

Serious intra-articular problems are probable in the presence of any of the following:

- A large, rapidly developing effusion
- Complete inability to weight-bear
- Demonstrable collateral or cruciate laxity.

> If the patient can lie with the joint fully extended so that the back of knee is on the couch while the heel is a few centimetres off it, and also squat down with the knee fully flexed, then serious injury is extremely unlikely.

Effusions in the knee joint: the speed of onset of an effusion is as important as the size. Rapid collection suggests the presence of blood and thus damage to vascular structures such as the bone or ligament. The

Box 7.6 A method of examining the knee joint

- Watch the patient climb on to the couch
- Look for scars, sinuses, muscle wasting and joint swelling
- Ask patient to point to the site of the pain
- Test for the presence of an effusion or haemarthrosis (→ *p. 96*)
- Palpate bony landmarks for irregularities and tenderness
- Confirm the ability of the quadriceps mechanism to extend the joint
- Check for the ability to hyperextend the knee so that the heel lifts off the couch while the back of the knee remains in contact with it. This usually signifies that the joint is not severely injured
- Determine the range of true extension and flexion and compare this with the normal side
- At 90° flexion (or as near as the pain allows) rotate the tibia on the femur by twisting the foot. Pain at the joint line suggests meniscal injury. Repeat this test with the patient prone, applying compression along the tibia. This increases pain of meniscal origin and lessens the pain of a collateral ligament lesion
- Keeping the joint at 90°, sit on the foot and attempt to pull and push the upper tibia on the femur to test the cruciate ligaments. The hamstrings must be flaccid; assess this by having the index fingers up against them while pulling forward. There is considerable variation in cruciate laxity between patients, but not between their two knees
- Test collateral ligament integrity at 10° flexion. Stand facing the supine patient, put the foot in your axilla and hold the leg just below the knee in both hands. All muscles must be flaccid while you attempt to shake the knee sideways. Normally, there will be painless – if alarming – clunks at the limits of valgus and varus stressing. A 'rubbery', painful end-point suggests collateral ligament injury. Complete rupture may be less painful than partial rupture
- Move the patella sideways on the femur with the knee fully extended. If lateral pressure causes anxiety and pain, consider potential dislocation. If downward pressure is painful consider chondromalacia

Box 7.7 Indications for radiography of the knee after injury

Any of the following:

- History of fall, blunt trauma or penetrating injury
- Age <12 years or >55 years
- Obvious deformity
- Severe swelling of rapid onset
- Tenderness at the head of the fibula
- Isolated tenderness of the patella
- Inability to flex to 90°
- Inability to straight leg raise
- Inability to walk four weight-bearing steps unaided in the ED
- Atypical features
- Return visit with no improvement.

Box 7.8 Knee problems that need immediate referral

- Haemarthrosis
- Ligamentous instability
- Locked knee
- Complete failure to straight leg raise
- Fracture on radiograph
- Possibility of septic arthritis
- Penetration of the joint

most common cause of a haemarthrosis is a partial tear of the anterior cruciate ligament. Fractures of the lower femur and upper tibia may extend into the joint and produce a haemarthrosis. Onset of swelling over 24 h is typical of a synovial response, commonly associated with damage to the avascular menisci or trauma to an osteoarthritic knee.

- Modest effusions can be detected by balloting the patella against the femur (patellar tap).
- Large effusions will prevent bony contact, but are obvious.
- Small effusions are best detected by emptying the suprapatellar pouch with one hand and testing for lateral fluid shift with the other. The normal concavity on either side of the patella is obliterated by quite small amounts of fluid. Pressure on one side of the patella will push fluid to the opposite side and increase the parapatellar convexity there.

Meniscal injury: injury to the medial or lateral meniscus of the knee is suggested by the ability to walk immediately after the incident followed by a gradual onset of swelling with increasing pain. Tenderness is maximal at the joint line. The knee may lock or give way days later. Damage will have been inflicted by tibial rotation on the partially flexed joint and pain at the joint line can be reproduced by recreating these stresses. The medial meniscus is the more commonly injured of the two because it has more restricting peripheral attachments than the lateral meniscus and is therefore subjected to greater shearing forces.

Collateral ligament injury: spraining of a collateral ligament in the knee is common and usually results in a very similar picture to meniscal injury. There may be pain on valgus or varus stressing but no demonstrable laxity. More significant tears or complete rupture of a collateral ligament may, paradoxically, leave the patient with very little pain. There will, however, be obvious laxity on valgus or varus stressing. The consequent instability of the knee may necessitate surgical repair.

Cruciate ligament injury: this is a major injury with long-term consequences. The anterior and posterior cruciate ligaments are very strong; their rupture is usually caused by significant trauma and is associated with damage to other structures, particularly the collateral ligaments and the menisci. Swelling is immediate and pain and loss of function are evident. If pain permits, excessive movement will be found on attempting to move the upper tibia back and forth on the femur when the joint is at right angles (→ *Box 7.6*). Radiographs may show an avulsed tibial spine. Immediate referral to the orthopaedic team is essential.

XR Radiological examination is usually unrewarding, but must be carried out to exclude intra-articular fracture. There may be an avulsion injury at the site of attachment of collateral or cruciate ligaments. An MR scan (or arthroscopy) is the definitive investigation.

Tx
Knee problems that require immediate referral → Box 7.8.

Early arthroscopy is increasingly used to aid diagnosis and to give appropriate treatment. Minor meniscal and collateral ligament injuries can be treated on an outpatient basis. A support bandage should be applied and crutches and analgesia given as necessary. Follow-up must be arranged and physiotherapy may be very helpful.

Withdrawal of fluid from the knee may relieve the pain caused by a tense swelling, facilitate examination, and distinguish between blood and serous

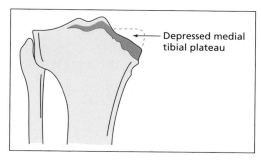

Figure 7.3 Fracture of the medial tibial plateau.

effusion. However, aspiration of an effusion should not be attempted in an unsuitable environment by an inexperienced doctor.

Fractures of the tibial condyles

Fractures of the upper tibia may occur after a forcible valgus or varus strain (e.g. knee hit by a car bumper). The patient is in pain, unable to walk and has an obvious haemarthrosis. However, the tibial plateau may be depressed to a lesser degree in elderly patients after relatively minor trauma, in which case the knee is not very swollen and the patient is able to walk. There is:

- localised pain and tenderness at the joint line
- a modest effusion
- a reasonable amount of movement of the knee
- pain on valgus/varus stressing (→ *Figure 7.3*).

XR Minor degrees of depression of the tibial plateau are often overlooked on a radiograph. The AP radiograph requires especially careful scrutiny. Osteoporotic bone is often present as a causative factor. The radiological appearance of osteoarthrosis may obscure the fracture.

Tx Patients with tibial condyle fractures generally require referral for surgical fixation. Some minor crush fractures of the tibial plateau may be treated on an outpatient basis in a plaster cast, but most patients will need to be admitted.

Fracture of the neck of the fibula

This injury may be associated with damage to the common peroneal nerve (causing drop-foot, paralysis of ankle everters and loss of sensation over the lateral aspect of the lower leg). It may be an isolated injury or accompany rotational injuries of the ankle (Maisonneuve's fracture).

XR Radiographs of this area are indicated when there is direct injury or tenderness accompanying an obvious ankle injury.

Tx The uncomplicated injury may be treated with an elastic bandage, analgesia, crutches and fracture clinic follow-up. Other variants require immediate referral.

Diffuse inflammation of the knee

Also → p. 405 in Chapter 21.

Septic arthritis may be florid, with acute joint pain, fever and systemic illness, or more insidious with only modest pain and some joint movement. Be alert to this possibility in elderly patients and those with rheumatoid disease. Also consider the diagnosis of gonorrhoea.

Crystal arthropathy may present with exquisite local pain and joint stiffness.

Deformity secondary to osteoarthrosis and bone destruction decreases locomotor efficiency. Muscle work is increased and the patient complains of fatigue as well as joint pain. The joint line is prominent and irregular as a result of osteophytes and there are usually a few degrees of fixed flexion. Collateral ligament instability follows tibial condyle collapse and instability predisposes to trauma. Osteoarthrosis extends recovery time after injury.

XR Radiographs may show calcified menisci or non-specific changes.

Tx Referral to an orthopaedic surgeon or rheumatologist should be decided by the most likely diagnosis. Diagnostic tap may be indicated.

Loose bodies in the knee joint

Intra-articular fragments may arise from an area of osteochondritis dissecans (→ *Figure 7.4*), degenerate menisci, osteophytes or the synovium. The patient complains of intermittent locking of the knee, typically in a different position each time. There may be a small effusion.

XR The loose fragments are usually easily seen on a radiograph.

Tx If the knee is locked, no attempt should be made to manipulate it but orthopaedic advice should be sought. In other cases, the patient is given a tubular support bandage and referred to the next orthopaedic clinic.

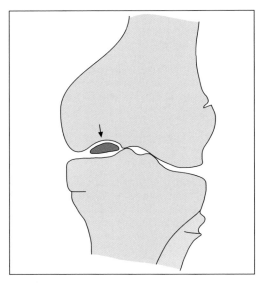

Figure 7.4 Osteochondritis dissecans (arrow).

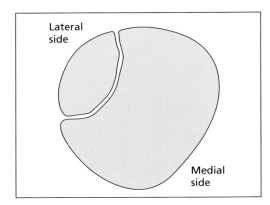

Figure 7.5 Bipartite patella.

Fracture of the patella/quadriceps injury

The patella may be fractured by a direct blow or fall or by sudden quadriceps contraction. Indirect traction force can break the quadriceps mechanism at different levels. The older the patient the higher the lesion:

- *Young*: patellar tendon
- *Middle-aged*: across the patella
- *Older*: rectus femoris muscle.

The action of the quadriceps muscle should be assessed by active knee extension; failure to straight-leg raise suggests a significant injury.

XR Occasionally, the patella is bipartite. The upper lateral part is separated from the rest of the patella by a curved line mimicking a fracture (→ *Figure 7.5*). This is a normal variant, but may not be present in both knees.

Tx Refer for specialist care. Comminuted fractures are excised. Minimally displaced fractures may be wired together. Undisplaced fractures are treated in a plaster cylinder. Transverse fractures of the patella, which extend laterally to involve the quadriceps expansion, require surgical repair, as do serious injuries of quadriceps.

Dislocation of the patella

The patella may dislocate laterally during active quadriceps action. Teenage girls are most often affected. All knee movements are painful and the deformity is obvious. If spontaneous reduction has occurred, the diagnosis can be confirmed by a positive patellar apprehension test: pushing the patella laterally (usually in either knee) causes pain and a feeling of imminent dislocation.

XR Radiographs should be taken to exclude bony injury.

Tx Reduction under sedation may be undertaken in the ED. This entails a gentle straightening of the leg by the application of distal traction. A plaster cylinder or other suitable straight-leg splint is then applied and the patient referred to the next fracture clinic, non-weight-bearing on crutches. Patients with a clear history of dislocation of the patella in whom spontaneous relocation has occurred should be treated in the same way.

Patellofemoral osteochondritis

Pain behind the patella is a common cause of knee pain in young women. Trivial direct trauma may be implicated. Symptoms are exacerbated by exercise, especially going down steps. Pain is reproduced by pressing on the patella. There may be a small effusion but the knee joint is otherwise normal.

XR Radiographs are usually normal.

Tx A support bandage and physiotherapy (to prevent wasting of the quadriceps muscles) are indicated. The condition is self-limiting and rarely requires surgical intervention. Initial referral to the patient's GP is usually appropriate.

Peripatellar bursitis

Both the prepatellar and infrapatellar bursae may become inflamed and then secondarily infected after repeated minor trauma. Colloquial names for these conditions, namely housemaid's and clergyman's knee, respectively, were derived from the most commonly affected professions and their differing kneeling positions. Nowadays – because of changing priorities in society – carpet fitters, electricians and plumbers are the people most prone to these conditions. The affected area is red, swollen and tender. Pain may limit full movements but there is no communication between the bursa and the knee joint.

Acute traumatic bursitis may follow a direct blow or fall. In this case, the prepatellar area is very tender and swollen. There often appears to be a fluid-filled area that could be aspirated but attempts to do this are usually unsuccessful.

XR After severe direct trauma, the knee should be have a radiograph taken to exclude an underlying fracture of the patella.

TX When there is no clinical evidence of infection (as indicated by body temperature), the patient can be treated with an elastic bandage, non-steroidal anti-inflammatory drugs (NSAIDs) and follow-up. The condition usually resolves spontaneously but occasionally the bursa has to be removed. Any suspicion of knee joint involvement demands immediate orthopaedic referral. If there is an acute localised infection of the bursa alone, incision and drainage under a general anaesthetic should be carried out by the orthopaedic team.

Rupture of a Baker's cyst

Bursae in the popliteal fossa may be connected to the knee joint. An enlarged and isolated popliteal bursa (Baker's cyst) is associated with rheumatoid involvement of the knee. If it ruptures, there is sudden pain in the upper calf as the synovial fluid is squeezed between the calf muscles. The condition is often misdiagnosed as either a tear of the calf muscles or a DVT (→ *pp. 101 and 108*).

Figure 7.6 Osgood–Schlatter disease (arrowed).

XR Arthrography is diagnostic.

TX Advice should be sought from the orthopaedic or rheumatology departments.

Osgood–Schlatter disease

Adolescents may experience pain around the insertion of the patellar tendon after exercise. This is caused by inflammation around the epiphysis. Knee movements are normal but resisted extension is painful.

XR Radiographs are diagnostic, showing break-up of the tibial epiphysis (→ *Figure 7.6*).

TX A tubular support bandage will provide symptomatic relief until an early orthopaedic outpatient consultation. Sport should be prohibited. Local injection of steroid may help but should be prescribed by and injected by a specialist. The condition always resolves when the epiphysis fuses just after puberty. **Sindig–Laarson disease:** This is of similar aetiology and involves the lower pole of the patella. Treatment is as for Osgood–Schlatter disease.

Exclude a popliteal aneurysm before considering other extra-articular swellings.

Tumours and sepsis may occasionally present with knee pain, especially in children.

THE LOWER LEG

Two anatomical features provide potential complications for injuries to the lower leg:

1 The skin, thinly stretched over the tibia anteriorly, has a poor blood supply.
2 The muscles are enclosed in a rigid fascial envelope.

Consequently:

- Many fractures of the tibia and fibula are compound.
- Wounds of the skin in this area are slow to heal.
- Muscle contusion or vascular damage in the calf may raise interstitial pressure sufficiently to occlude the circulation.

Fracture of the shaft of the tibia

Tibial shaft fractures follow a considerable amount of direct or indirect force. They are generally extremely painful injuries and render walking impossible. The fibula is usually also fractured, although a direct blow may break the tibia only. In the latter case there will be minimal deformity and occasionally the patient is able to weight-bear with difficulty. Vascular damage should be suspected in all lower limb injuries, especially if there is either a crush or high-speed mechanism of injury. If present, early recognition and referral are essential.

XR The diagnosis is usually evident clinically. Radiographs follow splintage and will show the fracture in adults but can be difficult to interpret in young children (→ below).

TX
Initial splintage → Box 7.9.

Most patients with a fractured tibia need admission, observation and internal fixation. Compound fractures must be debrided in theatre as soon as possible.
　　Some closed fractures can be managed on an outpatient basis but the decision should be left to the orthopaedic department. The application of a well-padded, above-knee plaster cast should not be delegated to inexperienced staff. 'Check radiographs' in plaster are essential, even if the fracture initially appeared stable and undisplaced. Displacement can occur during application of plaster. Crutches and analgesia will be required as will early orthopaedic follow-up.

> **Box 7.9 Splinting the lower leg**
>
> - Apply splintage under appropriate analgesia after removal of clothing and footwear but before radiography
> - Confirm the presence of foot pulses and toe movements
> - If there is gross ankle deformity, give morphine and nitrous oxide and quickly reduce the dislocation. This prevents pressure necrosis of overlying skin
> - If there is a compound fracture, remove gross contaminants and take an instant photograph before applying sterile iodine-soaked pads. Do not allow repeated examination – show the photograph instead. Start antibiotics
> - Apply an L-shaped splint or box splint
> - Check the pulses again and review the analgesia
> - Arrange for radiographs

Tibial fractures in children

Children with these injuries present with a limp or failure to weight-bear. A history of trauma is by no means inevitable. There may be no swelling or deformity and tenderness, although present, may be difficult to localise. Knee and ankle flexion are usually unaffected, although ankle rotation may be painful. The diagnosis is thus elusive and if there is any doubt follow the procedure for the limping child as described in *Box 7.3*.

XR Radiographs may not show an obvious fracture. Look at both films for a faint, long, oblique, black line. In the so-called toddlers' fracture, radiographs are initially normal and the characteristic periosteal elevation is not seen for several days.

TX Obvious fractures should be immobilised in an above-knee cast. The child will need analgesia and fracture clinic follow-up. Toddlers' fractures can be treated with rest and either an elastic support bandage or a below-knee plaster of Paris cast depending on the degree of pain and discomfort. In cases of doubt, arrange for a second opinion as soon as possible.

Fracture of the shaft of the fibula

The shaft of the fibula may be broken by direct trauma. Although there is localised pain and tenderness, there is little swelling and the patient can weight-bear. Consequently, the injury is often missed.

Xʀ The radiograph is diagnostic.

Tx The shaft of the fibula functions as a muscle anchor rather than a weight bearer so a plaster cast is unnecessary. The patient requires an elastic bandage, analgesia, crutches and a fracture clinic follow-up.

Pretibial pain

Shin pain may develop acutely in athletes. The patient complains of intermittent discomfort over the front of the lower leg. There may be local tenderness, but the diagnosis is made chiefly from the history of gradually increasing pain associated with exercise. 'Shin splints', as the condition is known, is probably caused by oedema within the anterior compartment.

Other possible diagnoses are chronic or acute osteomyelitis, bone tumour or hyperplasia of the anterior tibial cortex. This last condition occurs in footballers subjected to repeated shin injury and subperiosteal haematoma.

Xʀ Radiographs may show cortical thickening in some cases, but only a bone scan is diagnostic; this will also identify a stress fracture.

Tx Management of these patients depends on symptoms and diagnosis. A referral to a physiotherapist or a sports injury clinic may be appropriate. Stress fractures should be immobilised in a cast. All patients should have follow-up arranged.

Calf muscle strain or tear

Disruption within the calf muscles or at the junction with the tendon may be caused by overuse or sudden stretching. There is acute localised pain, usually towards the medial side of the gastrocnemius muscle. Weight-bearing is painful as is passive ankle dorsiflexion. It is important to exclude rupture of the Achilles tendon, which gives a similar clinical picture. DVT and ruptured Baker's cyst must also be considered (→ *pp. 99 and 108*).

Tx Patients require an elastic bandage, analgesia and crutches. Follow-up should be arranged, as should early physiotherapy.

Achilles tendonitis (tendonosis)

The Achilles tendon is the largest tendon in the human body but is prone to injury, inflammation and degeneration. Problems are usually due to a combination of repetitive stress injury and age-related degeneration, the exact proportions of each depending on the individual patient. Sudden increases in exercise, tight calf muscles and congenital or acquired calcaneal spurs are also implicated in the pathogenesis of the condition. Two main types are described:

1 *Non-insertional Achilles tendonitis*: fibres in the middle portion of the tendon develop tiny tears and then become swollen and thickened. This is more common in younger, active people including distance runners.
2 *Insertional Achilles tendonitis*: calcified fibres in the lower part of the Achilles tendon (at the junction with the calcaneum) become oedematous and inflamed. A bony spur may form on the heel and rub against the tendon. This type of tendonitis usually occurs in older, less active people.

Features of Achilles tendonitis include:

- Pain behind or above the back of the heel that gets worse during or after activity (sometimes on the following day)
- Pain in the region of the tendon that is worse in the morning
- Pain with ankle flexion (relatively unusual)
- Tenderness and thickening of part of the tendon.

Xʀ Plain radiographs may show calcification of part of the tendon or a calcaneal spur. An MR scan can demonstrate the exact amount of degeneration and inflammation of the tendon.

Tx Initial treatment includes NSAIDs and rest, including abstinence from high-impact exercises and strenuous work. Crutches or even a below-knee cast may be required. Early physiotherapy and graduated stretching exercises are helpful and heel pads often give considerable relief. Steroid injections may precipitate rupture of the tendon. Cases that fail to resolve after a few months may be referred for possible surgery. There are several recommended procedures but there is a high incidence of postoperative pain and infection after all of them.

Rupture of the Achilles tendon

Surprisingly, acute rupture may at first be dismissed by the patient as a trivial injury. The usual history is of sudden calf pain thought to have been caused by an object hitting the back of the leg. The acute pain subsides and the patient is able to walk flat-footed with difficulty but cannot run. On examination there is a palpable gap in the tendon, although this may be filled with inflammatory exudate. Plantar flexion is possible using the toe flexors, but is weak. Squeezing the calf fails to cause plantar flexion of the foot and is painful. This test is most accurately performed with the feet of the prone patient extending over the end of the couch and is always compared with the normal side.

Tx Refer the patient to the orthopaedic department immediately. Most patients will undergo early primary tendon repair, although immobilisation in equinus in a cast is another option. Recovery is often delayed because of pre-existing degenerative changes.

Rupture of the musculotendinous junction of the Achilles tendon: injuries that are in this area also require an immediate orthopaedic opinion.

Partial rupture of the Achilles tendon: sometimes patients present with the hallmarks of acute rupture and a normal, but painful, calf-squeeze test. This may be caused by partial rupture of a degenerate tendon. Ultrasonography or MRI may be required to confirm the diagnosis. Management is similar to that described for a complete rupture of the Achilles tendon.

THE ANKLE

Inversion sprains

Sprained ankles are the most common injuries seen in an ED, resulting in the attendance of around 2.5% of the UK population every year! They result from stretching and tearing of the lateral ligament and tendon complex of the ankle, and so are seen in a number of different varieties, depending on the particular structures torn and the severity of the damage (→ *Figure 7.7*):

- Grade 1 sprain = stretching of the ligament complex
- Grade 2 sprain = partial tearing of the ligament complex
- Grade 3 sprain = complete rupture of the ligament complex.

Some sprains will resolve quickly without treatment, many will heal more slowly and need routine outpatient care, and a few require specialised management from the outset. It is important, but not always easy, to assign the patient to the appropriate treatment category as soon as possible.

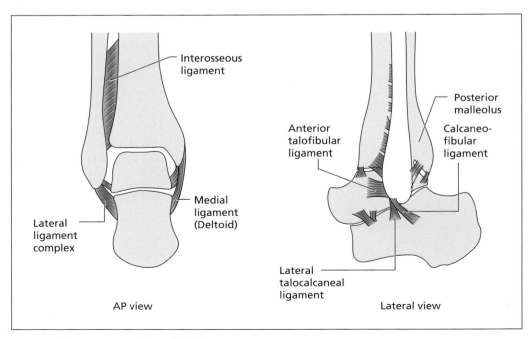

Figure 7.7 Ligaments around the ankle joint.

Ask the patient about:

- history and mechanism of injury
- extent and speed of appearance of pain and swelling
- mobility
- occupational and recreational demands.

The usual history is of ankle inversion while running, playing sports or slipping down a step. A crack may have been heard but this does not inevitably indicate bone injury. The initial pain settles and then gets worse again over the next few hours, causing difficulty in weight-bearing. This sequence is typical – but not diagnostic – of a soft-tissue injury.

Swelling and pain are often focused just anterior to the lateral malleolus – caused by injury to the anterior talofibular ligament – or over the side of the foot. Exclude ankle mortise instability by gripping the heel with one hand and the lower leg with the other. There should be no pain or movement when a sideways force is applied to the heel. In contrast, the patient will have acute pain on attempted inversion of the foot.

After examining the lateral side of the ankle, there are six other places to feel for related injuries:

1 The medial malleolus and medial ligament complex
2 The base of the little (fifth) metatarsal bone
3 The calcaneum
4 The Achilles tendon
5 The neck of the fibula
6 The midtarsal region.

The ankle must be palpated all around for bony tenderness, not just the swollen lateral side. Pain over the styloid process of the fifth metatarsal base may be caused by ligament or bone avulsion – a variation of ankle inversion injury. Fracture of the calcaneum and rupture of the Achilles tendon are injuries that are often wrongly diagnosed as ankle sprains on first presentation. The neck of the fibula should be examined because of its involvement in rotational injuries of the ankle (→ p. 104). Fracture dislocation at the tarsometatarsal junction (Lisfranc's fracture) causes significant pain over the dorsum of the foot, especially medially.

Xʀ If indicated, plain radiographs of the ankle are taken to exclude significant fractures of the malleoli. They should be supplemented with other films (e.g. knee, heel and foot) if there are atypical findings on clinical examination.

Indications for ankle radiographs → Box 7.10.

Ankle sprains may be associated with an avulsed flake from the lateral malleolus or the dorsum of the talus. New flake fractures have a sharp, irregular outline

Box 7.10 Indications for radiology of the ankle after injury

Any of the following:

- History suggesting severe injury
- Severe pain
- Age >55 years
- Inability to walk four steps unaided
- Obvious deformity
- Severe swelling of rapid onset
- Bony tenderness of the lateral malleolus especially posteriorly – anterior bone pain is common without a fracture
- Atypical features
- Return visit with no improvement

The corollary of these indications is that a radiograph is not needed in:

- a younger patient
- with a history of a simple inversion injury
- who can partially weight-bear, and
- who has tenderness and swelling over the lateral ligament area (dorsolateral foot) only

without a complete marginal cortex. Do not forget to look at the calcaneum. Lisfranc's fracture may be difficult to diagnose on standard radiographs.

Some patients continue to have severe symptoms and signs despite normal initial radiographs. These patients should be reviewed by a senior doctor after 7–10 days; further radiographs may be required. Stress views or an MR scan may be indicated to help choose optimum treatment.

Tx If the patient has a classic mild inversion sprain and is able to weight-bear, then treat with:

- a compression bandage, ice packs and analgesia
- initial rest and elevation, leading to graduated exercise
- GP follow-up.

However, if the patient is unable to weight-bear or has an obviously more severe injury, add:

- crutches (partial weight-bearing)
- early physiotherapy
- review after about 2 weeks to ensure satisfactory progress (physiotherapist or clinic).

In these patients, consideration should be given to offering immobilisation of the injured ankle in a below-knee walking cast for between 10 and 14 days.

This has been shown to be associated with less pain and discomfort during the 4 weeks after the injury, and better ankle function, activity and quality of life after 3 months. The cast should be applied after the initial swelling has subsided; this will necessitate a clinic appointment after 3–7 days. A purpose-made ankle brace is less effective than a cast but better than an elastic support bandage in effecting a speedy recovery and a cost-effective return to work. After 9 months, patients receiving any of these three methods of ankle support have similar symptoms and the same level of functioning.

Flake fractures represent variants of ligament injuries and should be treated in the same way. However, their detection is useful because they often indicate that a more severe injury has occurred. The patient should be told of their presence to prevent a later misunderstanding.

Most patients with mild ankle sprains can expect a marked improvement after 10–14 days and to be weight-bearing almost normally within 2–3 weeks.

Eversion sprains

These injuries produce pain and swelling below the medial malleolus. They are uncommon but may produce an unstable ankle joint.

XR Radiographs should be taken unless the patient can bear full weight without pain and has very little local swelling.

Tx Evidence of fracture or incongruity of the ankle joint is an indication for orthopaedic referral. Less severe injuries usually resolve with a support bandage and a short course of physiotherapy or a below-knee walking cast (→ *above*). Analgesia and crutches may be necessary.

Ankle fractures

A fracture of the ankle may follow a mechanism of injury similar to a sprain. There is usually significant pain and swelling, although some patients may be able to weight-bear. Examination must again include the knee, calf, ankle, heel and foot.

Two or more separate lesions, whether of bone or ligament, will produce a potentially unstable joint and require specialist attention. Isolated fracture of the lateral malleolus, for example, may render the ankle mortise unstable if there is concurrent rupture of the deltoid ligament (between the medial malleolus and the calcaneum). Fracture of the medial malleolus may be associated with a spiral fracture of the neck of the fibula (Maisonneuve's fracture).

XR Radiographs of the ankle are usually diagnostic but should be supplemented with views of the knee, leg, heel and foot, as clinically indicated. Vertical fractures of the posterior part of the tibia (seen on the lateral view and extending down to the ankle joint) are conveniently (but inaccurately) termed fractures of the posterior malleolus. Thus a fracture may be described as bimalleolar or even trimalleolar.

Tx Stable, undisplaced fractures of the lateral malleolus may be treated on an outpatient basis in a below-knee plaster cast. The patient should be seen at the next fracture clinic.

Unstable or displaced lateral malleolar fractures and all fractures involving the medial malleolus or distal fibula should be referred for an immediate orthopaedic opinion.

Posterior displacement of the lower tibial epiphysis

This may occur in children. Reduction under general anaesthesia is straightforward but overnight admission is usually required.

Dislocation of the ankle

The talus, and with it the foot, may be completely dislocated after severe local trauma. Usually, the skin remains intact but is stretched tightly over the bone. An accompanying fracture is common.

XR Radiographs should be delayed until after reduction.

Tx Immediate reduction is essential to reduce pain and minimise the risk of tissue necrosis.

- Give IV analgesia and supplement it with nitrous oxide or midazolam during the procedure
- Reduce the ankle with axial traction
- Check the skin circulation and foot pulses
- Apply a splint or cast
- Obtain radiographs
- Refer the patient to the orthopaedic team.

THE FOOT

Relative positions of the bones of the foot → Figure 7.8.

Fracture of the talus

Talar fractures present in a similar way to ankle injuries. They often produce long-term disability because

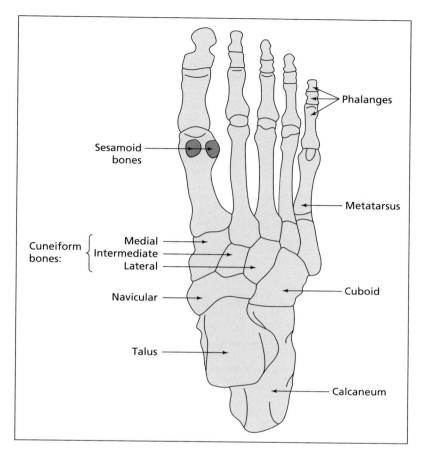

Sesamoid
bones

Phalanges

Metatarsus

Cuneiform
bones: {
Medial
Intermediate
Lateral

Navicular

Cuboid

Talus

Calcaneum

Figure 7.8 The bones of
the foot.

of disruption of the subtalar joint; sometimes avascular necrosis occurs.

Xʀ These fractures can be missed on radiographs unless the area is carefully inspected.

Tₓ The patient should have analgesia and orthopaedic referral.

Fracture of the calcaneum

Calcaneal fracture is usually caused by a direct fall on to the heel from a height such as a roof or a ladder. There is:

- pain and difficulty in weight-bearing
- local tenderness and sometimes bruising
- a possibility of associated, and perhaps masked, injuries elsewhere (e.g. lumbar spine).

A fracture of this region may also occur in osteoporotic bone, following relatively minor trauma. In this case, it may superficially mimic a soft-tissue injury of the ankle.

> The calcaneum is like an egg – it can be cracked, dented or completely smashed!

Xʀ Radiographs should be obtained of the ankle, heel and foot. The radiograph shows a normal ankle mortise. Single or multiple fracture lines through the cancellous os calcis are often missed. The flattening of Böhler's angle is an important radiographic sign (→ *Figure 7.9*). A CT scan may be required to assess the degree of injury and the consequent need for internal fixation.

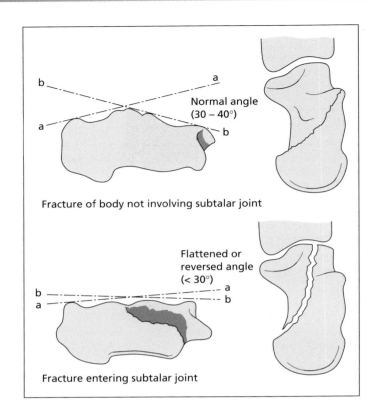

Normal angle
(30 – 40°)

Fracture of body not involving subtalar joint

Flattened or
reversed angle
(< 30°)

Fracture entering subtalar joint

Figure 7.9 Loss of Böhler's angle.

Tx Exclude associated injuries. Patients with this fracture require strong analgesia and orthopaedic referral. Weight-bearing is impossible; a thick wool and crepe bandage with crutches allows temporary mobility.

Tarsal fracture and tarsometatarsal dislocation

Fractures of the tarsus may be produced by crushing and twisting forces. Pain and swelling are usually prominent. The term 'Lisfranc's fracture' covers a variety of ligament and bone injuries at the junction of the mid- and forefoot. Trapping the foot in a stirrup when thrown from a horse is a typical cause. Although rare, it is difficult to diagnose and inadequate management leads to significant disability. There is usually a dislocation at the tarsometatarsal junction with associated fractures, commonly at the second metatarsal base but also at the metatarsal neck.

XR Tarsometatarsal dislocation with fracture of the second metatarsal base (Lisfranc's fracture) is important to recognise but may be overlooked on standard radiological views. A true lateral view of the area will reveal dorsal displacement.

Tx Open reduction may be necessary. Specialist advice should always be sought.

Pain in the foot

Plantar fasciitis

The patient complains of pain on the sole of the foot, often worst in the morning and after exercise. Pain is exacerbated by the heel striking the ground. There is tenderness localised to the anteromedial part of the os calcis about 5 cm below and 1 cm in front of the medial malleolus. The condition is caused by degenerative changes in or overuse of the plantar fascia, as with jogging and military training. This results in partial avulsion of the fascia from the os calcis. Chronic symptoms may be associated with a calcaneal spur. Radiographs are taken to exclude a fracture and identify a spur. Most cases of plantar fasciitis can be effectively treated by prescribing an excavated heel cushion or a pad composed of an energy-absorbing hydrogel. NSAIDs and physiotherapy may

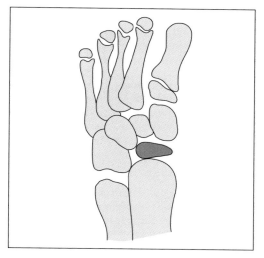

Figure 7.10 Avascular necrosis of the navicular bone.

Fractures of the forefoot

Metatarsal fractures are common but are only of importance when there is gross disruption or the bones of the first ray are involved. Most forces through the forefoot are transmitted along the first metatarsus. A stress fracture (March fracture) is most commonly seen in the index (second) metatarsal neck.

XR Stress fractures may not be visible on a radiograph until callus formation has occurred. A bone scan may be diagnostic.

Tx Multiple fractures of the metatarsal bones may require internal fixation. Patients with significant fractures of the first metatarsus should also be referred for an orthopaedic opinion. For most other metatarsal fractures, a below-knee plaster cast can be applied on an outpatient basis. The patient will require analgesia, crutches and follow-up in the fracture clinic.

Fractures of the toes

Fractures of the toes are common and usually result from a kicking or stubbing injury.

XR A radiograph is usually not necessary except where there is clinical deformity or the proximal phalanx of the big toe is involved.

Tx Fractures of the proximal phalanx of the big toe may need a below-knee walking plaster and fracture clinic follow-up.

Angulated toes should be straightened under ring block and then neighbour strapped. Check radiographs should be obtained and follow-up arranged.

Other toe injuries are treated symptomatically irrespective of the presence of a minor undisplaced fracture. Neighbour strapping is helpful. Pain around the metatarsophalangeal joints may be helped by the application of a metatarsal pad. Bulky dressings prevent the use of normal footwear and should be avoided. Follow-up is not necessary if the patient is advised on care of the strapping and told that symptoms will abate over the ensuing month.

be helpful. Local infiltration with a steroid is often effective but should be left to the discretion of the orthopaedic department. The presence of a calcaneal spur is not an indication for surgery, although its removal is occasionally necessary.

Köhler's disease

Osteochondritis of the navicular bone occurs mostly in teenage boys. They present with chronic pain on exercise. There may be a history of minor trauma. Midtarsal and subtalar joint movements are restricted. Radiographs show a collapsed sclerotic bone ($\rightarrow$ *Figure 7.10*). The patient should be given a support bandage and referred to the next orthopaedic clinic.

Prominent navicular bone

Teenagers (most often girls) may complain of pain over the inner aspect of the foot and relate the symptoms to exercise or injury. Anxious parents point to the prominent medial end of the navicular bone as the cause of the pain. If examination of the foot is otherwise normal they should be reassured. Periosteal inflammation may indeed make the bone appear prominent but most cases settle spontaneously. Attention should be directed to appropriate footwear.

Metatarsalgia

Pain under the metatarsal heads is often chronic and degenerative in origin. It may be relieved by providing a metatarsal gel pad. This should extend almost up to, but not under, the prominent bone.

VASCULAR CONDITIONS OF THE LOWER LIMB
Arterial embolism

Thrombi, which embolise to peripheral arteries, may arise from several sites:

1 The left atrial appendage (usually in the presence of atrial fibrillation)

2 The left ventricle (invariably on an area damaged by a recent myocardial infarction)
3 An atheromatous plaque
4 An aortic aneurysm
5 A thrombosis in a deep vein in a patient with a patent foramen ovale (paradoxical embolism).

All of these possibilities should be considered, although the first two are by far the most common.

Emboli tend to lodge at the sites of bifurcation of arteries. Their effects depend on the extent of the occlusion of the circulation and the degree of collateral circulation that exists. The following are common sites that involve the lower limb:

- The aortic bifurcation (bilateral ischaemia to the level of the knees)
- The origin of the deep femoral artery (ischaemia to the midcalf)
- The bifurcation of the popliteal artery (ischaemia of the foot).

Sudden occlusion of the femoral artery causes the six 'Ps':

1 Pain
2 Pallor
3 Pulselessness
4 Paraesthesia
5 Paralysis
6 Perishing cold.

Tx Embolism must be treated within 6 h of the onset of symptoms or else propagation of thrombus distal to the embolus will greatly worsen prognosis. Treatment includes:

- oral aspirin (300 mg)
- IV analgesia
- IV fluids
- referral to a vascular surgeon. Embolectomy or thrombolysis may be required.

Intra-arterial injection

Irritant substances may cause critical ischaemia if injected into an artery. IV drug abusers are the most common sufferers from this problem and temazepam gel is the drug most usually involved. The ischaemia results from a mixture of vasospasm and multiple small emboli. Severe pain is the prominent symptom but the other signs described above (the six 'Ps') may be absent.

Tx This is similar to the treatment described above for arterial embolism. Drugs that cause arterial dilatation may be considered.

Venous thrombosis

Thrombosis of the deep veins of the lower limb or pelvis (DVT) may be caused by changes in any of the following:

1 Blood coagulation (smoking, hormonal contraception, malignancy, recent surgery or major illness)
2 Blood vessels (pregnancy)
3 Blood flow (immobility, long-haul air or road travel, plaster casts).

> Thrombosis of veins distal to the popliteal vein ('below-knee DVT') is particularly common because of the venous sinuses present in the soleus muscle of the calf. At least 5% of below-knee DVTs spread to the proximal veins and half of all above-knee venous thromboses embolise to the lungs.

The classic clinical features of DVT are:

- swelling and oedema distal to the occlusion
- warmth, redness and deep tenderness of the thigh or calf.

These signs depend on venous occlusion. In contrast, there may be no signs in the presence of an extensive, non-occlusive but potentially lethal thrombus. Moreover, there is some evidence that non-occlusive thrombi float in the middle of the vein and thus break free very easily.

> Homan's sign cannot be relied on – it is positive in less than 20% of patients with DVT of the leg.

The following conditions may be mistaken for DVT:

- Chronic venous obstruction (→ *p. 110*)
- Superficial phlebitis (→ *p. 110*)
- Post-thrombotic syndrome
- Acute or subacute arterial ischaemia (→ *above*)
- Cellulitis of the leg (→ *p. 406*)
- Calf muscle tear (→ *p. 101*) or other soft-tissue injury
- Ruptured Baker's cyst (→ *p. 99*)
- Fracture of the lower limb
- Lymphoedema
- Hypoproteinaemia.

Table 7.2 Relative risks of deep vein thrombosis (DVT) and pulmonary embolism (PE) for women taking combined oestrogen and progestogen contraceptive pills

	Incidence of DVT or PE	Relative risk
No combined pill	5 per 100 000 women	1
Second-generation combined pill	15 per 100 000 women	3
First-generation combined pill	25 per 100 000 women	5
Pregnancy	60 per 100 000 women	12

In the UK, about a quarter of all women aged between 16 and 49 years (and almost half of all women in their 20s) use regular hormonal contraception. *For the relative risks of DVT and pulmonary embolism (PE) with combined oestrogen and progestogen contraceptive pills → Table 7.2.*

Table 7.3 Well's scoring system for clinical deep vein thrombosis (DVT)

Clinical feature	Score
Cancer treatment ongoing or within last 6 months	+1
Immobilisation of lower limb	+1
Bedridden for more than 3 days	+1
Major surgery in last 4 weeks	+1
Entire leg swollen	+1
Calf swelling >3 cm in diameter	+1
Increased pitting oedema in symptomatic leg	+1
Superficial collateral veins visible	+1
Alternative diagnosis as likely or more likely	−2
Total score ≤0	Low probability of DVT
Total score = 1–2	Moderate probability of DVT
Total score ≥3	High probability of DVT

Investigations: The Well's scoring system for clinical DVT may be used to stratify patients into low, moderate or high-risk groups (→ *Table 7.3*). Those patients with a low risk may be further subdivided by requesting a D-dimer blood test. (This protein is a cross-linked fibrin degradation product that is released into the bloodstream from active blood clots and sites of wound healing.) A negative D-dimer has >95% negative predictive value for DVT whereas a positive result has <70% positive predictive value. D-dimer is therefore a good test to rule out DVT in low-risk patients but is not a useful method of diagnosis.

First-line imaging depends on local availability. Doppler ultrasound studies have replaced the traditional venogram in most centres. If neither investigation is immediately available the patient must be treated on clinical grounds alone. Pelvic imaging may be required at a later date to look for causative factors.

Tx Once the diagnosis has been confirmed or provisionally suspected, most patients will be treated by rapid anticoagulation (usually as an outpatient). This may be achieved with either an IV infusion of standard unfractionated heparin (in hospital) or preferably, with a low-molecular-weight heparin (LMWH) given subcutaneously, e.g. enoxaparin 1.5 mg/kg once a day. This should be altered to 1 mg/kg twice a day in pregnant patients (based on weight in early pregnancy) and 1 mg/kg once a day in patients with severe renal impairment. Fondaparinux (a synthetic pentasaccharide that inhibits activated factor X) is an alternative to heparins. Parenteral anticoagulation will be required for at least 5 days and consequently effective community liaison is essential for outpatients. Follow-up in a clinic should be arranged to occur within 48 h. Oral anticoagulants are substituted for the heparin as soon as possible and are usually continued for about 3 months. In some cases of rapidly progressing or life-threatening DVT, thrombolysis (with streptokinase) may be considered.

Diagnosis and management of suspected PE → *pp. 190 and 214.*
Risk factors for venous thromboembolism → Box 13.13 on p. 215.

Phlebitis

Inflammation of the long or short saphenous vein usually occurs in patients with varicose veins or those who have had IV therapy. The vein is red, hot and tender.

Tx Phlebitis usually settles with topical therapy and oral NSAIDs. If there is a systemic pyrexia, an antibiotic (e.g. co-amoxiclav) can be added.

Venous disease in IV drug abusers

Repeated injection into the femoral vein causes chronic venous obstruction. There is swelling and oedema of the whole lower limb and dilatation of the superficial vessels; injection sinuses are often found in the groin. Thrombosis may occur, in which case the limb becomes hot, red and painful. This type of widespread DVT is potentially life threatening.

Acute compartment syndrome

A compartment is defined as a closed tissue space where muscle, neural or other soft tissue is surrounded by a layer of inelastic fascia (or bone). There are 46 such compartments in the human body, 38 of which are found in the upper and lower extremities.

Closed compartment syndrome of the limbs is caused by swollen, contused muscle or bleeding inside a rigid fascial envelope. As the intracompartmental pressure rises, there is venous obstruction and further swelling. When capillary perfusion pressure is exceeded, ischaemia and tissue necrosis begin to occur. Eventually, there is irreversible injury to both nerves and muscles (e.g. Volkmann's ischaemic contracture). The most common cause is trauma, usually with a fracture, and male patients aged <35 years are the most frequently affected. Anticoagulant drugs increase the likelihood of developing compartment syndrome.

Compartment syndrome can easily develop unseen under a plaster cast or below an eschar from a burn. The most common site to be affected is the lower leg (which has four anatomical compartments) but the syndrome is also seen in the forearm (three fascial compartments), the foot and the hand. The anterior compartment is the most commonly affected area of the leg whereas, in the forearm, it is the flexor compartment. Compartment syndrome is reported to occur in between 2% and 5% of patients with tibial fractures, often after comparatively low-energy mechanisms of injury.

The onset of compartment syndrome may be delayed after injury and insidious. Early symptoms are severe pain – aggravated by muscle stretching – and paraesthesia. The affected part may also, but not inevitably, be pale and cool with a slow capillary refill. Ischaemia results from compression of small blood vessels and so the presence of distal pulses is of no help in excluding the diagnosis. Venous outflow from the compartment is usually obstructed long before the entry of arterial blood is impeded.

In compartment syndrome, the limb may not be broken, distal pulses may be present and pulse oximetry may be normal. Worsening pain is an important sign.

XR Arteriography will reveal arterial lesions but will not demonstrate compartment syndrome.

Tx Suspicion of compartment syndrome is an indication for an immediate orthopaedic referral. Manometry is useful, particularly in patients with a depressed level of consciousness. Compartment pressures of over 40 mmHg or within 30 mmHg of diastolic blood pressure are highly suggestive of compartment syndrome. (The normal intracompartmental pressure is 10–12 mmHg.) There are four compartments in the lower leg and all may require extensive decompressive fasciotomy. This will produce significant fluid loss and blood transfusion may be necessary.

Elevation of the affected limb may increase ischaemia.

The upper limb

General principles of the management of limb injuries → p. 86.

Think about analgesia, support and splintage (→ *Box 8.1*) before starting your assessment.

THE SHOULDER AND UPPER ARM

> If the patient can put his or her hand behind the head and into the small of the back without pain, then the shoulder on that side is unlikely to be significantly injured.

Fracture of the clavicle

The clavicle provides the only skeletal continuity between the upper limb and trunk. It is occasionally broken by direct trauma but usually breaks in the middle two-thirds as a result of transmitted violence from a fall on to the upper limb. Damage to adjacent neurovascular structures is very rare except with posterior sternoclavicular dislocation. In adults, fractures cause well-localised symptoms with obvious deformity and tenderness.
Children: greenstick fractures are common after childhood falls. There may be little deformity and remarkably good movement of the arm and shoulder girdle. Alternatively, the child may refuse to use the whole arm on the affected side and thus mimic a pulled elbow *(→ p. 117)*.

XR An anteroposterior (AP) radiograph confirms the diagnosis.

Tx The weight of the arm should be supported in a broad arm sling. Figure-of-eight bandages, applied to achieve reduction, are usually more painful and do not succeed in their objective. Most displaced fractures settle to produce an acceptable cosmetic result. Prescribe appropriate analgesia and refer the patient to the next fracture clinic. Very painful, comminuted fractures may rarely require initial inpatient care, as do the occasionally occurring compound fractures.

Sternoclavicular joint disruption

This is rare and is the result of considerable indirect violence applied to the shoulder. Usually anterior dislocation with prominent bone is seen; posterior displacement is even rarer and may involve damage to major blood vessels, the trachea or the oesophagus.

XR Radiological confirmation is difficult. A CT scan may be helpful.

Tx This can be a major injury with potentially serious consequences. Orthopaedic advice should be sought.

Acromioclavicular joint disruption

This is much more common than the sternoclavicular joint disruption. The outer end of the clavicle is elevated at its articulation with the acromion. The weak fibres of the acromioclavicular joint are readily ruptured. The joint's normal stability is maintained by the conoid and trapezoid ligaments, binding the outer fifth of the clavicle down to the coracoid process of the scapula. It is the complete or partial rupture of these strong ligaments that results in an acromioclavicular dislocation or subluxation. Direct downward pressure will reduce the deformity rather

Emergency Medicine Lecture Notes, Fourth Edition. Chris Moulton and David Yates.
© 2012 Blackwell Publishing Ltd. Published 2012 by Blackwell Publishing Ltd.

painfully and only transiently. Shoulder movements are restricted because of pain.

XR Radiographic confirmation, if required, is obtained by taking a wide-angled erect AP film to show both acromioclavicular joints with the patient holding weights in both hands. Slight subluxation may occur normally.

Tx The raised outer end of the clavicle is accepted as a minor disability by most patients. Reduction is very difficult to maintain by closed methods and internal fixation, although successful, may leave an ugly prominent scar. A sling and analgesia are provided until the pain has settled. The shoulder will remain weak for some months. Manual workers may notice a very slight but permanent loss of power in the affected limb.

Supraspinatus tendinitis/ subacromial bursitis

These two conditions are very difficult to separate. Both are caused by a combination of soft-tissue degeneration and a modest increase in activity. The patient presents with an injured shoulder often following an event such as lifting. Symptoms may occur suddenly or be more gradual in onset. Movements are restricted, particularly abduction and forward flexion. Classically, there is a painful arc from about 20° to 90° of abduction, but initially the pain may be intense and affect all movements. There may be specific tenderness in the supraspinatus fossa laterally.

XR Radiographs sometimes show calcification within the tendon, near its attachment to the joint capsule.

Tx A sling and non-steroidal anti-inflammatory drugs (NSAIDS) should be prescribed. In severe cases, a short course of oral steroids can give dramatic relief. Patients should be reviewed within a week, when physiotherapy and orthopaedic referral may be considered. Surgical decompression may help in chronic cases.

Rotator cuff injury

The glenohumeral joint is stabilised by four muscles that surround it – the rotator cuff:

1 *Subscapularis* – a medial rotator
2 *Supraspinatus* – which initiates abduction
3 *Infraspinatus* – a lateral rotator
4 *Teres minor* – another lateral rotator.

The rotator cuff muscles may be acutely injured or chronically inflamed or both. This causes pain with shoulder movements, sometimes of the painful arc type. There may be a tender area anteriorly. The tendons of all the rotator cuff muscles may rupture or degenerate in a similar manner to the supraspinatus tendon (→ *above*).

Frozen shoulder → *p. 115.*

Tx Analgesia, together with rest in a sling, is required for a few days. Early physiotherapy is essential. The condition can be very slow to settle (up to 2 years), especially in older patients and in those with an acute onset.

Rupture of the long head of biceps

This is caused by a combination of tendon degeneration and powerful elbow flexion. The patient presents with the sudden appearance of a painless lump reminiscent of Popeye's biceps.

Tx This is usually symptomatic, but a specialist opinion should be sought at the next fracture clinic.

Dislocation of the shoulder joint

This may occur after trivial injury in a predisposed individual or follow major violence to the shoulder girdle and be associated with other bone and soft-tissue injuries.

A full examination is mandatory to exclude associated injuries and distal neurovascular complications.

The dislocation is usually anterior and easily detected clinically and radiologically (→ *Figure 8.1*). Posterior dislocation is rarer and associated with the muscle contraction that occurs during fits and electric shocks. Inferior dislocation *("luxatio erecta")* is very rare – the patient presents with the arm erect. A fracture of the greater tuberosity or neck of the humerus may accompany a dislocation.

Xr Radiographs must be taken before reduction is attempted. Lateral radiographs are difficult to interpret; modified axial views are more useful. *Figures 8.2* and *8.3* demonstrate the normal appearances of the shoulder joint on lateral and apical radiographs.

> Posterior dislocation of the shoulder may not be obvious clinically and can easily be missed on the AP radiograph (→ *Figure 8.4*).

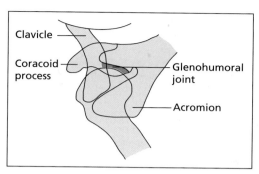

Figure 8.2 The normal appearance of the shoulder joint (apical view).

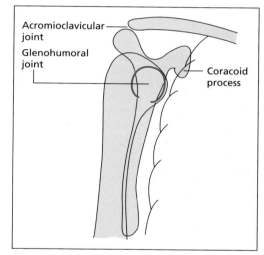

Figure 8.3 The normal appearance of the shoulder joint (lateral view).

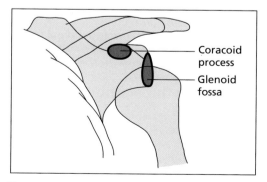

Figure 8.1 Anterior dislocation of the shoulder joint.

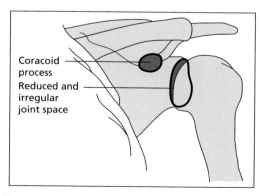

Figure 8.4 Posterior dislocation of the shoulder joint.

Box 8.2 Reduction of a dislocated shoulder

- Explain the procedure to the patient
- Ensure that adequate sedation and analgesia are achieved and appropriate resuscitation facilities are available
- Gently hold the wrist on the dislocated side in both hands. Countertraction, if required, may be applied by a second person supporting the patient with a towel sling around the shoulder or by the operator's (unshod) toes in the axilla. The latter (Hippocratic) method requires the operator to stand on a low stool
- Slowly (over a minute or two) abduct the arm out to 90°, keeping the elbow extended. As the arm is abducting, rotate it externally (i.e. so that the palm is facing upwards)
- Apply firm, constant traction along the patient's abducted, rotated arm. The shoulder joint is approaching its most unstable position. Gentle, uninterrupted traction with reassurance to maintain muscle relaxation is the key to success. Do not use excessive force because it may damage the axillary neurovascular structures. By slightly varying the angle of pull and the axial rotation of the arm, the joint will usually relocate within about 5 min with minimal patient discomfort

Tx The patient will need early parenteral analgesia. Reduction can be achieved without general anaesthetic by using one of a number of techniques to overcome muscle spasm. Prior analgesia helps but large amounts should not be necessary if the technique is good. The method of sedation will depend largely on the experience of the staff involved (→ p. 15). Many methods of reduction can be equally successful; a simple technique for anterior and posterior dislocations is described in *Box 8.2*.

Inferior dislocations usually reduce easily; the arm is gently brought down to a partially abducted position and then treated as an anterior dislocation.

Fracture of the greater tuberosity may accompany a dislocated shoulder. It will usually relocate easily as the shoulder dislocation is reduced.

Patients with a dislocation and a co-existing fracture of the neck of the humerus need immediate orthopaedic referral as do patients with a dislocation that is more than 24 h old.

After reduction, the arm is immobilised in a sling and a body bandage is applied to prevent abduction and external rotation. Radiographs are then repeated to confirm reduction and the arm is again examined to exclude neurovascular damage. The patient is then referred to the next fracture clinic with instructions to keep the wrist and hand mobile. Physiotherapy and gradual mobilisation will be necessary at a later date, possibly followed by surgical repair of the lax shoulder joint capsule if there has been recurrent dislocation.

Brachial plexus injury

These injuries are caused by sudden traction on the arm (e.g. a window cleaner grasping the window ledge as the ladder slips) or by direct violence to the shoulder region (e.g. a motor cyclist struck from in front by an oncoming vehicle). They may also be seen in patients who have sustained prolonged pressure on the axilla while under the influence of alcohol. Proximal injuries may avulse the nerve roots from the spinal cord. Differing amounts of damage occur. There may be any of the following:

- *Complete section* – neuroptmesis
- *Axonal damage* – axonoptmesis
- *Failure of transmission only* – neuropraxia
- *A combination of the above.*

Neurological examination determines the areas involved. The presence of Horner's syndrome indicates preganglionic damage. A histamine test on anaesthetised skin distinguishes lesions proximal (triple response) and distal (no response) to the dorsal root ganglion.

XR Radiological examination should include the shoulder, cervical spine and thoracic outlet.

Tx Early specialist referral will be required. Axonal regeneration down intact sheaths occurs at a rate of about 1 mm/day (or 1 inch/month). Surgical repair is rarely attempted and then mainly for distal lesions. No regeneration or repair is possible if part of the plexus has been avulsed from the spinal cord.

Fracture of the scapula

Fractures of the scapula are relatively uncommon and usually the result of direct trauma. Significant force is required to break the scapula and so accompanying injuries must be excluded. Any part of the bone may be fractured, including the body, spine, neck, acromion process and coracoid process. Local pain and tenderness are the main clinical features; shoulder movements may be relatively intact.

XR Fractures of the scapula are often missed on radiographs. An oblique view of the shoulder (to show the scapula more clearly) may be requested in cases of doubt.

Tx Displacement of a fracture of the spine or blade is rarely significant and management is conservative. The patient should be given a broad arm sling and analgesia, and then referred to the next fracture clinic. The scapula has an excellent blood supply and usually heals very well.

Fracture of the humoral neck

This can occur at all ages, but is particularly common in elderly people. It is usually an isolated injury, caused by a low-speed impact. Displacement is common and may be gross, but is usually unimportant.

A full examination should be made to exclude other injury, particularly at the wrist. The axillary nerve may be damaged, causing deltoid paralysis and an area of anaesthesia over the outer aspect of the shoulder. The joint may sublux inferiorly because of this deltoid paralysis. The nerve will recover spontaneously over a period of a few weeks. Bruising is often very extensive and may extend down to the mid-forearm over the first few days. The patient should be warned that this rather frightening but harmless phenomenon might occur.

XR An AP radiograph may be sufficient, but if shoulder dislocation is suspected an axial view will be required. In children, it is necessary to distinguish a greenstick fracture, with buckled cortex, from the normal epiphyseal line.

Tx A sling, analgesics and reassurance are all that are required initially. Fracture clinic referral is arranged; physiotherapy should follow.

Frozen shoulder

Adhesive capsulitis of the shoulder joint is most commonly seen in older patients. It may be spontaneous or follow the disuse associated with any type of upper limb injury. Early mobilisation after injury will help to prevent its development (e.g. for patients with Colles' fractures remove the sling every few hours so that the arm can be moved behind the back and the neck). Patients with established disease and no recent history of trauma may present to the ED. Cervical and thoracic outlet problems must be excluded.

The patient often complains of pain at the deltoid insertion but is actually tender over the anterior capsule. Abduction and internal rotation are particularly restricted.

> When assessing glenohumeral movement, always put one hand on the scapula to exclude the scapulothoracic contribution to shoulder mobility.

XR Radiographs may show an area of calcification in the shoulder joint capsule.

Tx This condition may be very slow (up to 2 years) to resolve spontaneously. The other shoulder may be affected just as the first is recovering. Physiotherapy is the mainstay of treatment. Steroid injection – particularly into calcified areas of the capsule – and NSAIDs may be helpful. Manipulation under anaesthesia may sometimes be needed.

Thoracic outlet obstruction

The neurovascular outflow from the thorax and spine to the upper limb is constrained by a narrow-based triangle above the first rib. The lower parts of the brachial plexus and the subclavian artery may be compressed here if the shoulders are depressed by heavy backpacks or unaccustomed lifting. Symptoms are more likely if the brachial plexus is post-fixed (i.e. arises from the spinal cord more caudally than usual) or if there is a cervical rib. A tumour at the apex of the lung can spread upwards to involve the lower part of the brachial plexus.

The patient complains of a gradual onset of diffuse shoulder girdle pain, made worse by carrying shopping bags, etc. Symptoms can be reproduced by pulling down on the arm with the patient standing. The radial pulse may be obliterated if the arm is abducted to 90° and the patient turns his or her head to the opposite side. There may be weakness of the small muscles of the hand and paraesthesia in the hand extending up the inner border of the arm.

XR Radiographs are taken of the cervical spine, thoracic inlet and chest.

Tx Always seek advice about management. If more sinister causes have been excluded, slow recovery usually occurs if traction on the shoulder can be avoided. Physiotherapy may help. Resection of the first rib may be necessary in severe cases.

Referred pain at the shoulder

Diaphragmatic irritation may produce shoulder-tip pain. Causes include cholecystitis, splenic injury, subphrenic abscess and pleurisy. Cardiac pain may present initially with a generalised ache in the shoulder joint.

Fracture of the humoral shaft

This fracture is unstable and painful and thus requires immediate splintage. The mechanism of injury and the possibility of damage elsewhere should always be considered. If little force was involved, pathological fracture is a possibility. The radial nerve is often damaged, but rarely divided, as it winds around the humoral shaft in the spiral groove; ensure ability to extend the wrist and fingers. The radial pulse should also be checked because brachial artery injury may sometimes occur.

XR Radiographs should include the shoulder and elbow joints.

TX Provide support and analgesia. Orthopaedic referral is indicated. Internal fixation is usually undertaken but external splintage with a U-slab of plaster and a collar and cuff is an alternative.

THE ELBOW

The elbow may be injured by a direct blow or by transmitted forces. In children, the constantly changing epiphyses make the interpretation of radiographs rather difficult (→ *Box 8.3 and Figure 8.5*).

> Full extension of the elbow (to a bony block) without pain makes the presence of a fracture very unlikely.

 Box 8.3 Elbow radiographs in children

Interpretation may be difficult in children but is aided by a knowledge of the times of appearance and fusion of secondary ossification centres (*also → Figure 8.5*):

C	2: capitellum – present by age 2 years
R	4: radial head – appears at 3–5 years of age
I	6: internal or medial epicondyle – present by age 6 years
T	8: trochlea – appears at age 7–9 years
O	10: olecranon – appears at age 9–11 years
E	12: external or lateral epicondyle – present by age 11–14 years

- The epiphyses of the capitellum, trochlea and lateral epicondyle become one centre in the early teenage years
- All the epiphyses fuse in teenage, usually a year or two later in boys than in girls
- Comparative views of the other elbow, taken at the same angle, are occasionally helpful but should not be requested unless absolutely necessary (and then usually after discussion with a radiologist)

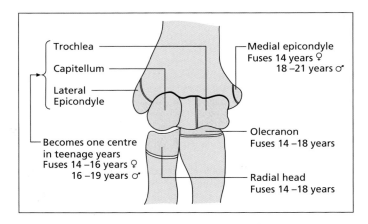

Figure 8.5 Secondary ossification centres around the elbow.

Pulled elbow

Sudden traction on a young child's arm may sublux the radial head through the soft annular ligament. A history of pulling may not be forthcoming. A fall may have occurred but picking the child up afterwards is more likely to have caused the problem than the fall itself. The diagnosis should be suspected in a child who:

- is between 1 and 4 years old
- has no history of significant trauma
- is unwilling to use one arm
- holds that arm limply by his or her side with the elbow semiflexed in mid-pronation
- has no obvious swelling, bruising or tenderness
- cries at attempts to elevate the arm.

XR Radiographs are unnecessary if you are confident in the diagnosis of a pulled elbow.

Tx The subluxation is reduced by gentle but determined supination of the forearm with the elbow at 90° and a thumb over the radial head. A palpable click indicates success. Final reassurance for the doctor, and doubting parents, is obtained by letting the child play and watching normal movements return. This may take some time. Arms that have been immobile for several hours can be slightly swollen and more difficult to reduce.

> Do not attempt to reduce a pulled elbow if you are in any doubt about the diagnosis. You will probably not do any harm but the child's parents may be upset if you discover a fracture sometime later!

If the above procedure is unsuccessful at any stage, the whole arm should be re-examined and radiographed. If nothing abnormal is found, a collar and cuff should be supplied and the child reviewed within 48 h. Most cases settle spontaneously in a few days.

The parents can be reassured that, although the condition may recur (in either arm), the ligaments will stiffen up after the age of 5 years and put an end to the problem (*also → Box 8.4*).

Supracondylar fracture

This injury occurs in older children (peak incidence at age 8 years) who fall on the outstretched arm. Severity varies from a hairline fracture to gross displacement, usually of the distal fragment posteriorly.

Box 8.4 The management of the child who is not using an arm

- Get a clear history
- Watch the child playing with toys and the interaction with the parents
- Look for bruising, swelling or tenderness. Do not forget to examine the clavicle and wrist
- Decide where the problem areas are. If there are no immediately obvious areas and the arm is held limply by the side, consider pulled elbow or fractured clavicle
- Obtain radiographs of the whole arm, including the clavicle. If they seem normal, look again for buckle fractures of the wrist or clavicle and effusions of the elbow. Consider plastic bowing fractures (→ *p. 121*)
- In all other cases, prescribe analgesia and a collar and cuff, reassure the parents and arrange for the child to be reviewed within 2 or 3 days

All displaced fractures are associated with the risk of brachial artery injury; check distal pulses.

Fractures of this area in adults are often comminuted and involve the articular surface. The elbow is swollen and movement very restricted. Neurovascular damage may occur.

Tx Reduction under general anaesthesia by the orthopaedic team and subsequent monitoring of distal neurovascular function is essential. Failure to do this may result in Volkmann's ischaemic contracture of the forearm muscles, with permanent disability in the hand. Internal fixation is often required especially if the articular surface is implicated. Some undisplaced fractures may be treated on an outpatient basis, but this decision should be left to the orthopaedic staff.

Fractures of the medial and lateral epicondyles

These fractures are caused by a varus or valgus strain at the elbow. Swelling may not be a major feature, but there is always a restriction of elbow extension and local bony tenderness. The medial epicondyle may be trapped in the joint; ulnar or median nerve injury may occur.

XR Radiographs may show little more than an effusion (→ *Figure 8.6*). Avulsion of an epicondyle in a

Figure 8.6 Lateral radiograph of the elbow joint showing anterior and posterior effusions (shaded) and fracture of the radial head (arrowed).

 Box 8.5 **Management of an injured elbow with a radiograph showing effusion but no fracture**

A joint effusion seen on the lateral radiograph (→ *Figure 8.6*) usually indicates a significant injury – radial head fracture in an adult or epiphyseal injury in a child. If there is an effusion but no visible fracture then:

- re-examine the injured limb
- reconsider the possibility of a fracture of the head of the radius
- discuss the problem with a senior colleague and consider the need for further (oblique) radiographs
- explain the situation to the patient
- support the elbow in a collar and cuff
- prescribe analgesia
- arrange for review in 5–10 days

child involves much more of the joint than the radiographs suggest, because most of the structure is cartilaginous.

Tx An orthopaedic opinion is essential.

Fracture of the olecranon

This is sustained by falling on the point of the flexed elbow. Triceps action will distract the bone ends and a gap can usually be felt beneath the rapidly developing haematoma and oedema. Active elbow extension is impossible. In the absence of an associated elbow dislocation, other movements, particularly supination and pronation, are often quite good and pain free.

Tx The patient is given a sling while awaiting specialist advice. Inpatient care and internal fixation will be necessary.

Fracture of the head or neck of the radius

This common fracture is usually sustained by a fall on the outstretched arm. Elbow flexion may be full but extension is restricted. There is pain on palpation of the radial head, which is exacerbated during forearm rotation. Injury to the posterior interosseous nerve – which winds around the neck of the radius – is rare.

XR Radiographs usually show an effusion (→ *Figure 8.6*) but the fracture may be elusive. Further oblique views may be necessary.

Radial head fracture is one of the most commonly missed limb injuries. It should be diagnosed clinically when there is:

- an appropriate history
- local tenderness
- reduced extension and supination
- a positive 'fat pad sign' on radiograph (anterior effusion).

Tx Minor undisplaced fractures are treated conservatively with early mobilisation. The patient will need analgesia, a collar and cuff, and referral to the next fracture clinic. More significant injuries may require internal fixation or excision of the radial head and should be referred immediately for specialist advice (*also* → *Box 8.5*).

Dislocation of the elbow joint

This requires considerable force. Consequently, there are usually associated fractures of the coronoid process, olecranon, capitellum or trochlea. There may also be damage to the brachial artery, or ulnar, median or radial nerves.

Tx Analgesia and splintage should be provided before taking a radiograph and the radial pulse must be monitored. Reduction may be carried out in the ED by suitably experienced staff. Under sedation, axial traction is applied to the elbow while it is in about 30° of extension. Subsequent care is carried out by the orthopaedic department.

Epicondylitis: tennis elbow and golfer's elbow

'Tennis elbow' causes pain around the lateral epicondyle of the humerus. The underlying 'epicondylitis' is most common between the ages of 40 and 60 years, and is usually caused by repetitive hand and wrist movements. There is inflammation and sometimes partial avulsion of the common extensor origin, which may be tender. Nerve entrapment is occasionally responsible for the symptoms. Movements of the elbow joint are not usually reduced, although there may be slight restriction of pronation. Sudden passive flexion of the wrist, especially from the extended position, may reproduce the pain, as may gripping and twisting movements.

'Golfer's elbow' refers to a similar inflammation of the common flexor origin at the medial epicondyle of the humerus. There is chronic pain, which is worse on gripping.

XR A radiograph may be taken to exclude fracture or bone disease. An ultrasound scan may be helpful.

Tx The inflammation is usually self-limiting although symptoms may persist for many months. In mild cases, an oral NSAID together with advice to modify activity at work or sport may be sufficient. A wrist brace may provide some symptomatic relief. Physiotherapy is of some value and local injection of steroid often helps. Surgical division of part of the extensor (or flexor) origin is occasionally necessary.

Degenerative disease of the elbow joint

Chronic osteoarthrosis of the elbow is usually secondary to imperfectly reduced fractures involving the articular surfaces. Symptoms may begin spontaneously or be triggered by further minor trauma. The main complaint is of an inability to extend the elbow fully with some restriction of forearm rotation. Loose bodies may cause locking. If the fracture occurred during childhood, inequalities of growth may have resulted in marked deformity. A traction injury to the ulnar nerve may develop if cubitus valgus occurs after a lateral epicondyle fracture.

XR Radiographs may reveal more joint destruction than might be expected from clinical examination.

Tx The elbow should be rested in a sling for a few days to allow any inflammation to settle. NSAIDs may also help. Physiotherapy often exacerbates elbow stiffness, whatever the aetiology. The patient should be referred to the orthopaedic department either directly or via the GP.

Olecranon bursitis

The patient presents with a large swelling over the olecranon, often after minor trauma. The elbow joint is not affected and is clinically normal except for pain on movement. The lump may be soft and fluctuant or tense and very painful if secondarily infected. Occasionally, the cause will be a crystal arthropathy.

XR Radiographs may reveal an underlying bony spur.

Tx The inflammation usually settles with an elastic support bandage and NSAIDs. Antibiotics should be prescribed if there is evidence of spreading infection or if the patient is pyrexic. Rarely, incision and drainage will be required under adequate anaesthesia. The patient should be reviewed at a clinic after a few days. When the acute episode has resolved, consideration should be given to referring the patient for formal excision of the bursa and underlying spur. If crystal arthropathy is thought to be a possibility, then the patient should be discussed with a rheumatologist.

THE FOREARM AND WRIST

Wounds to the forearm and wrist

Lacerations in this area frequently involve deep structures; accurate diagnosis is essential. The history is usually helpful, although many injuries are either self-inflicted or sustained while intoxicated, so the patient's account may be misleading. Penetrating glass can cause nerve and tendon damage at a distance from the puncture wound; casual exploration under local anaesthesia will fail to reveal deep injuries.

A full assessment of distal neurovascular function is essential. Test all tendons and nerves individually ($\rightarrow$ Box 8.6). Any positive finding of deep structure involvement must be discussed with a senior colleague at once. Further exploration must be carried out:

- in an operating theatre
- under adequate anaesthesia (usually general)
- with a bloodless field
- by an experienced surgeon.

Box 8.6 Median and ulnar nerve supply to the muscles that are involved in movements of the hand

Muscles of the anterior forearm
Ulnar nerve → 1 flexor carpi ulnaris
→ 2 medial half of flexor digitorum profundus
Median nerve supplies all the rest.

Intrinsic muscles of the hand
Median nerve → 1 lateral two lumbricals
→ 2 opponens pollicis
→ 3 abductor pollicis brevis
→ 4 flexor pollicis brevis
Ulnar nerve supplies all the rest.

A divided nerve may continue to conduct some sensation for several hours if the nerve ends are touching.

Abductor pollicis brevis is paralysed in T1 root lesions but not in ulnar nerve lesions. To test this muscle the thumb is moved vertically upwards against resistance with the hand in a supine position.

Fractures of the midshafts of the radius and ulna

These injuries are of three types:

1 A direct blow to the forearm produces a transverse fracture of either the ulna or both bones at the same level.
2 Rotational or transmitted forces produce a spiral fracture of each bone at different levels.
3 Rotational forces produce a fracture of one bone and a dislocation of the other at either of the radioulnar joints (→ *Figure 8.7*).

Clinical and radiological examination must thus include the elbow and wrist joints and neurovascular status must be carefully assessed. All of these forearm fractures are potentially unstable.

XR One long X-ray plate, including both joints with the forearm bones, is inadequate because it produces oblique, atypical views of the joints, which are difficult to interpret. Standard films of adjacent joints should be obtained.

Galleazzi fracture   Monteggia fracture
of radius   of ulna

Figure 8.7 Fracture dislocations of the radius and ulna. *Galleazzi fracture dislocation*: fracture of the radial shaft with dorsal dislocation of the lower ulna from the inferior radioulnar joint. *Monteggia fracture dislocation:* fracture of the ulnar shaft with volar dislocation of the radial head into the antecubital fossa.

Tx Analgesia and splintage should precede orthopaedic advice. Closed manipulation of some fractures under general anaesthetic may be successful, but this should be carried out in a fully equipped operating theatre so that failure can be quickly followed by open reduction and internal fixation under the same anaesthetic.

Forearm fractures in children

Children commonly sustain greenstick fractures of both forearm bones, in which case:

• there may be very little angulation
• there is usually only a modest amount of pain
• forearm rotation is always restricted
• elbow and wrist movements may be full
• neurovascular complications are unlikely.

For these reasons the fracture may be overlooked.

Tx Management must be discussed with an experienced colleague. A well-padded, above-elbow plaster cast, a sling, oral analgesics and outpatient follow-up may be acceptable, but significant displacement demands manipulation under general anaesthesia. This can be difficult. The greenstick fracture may have to be converted to a complete fracture before reduction can be achieved. Subsequent swelling caused by oedema formation and haematoma from the bone and damaged muscle always makes a second attempt technically more difficult. It is essential that the first attempt is successful and that the child is kept in hospital for 24 h with the arm elevated and the peripheral circulation carefully monitored.

Plastic bowing fractures of the radius and ulna

These relatively uncommon injuries are seen only in children between the ages of 2 and 5 years. The bending deformation is caused by a continuously applied longitudinal force, usually a fall on an outstretched arm. The most common variety occurs with the forearm pronated and involves bowing of the ulna with an angulated greenstick fracture of the radius. Conversely, a fall on a supinated forearm may fracture the ulna and bow the radius. Plastic bowing of both bones is the easiest variety to miss: although the child complains of pain and inability to use the arm, tenderness is difficult to localise and deformity may not be immediately obvious. Narrowing of the intraosseous space may cause pain on pronation and supination.

XR The affected bone appears bowed but with no actual fracture visible. (Microscopically, there is a series of microfractures on the concave aspect of the bone with intact cortex on the convex side.) Bowing is best seen on the lateral view. Ulnar bowing is usually convex posteriorly whereas bowing of the radius causes an anterior angulation.

Tx Orthopaedic management is required. In children aged <4 years, angulations of less than 20° that are not restricting movements can be left to remodel. Other plastic bowing fractures should be manipulated under general anaesthesia.

> Plastic bowing fractures may also occur in the fibula, femur and clavicle.

Fracture of the distal radius

Fractures of the distal radius mostly occur in osteoporotic bone and so are most common in older women. These fractures are usually sustained by falling on the outstretched hand and consequently

> **Box 8.7 The six characteristic features of displaced Colles' fracture**
>
> 1 Dorsal displacement
> 2 Anterior angulation
> 3 Impaction
> 4 Lateral (radial) displacement
> 5 Ulnar angulation
> 6 Rotational deformity
>
> Avulsion of the ulnar styloid is a common accompanying feature.

injuries higher up the arm should always be excluded. In adults, impaction of cancellous bone imparts some stability compared with the obvious instability of midshaft fractures. However, pain and deformity are usually obvious and supination is always restricted.

Colles' fracture is actually defined as any fracture of the radius within 2.5 cm of the wrist joint but the term is usually taken to mean a wrist fracture with either dorsal displacement or anterior angulation.

Management of fractures of the distal radius with volar displacement of the distal fragment → p. 122. The six characteristic features of a Colles' fracture → Box 8.7.

XR The degree of displacement or angulation, and therefore the need for reduction, can be estimated from the radiographs. The malposition is significant if either of the following occurs:

1 The articular surface of the distal radius on the lateral radiograph is not angulated in a volar direction, i.e. if angle ABC, as seen in *Figure 8.8*, is <90°.
2 Radial shortening is seen on the AP view such that the ulnar articular surface is >2 mm distal to the radial articular surface.

Tx For the purposes of management in the ED, there are three main types of Colles' fracture of the distal radius:

1 *Fracture with minimal or acceptable displacement in an older patient with osteoporotic bone:*
   – confirm acceptable position (→ *Figure 8.8*)
   – exclude other injuries
   – exclude medical cause of fall
   – apply padded forearm backslab
   – provide sling and analgesia
   – encourage shoulder and hand mobility
   – ensure adequate domestic support
   – refer to fracture clinic on the following day.

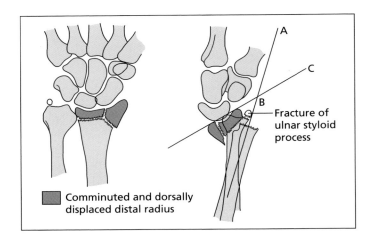

Fracture of
ulnar styloid
process

Comminuted and dorsally
displaced distal radius

Figure 8.8 Comminuted Colles'
fracture (with angle ABC identified).

2 *Displaced/angulated fracture in an osteoporotic wrist:* Treatment is as described in (1) above, but the fracture must be reduced under appropriate local, regional or general anaesthesia. *For one method of local anaesthesia → Box 8.8.* In some hospitals this will take place in the ED. Satisfactory home circumstances are then of even greater importance if post-operative discharge is anticipated.

Reduction is achieved by traction and slight hyperextension (to disimpact the fracture) and then flexion and ulnar deviation. Countertraction is applied by a colleague holding the upper arm. Unfortunately, the poor-quality dorsal cortex often allows the fracture to redisplace over the next 2 weeks. Re-manipulation may then be necessary. Good function is more important than good anatomical and radiological reduction, but this fact should not influence initial attempts to obtain perfection. The manipulated fracture is held in its reduced position by a plaster backslab, which extends from the metacarpal heads to the antecubital fossa, over the dorsoradial aspect of the forearm. Radiographs must be taken after reduction but before ending the anaesthetic, so that an inadequate manipulation can be corrected immediately (→ *Figure 8.8*). As a result of the difficulty in maintaining a good position after reduction, many orthopaedic surgeons prefer to manipulate these fractures in theatre and then fix the bones in position with wires.

3 *Fracture in a younger patient:* After providing temporary splintage and analgesia, refer the patient to the orthopaedic team for reduction and plating of the fracture under general anaesthesia.

 Box 8.8 Haematoma block for reduction of Colles' fracture

- Use an aseptic technique; clean the skin thoroughly
- Inject a maximum of 20 mL 0.25% prilocaine into the fracture haematoma. Approach from the dorsal aspect; the fracture site lies more proximally than you might expect
- Also inject some local anaesthetic around the ulnar styloid

Smith's fracture: A 'reversed Colles' fracture' in which the distal radial fragment is displaced in a volar direction and tilted anteriorly (i.e. there is posterior angulation). It usually results from a fall onto the back of the hand. All such fractures should be discussed with the orthopaedic department.

Barton's fracture: A type of Smith's fracture in which only the anterior portion of the distal radius is involved. It should be referred to the orthopaedic team for fixation.

Significant injury to the wrist is very unlikely following minor trauma if:

1 full supination is possible without pain
2 there is no tenderness in the anatomical snuff box

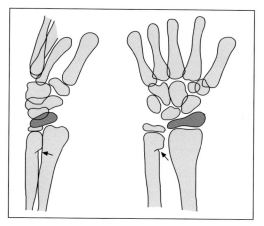

Figure 8.9 Posterior displacement of distal radial epiphysis (shaded) with buckle fracture of the ulna (arrowed).

Figure 8.10 Metaphyseal (pronator quadratus) fracture of the distal radius and ulna.

Wrist fractures in children

In children three types of wrist fracture are commonly seen:

Slipped (distal radial) epiphysis

The distal radial epiphysis may slip dorsally, usually taking with it a flake of metaphysis (→ *Figure 8.9*).

Tx Reduction is easily achieved by the orthopaedic staff under general anaesthetic and maintained by a forearm plaster backslab. Outpatient follow-up is appropriate. The patient is given a sling and oral analgesic.

Fracture of the distal radius

A complete or greenstick fracture may occur through the distal radial metaphysis, often with significant displacement of the distal fragment (→ *Figure 8.10*).

Tx Reduction can be difficult and may even require open operation. Refer for orthopaedic advice.

Buckle fracture of the distal radius

A buckle (or torus) fracture of the lower radial metaphysis may be easily overlooked. The child always has limitation of supination by at least 10° and is tender over the lower radius. There may be no visible swell-

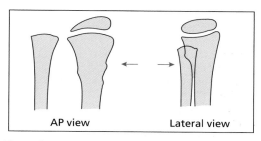

AP view   Lateral view

Figure 8.11 Buckle fracture of the distal radius (arrowed).

> All children with wrist pain need a radiograph, even if their wrist looks normal.

ing or bruising. In addition, the radiological abnormality is often minimal (→ *Figure 8.11*).

Tx These fractures rarely require manipulation and can be managed on an outpatient basis in a forearm plaster cast or wrist brace and sling.

Fracture of the radial styloid

This injury may mimic an undisplaced Colles' fracture or a scaphoid injury.

Tx A Colles-type plaster should be applied and the patient followed up in the fracture clinic.

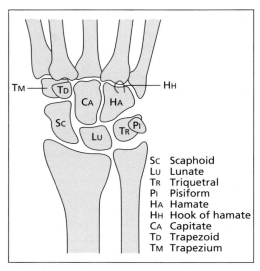

Figure 8.12 The carpal bones (AP view).

Sc Scaphoid
Lu Lunate
Tr Triquetral
Pi Pisiform
Ha Hamate
Hh Hook of hamate
Ca Capitate
Td Trapezoid
Tm Trapezium

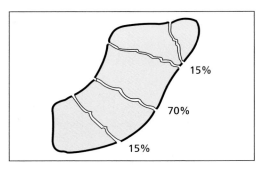

Figure 8.13 Sites of fracture in the scaphoid bone.

Small chip fractures of the carpus

These are commonly seen after hyperextension or flexion injuries of the wrist.

X℞ The bone of origin is not always obvious. MR scan may be required to demonstrate ligamentous injuries.

Relative positions of the carpal bones → Figure 8.12.

T℞ The wrist usually needs support in a cast or splint for 3 or 4 weeks.

Fracture of the scaphoid bone

The carpal bones lie in two rows but the scaphoid bone straddles both rows on the radial side. During trauma, considerable force may be transmitted through it, thus making it the most commonly fractured carpal bone (70% of all carpal fractures).

Sites of fracture in the scaphoid bone → Figure 8.13.

Fracture of the scaphoid bone is most common in men aged between 20 and 50 years. The relative compressibility of the bone in children makes fracture uncommon under the age of 14 years, although it can occur in children as young as 8 years. Early and accurate diagnosis of fractures of the scaphoid bone is essential to avoid the complications of avascular necrosis, non-union and radiocarpal arthrosis. The

diagnosis should be suspected if there is a combination of the following:

1 An appropriate mechanism of injury – usually a fall on to the outstretched hand or a direct blow to the scaphoid area.
2 Tenderness in the anatomical snuffbox between the long and short extensors of the thumb, and also on the dorsal and volar aspects of the scaphoid bone. In particular, the scaphoid tubercle may be tender when palpated on the palmar aspect of the wrist in radial deviation. Accompanying swelling is usually minimal.
3 A well-preserved range of movements. Forced thumb abduction and extension are usually painful as are pronation and ulnar deviation of the wrist.
4 A positive compression test (hold the thumb and apply pressure along the thumb metacarpus; a positive test causes wrist pain).

Unfortunately, many soft-tissue injuries, fracture of the radial styloid process and osteoarthritis of the carpometacarpal joint may present a similar clinical picture.

> The extensive articular surface of the scaphoid bone restricts the sites of vascular supply. Consequently, avascular necrosis – and long-term disability – may follow a missed fracture. This can cause more long-term morbidity than many major trunk injuries.

X℞ Two special radiographs of the wrist (i.e. scaphoid views = oblique and AP in ulnar deviation) should be obtained in addition to the standard two films. Even so, radiological evidence of the fracture may be elusive until bone resorption at 10–14 days has widened the fracture line. (The sensitivity of the first series of radiographs is only 65%.) Displacement of the fragments is uncommon. MRI is now replacing technetium bone scanning (scintigraphy) as the definitive diagnostic modality for carpal pathology.

Tx Patients with definite fractures should have their wrists immobilised in a cast (extending from the thumb interphalangeal joint to the elbow) with specialist follow-up at 2 weeks. Prolonged immobilisation (up to 3 months) will be required until there is both clinical and radiological proof of union.

If the fracture has not been confirmed on radiograph, patients should be treated according to the severity of their symptoms. For most, this will entail support of the wrist in a splint but patients with severe pain will still require a cast. After 2 weeks, the wrist should be re-examined and further radiographs taken. Patients who have negative radiographs but are still symptomatic must be reviewed at 2-week intervals. MRI or scintigraphic imaging may be required to reach a diagnosis.

Carpal dislocation

This uncommon problem is often missed on radiographs, although clinically there is obviously something wrong because swelling and pain are usually considerable. The lunate may be dislocated into the palm (anterior dislocation of the lunate) or the entire distal carpal row may dislocate dorsally (perilunar dislocation). In the latter, there is often an associated fracture of the scaphoid. Other variations are also described. Median nerve signs may occur as a result of direct compression in the carpal tunnel.

XR The lateral radiograph is diagnostic (→ *Figure 8.14*).

Tx Immediate specialist referral is essential. Closed reduction under general anaesthesia may be successful. The injured part must be elevated and distal neurovascular function assessed.

Wrist sprain

Diffuse pain may follow either a fall on to the outstretched hand or a hyperflexion injury. Tenderness is usually maximal over the dorsum of the carpus or at the inferior radioulnar joint. The degree of swelling is variable.

XR Scaphoid views should be requested but will be normal in the presence of a sprain.

Tx Suspicion of scaphoid injury should be treated accordingly. Most patients with a sprained wrist settle

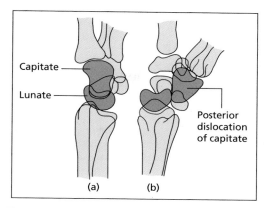

Figure 8.14 Lateral views of the wrist: (a) normal left and (b) abnormal right with perilunar dislocation.

spontaneously if provided with a wrist brace for 10–14 days. However, occasionally significant ligamentous damage will have been sustained leading to carpal instability and long-term disability. When symptoms are not resolving after 2 weeks, the patient should be referred for specialist advice. Arthroscopy or MR scan may identify lesions that are amenable to surgical repair.

Carpal tunnel syndrome

The median nerve may be compressed because its tunnel has become smaller (e.g. after a carpal fracture) or the nerve has become larger (e.g. in leprosy). However, the usual cause is that the contents of the carpal tunnel have expanded and the most common reasons for this are:

- interstitial fluid retention in pregnant and middle-aged women
- rheumatoid disease
- myxoedema
- acromegaly.

The condition is unusual, but not rare, in men. It may be bilateral.

The patient complains of paraesthesia in the hand and arm. The distribution varies but commonly includes the forearm and excludes the little finger. Symptoms classically awaken the patient in the early hours of the morning and are relieved by hand exercises or by hanging the arm out of bed. Examination reveals anaesthesia and thenar muscle wasting in advanced disease; otherwise, there is merely subjective impairment of touch. Pressure applied over the carpal tunnel may increase the symptoms. The upper limb should be examined to exclude pathology of the elbow, shoulder, thoracic outlet and cervical spine because nerve entrapment at these points can produce similar symptoms.

XR Radiographs are taken to exclude previous carpal fracture.

TX Temporary relief of symptoms may be achieved by splinting the wrist with a removable brace in partial flexion at night. This is particularly useful in pregnancy. Other patients should be referred to the orthopaedic clinic for surgical release.

Peritendonitis crepitans

This condition is more common than de Quervain's tenosynovitis and involves the more proximal part of the extensor tendons where there is no synovial sheath. The patient, usually male, presents with pain on moving the wrist. There may be a recent history of unaccustomed or repetitive wrist movements. On examination there is a fusiform swelling over the radial side of the forearm, over which crepitus may be felt when the wrist is moved.

TX The wrist should be rested in a removable splint during the day and NSAIDs should be supplied. With this treatment the condition usually settles within a few days. In prolonged cases, physiotherapy with ultrasound treatment is helpful.

De Quervain's tenosynovitis

Inflammation of the tendon sheaths of extensor pollicis brevis and abductor pollicis longus (at the volar side of the anatomical snuff box) produces acute local tenderness. Pain extends over the dorso-lateral aspect of the forearm and is made worse by thumb movements.

TX Immobilisation (thus stopping repetitive hand and wrist movements) will allow most cases to settle spontaneously. A replaceable splint is suitable. Referral back to the patient's GP is appropriate but some resistant cases may require steroid injection or surgical division of the stenosing tendon sheaths.

Avascular necrosis of the lunate

This condition is thought to be a long-term complication of minor wrist trauma without fracture. The patient presents with diffuse pain, which is worse on exercise; there is no recent history of injury.

XR The radiograph is diagnostic, showing a relatively dense lunate in a porotic carpus.

TX A wrist splint should be supplied and an orthopaedic clinic appointment made; excision of the lunate bone may be necessary.

Osteoarthrosis of the wrist

This commonly involves the carpometacarpal joint of the thumb in older patients. It is often asymptomatic until minor trauma to the wrist causes pain in the joint. Symptoms suggest a scaphoid fracture, but this is unusual in elderly people.

XR Degenerative changes in the joint are obvious on radiographs.

TX Symptoms are treated with a support bandage and NSAIDs, and the patient is referred to the GP.

Sudek's atrophy

This syndrome is characterised by vasomotor disturbance. It is a rare consequence of an often quite trivial wrist injury. Of unknown aetiology, it may be related to inadequate mobilisation after injury. Pain is the dominant symptom throughout. The skin is hot and dry at first and the hand and forearm are swollen. These signs settle after a few weeks but the patient continues to complain of discomfort.

XR The affected areas may appear osteoporotic on plain radiographs.

TX The condition usually resolves spontaneously after many months. Physiotherapy gives symptomatic relief. Orthopaedic referral is essential.

VASCULAR PROBLEMS IN THE UPPER LIMB

Compartment syndrome in the forearm or hand →
  p. 110.

Deep vein thrombosis of the upper limb

Although uncommon, thrombosis of the axillary or subclavian veins may occur in the same way as deep vein thrombosis (DVT) of the leg. There may be a history of repetitive movements such as weight lifting or ten-pin bowling. Neoplasia is another predisposing factor. The patient complains of non-traumatic swelling of the arm, usually with some discoloration of the skin. There is no pain or tenderness although some aching with movements may be present. DVT of the upper limb should not be confused with lymphoedema of the arm, which may follow infiltration or surgical clearance of the axillary lymph nodes in carcinoma of the breast.

Treatment of DVT → p. 108.

Ischaemia of the hand

Acute or subacute loss of blood supply to the hand may occur after accidental arterial injection of impure or insoluble substances (such as temazepam gel or plaster dust) into the arm, invariably by intravenous drug abusers. Any pallor or discoloration of the hand that cannot be attributed to Raynaud's syndrome requires an immediate opinion from a vascular surgeon (*also → pp. 107 and 108*).

9

The hand

The hand is a vital organ of function and is also important cosmetically. Its role in operating machines and using tools places it at a high risk of injury; 10–15% of all patients attending an emergency department (ED) have injured their hands.

Immediate assessment and management

- Check the patient's general condition – ABCs
- Make a quick local assessment
- Stop major bleeding by applying direct pressure
- Remove rings and bracelets
- Detect and document sensory loss
- Inject local anaesthetic if necessary
- Take a history of the injury
- Take a brief past and social history
- Ask which is the dominant hand
- Begin a detailed examination
- Obtain radiographs.

Swelling

Swelling, which accompanies soft-tissue injury, will produce venous occlusion under constricting bands. This can lead to interruption of arterial supply. Early removal of rings (and sometimes bracelets) is essential, using ring-cutters if necessary.

Pain

Pain may be severe. It heightens anxiety. Early injection of local anaesthetic (after examination of sensation) brings immediate relief. Subsequent cleaning and clinical and radiological examination can be carried out more carefully and therefore more accurately.

Cleaning

Cleaning can often be started by the patient. Industrial hand injuries are often extremely dirty. There is little point in applying a clean dressing to an oasis of sterile sutured skin that is surrounded by grease and grime. Make sure that the rest of the hand and forearm is cleaned. This may not be possible once a dressing has been applied.

History

The history may give important information on the extent of occult injury, e.g. contusion and devitalisation caused by crushing, direction of wounding, retained foreign bodies or injection of material through high-pressure hoses.

> Examination of the hand should follow the usual sequence of four four-letter words: **look, feel, move, X-ray**. Findings should be recorded with the aid of drawings. Digits must be identified by name, i.e. **index, middle, ring** and **little** – never by number.

WOUNDS TO THE HAND

General management of wounds → p. 391.
Small wounds and localised infections → Chapter 21 on p. 391.

In the hand, skin is at a premium and must be handled gently and conservatively; toothed forceps should be

Emergency Medicine Lecture Notes, Fourth Edition. Chris Moulton and David Yates.
© 2012 Blackwell Publishing Ltd. Published 2012 by Blackwell Publishing Ltd.

avoided. The main obstacles to sound healing are haematoma, infection and tension.

- Dead tissue must be excised, but the normal blood supply is good and may maintain flaps that would die elsewhere.
- Cleaning must be thorough. Gentle use of a tooth-brush or a scrubbing brush is effective.
- Lacerations over the dorsum of the hand, sustained in a fight, are often inflicted by the opponent's teeth. They are human bites and must be treated accordingly ($\rightarrow$ p. 399).
- Patients with compound fractures should be given systemic antibiotics and referred for specialist care. Osteomyelitis or septic arthritis may not be apparent on a radiograph for the first 10 days after infection.
- All patients with hand wounds must be protected against tetanus. ($\rightarrow$ p. 394).
- The median nerve motor supply to the thenar muscles ($\rightarrow$ Box 8.6 on p. 120) is very superficial and may be damaged by apparently minor wounds to the radial side of the palm.
- Adhesive, reinforced paper skin closures are not suitable for hand and proximal finger lacerations because they either restrict movement or impair blood supply – and they usually come off!
- Sutures to the palm that are too large (or badly placed adhesive strips) may cause skin overlap and a final, unacceptable, proud wound.

Injection injuries to the hand

EpiPen injection injuries: as more patients are issued with self-injecting devices to treat anaphylaxis, accidental injections have become more common. Anti-allergic 'pens' (such as EpiPen) contain either 0.15 mg or 0.3 mg adrenaline and so subcutaneous injection is rarely systemically dangerous. However, accidental injection into a digit may cause intense vasoconstriction and even irreversible tissue ischaemia. The affected finger may be pale and white with reduced sensation. Local injection of phentolamine (1.5 mg with 1 mL 2% lidocaine) may be effective in reversing the adrenaline-induced vasoconstriction for up to 13 h after the accidental injection. An opinion from a vascular surgeon may be required. Intravenous infusions of the prostacyclin analogue, iloprost, have also been used in this situation, as has stellate ganglion blockade. Calcium channel blockers and nitrates are ineffective.

High-pressure hose injection injuries: high-pressure hoses containing air, water, oil, grease and paint are used in many industries. Injection injuries from these tools can cause delayed but extensive soft-tissue damage. Skin penetration occurs easily (and often relatively painlessly) leaving minimal superficial injury and a normal-looking hand or finger. Initially, the injury may appear trivial but, within 24 h swelling, paraesthesia and loss of function are apparent. Tissue necrosis follows and damage to deeper structures is often widespread. Radiographs may reveal particles or an air track. All of these injuries must be referred for inpatient treatment at the time that they are first seen. Laying open the track and removal of injected particulate matter are often required. Tetanus prophylaxis is essential.

Oil-based veterinary vaccine injection injuries: accidental self-inoculation of oil-based veterinary vaccine fluid leads to intense local pain. The wound may appear trivial but can lead to widespread necrosis. Orthopaedic referral is essential for observation, debridement and decompression, if required.

Crush injuries of the hand

Inspection may not be a reliable guide to the extent of crushing. The history can give valuable additional information.

X_R This is almost always indicated.

T_X If the whole hand has been crushed, e.g. between rollers, admission and elevation are necessary even if the initial examination does not reveal extensive injuries.

Less extensive crushing injuries can be treated in the ED by:

- excluding injury to deep structures (radiological and clinical examination)
- providing local anaesthesia
- cleaning thoroughly (scrubbing brush or toothbrush)
- delaying closure for 3–5 days until the oedema has settled.

Amputations of the fingers

These are common in many industries. Distinguish between crisp sharp injuries where the damage is usually immediately evident and crush or tearing injuries, where the damage is often hidden and complications delayed.

X_R This is necessary to exclude bony damage.

T_X Amputation of the digits proximal to the distal interphalangeal (DIP) joint may be suitable for reimplantation ($\rightarrow$ p. 394).

Loss of more than the tip of the phalanx requires an orthopaedic opinion. Clean amputations through the terminal phalanx are best treated by primary closure. It may be necessary to trim the bone to allow flaps to be prepared without tension. The volar flap should be the longest, to achieve a dorsal suture line. Crush injuries producing amputation at this level must be left open.

Amputations through the fingertip can be left to close spontaneously. Cleaning must be vigorous and all dead tissue and dirt must be removed. The wound should then be covered with a non-adherent dressing and inspected not more than twice weekly. Antibiotics are not required unless there is bony involvement or infection is evident at the first dressing change. Exposed bone is best treated by referral for trimming.

Figure 9.1 Crush–flexion injury to the fingertip.

> Fingertip injuries that remain red, tender or swollen for more than 10 days may be developing osteomyelitis or septic arthritis. A radiograph may show early destruction of bone or loss of the joint space.

Partial avulsion of the fingertip

A combination of crushing and flexion of the fingertip (e.g. finger trapped by a door) may partially avulse the proximal end of the nail. There may be an associated crush fracture of the terminal phalanx ($\rightarrow$ *Figure 9.1*). This injury is very common in children.

XR This should be obtained in all cases.

Tx
- Obtain adequate conditions for the repair. General anaesthesia may be necessary but local anaesthesia with a ring block is usually adequate in adults ($\rightarrow$ *Box 21.2 on p. 392*). *For sedation of children $\rightarrow$ p. 352.*
- Clean the area thoroughly.
- Restore the normal alignment of the finger. It may sometimes be possible to replace a nail with a firm distal attachment under the proximal skinfold; otherwise remove it. Do not leave the nail in an avulsed position because it will splint the bone and/or finger pulp in the same position.
- Maintain the alignment with sutures to the lateral lacerations if needed but do not suture the nail bed ($\rightarrow$ *Figure 9.2*).
- Dress the finger with a non-adherent, antiseptic dressing.
- Provide adequate splintage. A Mallet splint may be slit dorsally for this purpose.
- Arrange follow-up.

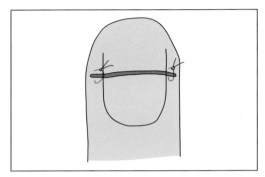

Figure 9.2 Position of sutures after removal of nail in crush–flexion injury.

The tip of the finger will swell but decompression will occur through the laceration.

Tendon injuries in the hand

Injuries to the tendons of the hand are common and often overlooked. Even the smallest wound to the skin may sometimes have allowed sufficient penetration to damage a tendon. Wounds involving glass are particularly sinister in this respect. Loss of function is the only reliable sign. Extensor tendon division is relatively easy to diagnose. *For the detection of flexor tendon damage $\rightarrow$ Box 9.1.* Also note the following:

- In the relaxed hand, the fingers tend to be held in increasing flexion from index to little finger. A pointing finger, which is out of line with this trend, suggests a flexor tendon or nerve injury.
- Partial division of a tendon may be overlooked initially but subsequent rupture may occur. Suspicion of a tendon injury warrants referral for exploration.
- The relationship between a tendon and the overlying skin varies with joint position. This means that

> **Box 9.1 The detection of flexor tendon injuries**
>
> *Anatomy:* flexor digitorum superficialis is used for fine movements. It has four fairly distinct muscle bellies. Each tendon inserts into the base of a middle phalanx. Flexor digitorum profundus is used for power grip. It arises as one muscle and is variably divided towards the musculotendinous junction. Each tendon inserts into the base of a distal phalanx.
>
> *Theory:* hyperextension of one fingertip will stretch the entire profundus belly and preclude it from initiating flexion of any of the other fingers. Flexion of the unrestrained fingers can be achieved only at the proximal interphalangeal (PIP) joint by action of the more independent superficialis tendon.
>
> *Testing:* for profundus assess active flexion at the DIP joint. For superficialis assess active flexion of the whole finger while the other fingers are hyperextended. Normally, flexion will occur at the PIP joint with the DIP joint remaining flaccid (profundus inactivated). If superficialis is divided, the whole finger will be flaccid.

the damage to a tendon may not be immediately visible through a skin wound. The tendon must therefore be inspected during finger or wrist movements.

XR All wounds involving glass must have a radiograph taken.

TX Extensor tendons on the back of the hand may be repaired in the ED if a clean theatre and appropriate skill are available. Patients with other tendon injuries must always be referred. Minor degrees of tendon damage, involving less than a third of the diameter of the tendon, may be managed conservatively but this needs experienced judgement.

Digital nerve injuries

Similar to tendon injuries, nerve injuries may not be immediately apparent. In both cases, deceptively small wounds can be sufficiently large to allow underlying damage. Distal sensation should always be tested and any complaint of changed sensation taken seriously. Sometimes the patient complains of paraesthesia in the affected digit but retains crude awareness of touch as a result of apposition of the severed nerve ends. The affected skin becomes dry 24 h later and is evidently anaesthetised. Patients often describe the sensation of absent nerve conduction in terms of their last experience of it – as being injected by the dentist with local anaesthetic.

TX Neural injury distal to the PIP joint rarely warrants repair. Any resulting area of anaesthesia will become smaller with the passage of time as in-growth occurs from other nerves.

The digital nerve is more commonly damaged in its superficial position near the metacarpophalangeal (MCP) joint. Repair is indicated, especially if the anaesthesia is on the ulnar border of the little finger, the radial aspect of the index finger or the thumb. If in doubt, the patient should be referred for a specialist opinion.

METACARPAL FRACTURES

Spiral fracture of the shaft of the metacarpus

This injury is produced by rotational forces on the finger. Rarely, it may be compound or multiple. The fracture is stable and usually undisplaced as a result of the integrity of the transverse metacarpal ligaments. Tendon and neurovascular damage is rare.

XR Anteroposterior and oblique views of the hand usually show the fracture clearly. Overlapping soft-tissue shadow or nutrient artery may be misinterpreted as an undisplaced spiral fracture.

TX Encourage movement but give a little support initially to alleviate pain. Follow-up should be in the fracture clinic.

Very rarely, rotational instability will result in persisting rotation of the finger, which is more easily detected on clinical than radiological examination – when the finger is fully flexed the tip is clearly maligned. An immediate orthopaedic opinion is then necessary.

Transverse fracture of the shaft of the metacarpus

This injury is the result of direct trauma. It is often multiple and may be compounded with extensive soft-tissue damage. The inherent stability of the metacarpal arch is lost and so displacement is common.

XR Epiphyseal lines may be partially developed at the proximal end of the index finger metacarpus and are commonly misinterpreted as linear fractures.

Tx This fracture requires immediate specialist attention. Internal fixation may be necessary to achieve stable reduction.

Fracture of the neck of the metacarpus

This is often termed the boxer's fracture, although most patients do not admit to fighting or, more usually, to missing their opponent and hitting a brick wall. The fracture is usually of the little metacarpus but injury to the ring or other metacarpal bones may also be seen.

> If the overlying skin is injured, it should be assumed that this is caused by contact with the opponent's teeth. This compound fracture has the potential to develop the serious complications of a human bite (→ p. 399).

In the absence of a bite injury, associated damage to deep structures is unusual. The metacarpal head may be angulated into the palm by up to 90°. Pain and angulation cause an associated lag in extension of the corresponding finger.

XR The fracture is confirmed on oblique films of the hand, but may be missed on an anteroposterior (AP) film.

Tx Various manoeuvres have been described to achieve reduction of the displaced metacarpal head. These usually fail to maintain a good position and, indeed, are unnecessary because remodelling will achieve good long-term function despite gross initial displacement. The patient should be warned that inability to extend the affected finger fully will persist for a few months, but that normal function can be guaranteed if the joints are mobilised as soon as possible. This explanation is an important part of the treatment. Most long-term complications are a direct result of immobilisation.

A crepe bandage and oral analgesia are supplied for use in the first few days and the patient should then be reviewed to ensure appropriate mobilisation.

BONE AND JOINT INJURIES OF THE FINGERS

Dislocation of the MCP joint

Dislocation without fracture may occur in either direction. Importantly, the metacarpal head may

'button hole' through the articular capsule, which then shrinks around the metacarpal neck and prevents closed reduction.

Tx This dislocation should be referred for specialist advice. Open reduction may be necessary. The prognosis is usually good.

Ligament injuries of the MCP joint

Sudden sideways forces may cause ligamentous injuries at the index and little finger MCP joints.

XR Such injuries may be associated with minor flake fractures of the proximal phalanx – representing avulsion of the attachment of the collateral ligament – or with fractures of the base of the phalanx (→ *below*).

Tx These injuries resolve with conservative management unless the joint is grossly unstable, when open repair is indicated. Strapping the finger to its neighbour is sufficient. This allows flexion but prevents abduction. Follow-up by the orthopaedic department is advisable.

Fracture of the proximal phalanx

Proximal phalanx fractures may occur through the base, shaft or neck. When compound, they must be referred immediately for specialist treatment. Antibiotics should be started in the ED and antitetanus cover provided. Fractures into the joint also require orthopaedic care.

Spiral fractures: these may produce rotational deformity, which is not always evident on a radiograph. Rotation is best detected clinically by noting the relative positions of the fingernails when the fingers are fully flexed into the palm. All the nails should lie in approximately the same plane with the fingertips pointing towards the palpable part of the radial artery. Rotational deformity, if found, requires orthopaedic correction.

Fracture of the base of the proximal phalanx: this is most commonly seen, as a greenstick or buckle injury, in the little finger of children (→ *Figure 9.3*). The fracture is easily (and often) overlooked on a radiograph. Reduction may be achieved under local anaesthesia by inserting a pencil into the cleft between the little and ring fingers and pushing the little finger towards the ring finger. A post-reduction radiograph is essential. Neighbour strapping is then applied and follow-up arranged.

Other metaphyseal fractures: fractures at the metaphyses through cancellous bone are usually stable

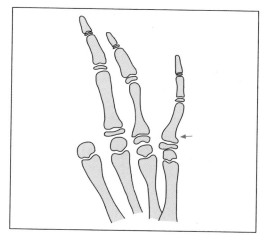

Figure 9.3 Greenstick fracture of the base of the proximal phalanx of the little finger.

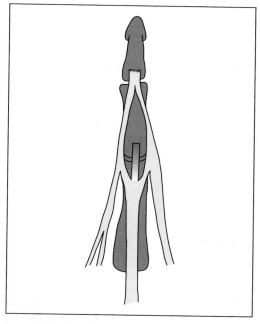

Figure 9.4 The extensor tendons of the finger. The central slip to the middle phalanx is shaded.

and, if not significantly displaced, can be treated conservatively by neighbour strapping. Displaced metaphyseal fractures may be reduced under local anaesthetic by manipulation over a pencil.

Fractures in the cortical diaphysis: these are more often displaced and very unstable. Delayed displacement of apparently stable fractures may occur. They may require internal fixation and should be referred immediately to the orthopaedic department.

Proximal interphalangeal joint injuries

The PIP joint deserves careful consideration because:

1 It has the largest range of movement.
2 Long-term stiffness is a major disability.
3 Initial injury is often overlooked.
4 Delayed displacement of the extensor tendon can occur.

The extensor hood, volar plate and collateral ligaments may all be damaged without joint dislocation and assessment can be difficult.

> The ability to extend fully, or even slightly hyperextend, all of the joints (especially the PIP joint) of an injured finger is associated with good recovery. Failure to achieve a straight finger must be followed up because the flexion may become permanent.

Xʀ Initial radiographs may look normal, even in the presence of a serious injury. Volar plate fractures are often missed.

Tx A patient with a PIP joint that is swollen or has a reduced range of movements should be followed up in clinic. Swelling can take several months to settle.

The boutonnière deformity

Extensor hood and central slip rupture may go unrecognised (→ *Figure 9.4*). Extension may be possible initially because the lateral bands remain intact but, if the finger is not splinted, these gradually migrate laterally and, within a few days, lie anterior to the axis of the joint. The extensor mechanism now flexes the proximal joint, and by a compensatory device hyperextends the distal joint. This is a boutonnière deformity. To prevent this serious complication all significant PIP joint injuries should be immobilised in extension and advice sought.

Dislocation of the PIP joint

Dislocation may occur in either direction. Buttonhole entrapment of the head of the proximal phalanx in the disrupted volar plate (capsule) is particularly difficult to reduce and requires expert surgical skill to repair.

XR Radiographs should always be taken before reduction of any finger dislocation.

Tx Manipulation may be attempted under local anaesthesia but, if the dislocation does not reduce easily on the first attempt, specialist advice must be sought. Repeated attempts at closed reduction will increase soft-tissue damage and make open repair more difficult. If closed reduction is immediately successful and examination does not reveal major ligamentous instability, the finger is held fully extended in a volar splint and strapped to its neighbour. The MCP joint must be left free to allow 90° of flexion. The patient is referred to the next fracture clinic.

Fracture of the intermediate phalanx

Fractures of the middle phalanx often extend into either joint and thereby produce an inherently unstable finger with a tendency to increasing deformity.

Tx These injuries must be referred for specialist advice, however small the fracture and however minimal the apparent displacement.

Dislocation of the DIP joint

The DIP joint has a smaller range of movement than the more proximal joints and injury to it is less often associated with major disability.

Dislocation of the DIP joint may be accompanied by a flake fracture from adjacent bone. This may indicate collateral ligament injury if it is lateral, or long-tendon avulsion if more central.

XR Radiographs must precede attempts to reduce the dislocation and repeat clinical examination must follow successful reduction.

Tx Reduction is achieved by axial traction, without excessive force. Follow-up is required to ensure return of full movement.

Mallet finger

Extensor tendon avulsion from the terminal phalanx produces a Mallet deformity. Passive movements are full and pain free, but there is no active extension at the DIP joint.

XR Radiographs should be taken to exclude other fractures. The presence of a small dorsal flake fracture improves the prognosis – the repair potential of bone is better than that of the extensor tendon.

Tx The patient should be referred to the next fracture clinic where a purpose-made hyperextension splint will be fitted (often under the auspices of an occupational therapist). In the meantime, the DIP joint must be held continuously in full extension by a temporary plastic (Mallet) splint; the DIP joint can be left free.

The splint may be changed occasionally to allow skin cleaning but the finger must not be allowed to flex while unsplinted. After 6 weeks the splint is worn only at night and during heavy manual work for a further month. Full return of active extension cannot be guaranteed. Functional disability is usually minimal even if no treatment is given, although there is also a cosmetic consideration. Some patients prefer to accept this outcome rather than suffer the restrictions imposed by a finger splint.

Fracture of the distal phalanx

These fractures are usually produced by crushing forces and are often comminuted. They may cause problems at the DIP joint when they extend across the articular surface but this is unusual. Bleeding is restricted by the fibrous loculi of the pulp space and by the nail to produce a subungual haematoma. Interstitial pressure quickly rises and the pain is severe.

Tx Trephining the nail with a red-hot paper clip brings instant relief to the patient who has a haematoma under the nail. It is not contraindicated in the presence of a fracture. The nail is insensitive and the blunt paper clip produces a wide sterile hole compared with that produced by the tip of a drill.

A simple fracture of the terminal phalanx can be treated in a Mallet splint for 2–3 weeks until the pain has settled. More commonly, there is a soft-tissue injury, which demands more careful attention (→ *p. 130*).

THUMB INJURIES

Thumb injuries produce greater disability than similar injuries to the other digits because of impairment of pinch and grip. Principles of treatment are similar, but particular attention is given to maintenance of length after terminal injury and the ability to oppose and rotate the thumb against the other fingers.

> A thumb that can be flexed to touch the palm of the hand at the base of the little finger is unlikely to be severely injured.

Fracture of the thumb metacarpus

These fractures are often the result of an oblique abducting force and may be disabling. They usually occur through the proximal part or the base of the metacarpus. There is a painful swollen deformity at the base of the thumb but associated, deep, soft-tissue injuries are uncommon.

XR Epiphyseal lines may be partially developed at the distal end of the thumb metacarpus and are commonly misinterpreted as linear fractures.

Tx If the fracture enters the carpometacarpal (trapezometacarpal) joint (Bennett's fracture), displacement is significant and reduction is then difficult. The patient should be referred to the orthopaedic department because internal fixation may be necessary. Closed manipulation may succeed but must be carried out by an experienced doctor. The fracture is usually held in a modified scaphoid plaster cast with the thumb abducted.

The more usual fracture through the metacarpal base, not involving the joint, is adequately treated in a scaphoid plaster cast. Reduction is not usually necessary.

Ligament injuries of the thumb MCP joint

Injury to the MCP joint of the thumb may be incapacitating, because functional impairment is associated with thumb instability. The collateral ligaments or the MCP joint capsule may be extensively torn by forced extension or abduction. The ulnar collateral ligament is the most frequently damaged structure.

Chronic injury to this ligament was common in gamekeepers. Nowadays skiers sustain an acute injury by pulling the thumb back in the ski-stick strap or artificial ski-slope matting during a fall – hence the term 'skier's thumb'.

Examination reveals specific tenderness over the palmar and web aspects of the MCP joint and pain on attempted abduction. There is usually a haematoma in the thenar area. The laxity of the joint may be compared with that of the opposite thumb. Instability is not always apparent because of the protective action of the thenar muscles.

XR Stress views may show subluxation of the joint. Local anaesthetic around the metacarpus may be required to enable this procedure.

Tx Surgical repair or plaster cast immobilisation may be indicated for significant ligamentous injury; specialist advice should be sought. Injuries to the MCP joint without either laxity or haematoma can be treated with a bandage thumb spica and review in clinic.

Other injuries to the thumb

Dislocation of the MCP joint: the dislocation may be reduced by axial traction under metacarpal ring block. The patient should then be referred to the orthopaedic department because ligamentous instability or capsular damage may accompany the dislocation. A bandage thumb spica will give temporary support.

Fractures of the proximal phalanx: unstable or angulated fractures should be referred for reduction and fixation. This will include all fractures of the shaft. Undisplaced fractures of the base of the proximal phalanx can be treated with a bandage thumb spica and clinic review.

Dislocation of the interphalangeal joint: this can be reduced with axial traction under a ring block. A Mallett splint is then applied and fracture clinic review arranged.

Fractures of the distal phalanx: these fractures usually follow a crushing type of injury. Associated soft-tissue injury predominates. The treatment is the same as that for distal phalangeal injuries of the other fingers (→ *p. 134*).

10

Burns, contamination and irradiation

LARGE BURNS

The skin is the largest organ of the body and constitutes a vital barrier against disease. It is also a major sense organ and one of the main determinants of beauty. Its damage is thus dangerous, painful and distressing. Thermal injuries may also involve the respiratory tract and lead to disturbances of metabolism and thermoregulation.

Immediate assessment and management

- Ensure an adequate airway. Give a high concentration of oxygen.
- Remove the source of the burn. Cut off clothes. Flood the affected area with cold water if there is still evidence of heat transfer.
- Look for evidence of inhalation injury (→ *later*). If there is wheezing, give nebulised salbutamol.
- Measure the arterial blood gases and carboxyhaemoglobin level.
- Estimate the extent of the burn (→ *p. 137*). If more than 15% of skin area (or more than 10% in a patient <10 or >70 years), set up an intravenous (IV) infusion and take blood for haemoglobin, PCV (packed cell volume), urea and electrolytes (U&Es), and glucose.
- Monitor the pulse, BP (blood pressure) and SaO_2 (arterial O_2 saturation).
- Assess the level of consciousness; if depressed consider carbon monoxide poisoning → *p. 292*.
- Obtain brief details of the incident and the patient.
- Give adequate IV analgesia.

- Assess the depth of the burn (→ *p. 137*). If there are extensive, deep burns, cross-match blood and consider colloid infusion.
- Cover burns with sterile towels, dry dressings or Clingfilm.
- Insert a urinary catheter and measure the output of urine.
- Consider the possibility of other injuries.

Inhalation injury

Inhalation of hot smoke and fumes is common in patients exposed to house fires. This may cause:

- direct thermal injury to the respiratory tract
- bronchospasm
- delayed pulmonary oedema
- systemic poisoning.

Direct thermal damage to the respiratory tract is uncommon in the otherwise minimally injured victim of a fire. In a more seriously burned patient, it may lead to severe oedema and a rapid onset of airway obstruction. This may also result from delayed sloughing of tracheal or bronchial mucosa. Such patients may need fibreoptic bronchoscopy.

Fumes may contain gases that impair surfactant activity and irritate the respiratory mucosa. Early bronchospasm may occur but there may be no obvious evidence of damage until pulmonary oedema develops some hours later.

Incapacity, which occurs quickly in domestic and industrial fires, is caused by a combination of hypoxia, carbon monoxide poisoning (caused by incomplete combustion) and hydrogen cyanide poisoning. Soft

Emergency Medicine Lecture Notes, Fourth Edition. Chris Moulton and David Yates.
© 2012 Blackwell Publishing Ltd. Published 2012 by Blackwell Publishing Ltd.

furnishings are a particular hazard, producing many toxic substances, including highly irritant and lethal hydrogen chloride.

Inhalation is likely to have occurred if two or more of the following apply:

- History of exposure to fire in enclosed space
- Decreased ability to respond to fire, as with small children, or handicapped or intoxicated patients
- History of impaired consciousness or confusion at any time
- Symptoms or signs of respiratory distress, including irritation of mucous membranes
- Stridor, hoarseness or aphonia
- Production of carboniferous (black) sputum
- Burns around the lips, mouth, throat or nose, including singeing of nasal hairs.

Tx Consider the need for early intubation – before oedema of the upper airway makes this difficult or impossible. Request anaesthetic advice. Endotracheal tubes should be left long and uncut to allow for swelling of the face and airway.

> Suxamethonium may cause a dangerous rise in serum potassium in patients with burns.

- Give high-concentration oxygen
- Give nebulised salbutamol for wheezing
- Estimate arterial blood gases and carboxyhaemoglobin

> Beware of conventional blood gas analyser readings in patients who may have high carboxy- or methaemoglobin levels. The oxygen electrode measures oxygen dissolved in plasma only and O_2 saturation is then calculated assuming all haemoglobin to be normal. Arterial O_2 pressure (PaO_2) and O_2 saturation may thus appear to be satisfactory despite very low total blood O_2 content.

- Save blood for forensic tests
- Request a chest radiograph
- Admit for 24 h observation even if burns appear minimal.

Carbon monoxide poisoning → *p. 292.*
Cyanide poisoning → *p. 296.*

Assessment of a burn

Extent

The extent of a burn is estimated by using the rule of nines in adults (→ *Figure 10.1*). In children, the Lund–Browder chart is used to take account of the relatively larger head and smaller legs (→ *Figure 10.2*). As a useful guide, the surface area of the patient's own outstretched hand is around 1% (or more exactly 0.8%) of the total body surface area.

> Do not take areas of superficial erythema into account when calculating the area of a burn. Make a note of these areas separately.

There is only a slight difference between the volume of fluid lost through partial-thickness and that lost through full-thickness burns, although the extent of erythrocyte destruction is greater in the latter.

Depth

The depth of a burn is a function of:

1. the temperature of the agent causing the burn
2. the length of time that it is in contact with the skin (i.e. the amount of energy transferred). Scalds are associated with a water temperature >50°C.

> It is often very difficult to estimate confidently the depth of a burn in the first few days.

The circumstances leading to the cause of the burn may help. A motorbike exhaust pipe burning through a leather boot may only inflict a superficial burn. Someone with epilepsy or alcohol problems who falls into a fire will sustain deep burns. Elderly patients and those with peripheral neuropathy (e.g. people with diabetes) are at especial risk. Electrical burns are usually very deep.

Clothes closely applied to the skin, such as underwear, socks, belts and collars, tend to trap fluids and potentiate the severity of the burn locally.

Superficial burns expose intact nerve endings and are painful. Deep burns destroy nerve endings and are painless – testing the response to a pinprick may be helpful but is not always reliable. The skin often resembles thick, dry, cream-coloured parchment, unlike the red, angry skin of a superficial burn.

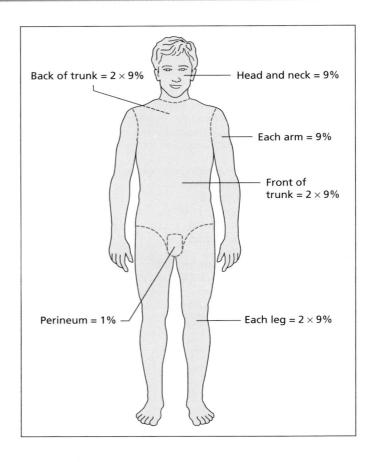

Figure 10.1 The 'rule of nines'.

Back of trunk = 2 × 9%

Head and neck = 9%

Each arm = 9%

Front of trunk = 2 × 9%

Perineum = 1%

Each leg = 2 × 9%

> Infection can easily convert a partial-thickness burn into a full-thickness injury.

Treatment of burns

Flooding with cold water

The damage inflicted by hot fluids may be diminished by flooding the affected part with cold water. Pain is simultaneously reduced. Immediate irrigation for up to 5 min may limit the extent of the burn, but beware of hypothermia, especially in small children.

> Never apply neutralising fluids to acid or alkali burns – the resulting chemical reaction is exothermic.

Analgesia

Analgesia should be given early and always before transfer to another unit. It is usually under-prescribed. The beneficial effects of morphine in small children greatly outweigh any haemodynamic side effects, but it is essential to calculate the initial dose using the patient's weight. Do not be afraid to give further doses as dictated by the state of the patient (→ *p. 13*).

> Most significant burns need IV analgesia.

Intravenous fluids

If the burn involves more than 15% of the skin (10% in children and elderly people) or involves the face (making oral feeding difficult), an IV line must be set

Ignore simple erythema

Partial thickness loss (PTL)
Full thickness loss (FTL)

Region	% PTL	FTL
Head		
Neck		
Anterior. trunk		
Posterior. trunk		
Right arm		
Left arm		
Buttocks		
Genitalia		
Right leg		
Left leg		
Total burn		

Relative percentage of body surface area affected by growth

Area	Age 0	1	5	10	15	Adult
A = 1/2 of head	9 1/2	8 1/2	6 1/2	5 1/2	4 1/2	3 1/2
B = 1/2 of one thigh	2 3/4	3 1/4	4	4 1/2	4 1/2	4 3/4
C = 1/2 of one leg	2 1/2	2 1/2	2 3/4	3	3 1/3	3 1/2

Figure 10.2 The Lund–Browder chart.

up. It will be required for a few days and must be reliable and easy to maintain. Reduced immunological competence increases the risk of infection after burns. An aseptic technique must be used.

The initial fluid should be Hartmann's solution; later on, a colloid may be used. The choice includes synthetic sugars, gelatin and starch, albumin, plasma protein fraction and reconstituted plasma. Most departments use a gelatin solution initially but check the local burns unit's preference. Whole blood will be required if there is a significant element of full-thickness skin loss.

Calculation of fluid requirements → Box 10.1.

Calculated fluids are required in addition to normal metabolic requirements. Fluid loss begins at the time of the burn.

Definitive care of large burns

Patients with large burns must not be kept in the ED for longer than it takes to:

- initiate resuscitation
- exclude, or treat, other major injuries

Box 10.1 Fluid replacement for burns

- Intravenous fluids are required if more than a 15% surface burn (10% in those <10 or >70 years). Hartmann's solution should be used. An initial 10–20 mL/kg can be given whilst awaiting formal calculations
- Isolated areas of erythema are not included in the calculation but cannot be ignored
- No distinction is made between areas of full- and partial-thickness loss at this stage
- Patients who have inhalational injuries in addition to skin burns initially require up to 40% more fluid
- Fluid to be given must be calculated from the time of the burn rather than the time of arrival at hospital
- The Parkland formula is used to calculate the amount of Hartmann's solution required in the first 24 hours following the burn:

$$\text{Weight (kg)} \times \text{Percentage burn} \times 4 \text{ (mL)}$$

Half of this volume should be given during the first 8 hours and the remainder over the following 16 hours.

- An additional amount will be required to satisfy the patient's normal fluid requirements (about 1500 mL/day for a 70-kg man). This will be raised if there is pyrexia
- Urinary output is the best way of monitoring fluid replacement. Plasma substitutes and blood will be required later on if there is a significant element of full-thickness burning

- establish monitoring and investigations
- agree a treatment plan with the local burns unit
- prepare for controlled transfer to the appropriate area.

The indications for admission are based on the extent and site of the burns:

- Burns >15% (>10% in children and elderly people) produce haemodynamic changes, which demand inpatient treatment.
- Burns to the perineum, around the mouth and to the airway will require specialised nursing care.
- Some small burns can be managed safely and effectively only if the patient is in hospital. These include circumferential limb burns and full-thickness loss around the eyes, nose and ears (these are discussed in the next section).

Local arrangements will influence whether admission is to a general surgical ward, an intensive care unit or a specialised burns unit. The last is often some distance from the ED and usually has a limited number of beds. It is inappropriate to refer very severely burned elderly patients to specialised (and often distant) burns units when it is clear that they will die.

> If age + percentage burn ≥100, survival is most unlikely even with optimum care.

Before transfer check the following:

- The airway control is immaculate, and unlikely to deteriorate.
- IV access is adequate and cannula fixed well in place.
- Fluid regimen is agreed and running.
- Monitoring equipment is suitable.
- Charts, notes and laboratory results are with the patient.
- Analgesia is satisfactory and can be topped up.
- Level of nursing/medical care required en route has been considered.

SMALL BURNS

Most burns under 10% of the body surface area can be managed on an outpatient basis. *Exceptions are discussed under Special burns* → p. 142.

Initial assessment and management

Initial action includes:

- the removal of the source of the burn
- flooding with cold water
- analgesia
- assessment of size, site and depth (a drawing is useful) → p. 137.

A temporary dressing, without medication, is applied once the burn area has been exposed and the patient is waiting for definitive care. Analgesia must be given as soon as possible, especially to children.

> Simple erythema is extremely painful. Even patients expected to go home after treatment may need parenteral analgesia.

Box 10.2 **Features of a burn that suggest non-accidental injury**

- Glove or stocking distribution, especially if bilateral
- Involvement of buttocks or perineum
- Scalds with a clearly demarcated edge with no peripheral splash marks
- Small, even, rounded (cigarette tip) burns
- General features of history and presentation suspicious of abuse

Dressing and follow-up of simple superficial burns

Skin debris and foreign material are removed with dilute antiseptic and cotton-wool balls.

> Small blisters should be left alone. Large ones can be slit open at the dependent edge to allow drainage. Complete deroofing is unnecessary and leaves a painful base.

The pattern of burning should be considered in the light of the history available. A scald from spilt water will produce a cascade effect, with streaks of burnt skin following the path of the falling fluid, possibly with increasing depth of injury where its flow has been held up by constricting clothes such as waistbands or socks. A scald with a glove or stocking distribution is unusual; either the patient has impaired peripheral or central pain perception or the limb was held under water. In children, this type of appearance suggests abuse ($\rightarrow$ *Box 10.2* and p. 353).

The depth of the burn influences long-term treatment and should be determined as soon as possible. Superficial erythema is initially painful whereas full-thickness burns will be insensitive because the nerve endings have been destroyed. Most areas of most burns fall between these extremes and are termed partial-thickness burns.

If most of the dermal papillae and all of the skin appendages (hair follicles and sweat glands) are intact, there is a very good potential for spontaneous regeneration. The term 'deep dermal' is used to describe partial-thickness burns with only a few epidermal remnants remaining – usually around the necks of sweat glands and hair follicles. If the wound becomes infected, these cells may die, resulting in full-thickness skin loss. Prevention of infection is thus of paramount importance in deep dermal burns.

There is frequently a combination of partial- and full-thickness burning. The patient may consider the whole area sensitive and it is often difficult to determine depth at the first examination. However, the distinction is usually unimportant in the very early stages of treatment. Most areas of full-thickness loss that require grafts are evident by 5–10 days. Electrical burns may be suitable for the specialised technique of immediate excision and grafting.

A sterile, non-adherent dressing is then applied. Antiseptic substances are not needed for most burns but are often used (e.g. silver sulfadiazine or mupirocin cream). Healing will occur more rapidly in a moist environment, but excess exudate should be kept away from the wound surface. A moist wound surface reduces damage to the new epithelium when the dressing is changed and is less painful. Specialised dressings are available that retain excess exudate and allow gas exchange but they are expensive. Technique and experience are as important as dressing material.

The wound dressing is covered with a more robust gauze for added protection. Limb burns should be elevated, but the patient encouraged to move the burned part as much as possible. Stiffness will develop quickly and is slow to resolve once established. Routine prophylaxis with antibiotics is not indicated.

The burn should be reassessed within 36–48 h. Dressings should be changed no more than three times in the first week and less frequently thereafter. Most patients can be taught to dress small burns at home. Elderly patients can be treated at home by the district nurse or at the local health centre. All burns to special areas and full-thickness burns should be reviewed in the ED.

Once the wound has fully epithelialised, and has thus become dry, it should be exposed to a clean environment but protected from dirt and friction by temporary dry dressings. A moisturising cream can be applied to replace the sweat gland secretions, which are often deficient for some months after burning. The patient should be warned that the skin will be especially sensitive to ultraviolet light throughout the following summer.

Skin grafting of burns

Some electrical burns are most effectively treated by initial excision and early grafting and are best referred immediately to a burns unit. However, most small, simple burns treated on an outpatient basis in an ED should be managed conservatively for at least the first 5 days.

Wounds under 2 cm in diameter usually contract and close spontaneously, even if there is full-thickness skin loss. Larger wounds will show evidence of marginal and focal epithelialisation. It should be possible to distinguish deep-dermal from full-thickness burns within 10 days of the injury. If the former remain sterile, thereby avoiding destruction of the epithelial remnants, they will heal spontaneously. The latter will require split-skin grafts. *The technique is described on p. 395.*

SPECIAL BURNS

Burns to the face

Inhalation burns must be excluded ($\rightarrow$ *p. 136*). The patient may have deceptively good function when first assessed but can deteriorate over 24 h. Swelling is a major problem:

- Patients with burns to the eyelids and cornea must be admitted to a specialised eye unit. Lid retraction may cause major problems. Apply an antibiotic (e.g. chloramphenicol) eye ointment before transfer.
- Burns around the mouth cause feeding problems. Inpatient care is usually required. The burns unit should be contacted for advice.
- Deep burns involving the nose and ear may destroy underlying cartilage and should always be referred for specialised care.
- Partial-thickness burns of other areas of the face can be adequately treated on an outpatient basis. Silver sulfadiazine cream is applied very sparingly and repeated by the patient at home, once or twice per day. The area may blacken and be unsightly, but this is not harmful. No other dressing is required. Chloramphenicol ointment should be prescribed if the burns have encroached on the periorbital area.

Burns to the hands

The fingers quickly stiffen up and conventional bandages become very dirty, with an increased risk of infection. These complications are avoided if plastic gloves are used initially instead of standard dressings. Silver sulfadiazine cream is applied and a loosely fitting examination glove is fitted in place with tape around the wrist. The gloves tend to burst, so patients must be given a supply to apply by themselves.

Patients are encouraged to move the hand as much as possible. The skin becomes macerated and the exudate and silver sulfadiazine produce an aesthetically unpleasant sight. Coloured gloves overcome some of the patient's understandable anxieties but reassurance should be given that the maceration will resolve rapidly once the glove is removed.

Burns to the perineum

The perineum must be examined carefully. It is a common site for non-accidental burns. Any burns to the top of the thighs or on the buttocks, which cannot be adequately dressed, and all those nearer the perineum, which cannot easily be kept clean, must be managed in hospital. A short-stay ward may be appropriate, but extensive or full-thickness burns should be referred to the burns unit.

Circumferential burns

If a partial- or full-thickness burn extends completely around a limb the distal circulation may become impaired. Minor degrees of venous obstruction can be treated by admission and elevation. Deep burns, which will quickly contract, may cause more serious obstruction. Similar complications may occur on the trunk causing respiratory distress. Escharotomy may be required. This is associated with significant fluid loss and must not be undertaken without expert advice.

Chemical burns

Acidic solutions produce painful coagulation burns, which are often self-limiting and superficial with destruction of the surface epithelium and submucosa only. Concentrated and corrosive acids such as phenol and hydrofluoric acid ($\rightarrow$ *p. 143*) may cause deep burns with systemic absorption. Alkaline solutions produce deep, full-thickness liquefaction burns that can be surprisingly pain free at first. However, there is extensive damage that is due to solubilisation of proteins such as collagen, saponification of lipids and dehydration of tissue cells.

Tx No attempt should be made to neutralise chemicals on the skin (*except hydrofluoric acid* $\rightarrow$ *p. 143*). Most neutralising reactions are exothermic and would cause an additional thermal injury. Dilution by continuous irrigation with water for at least 10–15 min (or until the pH of the burned area is normal) is the mainstay of treatment. Prolonged irrigation with cold water also reduces pain significantly. Caution must be exercised with young children who quickly become hypothermic. Systemic absorption of some chemicals (e.g. phenol) may be significant. Toxicological advice should be sought.

Hydrofluoric acid burns

Hydrofluoric acid (hydrogen fluoride) is used extensively in industry and horticulture. Skin contact causes severe local tissue damage with a great deal of pain. The burn is deep and slow to heal. With solutions containing less than 50% hydrofluoric acid there may be a delay until the burn develops as follows:

- Anhydrous or >50% concentrations – immediate damage
- 20–50% concentrations – up to 8h delay
- <20% concentrations – up to 24h delay.

Even concentrations of acid as low as 2% may cause burns after prolonged skin contact.

Investigations: Significant absorption of fluoride ion through the skin may cause hypocalcaemia. Cardiac arrest may occur in the extensively burned patient. The serum calcium should be checked in all patients with larger burns resulting from contact with hydrogen fluoride.

Tx Immediate irrigation of the contaminated area is essential and may be very effective. Pain, tissue destruction and hypocalcaemia can be reduced by converting the acid to its calcium salt. This is achieved by repeated application of calcium gluconate gel (marketed as hydrofluoric acid burn jelly). There is no exothermic reaction. The injection of 10% calcium gluconate around and under the burn is sometimes advocated for persistent pain in well-localised lesions.

White phosphorus burns

White (or yellow) phosphorus is commonly used in incendiary devices and so may cause severe burns. Exposure to phosphorus can lead to hypokalaemia, hypocalcaemia and hypophosphataemia. In addition, toxic phosphorus pentoxide gas can be released, which is irritant to the lungs.

Tx Injuries and burns that are contaminated with white phosphorus require special and unique management:

- The burned area should be lavaged copiously to remove identifiable particles (which should be placed in water to prevent spontaneous combustion). A Woods lamp (in a darkened room) may help to identify phosphorus particles. The burned area

must be kept covered with saline-soaked gauze to prevent further combustion.
- Definitive treatment consists of a rinse using 1% copper sulphate ($CuSO_4$) solution to aid removal of the particles of phosphorus. Copper sulphate combines with phosphorous to create a blue–black cupric phosphide coating. This impedes further combustion and makes phosphorus particles easier to find. The burn is irrigated with copper sulphate solution, particles are removed and then the copper sulphate is lavaged away with saline. Excess copper sulphate absorption can cause intravascular haemolysis and renal failure.

Chemical burns from giant hogweed

The plant *Heracleum mantegazzianum* – better known as giant hogweed – is a public health hazard and an environmental nuisance. In addition to its toxicity, this aggressive foreign invader prevents native plant species from growing and increases soil erosion. Under the Wildlife and Countryside Act 1981 and the Wildlife (Northern Ireland) Order 1985, it is an offence to 'plant or otherwise cause giant hogweed to grow'. Despite this, the species is common in the British Isles and is found alongside roads, railway lines, rivers and footpaths, often in areas of wasteland. The plant is characterised by its size. Over a period of 4 years, it may grow up to 5m in height and looks rather like an overgrown cow parsley. It has a reddish-purple stem and spotted leaf stalks with fine spines that make it appear furry. The leaves may be up to 1.5m in width with large flowering heads. These characteristics make the giant hogweed plant irresistible to children who make swords and umbrellas from it.

Unfortunately, giant hogweed exudes a clear watery sap from its leaves and also from the stem in even greater quantities. This sap contains a glucoside called furanocoumarin, which renders the skin photosensitive to ultraviolet (UV) light. Exposure to sunlight after contact with the sap results in large painful blisters, burns and linear inflammation. This reaction usually appears within 15–20h of contact although it can occur up to 48h later. Damaged skin heals very slowly over at least 2 weeks, leaving residual pigmentation that can develop into chronic phytophotodermatitis. Inflammation may recur in sunlight for many months.

Tx In the event of contact with giant hogweed sap, the skin should be washed immediately with soap and water and then covered to reduce the exposure to sunlight. Application of topical steroids, if started early in the inflammatory process, can reduce the severity of the developing burns. Otherwise, partial-thickness lesions are treated with dressings and analgesia until healing occurs. Advice about subsequent UV light exposure should be given to all patients.

Burns from hot tar

Hot bitumen solidifies on contact with the skin. Water should be applied at the site to hasten hardening and limit heat transfer. Bitumen on blistering skin should be removed with the blister. Adherent bitumen should be left in place and covered with paraffin gauze. This will help to dissolve and separate it. Earlier excision would inflict more damage.

Sunburn

Unprotected exposure to UV radiation can cause extremely painful, blistering, oedematous skin. In general, the treatment is as for any other burn. However, the pain of the intense erythema that so often results can be greatly alleviated by the regular application of 1% hydrocortisone cream.

ELECTROCUTION

High-voltage injury (including lightning)

Injuries following a high-voltage electric shock may result from the following:

- Falling or being thrown to the ground, causing secondary injuries
- Tetanic muscle contraction, causing fractures of long bones, crushed vertebrae, torn muscles
- Spontaneous ignition of clothing, causing burns
- Conduction of electricity through the body, causing entry and exit wounds and internal injuries
- Current passing along the surface of the body to earth, causing very deep burns over a large area of skin
- Current jumping from one part of the body to another, causing secondary exit and entry wounds.

The patient may have a respiratory or cardiac arrest. If this is successfully reversed or if the patient presents without having had a life-threatening cardiac dysrhythmia, it is unlikely that one will develop subsequently. Supraventricular tachycardia has been reported, but more commonly the ECG shows right bundle-branch block and/or ST changes. These may last many weeks. Treatment is based on symptoms and clinical signs in the normal way.

Cardiac markers will be raised irrespective of cardiac damage and so their measurement is not helpful.

If the current travels through the body, it naturally follows the path of least resistance. Nerves and blood vessels are good conductors. Increasing resistance is offered by muscle, skin, tendon, fat and bone in that order. Structures with high resistance will generate the greatest heat but, clearly, some tissues are more readily damaged by heat than others. Nerves, blood vessels, muscles and skin sustain most of the injury.

The entry point is typically charred and depressed. It becomes swollen very quickly, with the accumulation of extracellular fluid. The exit point has an explosive appearance – round or oval grey craters with no inflammatory changes. These increase in size over the first few days.

In the peripheral nerves, axons are distorted and Schwann cells break down and coalesce. Spinal cord lesions are surprisingly common, often producing partial transections. Brain damage is unusual unless the head has been directly involved.

Blood vessels sustain endothelial damage and media degeneration. Thrombosis and late rupture can occur at sites distant from the entry point. Visceral lesions, which are often unrecognised, probably have a vascular aetiology.

Muscle involvement is typically patchy, with swelling, necrosis and the later development of deep sepsis.

Acute tubular necrosis is common. Inadequate volume replacement, myoglobinuria and direct damage to renal vessels probably all contribute to its development.

Cataracts are a well-recognised, late complication.

Late death is commonly caused by overwhelming sepsis. However, there is only a one in several million chance of being killed by lightning in the UK!

Characteristic signs in patients struck by lightning → Box 10.3.

Tx Treatment in the ED is directed towards stabilisation of any life-threatening dysrhythmia and the early transfusion of crystalloid. Fluid loss cannot be calculated by burns formulae. The volume required is titrated against central venous pressure (CVP), pulse and BP to maintain a high urine output. Blood gases and plasma U&Es (including creatinine) should be measured. Acidosis is common in patients with extensive electrocution injuries and bicarbonate is often required.

The care of all patients who have been electrocuted must be discussed with a senior member of staff. Extensive soft-tissue injuries will be assessed in the main theatre. Tissue loss can be minimised by very

Box 10.3 Characteristic signs of injury by lightning

- Damaged clothing
- Surface burns in linear or arborescent patterns (the latter describes a branching distribution sometimes likened to leaves on a tree)
- Tiny necrotic burns around the edges of the feet and toes
- Ruptured tympanic membranes

early fasciotomy and removal of dead tissue. However, because of the patchy nature of the muscle involvement, this process is not as easy as with muscle damage resulting from direct injury. Occult visceral damage must also be considered.

Antitetanus prophylaxis is required for all patients.

Low-voltage injury

Low-voltage burns of the type sustained from the domestic electricity supply are not usually associated with the above complications. However, the local burn is almost always full thickness and much deeper than it appears. The area of tissue necrosis may extend over the first few days. Senior advice should be sought. Early excision and grafting are often favoured by specialised burns units. Continuous ECG monitoring is not required.

CONTAMINATION AND IRRADIATION

Contamination by toxic chemicals

In the UK, the National Focus for Chemical Incidents (based at the University of Wales Institute in Cardiff) monitors and provides advice on all types of chemical incidents. There is a 24-hour emergency hotline.

Tx at the scene The senior fire officer is responsible for identification of the substance(s) involved and for deciding the level of protection appropriate for personnel and the environment. The fire service will usually carry out immediate decontamination using running water. The patient should be kept warm and removed to a well-ventilated and protected area. Resuscitation may need to precede decontami-

nation, in which case direct skin and mucosal contact with the patient should be avoided.

Tx in the ED The contaminated patient should be taken to a designated area. If volatile substances are involved, the hospital engineers must be alerted to prevent contamination of the air-conditioning systems. Staff should wear protective clothing; gloves and gown are usually sufficient. Further decontamination of the patient may be achieved by washing with soap and water or showering for 20 min. A special bath with a collecting tub for contaminated water should be used and movements of the patient in the department must be kept to a minimum. Some substances (e.g. phenol) may cause severe systemic poisoning by skin contact alone.

Contamination by radioactive substances

On average, there is one serious radiation incident – resulting in death or major radiation injury – in the world each year. In the last 50 years, there have been more than 200 incidents involving lost, stolen or misused sources of radiation. Recent anti-terrorist concerns include the possibility of exposure from a 'dirty bomb' (conventional explosive used to disperse radioactive material), a low-yield improvised nuclear device or a deliberately hidden source of radiation.

A person is contaminated when radioactive material is deposited on skin and/or clothing (external contamination) or into the body (internal contamination) by inhalation, ingestion or absorption via a wound.

Measurement of radioactivity and radiation → Box 10.5 on p. 146.
Types of ionising radiation → Box 10.4 on p. 146.

Symptoms and signs of external contamination

There may be no symptoms or signs although heavy contamination will provoke redness and burning of the skin. The patient must be informed about the importance of decontamination for both personal and public health reasons.

Box 10.4 **Types of ionising radiation**

Ionising radiation is a form of energy that is emitted spontaneously by radioactive materials. It is invisible, odourless and tasteless. Natural radiation is present all around us: in air from cosmic rays, in the earth and building materials, and in food and water. This comprises the background radiation to which we are all constantly exposed. Man-made sources of radiation and radioactive materials are used widely in medicine, scientific research, industry and radiographic detection systems.

- **Alpha particles** are heavy, highly charged and interact strongly with atoms. As a result, they lose momentum rapidly, can travel only very short distances and cannot penetrate human skin. Alpha emitters are hazardous only when inhaled, ingested, injected or absorbed through a wound
- **Beta particles** are also charged but interact less strongly with atoms than alpha particles. Consequently, they travel further and penetrate more: they can enter the skin. Clothing (including standard personal protective equipment [PPE]) provides some protection against them. Beta particles can cause radiation skin injury on prolonged exposure but are hazardous to internal organs only when inhaled, ingested, injected or absorbed through a wound
- **Gamma rays** and their man-made equivalent, **X-rays**, are uncharged and so do not interact directly with atoms. They travel many metres in air and can easily penetrate the human body and cause organ damage. Their effects can be attenuated by concrete or lead shielding
- **Neutrons** are uncharged particles that travel far and penetrate everything except thick layers of concrete and water. They are highly damaging but only likely to be produced in the very early stages of a nuclear detonation or accident

 Box 10.5 **Measurement of radioactivity and radiation**

Radiation is readily detectable with equipment, and contamination is easily measurable. Medical physics and nuclear medicine departments and frontline services all have equipment for detecting beta and gamma radiation and people trained to use it.

- **Radioactivity (and contamination by radioactive material)** is measured in becquerels (1 Bq = 1 disintegration/s)
- **The absorbed dose** of radiation (the amount of energy absorbed per unit mass of tissue) is measured in grays (1 Gy = 1 J/kg tissue)

Different types of radiation have different effects on human tissue. In equivalent dosages measured in grays, alpha particles and neutrons are more damaging than beta particles, gamma rays or X-rays in terms of the risks of cancer or of in heritable genetic defects. To account for this, the absorbed dosage is multiplied by a 'radiation weighting factor' to produce:

- **The equivalent dose** (of an organ or tissue) measured in sieverts (Sv). For X-rays, gamma rays and beta particles, the weighting factor = 1 and so 1 Gy = 1 Sv = 1000 mSv. Some organs are more radiosensitive than others (e.g. the bone marrow is more sensitive than the thyroid) and exposures are rarely uniform. Weighting the equivalent doses received by different organs and tissues during an exposure to allow for each organ's radiosensitivity, and then summing the results, gives the **effective dose**. An estimate of the **whole body dose** is helpful in estimating long-term cancer risk

Tx of external contamination at the scene

It is the responsibility of the police to seek advice and take appropriate measures to secure the scene.

Tx of external contamination in the ED

- The local radiation protection officer should be contacted for advice and to measure the level of radioactive contamination.
- A predetermined and separate entrance and treatment area for isolation and decontamination should be demarcated. This area must have a shower and water collection facility as detailed above. Floors of treatment and transit areas should be covered with disposable sheeting, as should non-disposable equipment. Air conditioning must be switched off and portable equipment removed.
- Involved staff must wear theatre suits, long plastic aprons, caps, overshoes and two pairs of gloves.

- Patients and staff must not eat, drink or smoke within the designated area.
- There must be a place to decontaminate staff on arrival from the scene and before leaving the designated area. All personnel involved must be checked by the radiation protection adviser and should have a shower before leaving this area.
- Resuscitation is still the first priority but efforts must be made throughout to limit the spread of radioactive particles.
- Levels of radiation should be measured before and after decontamination.
- All clothing, swabs and fluids should be handled carefully and collected in labelled bags and containers. Removal of clothing can reduce external contamination by as much as 90%!
- Areas of the body unprotected by clothing take priority. Hands and nails should be cleaned with running water and surgical scrub for 5 min. Hair must be washed (with any shampoo) in a similar way; showers should not be taken while the hair is contaminated. The face should be cleaned and ears and eyes irrigated. The nose must be blown and the mouth washed out. Vacuum cleaning is sometimes recommended. If radiation monitoring confirms residual contamination of skin, then cleaning should be attempted with 5% potassium permanganate solution for 5 min. The brown staining is removed by the application of 5% sodium bisulphite. This system gives a visual confirmation of coverage and removal.
- Wounds must be covered before surface decontamination and later cleaned by direct irrigation.
- A member of staff should be tasked with recording all patient movements around the department.

Symptoms and signs of internal contamination

In 2006, a man died in a London hospital after unwittingly ingesting a drink containing polonium-210. This naturally occurring radionuclide has a half-life of 138 days. It undergoes decay by emitting alpha particles, accompanied by very low intensity gamma radiation.

At high internal radiation doses, patients develop acute radiation syndrome ($\rightarrow$ *below*) and necrosis of internal tissues. However with substances that emit alpha particles (such as polonium-210) symptoms are more limited. The most common route for internal contamination is ingestion (often from contaminated hands), and then nausea, vomiting and diarrhoea are the initial symptoms. (These are also the early symptoms of classic radiation sickness.) Most ingested polonium-210 passes out of the body in the faeces but the urine and other body fluids will also be contaminated.

Measurement of radioactivity and radiation $\rightarrow$ *Box 10.5.*
Treatment of internal contamination by radioactive substances $\rightarrow$ *p. 149.*
Types of ionising radiation $\rightarrow$ *Box 10.4.*

It is important to distinguish between patients who have been contaminated by radioactive particles and those who have been irradiated. The former can spread radiation; the latter cannot. Some will be in both categories.

Exposure to radioactive substances (irradiation) and acute radiation syndrome

Radiation exposure occurs when all or part of the body is irradiated. Three key factors affect exposure: duration, distance and shielding. If the exposure time is halved, then the dose of radiation is halved. The inverse square law applies to distance: doubling the distance between the source and the body reduces the dose by a factor of four; trebling the distance between the source and the body reduces the dose by a factor of nine; and so on. In the same way that a patient who has had a radiograph presents no risk to others, radiation safety precautions are not needed for patients who have been exposed to radiation but are not contaminated.

At low doses of radiation that are equivalent to whole body doses of up to 1 Gy (equivalent to about 50000 chest radiographs) there are no acute symptoms. The hazard is an increase in the lifetime risk of cancer that is quite modest compared with the 'background' cancer risk.

Measurement of radioactivity and radiation $\rightarrow$ *Box 10.5 on p. 146.*
Types of ionising radiation $\rightarrow$ *Box 10.4 on p. 146.*

Many radiation accidents cause partial body injury: early erythema followed by bullae and, if severe, ulceration and necrosis (often of the hands). This may not necessarily progress to acute radiation syndrome (ARS). ARS follows a large, usually external exposure of all or most of the body to penetrating radiation (gamma rays, high-energy X-rays or neutrons) in a short time (seconds, minutes or hours). Symptoms of ARS occur in four phases: prodromal phase → latent period → illness → recovery or death. As the radiation dose increases, the prodromal and latent periods shorten and the severity of illness and the risk of mortality increase. Major trauma and radiation exposure interact synergistically on mortality.

> If there are no symptoms (such as nausea or vomiting) in the first 6 h after a suspected exposure, then serious acute radiation sickness is unlikely.

Features suggestive of significant penetrating irradiation that may progress to full radiation sickness include the following:

- A history of loss of consciousness (this suggests a high dose of radiation with a bad prognosis)
- Transient erythema after 24 h
- Early nausea, diarrhoea and vomiting (especially within 1 h of exposure)
- An early and dramatic fall in the white cell count.

Dose-related symptoms and signs of ARS → Box 10.6.

Tx

> Assume that all patients are contaminated until you know that they are not!

Initial symptoms of ARS are non-specific and rarely immediately life threatening; treatment of other injuries therefore takes priority.

- Commence standard resuscitation measures.
- Do not handle unfamiliar objects or embedded fragments directly.
- Relieve pain with morphine; give cyclizine or odansetron for nausea and vomiting.
- Obtain and record as much information as possible about the type and extent of the exposure in order to help assessment of the dose of radiation received.

Box 10.6 Dose-related features of acute radiation syndrome

<1 Sv: *usually asymptomatic*
- Mild symptoms in up to 10% of people of episodic nausea and vomiting for 48 h
- Slightly depressed white blood cell (WBC) count at 2–4 weeks post-exposure
- No fetal effects if the effective dose <100 mSv (100 000 mcSv) but counselling needed if pregnant and effective dose >100 mSv (100 000 mcSv)

1–8 Sv: *haematopoietic syndrome*
- Anorexia, nausea, vomiting and fatigue between 1 and 4 hours after exposure (the timing and severity are dose related)
- Latent period of between 2 days and 4 weeks and then
- Bone marrow depression (leukopenia and infection; low platelets and bleeding)
- Serial lymphocyte counts in the first 48 h predict the severity
- Hair loss after 2 or 3 weeks after a dose of >3 or 4 Sv
- Lethal dose (LD) 50/60 is around 4.5 Sv without treatment

>6 Sv: *gastrointestinal syndrome*
- Early nausea, vomiting, diarrhoea, anorexia and fatigue
- Latent period of up to 1 week and then
- Severe gastrointestinal (GI) symptoms (fever, abdominal pain, watery diarrhoea, GI haemorrhage, electrolyte imbalance and dehydration)
- Bone marrow depression (leukopenia and infection; low platelets and bleeding)
- LD 100 is about 10 Sv; death usually occurs within 2 weeks

>20 Sv: *central nervous system/cardiovascular system syndrome*
- Burning sensation on the skin
- Almost immediate projectile vomiting and explosive bloody diarrhoea
- Headache, collapse, agitation, confusion and loss of consciousness
- May be a lucid interval (hours) and then
- Convulsions, coma, hypotension, shock and death within 2–3 days

Figure 10.3 Comparative doses of radiation.

- Take routine blood samples including a baseline full blood count. Perform serial absolute lymphocyte counts every 3 or 4 h for the first 12 h after an acute exposure and then 6-hourly for the next 48 h.
- Arrange HLA typing and chromosome analysis (venous blood and nasal swabs).
- Test for internal contamination by faecal sampling or 24-hour urine collection.

Early expert advice (e.g. from departments of medical physics or nuclear medicine, the Health Protection Agency or the Ministry of Defence) is essential for formal radiation dose assessment and the management of internal contamination. The development of radiation sickness is a delayed phenomenon and at-risk patients should be referred to the nearest oncology or haematology unit after discussion with the local radiation protection adviser. A history of irradiation should not delay surgery. As a result of the immunosuppressive effect of the radiation, if the dose is more than 1 Sv, all surgery should be carried out as soon as possible and certainly within 36–48 h of the incident. If this is not possible, then recovery of the bone marrow must be awaited.

Comparative doses of radiation → Figure 10.3.

11

Cardiac arrest and cardiac dysrhythmias

This chapter covers the essential theoretical and practical aspects of cardiac arrest and dysrhythmia management. However, it does not claim to equip the reader with all the skills necessary for leading a resuscitation team. To achieve such competence, it is essential to have participated in an Advanced Life Support or similar course.

The protocols and algorithms used in this chapter are taken from the guidelines published in 2010 by the Resuscitation Council (UK). As such, they are consistent with the European Resuscitation Council (ERC) Guidelines for Resuscitation 2010 and are based on the current recommendations of the International Liaison Committee on Resuscitation (ILCOR).

Cardiac arrest in hypothermic patients also → p. 244.

Choking → p. 196.

Resuscitation Council (UK) algorithm for life support of the newborn infant → Figure 17.2 on p. 319.

Resuscitation Council (UK) algorithms for the treatment of choking in adults and children → Figures 13.1 and 13.2 on p. 197.

Resuscitation of the newborn infant also → Box 17.2 on p. 318.

CARDIAC ARREST

In 20% of people with cardiac arrest there is no previous history of ischaemic heart disease.

The heart is a pump with an electrical controlling system. Its power supply comes from burning fuel with oxygen. It stops functioning in three main ways:

1 Failure of the oxygen supply causes asystole (or extreme bradycardia). There is no electrical activity and no pumping.
2 Failure of electrical control causes ventricular fibrillation (VF) or pulseless ventricular tachycardia (VT). There is no effective electrical activity and no effective pumping.
3 Failure of the pump mechanism causes pulseless electrical activity (PEA) (formerly known as electromechanical dissociation or EMD). There is electrical activity but no pumping.

Asystole is the final rhythm in all cases. The underlying causes of the three arrest rhythms are described below.

Asystole

Similar to any other pump, the heart slows and stops when deprived of its power supply. This results from:

- hypoxia or
- a condition leading to hypoxia (e.g. hypovolaemia).

Tachycardia during hypoxia is the result of the influence of the autonomic nervous system. Left to its own devices, the hypoxic heart contracts more slowly (terminal bradycardia) and then arrests in asystole.

Ventricular fibrillation

Ventricular fibrillation is caused by direct damage or irritation of the heart. This may be because of:

Emergency Medicine Lecture Notes, Fourth Edition. Chris Moulton and David Yates.
© 2012 Blackwell Publishing Ltd. Published 2012 by Blackwell Publishing Ltd.

- myocardial ischaemia or infarction
- poisoning
- gross electrolyte imbalance
- hypothermia and near drowning
- electrocution
- penetrating trauma
- iatrogenic causes (e.g. cardioversion and cardiac catheterisation).

In adults VF is most commonly seen in patients with ischaemic heart disease whereas, in children, poisoning with tricyclic antidepressants should always be considered. Pulseless VT is a similar condition to VF in both causation and treatment. Unfortunately, these 'shockable' rhythms occur less than half the time, accounting for only 40% of prehospital cardiac arrests and 25% of arrests in hospital.

Pulseless electrical activity

Pulseless electrical activity is that state when the pump (the myocardium) is unable to function despite a relatively normal electrical stimulus (the ECG signal). This can be because of primary damage to the cardiac muscle including:

- extensive myocardial infarction
- ruptured cardiac aneurysm
- papillary muscle rupture
- extreme direct trauma

or because of various secondary causes (some of which may be treatable):

- tension pneumothorax
- cardiac tamponade
- pulmonary embolism (PE)
- hypovolaemia
- hypothermia
- poisoning
- electrolyte imbalance.

In adults, myocardial infarction (MI) is the most common cause of PEA, whereas hypovolaemia should be suspected in children. PEA should not be confused with an agonal rhythm ($\rightarrow$ *p. 161*).

> Many patients with a diagnosis of PEA will, in fact, have a very low output state rather than complete circulatory arrest.

The chain of survival

Survival from cardiac arrest is most likely if:

- the arrest is witnessed (and recognised!)
- the initial rhythm is VF (or VT).

Thereafter, the chain of survival depends on the patient receiving the following:

1 Basic life support (especially chest compressions) at scene
2 Defibrillation as soon as possible
3 Advanced life support from trained health professionals
4 Good post-resuscitation care.

Complete failure of the circulation for more than 3 or 4 minutes leads to irreversible brain damage.

There are only three interventions that are known to increase the survival from cardiac arrest: chest compression, defibrillation and airway management. The aim of life support must be to deliver these three treatments to the patient in the shortest possible time.

> Even after a cardiac arrest in hospital, less than 20% of adults will survive to go home

Cardiac arrest in children

Children's hearts usually arrest as a result of hypoxia secondary to respiratory distress or depression, or hypovolaemia (fluid loss or maldistribution). These conditions lead to asystole, which has a very poor prognosis. Coronary artery disease and thus VF are extremely uncommon in children.

Cardiac arrest protocols for children $\rightarrow$ pp. 153 and 156.
Drug and defibrillation dosages and equipment sizes for children $\rightarrow$ pp. 157, 158 and 159.
Intraosseous access $\rightarrow$ Box 18.4 on p. 332.

Basic life support

Choking and airway obstruction $\rightarrow$ p. 196.
Resuscitation Council (UK) algorithm for BLS for adults $\rightarrow$ Figure 11.1.
Resuscitation Council (UK) algorithm for BLS for children $\rightarrow$ Figure 11.2.

The manual methods of BLS (Schafer's, Silvester's and the Holger–Nielsen procedures) were replaced by exhaled air resuscitation in the late 1950s. In 1960, Kouwenhoven, Jude and Knickerbocker reminded the world of the efficacy of closed chest compression and thus modern BLS was born. There are four elements:

1 Initial assessment
2 Airway clearance and maintenance
3 Rescue breathing
4 Chest compression to support the circulation.

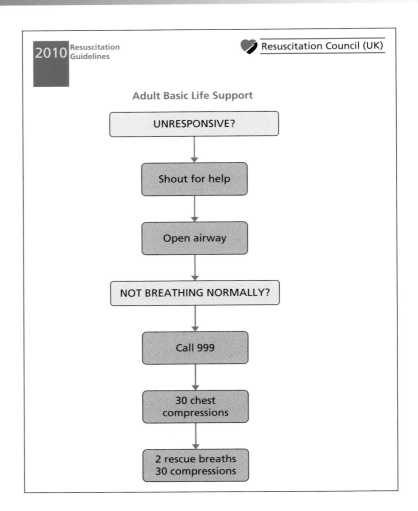

Figure 11.1 Basic life support for adults. Reproduced with the kind permission of the Resuscitation Council (UK).

Basic life support is not very effective – even optimal chest compressions do not achieve more than 30% of the normal blood flow to the brain and 15% of the normal coronary blood flow. It is thus essential to restart the heart within a few minutes (→ *The chain of survival above*).

In adults, arrest is usually a primary cardiac event and so most effort relates to obtaining a defibrillator as soon as possible, even if this means leaving a pulseless patient to go to a telephone before starting chest compressions. Minimally interrupted chest compressions are then the primary focus of BLS. In children, more attention is given to the correction of hypoxia and so resuscitation, starting with five rescue breaths, should be performed for about 1 minute before an isolated rescuer goes for help.

(The exception to this recommendation is a child with a sudden witnessed collapse when a shockable rhythm is more likely.) Adults who are victims of drowning should also be given five breaths and a short period of cardiopulmonary resuscitation (CPR) before seeking assistance. BLS for adults is now taught assuming one rescuer who will perform sequences of 30 compressions to 2 ventilations. Two-rescuer CPR (using the same compression:ventilation ratio of 30:2) is taught to professionals only. For children, the 30:2 ratio is taught to lay rescuers but two or more health professionals should use a 15:2 sequence. The only exception is neonates where a 3:1 ratio of compressions to ventilations is advocated. After successful endotracheal intubation, the synchronisation of compression and ventilation is

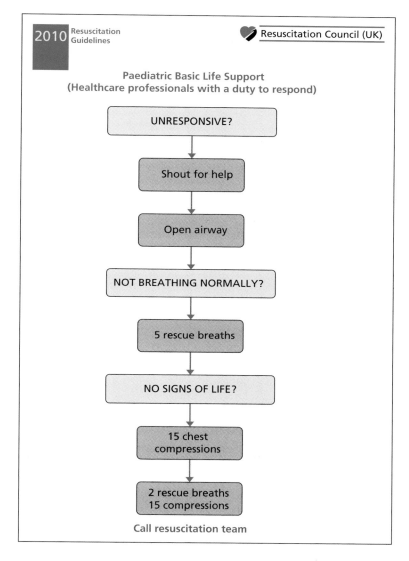

Figure 11.2 Basic life support for children. Reproduced with the kind permission of the Resuscitation Council (UK).

abandoned and the two operations are performed independently.

Initial assessment

- Make sure that the victim, any bystanders and yourself are safe.
- Shake and shout 'Are you alright?'.
- If the patient is responsive, leave them in the position found (or in the recovery position if safer), try to find out what is wrong and get help. Review the situation regularly.

- If the patient is unresponsive, call for help (or go for help if alone). Turn the victim on to his or her back, open the airway and, in less than 10 seconds, look for chest movements, listen at the mouth for sounds and feel for air flow on your cheek.
- If the patient is breathing normally, turn him or her into the recovery position, get help and continue monitoring the situation.
- If the patient is not breathing, call for help (or go for help if alone) and then start chest compressions.

Chest compression

> Chest compression is more important than ventilation in BLS and, as a single therapy, gives far better results than inactivity. (Chest compression-only CPR may be effective for up to 5 min!) The Resuscitation Council (UK) 2010 guidelines emphasise the importance of chest movements at the expense of rescue breathing.

Even the best external chest compression provides poor core circulation. Squeezing the chest results in cardiac valve deformation and incompetence which allows regurgitation of blood into the inferior vena cava. Retrograde flow up the superior vena cava is reduced by a valvular effect where the superior vena cava enters the chest. Forward flow to the brain is thus more likely to occur than forward flow to the trunk. In contrast, coronary artery perfusion, which normally occurs only in diastole against a closed aortic valve, is very poor during BLS. A coronary perfusion pressure <15 mmHg has been shown to be unlikely to lead to a return of spontaneous circulation and the average coronary perfusion pressure during manual CPR is only around 12.5 mmHg.

Mechanical chest compression → p. 161.

The mechanism by which BLS produces cardiac output remains unclear; there is probably a combination of direct cardiac compression and intrathoracic pressure fluctuations. Their relative importance may vary between individuals, depending on the shape and elasticity of the chest. At the current time, Resuscitation Council teaching assumes that direct cardiac compression is the most important factor – hence the emphasis on correct site and adequate depth. A compression rate of about 100/min is recommended for both adults and children. The weight of the resuscitator's body is transmitted through the arms to achieve a compression of 4–5 cm in normal adults or about a third of the depth of the chest in children. The compression:release ratio should be 1:1. The current guidelines aim to reduce the interruptions in chest compression that occur for 'rescue breaths' by advocating a compression:ventilation ratio of 30:2. Pauses for ventilation should be limited to 1 s/breath only. For children, the same ratio of 30:2 is appropriate for lay rescuers but a 15:2 sequence should be used when two or more health professionals are present. The only exception is neonates where a 3:1 ratio of compressions to ventilations is advocated. After successful endotracheal intubation, the synchronisation of compression and ventilation is abandoned and the two operations are performed independently.

Ventilation

Five initial 'rescue breaths' are recommended for children whereas, for adults, the 2 first breaths are given only after the first 30 chest compressions. Each breath should only take 1 second so as to maintain constant chest compressions. Mouth to mouth-and-nose ventilation is required for infants. A pocket mask may be used by occasional resuscitators to avoid direct patient contact; professional rescuers should use bag, valve and mask units initially but aim for endotracheal intubation as soon as practically possible. Airway adjuncts such as the oesophageal obturator airway and Combitube are not recommended – there are more disadvantages to their use than advantages. However, the laryngeal mask airway (LMA) is increasingly used by first responders.

Advanced life support

These protocols apply, by definition, to healthcare professionals trained in advanced life support techniques.

Resuscitation Council (UK) algorithm for ALS for adults → Figure 11.3.
Resuscitation Council (UK) algorithm for ALS for children → Figure 11.4.

A display of the ECG must be obtained as soon as possible to guide treatment. Monitoring via defibrillator pads (or paddles) may be adequate initially but should be replaced by adhesive chest electrodes once ALS is established. Endotracheal intubation must be achieved as soon as practically possible and early venous (or intraosseous) access is also desirable. Once the airway has been secured with a cuffed endotracheal tube, compressions should not be interrupted for ventilations. From then on, ventilation of the lungs should be performed asynchronously at a rate of approximately 10–12 breaths/min. To ensure effective chest compressions, the person responsible for this tiring part of the resuscitation should be changed every 2 min at least.

Intraosseous access → Box 18.4 on p. 332.
Mechanical chest compression → p. 161.

With the aid of the ECG rhythm, the algorithms divide patients into two categories: those who have VF or pulseless VT and those who do not have VF or VT. VF is not the most common arrest rhythm but is the

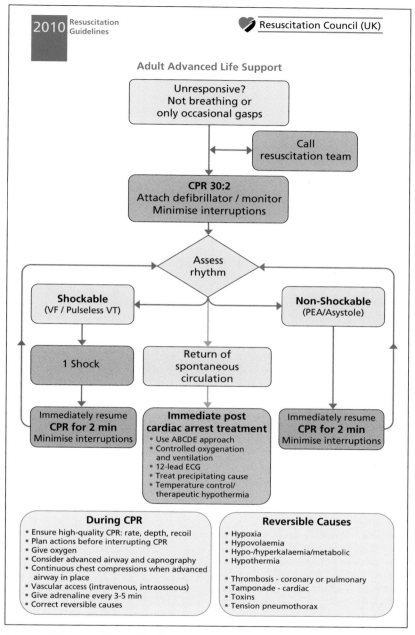

Figure 11.3 Advanced life support for adults. Reproduced with the kind permission of the Resuscitation Council (UK).

most survivable by far. The only effective treatment for it – defibrillation – was introduced into clinical practice by Zoll and colleagues in 1956. In almost all circumstances, no other intervention must take precedence over defibrillation.

Precordial thump

This supplies energy that may abort VT or even VF but in the unstable heart it may also possibly convert sinus rhythm into VF. Therefore, its use is

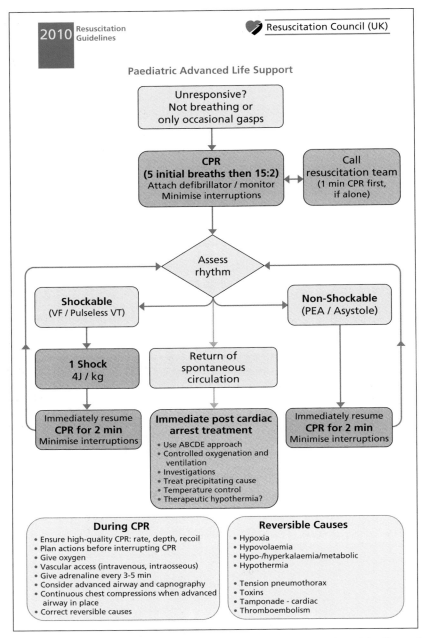

Figure 11.4 Advanced life support for children. Reproduced with the kind permission of the Resuscitation Council (UK).

recommended only in witnessed arrests when ALS skills are available.

Gastric decompression

Inflation of the stomach is inevitable during BLS. It causes splinting of the diaphragm and may impair cardiac output. For this reason, it is helpful to decompress the stomach with a large-bore orogastric (lavage-type) tube as soon as possible during all resuscitations. This should not be attempted until the airway is protected by intubation. The stomach may be emptied of both air and fluids in order to decrease the risk of aspiration. At postmortem examination, almost half of all patients who have died after attempted resuscitation are found to have full stomachs. Contamination of the respiratory tract is evident in 30%. Airway protection is ensured by early endotracheal intubation; the LMA is an effective alternative for first responders.

Relatives

Honest, accurate and frequent communication with relatives is essential throughout all resuscitations. Increasingly, relatives are being encouraged to come into the resuscitation room, even if it is only for a very short period. Staff may feel threatened by their presence but relatives are reassured by the experience; however cluttered and confusing the resuscitation area may appear, the reality is often less frightening than their imaginings. A dedicated member of staff should accompany relatives in the resuscitation room at all times.

Drugs in advanced life support

Adrenaline

The vasoconstrictor adrenaline is known to enhance both myocardial and cerebral perfusion, although there is no evidence that it increases the survival to hospital discharge in cardiac arrest. It has a very short half-life and so repeated intravenous (IV) doses (1 mg for adults) are given every 3–5 min during CPR. In children, the corresponding IV/intraosseous (IO) dose is 10 mcg/kg. Adrenaline should be given as soon as circulatory access is obtained in non-shockable rhythms and after the third shock (once chest compressions have been resumed) in shockable rhythms. Adrenaline may be contraindicated in arrests secondary to solvents, cocaine or other sympathomimetic drugs.

Amiodarone

Amiodarone is given for refractory VF/pulseless VT after the third shock (once compressions have been

Table 11.1 Doses of adrenaline and amiodarone for adults and children in cardiac arrest

	Adrenaline (to be given as soon as possible in asystole/PEA and after the third shock in VF/VT)	Amiodarone (to be given after the third shock in VF/VT)
Adult	1 mg every 3–5 min	300 mg
Child	10 mcg/kg every 3–5 min	5 mg/kg

All dosages are the same whether the drugs are given by the intravenous or intraosseous route.
10 mcg/kg of adrenaline = 0.1 mL/kg of 1 in 10 000 solution.
Peripheral IV or IO doses should be flushed in with saline.

resumed). It stabilises cell membranes and thus increases the duration of the action potential and refractory period in both atrial and ventricular myocardial cells. As an antiarrhythmic agent, it prolongs the Q–T interval and slows conduction through both the atrioventricular (AV) node and any accessory pathways. Amiodarone has less negative inotropic effects and fewer proarrhythmic actions than most similar drugs. An initial IV bolus of 300 mg should be given in adults; the equivalent IV/IO dose for children is 5 mg/kg. A further dose of 150 mg may be given for persistent or recurrent VF/VT, followed by an infusion of 900 mg over 24 h.

Atropine

Atropine is no longer recommended in cardiac arrest. Pulseless patients with extreme bradycardia or isolated P waves may benefit from pacing (→ p. 160).

Bicarbonate

Bicarbonate therapy is contraindicated in early resuscitation. Acidosis develops but aids oxyhaemoglobin dissociation; temporary buffering of pH is achieved by hyperventilation. Sodium bicarbonate is reserved for cardiac arrests that are associated with the following:

1 Hyperkalaemia (→ p. 248)
2 Poisoning with tricyclic antidepressants (→ p. 278).

The initial dose is 50–100 mmol (or 1–2 mmol/kg). *Further information about bicarbonate therapy → Box 14.24 on p. 252.* Prolonged arrest (i.e. over 20–25 min) causes profound intracellular acidosis and so may also be treated with alkalising agents, especially in children.

Lidocaine

Lidocaine reduces ventricular automaticity and ectopic activity and increases the threshold for the development of VF. However, it also causes an increase in:

- the energy required for defibrillation
- the incidence of post-shock asystole.

In addition, it is a negative inotrope. For these reasons, it is not routinely used for refractory VF/VT unless amiodarone is unavailable. The initial IV/IO dose for both adults and children is 1.0–1.5 mg/kg to a maximum total dose of 3 mg/kg in the first hour. Lidocaine and amiodarone should not be used together.

Magnesium

Magnesium is an important intracellular cation and co-factor. It should be given for refractory VT that could be associated with low serum magnesium levels, e.g. in a patient known to be taking potassium-losing diuretics. Similar indications include arrests after episodes of torsade de pointes or in patients with digoxin toxicity. The usual dose of magnesium sulphate is 8 mmol (2 g or 4 mL of a 50% solution). For children, the dose is 25–50 mg/kg by IV infusion over several minutes. These doses may be repeated after 10–15 min.

Further information about magnesium → Box 11.6 on pp. 174 and 250.

Calcium

Calcium influx occurs at the time of cell death and thus it is illogical to give calcium to patients in cardiac arrest. Exceptions occur during resuscitation from PEA or asystole when there is thought to be one of the following conditions:

1 Hyperkalaemia
2 Hypocalcaemia
3 Poisoning with calcium antagonists
4 Overdosage with magnesium (e.g. during treatment of eclampsia).

The initial IV dose in these situations is 10 mL of 10% calcium chloride (6.8 mmol calcium ions), repeated as necessary. For children the dose of 10% calcium chloride solution is 0.2 mL/kg. Calcium may form a precipitate if given in the same IV line as bicarbonate and is dangerous in the digitalised patient. Calcium channel blocking drugs have not fulfilled their early promise and do not improve outcome after cardiac arrest.

Further information about calcium → p. 249.

Drugs in cardiac arrest after hypothermia

Drug metabolism is reduced in hypothermia and toxic accumulation of drugs may thus occur. For this reason, it is usually recommended that adrenaline and other drugs are withheld until the patient's core temperature reaches 30°C. At this point, the interval between drug doses is doubled (adrenaline is given every 6–10 min) until a core temperature of around 35°C has been reached.

Defibrillation in cardiac arrest due to hypothermia → p. 159.
Hypothermic patients with no detectable cardiac output also → p. 244.

Ventricular fibrillation and pulseless ventricular tachycardia

In adults, VF/VT is the most treatable cause of cardiac arrest. Cardioversion by DC shock is most likely to be successful if carried out within 90 s of cardiac arrest. Thereafter, the chances of success decline at a rate of about 7–10%/min. Nevertheless, repeated shocks are delivered until sinus rhythm is established or resuscitation is abandoned. First and all subsequent shocks are delivered with an energy level of 360 J (or 4 J/kg) from a monophasic source. However, when using a modern biphasic defibrillator, fixed or escalating energies of between 150 and 360 J (4 J/kg for children) are recommended (→ Table 11.2).

The largest possible size of paddle (electrode) should be used for all DC shocks. There are three diameters currently available (→ Table 11.3). Size is limited by the two following criteria:

1 *The curve of the chest* – there must be good contact over the entire paddle area.
2 *The width of the chest* – the two paddles must be well separated.

Table 11.2 Doses of electricity for adults and children in VF or pulseless VT

	Monophasic all shocks	Biphasic first shock	Biphasic second shock
Adult (J)	360	150–200	150–360
Child (J/kg)	4	4	4

Table 11.3 Suggested paddle diameters for DC shock

Size of patient	Diameter of paddle (cm)
Infants (i.e. weight <10 kg)	4.5
Children aged <8 years (i.e. weight <25 kg)	8
Adults and children aged >8 years	13

Box 11.1 Potentially reversible causes of cardiac arrest ('the 4 Hs and 4 Ts')

Hypoxia
Hypovolaemia
Hypo- or hyperkalaemia, hypocalcaemia, acidaemia and other metabolic disorders
Hypothermia
Tension pneumothorax
Tamponade of the heart
Toxic substances
Thromboembolism (pulmonary embolus or coronary thrombosis)

Self-adhesive electrode pads are likely to replace defibrillator paddles completely in the near future.

Single shocks are given every 2 min. After administering a shock, there should be no delay in resuming CPR. It will not harm the patient if the defibrillation has been successful and the circulation has returned. The central pulse is checked only if the clinical condition of the patient changes or if the ECG shows a rhythm that is compatible with a cardiac output. (The carotid pulse is used in adults and children aged >12 months but in infants the brachial pulse is more appropriate.) After three unsuccessful shocks, adrenaline and amiodarone should be given. Further doses of adrenaline are given every 3–5 min throughout the resuscitation, immediately after alternate shocks (→ *Table 11.1*).

Potentially reversible causes of cardiac arrest must always be considered (→ *Box 11.1*). Underlying noncardiac causes of VF are more likely to be found in children than in adults. Magnesium should be considered if there is any suspicion of hypomagnesaemia (→ *p. 174*). If attempts at defibrillation remain unsuccessful, a change of paddle positions or a change of machine should be considered. Alternatives to the traditional anteroapical (AA) positioning of electrodes include anteroposterior (AP) and biaxillary (LL) placement. The latter positions (LL) should always be employed in patients with a pacemaker *in situ*.

After successful defibrillation

After successful defibrillation (if it has not already been utilised), amiodarone may be given to stabilise the myocardium and prevent a return to VF/VT. The IV dose is 300 mg over 20–60 min followed by an infusion of 900 mg over 24 h. Lidocaine (which also raises the fibrillation threshold) is a further option. The dose is 100 mg for an average adult followed by an infusion of 2–4 mg/min.

Safety of staff

This is paramount during attempts at defibrillation and requires:

• a good knowledge of the equipment
• a warning shout of 'stand clear' and a visual check before each discharge.

The use of adhesive electrode pads makes the procedure much safer and better controlled.

Defibrillation in cardiac arrest after hypothermia

VF may not respond to defibrillation if the patient's core temperature is <30°C. Thus it is usually recommended that, if there is no response to the first three shocks, subsequent attempts at defibrillation are delayed until the core temperature rises above 30°C.

Drugs in cardiac arrest due to hypothermia → p. 158. Hypothermic patients with no detectable cardiac output also → p. 244.

Developments in defibrillation

1 Conventional defibrillators produce a damped sinusoidal waveform but a biphasic discharge has both theoretical and empirical advantages, so almost all modern defibrillators incorporate this technology into their design. In practice, biphasic shocks delivered with an energy of 150 J seem to be more effective than monophasic currents with higher energies, although the optimal level for either type is uncertain. A biphasic shock crosses the heart and then returns along the same pathway as the phase inverts. This returning current catches the fibrillating myocytes that the first current

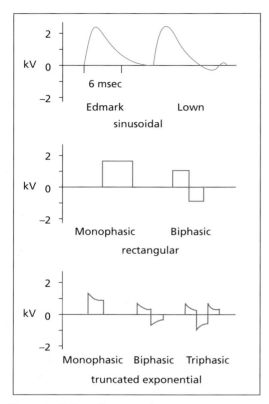

Figure 11.5 Defibrillator waveforms.

missed (in much the same way as a double-bladed safety razor removes stubborn remaining hairs with its second blade). There are three different biphasic waveforms that are commonly used. The two most effective are truncated exponential and rectilinear waves. *For some typical defibrillator waveforms → Figure 11.5.* The exact equivalence of biphasic and monophasic shocks depends on the waveform that is generated but, as a rough rule, 1 J of biphasic discharge equates to 1.5 J of monophasic discharge.

2 Successful defibrillation depends on the passage of an appropriate current through the chest rather than on the administration of a preset energy. This current is around 30 A for an average adult (about 0.4 A/kg). New current-preset defibrillators, which measure transthoracic impedance and then give a predetermined current, may replace traditional energy-preset machines in the future.

3 Myocardial current density is the ultimate determinant of both efficacy of defibrillation and cellular damage. The positioning of the treatment electrodes (paddles) is the main variable that can be

used to alter the distribution of the current in the chest and heart. Oesophageal electrodes, which can be positioned directly behind the heart, have been described; transoesophageal defibrillation may one day become accepted practice.

Asystole

Before a diagnosis of asystole is made, the leads, 'gain' control and switches on the monitor/defibrillator must be checked. 'Fine VF' is no longer an indication for defibrillation and has a poor prognosis. In confirmed aystole, 2-min cycles of CPR are performed between rhythm checks. Adrenaline is given during alternate cycles (*for doses → Table 11.1*). Potentially treatable causes for the arrest must be sought (→ *Box 11.1*). Cardiac pacing for asystole (see below) is only of benefit in cases with complete heart block where P waves are present.

> Most patients who present in asystole are dead, having been in VF for some time and having suffered irreversible hypoxic damage as a result. In a few cases, the primary rhythm change is extreme bradycardia and it is these patients who are most likely to respond to therapy.

Pulseless electrical activity

In PEA (also known as EMD), 2-min cycles of CPR are performed between rhythm checks. Adrenaline is given during alternate cycles (*doses → Table 11.1*). If the ECG changes and organised electrical activity continues, a central pulse should be checked. (The carotid pulse is used in adults and children aged >12 months but in infants the brachial pulse on the inner aspect of the upper arm is more appropriate.) Potentially treatable causes for the arrest must always be considered (the four Hs and four Ts → *Box 11.1*). *For further information about the reversible causes of PEA → p. 151.* The administration of IV fluids is particularly important for children.

Emergency pacing

External cardiac pacing is the method of choice in an ED; it is available as an additional feature on most advanced defibrillators. The external pacing electrodes must be placed on the front and back of the chest to ensure good contact. The pacing voltage is increased until capture of the ECG is obtained. While establishing pacing, the patient's general condition and central pulse should be monitored. 'Blind' transvenous pacing in the ED is rarely successful – there is a risk that the pacing wire may loop and knot in the right ventricle or the pulmonary artery. In the absence of any form of pacing equipment, external cardiac percussion (fist pacing) may sometimes maintain a satisfactory heart rate. Blows are delivered to the left central side of the chest at a rate of about 100/min.

Alternative techniques of cardiac compression

Several alternative techniques of external chest compression have also been described. None has found widespread acceptance yet in the UK.

Mechanical chest compression

This has been around for over 35 years, but, recently, there has been a long overdue resurgence of interest. Three main types of devices are now on the market:

1 Mechanical arms that directly compress the anterior chest (gas driven)
2 Pneumatic vests that inflate to squeeze the entire chest (electric)
3 Encircling bands that tighten around the mid-chest (electric).

Studies have shown that these machines give an increased cardiac output and are reliable and constant when compared with a human resuscitator, who generally tires after only a couple of minutes. Mechanical CPR is particularly desirable during transfers and for prolonged resuscitations. It is ideal for chest compression in the back of an ambulance.

Active compression/decompression

Active compression and decompression (ACD) of the chest can be achieved with a sucker attached to the precordium (the AMBU ACD device). The active decompression that occurs when the chest is pulled upwards by the suction device has been claimed to improve cardiac filling and hence cardiac output. However, the instrument is very tiring to use and in most controlled trials has not been shown to improve survival. It is more likely to be effective when coupled with mechanical CPR as in (1) above.

Internal cardiac massage

This achieves a much better output than external chest compression. Access to the pleural cavity is gained via a fourth left interspace thoracotomy; the pericardium may be left intact. The heart is squeezed up against the sternum with the extended fingers. (*Emergency thoracotomy* → p. 80.)

When to stop life support

> A person with a cardiac arrest should not be declared dead inside an ambulance at the door of the ED. The full cardiac arrest procedure should be initiated. The decision to abandon resuscitation can be made when there is no response and all of the relevant information is available.

The team leader must decide when it is appropriate to abandon attempts at resuscitation. This will require consideration of:

- the patient's past medical history
- the history of the current collapse and resuscitation
- the clinical and ECG findings
- the views of the other team members, including paramedics.

Recovery is very unlikely in asystole from a primary cardiorespiratory cause that does not respond to 15 min of ALS.

Medicolegal aspects of death → p. 385.

Agonal rhythm

The wide, rounded or M-shaped complexes that are characteristic of a dying heart are not capable of stimulating myocardial contraction (→ *Figure 11.6*). Thus, this agonal rhythm is not a form of PEA although the two are often confused.

Post-resuscitation care

Recovery from cardiac arrest depends on the maintenance of an adequate circulation to protect the brain and then on the restoration of spontaneous cardiac output as soon as possible. The arbiter of success is thus satisfactory tissue perfusion and not electrical activity on an ECG. Neurological recovery from cerebral ischaemia may take more than 24 h and so isolated signs such as the state of the pupils are of little prognostic value in the first few hours after cardiac arrest. Fits may occur in up to 25% of patients and are also unrelated to eventual outcome. On the whole, however, rapid return of normal function equates with a good outcome, especially regular spontaneous ventilation and improving level of consciousness.

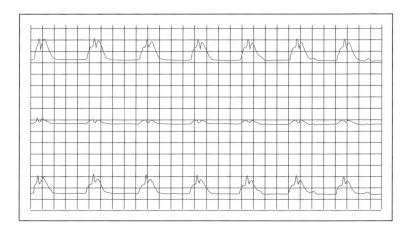

Figure 11.6 Agonal rhythm.

Coma persisting for more than 6 h post-arrest is associated with a high probability of severe neurological damage and only 10% of such patients will return to an independent existence. After 3 days in a coma, absent pupillary light reflexes and absent motor responses to pain are independent and specific predictors of a poor outcome (death or vegetative state).

Tx When spontaneous cardiac output returns 'reanimation' becomes 'resuscitation' and intensive care must begin. The patient has been effectively dead for a short period of time:

- Continue with oxygen therapy/ventilation.
- Ensure good venous access; usually both peripherally and centrally (*for central venous access → Box 11.2*).
- Consider therapy with amiodarone (or lidocaine) in order to prevent a recurrence of VF.
- Monitor pulse, BP, SaO₂ and ECG.
- Obtain a 12-lead ECG and a chest radiograph.
- Take blood for arterial blood gases, blood chemistry and FBC.
- Obtain a detailed history and perform a full examination.
- Catheterise the bladder and monitor the urinary output.
- Consider the possibility of immediate coronary reperfusion by either thrombolysis or percutaneous coronary intervention (*for reperfusion → p. 182*).
- Treat pyrexia with antipyretics and cooling. (Body temperatures >37°C worsen prognosis after cardiac arrest.)
- Control the blood glucose with an insulin infusion if necessary. (High blood glucose levels are strongly associated with a poor neurological outcome after cardiac arrest.)

- Arrange admission to a coronary care unit or intensive care unit. Ventilation will be necessary in the absence of adequate spontaneous breathing or satisfactory tissue oxygenation. Some authorities advocate at least 24 h of controlled ventilation for all post-arrest patients, irrespective of their respiratory state, although there is little evidence that this improves outcome.

Inotropic and vasopressor support may be required (→ *Box 14.11 on p. 238*) because haemodynamic instability is common after the return of spontaneous circulation. A BP >80–90 mmHg is necessary to maintain coronary perfusion, which occurs mainly during diastole. Intra-arterial BP monitoring is essential in this situation. Treatment may also be needed for pulmonary oedema (→ *p. 208*) and cardiac dysrhythmias (→ *p. 164*). The intensivist will aim for a pulmonary capillary wedge pressure (PCWP) of <18 mmHg, measured with a pulmonary artery (or Swan–Ganz) catheter. This may require the administration of IV fluids, vasodilators or diuretics.

Therapeutic hypothermia

Mild hypothermia (32–34°C) is thought to suppress many of the chemical reactions associated with reperfusion injury although the exact mechanism of cerebral protection is uncertain. A period of 12–24 h of hypothermia is sufficient and should be started as soon as possible after cardiac arrest for all comatose patients. Surface cooling techniques are usually adequate with accurate monitoring of temperature by an internal probe. Shivering must be avoided (by sedation and neuromuscular blockade) because it causes a marked increase in metabolic demands.

Box 11.2 Central venous cannulation

If possible, cannulation of central veins should take place under ultrasound guidance

- Position the patient slightly head-down to fill the veins and minimise the risk of air embolism
- Take whatever aseptic precautions are reasonable for the urgency of the situation
- Use a cannulation set that is familiar to you. A Seldinger-wire/long-line approach is ideal but a simple cannula over needle can be inserted more quickly
- Attempted cannulation of the right side is preferable because it avoids damage to the thoracic duct, which lies on the left, and the apex of the pleural cavity, which is more inferior on the right
- Local anaesthetic should be used in the conscious patient

Cannulation of the subclavian vein
Introduce the needle in the concavity below the clavicle, a third of the way along from the tip. Advance the needle under the clavicle while withdrawing on the attached syringe. Aim for an index finger placed in the suprasternal notch. The vein is usually entered about 4–6 cm from the entry point. Coughing suggests pleural penetration.

Cannulation of the internal jugular vein
Turn the patient's head away from the vein. Identify the triangle that is made by the bifurcation of the lower end of the sternocleidomastoid muscle into its two insertions. Insert the needle at the apex of this triangle. Palpate the carotid artery; the jugular vein lies lateral to it. Advance the needle towards the ipsilateral nipple at about 30° to the horizontal and the sagittal planes, while withdrawing the syringe. The vein lies about 2–3 cm from the skin.

- When blood is aspirated, slide the cannula into the vein and withdraw the needle simultaneously.
- Connect the cannula to a three-way tap and secure it in place.
- Request a chest radiograph to check the cannula position and to exclude pneumothorax.

Unsuccessful resuscitation

The care of bereaved people is as important as any other care in the ED (→ *below*). After some resuscitations, staff may be distressed and in need of either formal or informal support.

Brain-stem death → p. 386.
Notification of death to the coroner or procurator fiscal → p. 385.
Organ and tissue donation → p. 387.

Care of suddenly bereaved individuals

Death of a patient from a cardiac arrest is always sudden and thus is generally unexpected by the next of kin who may be ill prepared for it. The same is true of other, less common, causes of death in an ED such as trauma and sudden infant death syndrome (*for cot death → p. 356*). Certain principles of care may make this terrible experience more bearable:

- Relatives should be contacted promptly and dealt with as soon as they arrive at the ED. A designated (named) nurse should stay with the family throughout and act as a liaison with the rest of the medical and nursing team. In an on-going resuscitation, this nurse must make every effort to obtain up-to-date information for the relatives.
- Special facilities should be available for bereaved relatives, including a quiet, private room with a telephone, access to drinks and a toilet.
- Spiritual support may be needed for all denominations and religions. The hospital chaplains should be welcomed into the ED as part of the team.
- When bad news is broken, it should be imparted gently and honestly, avoiding euphemism and over-involved medical explanations. Presumptions as to the cause of death should not be made. The family can be left to assimilate the news but should have another opportunity to ask further questions later on. Although the medical staff must be involved in the contact with the relatives, the breaking of bad news can be undertaken by any experienced member of the team.
- Both verbal and written information must be provided for the relatives concerning:
  - what to do next
  - coroner's procedures and the possibility of a postmortem examination
  - helpful telephone numbers
  - a named contact in the ED with a phone number
  - details about any follow-up by a nurse or counsellor specialising in bereavement care (→ *p. 164*).

- Arrangements must be made for relatives to get home safely and for care for those who are alone.
- Other agencies must be informed including:
  - the deceased patient's GP
  - the next of kin's GP
  - the medical records department
  - the health visitor for a child aged <5 years and the school nurse for an older child.
- Staff support and training should be available. All staff need access to a staff care or counselling scheme; this may involve contact with the hospital chaplains or psychologists. Debriefing can include both clinical and emotional aspects. Feedback from the relatives should be reviewed.

The bereavement nurse

A person specialising in the care and counselling of suddenly bereaved people can be invaluable to an ED. Such a person, who is usually a specially trained nurse, can visit the next of kin soon after death to provide information, answer questions and offer comfort. This visit also serves to reinforce the caring nature of the ED's work and to provide an outlet for any anger or misunderstandings. A second visit, after about 6 weeks, serves the same purposes later on in the grieving process and may identify the emergence of long-term problems in the bereaved relative.

CARDIAC DYSRHYTHMIAS

Management of palpitations → p. 240.
Rhythms where the patient does not have a palpable pulse → cardiac arrest on p. 150.
Specific treatment of tachydysrhythmias due to tricyclic antidepressant poisoning → p. 278.

General principles

Treatment of all cardiac dysrhythmias should include:

- Attention to the ABCs
- High-concentration oxygen
- Venous access
- Monitoring of SaO_2, ECG and BP
- Obtaining a 12-lead ECG as soon as possible
- Observing the patient in a high-dependency area.

The ECG should be examined to determine:

1 The ventricular rate
2 Whether the QRS rhythm is regular or irregular (fast atrial fibrillation [AF] may look deceptively regular)
3 The presence of atrial activity (P waves may be hidden; atrial activity includes AF)

4 The relationship between atrial and ventricular activity
5 Whether the QRS complex is normal or prolonged.

The clinical condition of the patient, especially the presence of a central pulse, is the most important factor in any treatment decision. Pallor and sweating are always bad signs.

> In patients with otherwise normal hearts, serious symptoms and signs are unusual if the ventricular rate is >40 and <150 contractions/min.

Assessment and management of bradycardia

The need for emergency treatment depends on the following:

1 The presence of adverse clinical findings:
  - hypotension or shock (systolic BP <90 mmHg)
  - symptoms of low blood flow to the brain (dizziness, faintness or syncope)
  - symptoms of myocardial ischaemia (chest pain or heart failure)
  - heart rate <40 beats/min
  - presence of ventricular escape dysrhythmias that require suppression.
2 The presence of features that suggest that there is a significant risk of asystole:
  - previous asystolic episodes
  - Mobitz type 2 or fixed 2:1 AV block
  - ventricular pause >3 s
  - complete heart block (especially with a wide QRS complex or initial rate <40/min).

> Bradycardias with wide QRS complexes are likely to be caused by blocks below the level of the AV node. They are usually unresponsive to atropine and relatively unstable. An AV junctional ectopic pacemaker is more reliable and may provide a reasonable heart rate with a narrow QRS.

Tx Bradycardias that do not fall into the above criteria may be observed. Other bradycardias should be treated with IV atropine (in 500-mcg increments up to a maximum of 3 mg for an adult) and then expert advice sought immediately. Interim measures while awaiting emergency transvenous pacing ($\rightarrow$ *p. 160*) include the following:

- Transcutaneous external pacing
- Isoprenaline by IV infusion (at a rate of 5 mcg/min for an adult)
- Adrenaline by IV infusion (at a rate of 2–10 mcg/min for an adult)
- A range of other chronotropic drugs including aminophylline and dopamine. Glucagon is used for bradycardia in poisoning with β blockers and calcium antagonists. Glycopyrrolate is an alternative to atropine.

Resuscitation Council (UK) algorithm for the treatment of bradycardia in adults $\rightarrow$ *Figure 11.7.*

Bradycardia in children may be a pre-terminal finding secondary to hypoxia or hypovolaemia. It is treated with a combination of:

- resuscitation with oxygen and fluids
- atropine by IV/IO bolus (20 mcg/kg)
- adrenaline by IV/IO bolus (10 mcg/kg)
- adrenaline by IV infusion (0.05–2 mcg/kg per min).

Sinus bradycardia

Sinus rhythm with a heart rate of <60/min may follow:

- a myocardial infarction, usually inferior
- a vasovagal attack
- the use of some drugs (e.g. β blockers).

Hypotension, accompanied by symptoms of faintness and malaise, does not usually occur until the heart rate falls below about 40–45 beats/min.

Tx At heart rates above 40 in asymptomatic patients, the bradycardia can be observed without treatment. Below this rate, it can be corrected with small increments of IV atropine (i.e. doses of 100–200 mcg for an adult) depending on the response. Tachycardia may reduce coronary perfusion while increasing oxygen demand and is thus to be avoided.

Complete (third-degree) heart block

Impairment of conduction of electrical impulses from the atria to the ventricles (AV or "heart" block) is usually a result of:

- myocardial ischaemia
- poisoning (including digitalis)
- chronic heart diseases, especially aortic stenosis and congenital lesions
- some acute infectious diseases, including rheumatic fever.

In inferior infarction, complete AV block results from localised occlusion of the right coronary artery; the AV nodal artery is one of its branches. However, in anterior infarction, complete AV block usually represents massive septal necrosis with additional damage in the territory of the circumflex artery.

The heart rate is around 35–45 beats/min in complete heart block and thus symptoms are likely. However, if there is narrow complex junctional escape rhythm, there may be a heart rate that is both adequate and regular.

Tx The Resuscitation Council (UK) algorithm for bradycardia should be followed ($\rightarrow$ *Figure 11.7*) and the patient referred to a cardiologist for assessment and temporary pacing.

Chronic complete AV block causing Stokes–Adams attacks

This is usually caused by fibrosis around the bundle of His (Lenegre's disease). There is a widened QRS complex. Ventricular pauses (which lead to transient failure of the cardiac output and consequent syncope) may be hard to capture on ECG. Pacing abolishes symptoms and prolongs life.

> Lyme disease should be considered as a possible cause in a young person with a new onset of heart block. *Borrelia burgdorferi* may cause a myocarditis that involves the heart's conducting tissue, especially the AV node.

Incomplete heart block

This may be caused by ischaemic heart disease, acute myocarditis, drugs or metabolic disturbance.

First-degree heart block

This causes prolongation of the P–R interval so that it is >0.2 s (one large square). After myocardial infarction, 40% of patients with first-degree AV block will go on to develop second- or third-degree blocks, so close observation of these patients is required.

Second-degree heart block

This is said to exist when there is an intermittent failure of conduction through the AV node or the bundle of His. There are three variations:

1 *Wenckebach's phenomenon (Mobitz type 1 block):* there is progressive lengthening of the P–R interval, then a failure of conduction. This is followed by a

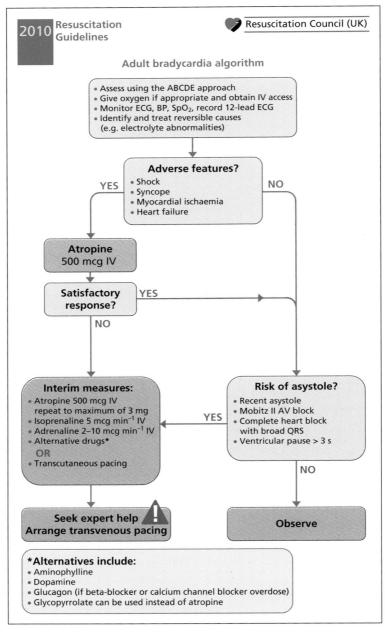

Figure 11.7 Algorithm for bradycardia in adults. Reproduced with the kind permission of the Resuscitation Council (UK).

conducted beat with a normal P–R interval, then the lengthening process starts again. The conduction deficit is in the AV node.

2 *Mobitz type 2 block*: the majority of beats are conducted with a normal and constant P–R interval but occasionally a P wave is not followed by a QRS complex – a dropped beat. The problem lies distal to the AV node.

3 *Fixed second-degree (2:1 or 3:1) block*: there are intermittent conducted and non-conducted atrial beats giving a ratio of P waves to QRS complexes of 2:1 or 3:1.

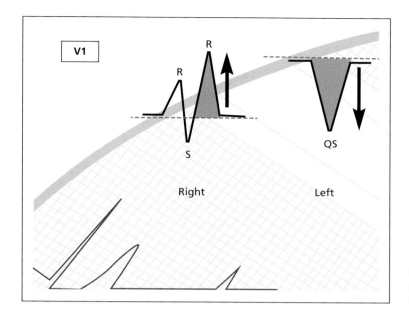

Figure 11.8 Differentiation of RBBB and LBBB using morphology of V1.

Tx Mobitz type 2 block and fixed 2:1 AV block may herald complete heart block and so require prophylactic pacing.

Wenckebach's phenomenon is usually benign and transient; it is caused by drug toxicity, high vagal tone or an inferior MI involving the AV nodal artery. The heart rate may be increased by atropine. When Wenckebach second-degree block occurs after an anterior infarction, temporary pacing is indicated.

Bundle-branch block

Bundle-branch block (BBB) of recent onset after MI is associated with a less favourable prognosis and, in the case of left BBB (LBBB), is an ECG indication for reperfusion therapy (→ p 182). As a rough guide, a broad RSR (M-shaped) pattern in V1 is caused by right BBB (RBBB) and a similar pattern in V6 indicates LBBB. (*For further information about the ECG diagnosis of BBB → Table 11.4 and Figure 11.8.*) The further interpretation of BBB requires an expert opinion.

Bifascicular block

This results when only half of one bundle branch is conducting normally. There is most usually a combination of RBBB with left anterior hemiblock, which appears as left axis deviation on the ECG. A quick way to check for this common type of bifascicular block is to look for a broadened M pattern in V1 and a deep S wave that is bigger than the R wave in lead

Table 11.4 ECG diagnosis of bundle-branch blocks (*also → Figure 11.8.*)

RBBB	LBBB
QRS >120ms	QRS >120ms
Secondary R wave in V1, V2 and V3	Broad monophasic R wave and absence of Q wave in I, V5 and V6
Wide S wave in I, V5 and V6	ST and T in opposite direction to QRS

II. This conduction disturbance may cause drop attacks in the same way as complete heart block. Patients with evidence of either trifascicular or bifascicular disease after MI may need to be prophylactically paced.

Intraventricular abnormalities of conduction

These may cause notching of the QRS complex but do not require treatment.

Supraventricular tachycardia

The main causes of supraventricular tachycardia (SVT) are:

- Ischaemic heart disease, often at the time of acute myocardial infarction or in the peri-arrest situation

- Congenital abnormalities of conduction (which cause paroxysmal attacks)
- Drugs
- Metabolic disturbances.

The two main types of SVT are outlined below.

1 Junctional tachycardias

Atrioventricular nodal re-entry tachycardia (AVNRT): This is the most common type of regular narrow-complex tachyarrhythmia and also the most common paroxysmal SVT. It often occurs in patients with otherwise normal hearts and is thus relatively benign. The cause is a re-entry circuit within the AV node. *Explanation of AV nodal re-entry circuits → Box 11.3.* The ECG is regular with no visible atrial activity.

Atrioventricular re-entry tachycardia (AVRT): Re-entry involves an accessory pathway such as the bundle of Kent in Wolff-Parkinson–White (WPW) syndrome. There is usually no visible atrial activity on the ECG. After resolution of the tachycardia, the ECG may show a short P–R interval and a delta wave (a slurred upstroke denoting pre-excitation) at the start of the QRS complex.

2 Atrial tachycardias

Atrial tachycardia: An ectopic atrial focus causes an atrial rate of 150–250 beats/min. Often the rate is between 160 and 170 beats/min with a 1:1 response but at faster rates 2:1 block may occur.

Atrial flutter: The atria flutter at around 300 beats/min and 2:1 or 3:1 block occurs to give rates of up to 150–160 complexes/min (→ *below*). It may be difficult to identify flutter waves on the ECG.

Atrial fibrillation: The heart rate is irregular.

Fast atrial fibrillation → p. 171.

> Haemodynamic disturbance accompanying tachycardia often suggests a ventricular origin for the dysrhythmia but does not exclude a supraventricular cause.

 Box 11.3 AV nodal re-entry circuits

In the normal AV node there are two pathways along which the atrial impulse can travel – a slow pathway with a short refractory period and a fast pathway with a longer refractory period. The two unite to become the bundle of His. During normal sinus rhythm, the atrial impulse travels along both pathways but completes its journey via the fast pathway only because the slow pathway has already become refractory. In AVNRT a premature atrial beat occurs at a crucial time and the impulse finds the fast pathway to be still refractory and so travels along the slow pathway. When it gets to the point where both fast and slow pathways join to form the bundle of His, the fast pathway has recovered from its refractory period and the impulse travels backwards up it. This establishes a re-entry circuit and is the mechanism in 90% of patients with AV nodal tachycardia. In the other 10% of patients, a premature ventricular beat is the source of the problem and a slow–fast circuit is set up – the reverse of the situation described above. As a result of the normal anatomy involved, affected individuals are often young and healthy with no detectable heart disease.

Irregular or broad-complex SVT

SVT usually appears as a narrow-complex tachycardia on ECG but, if there is aberrant (i.e. abnormal) conduction such as BBB, then broad complexes may be seen. In the peri-arrest situation, SVT may precipitate VF. An irregular narrow-complex tachycardia is most likely to be fast AF.

Infants with SVT

Infants with a tachydysrhythmia may present with a sudden onset of poor feeding, tachypnoea, pallor and lethargy. SVT is the most common non-arrest arrhythmia of infancy and may give rise to cardiogenic shock. Heart rates range from 220/min to as high as 300 complexes/min.

Tx of SVT

Resuscitation Council (UK) algorithm for the treatment of tachycardia in adults (with a pulse) → Figure 11.9.

Fast atrial fibrillation is a difficult situation requiring expert advice (→ *p. 171*).

- Vagal manoeuvres such as carotid sinus massage, orbital pressure, Valsalva's manoeuvre, iced water

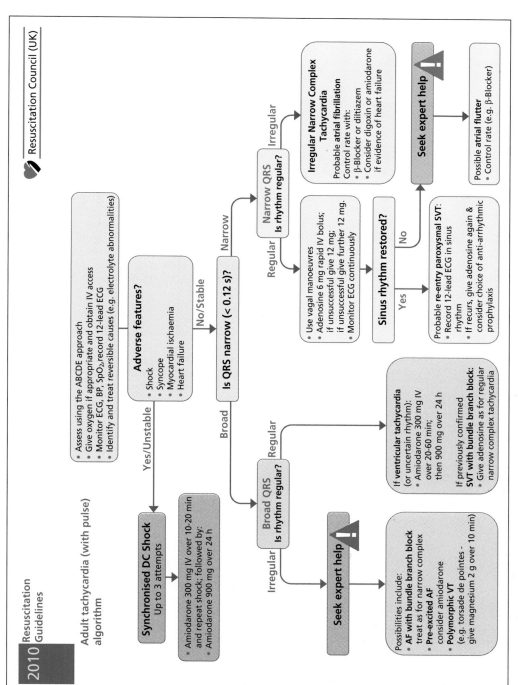

Figure 11.9 Algorithm for tachycardia (with a pulse) in adults. Reproduced with the kind permission of the Resuscitation Council (UK).

to the face can be attempted – with care – in most patients. Infants can have their faces immersed in iced water for 5 s.

- Adenosine is effectively a 'chemical shock' – immediate effect, short acting and relatively safe in both stable and unstable patients. The initial dose is 6 mg for an adult which is given as a rapid IV bolus. If this proves to be ineffective, up to two further doses (each of 12 mg) may be given at 2-min intervals. Patients after heart transplantation are very sensitive to the effects of adenosine and should be given an initial dose of 3 mg. Undesirable effects from adenosine may be seen in patients with WPW syndrome or in those who are taking dipyridamole or carbamazepine. Adenosine (or vagal manoeuvres) will terminate almost all AVNRTs or AVRTs within seconds. Failure to terminate a regular narrow-complex tachycardia with adenosine suggests the presence of an atrial tachycardia such as atrial flutter. Adenosine may be repeated if an arrhythmia recurs; an antiarrhythmic prophylactic drug should then be started.

Patients with signs of cardiac or cerebral compromise

For patients with adverse features such as:

- hypotension or shock (systolic BP <90 mmHg)
- symptoms of low blood flow to the brain (dizziness, faintness or syncope)
- symptoms of myocardial ischaemia (chest pain or heart failure)
- heart rate >200 beats/min

treatment consists of:

- *Sedation and synchronised cardioversion* (starting with 120–150 J biphasic or 200 J monophasic shocks)
- *IV amiodarone* 300 mg over 20–60 min followed by 900 mg over 24 h and repeated shocks if SVT persists.

Stable, alert patients

There is a choice of suitable drugs:

- *Verapamil* (IV, 5–10 mg): this is hazardous in WPW syndrome, some SVTs of childhood, ventricular tachycardias and in conjunction with β blockers. It must not be used in infants.
- *Esmolol*: this is an ultra short-acting cardioselective β blocker with a half-life of 9 min; it is contraindicated in shock, heart failure, heart block, asthma and after verapamil. In SVT, when time for

> **Box 11.4 Adenosine and synchronised DC shock for narrow-complex tachycardia in children**
>
> *Adenosine*
> 50 mcg/kg, then 100 mcg/kg and then 250 mcg/kg
> (To maximum total dosage of 500 mcg/kg or 300 mcg/kg for infants <1 month old)
>
> *Synchronised DC shock*
> 0.5 J/kg, then 1 J/kg and then 2 J/kg

titration is available, a loading dose of 40 mg (500 mcg/kg) is given intravenously over 1 min, followed by an infusion of 50–100 mcg/kg per min until the desired effect is achieved. Esmolol may also be used for the treatment of symptomatic sinus tachycardia.

- *Digoxin* (IV, up to 500 mg over 30 min, repeated if necessary).
- *Amiodarone* (IV, 300 mg over 20–60 min followed by 900 mg over 24 h).
- *Flecainide*: this is a potent sodium channel blocker which is indicated in the special SVTs associated with accessory pathways (e.g. WPW syndrome) and AF. The dose is 100–150 mg (2 mg/kg for children) given intravenously over 20–30 min.

Overdrive pacing is a further option (not for AF). In patients who have ventricular pre-excitation (due to WPW syndrome) together with AF or atrial flutter, drugs that block the AV node must be avoided because they cause an increase in pre-excitation. These drugs include adenosine, verapamil, diltiazem and digoxin.

Children with narrow-complex tachycardias

Children are treated along much the same lines as adults. *Doses of adenosine and electricity for children → Box 11.4*.

Atrial flutter

The atria flutter at a rate of between 280 and 320 contractions/min; 2 : 1 or 3 : 1 AV block occurs, resulting in a ventricular response of around either 150 or 100 beats/min. The ECG shows a characteristic saw-tooth pattern (best seen in lead II), which is accentuated by increasing the degree of AV block (e.g. by carotid sinus massage). An irregular narrow-complex tachycardia may result from atrial flutter with a variable AV block.

Tx An isolated attack of atrial flutter is best treated by cardioversion. It is the cardiac dysrhythmia that is most likely to convert to sinus rhythm. Only relatively small DC shocks are usually required: 70–120 J biphasic or 100 J monophasic. If necessary, the ventricular rate can be slowed with either β blockers or digoxin (→ *below*). Paroxysmal flutter is controlled with drugs.

Fast atrial fibrillation

> The human body responds to many different forms of illness with a tachycardia. If a patient has chronic AF, then he or she will develop fast AF rather than a sinus tachycardia.

AF is the most common sustained cardiac dysrhythmia. Its prevalence doubles with each advancing decade of life after the age of 50, rising to 9% in patients aged >80 years. It is also the most common dysrhythmia to cause hospitalisation. AF is associated with a 1.5-fold increase in mortality in men and a 1.9-fold increase in women. The fibrillation is a non-specific response to atrial distension, so may occur acutely in conditions such as:

- MI (AF occurs in up to 10% of cases)
- pulmonary embolism (PE)
- sudden and excessive ingestion of alcohol.

Chronic AF is seen with:

- ischaemic and hypertensive heart disease
- mitral valve disease
- ventricular failure
- cor pulmonale
- cardiomyopathy
- thyrotoxicosis.

Recurrent bouts of AF (paroxysmal AF) may also occur. There is usually no identifiable underlying cause and episodes settle spontaneously. In AF, chaotic depolarisation of the atria results in a loss of atrial contraction and a fast, irregular ventricular rhythm. There is a consequent reduction in cardiac output and a risk of systemic embolism. Symptoms of AF include palpitations, dyspnoea, fatigue and chest pain. The main need for treatment of AF in the ED arises when a fast heart rate is causing signs of haemodynamic disturbance or is contributing to left ventricular failure (LVF).

Tx
Resuscitation Council (UK) algorithm for the treatment of tachycardia in adults (with a pulse) → Figure 11.9.

For AF, there are three main treatment options:

1 Control of the ventricular rate by drugs
2 Control of the atrial rhythm by pharmacological cardioversion
3 Control of the atrial rhythm by electrical cardioversion.

It is important to treat the underlying causes of both the fibrillation and the tachycardia. In addition, some complications must be prevented (e.g. thromboembolism) and some must be treated (e.g. heart failure).

Paroxysmal AF usually reverts spontaneously to sinus rhythm within 48 h and so cardioversion is seldom required.

In patients with AF complicating heart failure, digoxin is used to slow AV conduction and thus control the ventricular rate. It has no effect on the underlying dysrhythmia. It may be given orally or intravenously depending on the urgency of the situation. A suitable IV dose of digoxin is 0.75–1 mg made up to 50 mL and infused over 2 or more hours. Too rapid infusion causes nausea and dysrhythmias. Oral digitalisation can be achieved by giving 1–1.5 mg digoxin in divided doses over 24 h.

> In AF, the optimum ventricular rate at rest is about 90 beats/min.

In a patient with AF complicating an acute illness, sinus rhythm usually returns spontaneously when the underlying disease, together with any aggravating factor such as hypokalaemia, resolves. Cardioversion is usually unnecessary unless AF is causing haemodynamic instability. Fast heart rates causing breathlessness or poor perfusion can be controlled with digoxin, amiodarone, diltiazem or β blockers, the choice of drug and the route of administration depending on the underlying condition and the urgency of the situation. Digoxin and amiodarone are preferable in patients with signs of heart failure.

Cardioversion for AF: Electrical cardioversion is usually successful in AF of recent onset (<48 h) and may be required urgently in the presence of chest pain or critical perfusion. Under sedation or general anaesthesia, synchronised DC shocks are delivered with escalating energies starting with 120–150 J (biphasic) or 200 J (monophasic). Following successful cardioversion, there are several drugs that can be used to maintain sinus rhythm; the choice depends on the underlying condition and is a matter for a cardiologist. However, amiodarone (300 mg given intravenously over 20–60 min followed by 900 mg over 24 h) is a safe and common choice.

If the anaesthetic skills needed for the administration of a DC shock are not available, then chemical cardioversion is also an option in acute AF of under 48 h duration. The best drug (for a relatively healthy heart) is probably IV flecainide 2 mg/kg (to a maximum of 150 mg) given over 20 min. Amiodarone can also be used (IV 300 mg over 20–60 min followed by 900 mg over 24 h) and is better than flecainide for a diseased heart. Both drugs may worsen haemodynamic disturbance and so should be administered only by the experienced practitioner. Patients who have been in AF for more than 48 h should not be cardioverted, either electrically or pharmacologically, until they have been anticoagulated for at least 3 weeks.

Anticoagulation for AF: Thrombi may form in the atria within 48 h of the onset of AF. They may also form after successful cardioversion because the atria may not empty well for several days due to 'atrial stunning'. All patients should therefore be considered for prophylactic heparinisation.

Ventricular tachycardia

This is a sign of a heart that is 'irritable' or has disordered conduction caused by intrinsic damage, electrolyte disturbance or drugs. High rates may cause a variable loss of cardiac output although this feature alone does not distinguish VT from SVT. The ECG shows a regular broad complex tachycardia (QRS >120 ms) at a rate of >120 beats/min. Independent P waves may be seen that are unrelated to the QRS complexes; fusion beats can also occur. VT may be monomorphic or polymorphic depending on the origin. Torsade de pointes is a form of polymorphic VT (→ *p. 173*).

Tx VT always has the potential to degenerate into VF and so treatment must not be delayed.

Magnesium therapy → Box 11.6.
Resuscitation Council (UK) algorithm for the treatment of tachycardia in adults (with a pulse) → Figure 11.9.

Patients with no pulse

VF and pulseless VT protocol → p. 158.

Patients with signs of cardiac or cerebral compromise

For patients with adverse features such as:

- hypotension or shock (systolic BP <90 mmHg)
- symptoms of low blood flow to the brain (dizziness, faintness or syncope)
- symptoms of myocardial ischaemia (chest pain or heart failure)
- heart rate >200 beats/min

management includes:

- *Sedation and synchronised cardioversion* (starting with 120–150 J biphasic or 200 J monophasic shocks)
- *Consider treatment for hypokalaemia* if the serum potassium is known to be low (with IV potassium and magnesium)
- IV *amiodarone* 300 mg over 20–60 min followed by an infusion of 900 mg over 24 h
- *Further shocks as required* and consider treatment with other drugs (e.g. lidocaine, procainamide, flecainide or sotalol) or overdrive pacing.

Stable, alert patients

- *Consider treatment for hypokalaemia* if the serum potassium is known to be low (with IV potassium and magnesium)
- IV *amiodarone* 300 mg over 20–60 min followed by an infusion of 900 mg over 24 h. An alternative is lidocaine (100 mg by slow IV bolus for an average adult, followed by an infusion of 4 mg/min for 30 min, then 2 mg/min for 2 h, then 1 mg/min). Intravenous lidocaine has a short duration of action (15–20 min). If an infusion is not immediately available, the initial IV bolus can be repeated once or twice at intervals of not less than 10 min.
- *Synchronised DC shock* if VT persists, then amiodarone and further shocks if necessary.

Broad-complex supraventricular tachycardia

This arises when SVT occurs in conjunction with delayed conduction through the ventricles (aberrant conduction). The most common causes of aberrant conduction are BBBs and pre-excitation from accessory pathways. Fast AF with pre-existing LBBB is especially easy to mistake for VT.

Broad-complex tachycardia of uncertain origin

Unlike verapamil, which may be dangerous, adenosine can be given to a patient with a broad-complex tachycardia of uncertain origin. This constitutes a useful diagnostic test – in SVT the ventricular rate will usually slow after adenosine whereas in VT the heart rate will continue unchanged. However, in fast AF or atrial flutter occurring in patients with an accessory AV pathway, there may even be a worsening of the tachycardia as the anomalous pathway is left unchallenged by normal conduction.

Broad-complex tachycardia that is irregular

This is most likely to result from AF with BBB or, in patients with WPW syndrome, AF with ventricular pre-excitation (→ p. 168). A third cause is polymorphic VT (e.g. torsade de pointes → below).

Children with broad-complex tachycardias

Children with broad-complex tachycardias are treated in much the same way as adults. Adenosine may be used as described above to determine the source of the tachycardia. It can sometimes be impossible to deliver a synchronised DC shock in VT because synchronisation relies on the ability of the defibrillator to recognise a QRS complex within the ECG signal. In many cases of VT, especially in children, there is no recognisable complex, so the defibrillator will not discharge while in the synchronised mode. For this reason, non-synchronous shocks are sometimes recommended for VT in shocked or otherwise unstable children. However, it is best to attempt to use synchronous shocks at first because these are less likely to produce VF than asynchronous ones. If the defibrillator fails to discharge, then it should be desynchronised immediately. *For doses of amiodarone, lidocaine and electricity for VT in children → Box 11.5.* Procainamide is sometimes used in stable children with VT (15 mg/kg given intravenously over 30 min).

Torsade de pointes

This is a variety of polymorphic VT where the fast ventricular complexes vary from beat to beat, as if the electrical axis is twisting around a fixed point (→ *Figure 11.10*). There is usually an underlying prolongation of the Q–T interval, caused by drugs (especially the selective serotonin reuptake inhibitor or SSRI group of antidepressants) or electrolyte disturbance (e.g. hypokalaemia). The condition may occur in patients who have taken the antihistamine terfenadine in overdose or in combination with any of the following interacting substances:

- Erythromycin, clarithromycin or related macrolide antibiotics
- Ketoconazole, itraconazole or related imidazole antifungal drugs
- Concentrated grapefruit juice.

Patients with cardiac or hepatic disease are especially at risk.

Tx Episodes of torsade de pointes are usually self-limiting but may progress to VF. Treatment is with IV

 Box 11.5 Amiodarone, lidocaine and DC shock for broad-complex tachycardia in children

Amiodarone
IV 5 mg/kg over 30 min

Lidocaine
IV boluses of 0.5 mg/kg and then 1 mg/kg followed by an infusion of 10–50 mcg/kg per min

DC shock
0.5 J/kg, then 1 J/kg and then 2 J/kg

Figure 11.10 ECG trace of torsade de pointes.

Box 11.6 Magnesium therapy

Intravenous magnesium may sometimes be helpful in the control of certain resistant ventricular dysrhythmias such as:

- VT secondary to hypokalaemia
- VT that is resistant to DC shock
- Torsade de pointes
- Some tachycardias that are secondary to the effects of drugs including digitalis, antiarrhythmics and occasionally tricyclic antidepressants

The dose is 4–8 mmol magnesium (diluted to 20 mL with saline) administered intravenously over 5–10 min; 1 g magnesium sulphate contains 4 mmol magnesium ion; a 50% solution contains approximately 2 mmol/mL. Transient flushing – sometimes accompanied by hypotension – is to be expected in almost all patients. The total dose of magnesium may be up to 16 mmol, followed by an infusion of 2.5 mmol/h.
Children: IV magnesium sulphate 25–50 mg/kg over several minutes; maximum dose 2 g.

 Box 11.7 Acquired causes of a long Q–T interval

- Drugs: antiarrhythmics, antidepressants, antihistamines, antimalarials, phenothiazines, organophosphates and high-dose methadone (the commonly used SSRI antidepressants citalopram and escitalopram are both associated with dose-dependent Q–T interval prolongation)
- Electrolyte disturbances: hypokalaemia, hypocalcaemia or hypomagnesaemia
- High protein liquid diets and other dietary factors
- Coronary ischaemia, myocarditis and severe heart failure

Table 11.5 Pacemaker code

Position of letter	Meaning of letter
First	Identifies chamber(s) paced (V = ventricle; A = atrium; D = dual)
Second	Identifies chamber(s) sensed (V = ventricle; A = atrium; D = dual; 0 = none)
Third	Describes the pacemaker's response to sensed impulses (T = triggered; I = inhibited; D = dual; R = reverse)
Fourth	Describes programmable functions
Fifth	Describes tachydysrhythmia control functions

magnesium (→ *Box 11.6*) or β blockers. Antiarrhythmic drugs such as lidocaine, quinidine, sotalol and amiodarone may further increase the Q–T interval and thus worsen the condition. Overdrive pacing may be required to prevent rapid relapse.

Long Q–T syndromes

A long Q–T interval may be acquired or, in very rare cases, congenital. *For the commonest acquired causes of a long Q–T syndrome → Box 11.7.* Consequent ventricular dysrhythmias may cause palpitations, syncope or even sudden death. The Q–T interval must be corrected for heart rate and is then called the QTc. This calculation is usually performed automatically by modern ECG machines. The normal QTc is 0.38–0.46 s. To make a confident 'eyeball' diagnosis, the Q–T interval should be around half a second (0.48 s or 12 small squares on the ECG).

Ectopic beats

During a 24-hour period, over 50% of apparently normal individuals will have ectopic beats within their ECG; in some cases these will be multifocal. The causes of extrasystoles include:

- fatigue
- anxiety
- excessive smoking, alcohol or caffeine intake
- idiopathic causes
- myocardial ischaemia
- heart diseases with atrial enlargement (→ *atrial fibrillation on p. 171*)
- digitalis and other drugs
- hyperthyroidism.

The treatment (if any) is dependent on identifying the likely causation. Multifocal ectopics, with differing waveforms, and runs of ectopic beats are more significant than isolated extrasystoles because they are more likely to develop into VT and VF.

Palpitations → p. 240.

Identification of pacemakers

The increasing complexity and diversity of pacemakers has necessitated the use of an identification system. An original three-letter code, which was agreed by the International Association of Pacemaker Manufacturers, has been expanded into a five-letter code to enable description of newer programmable units (→ *Table 11.5*). A simple pacemaker is described by the code VVI (ventricular pacing which is inhibited by sensed ventricular impulses).

12

Chest pain

Pain in the area of the chest is a worrying symptom for both the doctor and the patient. The patient knows that chest pain occurs in a heart attack. The doctor is aware that the symptoms of myocardial infarction (MI) and pulmonary embolism (PE) can be very different from the classic descriptions in the textbooks.

> Patients with chest pain account for more than 20% of all medical admissions in the UK.

Immediate assessment and management

- Assess ABCs as outlined in Chapter 1.
- Reassure the patient.
- Allow the patient to sit or lie in whatever position is most comfortable.
- Obtain a 12-lead ECG immediately (within 5–10 min of arrival) and interpret it at once. If there are changes that, when combined with the clinical picture, indicate the need for reperfusion therapy (ST-segment elevation MI, left bundle-branch block or posterior MI) treat without delay (→ p. 181).

In any case, if there are any immediately obvious symptoms or signs of serious illness or if the patient looks unwell:

- Administer a high concentration of oxygen by mask if the SaO_2 (arterial O_2 saturation) is <94% on air.
- Connect the patient to monitoring devices – ECG, BP and SaO_2.
- Obtain venous access and take blood for routine tests. Samples for cardiac markers should be taken at times dictated by local protocols (usually 12 h after the onset of pain for troponins) (→ p. 185).

- Request an urgent chest radiograph (CXR).
- Consider the need for early analgesia.

> Pallor and sweating usually indicate serious illness.
> Beware of the middle-aged man who wants you to make a diagnosis of indigestion.

Further assessment

Ask about

- Duration of pain
- Nature of pain including radiation and whether constant or intermittent
- Relationship of pain to breathing, coughing or moving
- Precipitating or relieving factors, including glyceryl trinitrate (GTN)
- Similarity of pain to previous events (e.g. MI or angina)
- Accompanying symptoms such as sweating, nausea, vomiting, flatus or general malaise
- Shortness of breath
- Collapse or blackout, however transitory
- Family and smoking history.

Look for

- Pallor, sweating or cyanosis
- Abnormal pulse or BP
- Raised jugular venous pressure (JVP) or dependent oedema
- Added heart sounds
- Changed respiratory rate and pattern
- Low SaO_2 on air

Emergency Medicine Lecture Notes, Fourth Edition. Chris Moulton and David Yates.
© 2012 Blackwell Publishing Ltd. Published 2012 by Blackwell Publishing Ltd.

- Reduced air entry and abnormal breath sounds
- Abdominal tenderness – especially epigastric and renal (which may mimic chest pain) and hepatic discomfort (congestive heart failure).

MI AND THE ACUTE CORONARY SYNDROMES

Coronary heart disease (CHD) is the most common cause of death and the single main cause of premature death in both men and women in the UK. It accounted for over a quarter of all deaths in England and Wales in 2010. By 2020, it is projected to be both the number one cause of death and the leading cause of life-years lost on a global scale. The three major risk factors for CHD are smoking, hypertension and hyperlipidaemia. The disease progresses faster in the presence of diabetes and obesity and doubles in incidence in those who are physically inactive. However, its victims are not all overweight, unfit individuals; MI strikes all shapes and sizes of people at almost all ages. Thirty per cent of people die from their first MI.

> Only 10% of the British population are free from all the major risk factors for CHD. Asians in the UK are at a particularly high risk. People with no obvious risk factors are still more likely to die of an MI than from any other cause.

CHD begins several decades before the acute event with the formation of atherosclerotic plaques. Seventy-five per cent of fatal coronary thromboses occur when there is a sudden rupture of the thin fibrous cap covering an inflamed, lipid-rich plaque. Mechanisms such as plaque erosion account for the rest. The initial flow obstruction is due to platelet aggregation followed by vasospasm. This process is accelerated by the secretion of substances such as thromboxane A_2, ADP and serotonin (5-hydroxytryptamine, 5HT) from entrapped platelets. Activation of the coagulation cascade then leads to the conversion of fibrinogen to fibrin, which is responsible for the subsequent stabilisation of the fragile thrombus. Within 30 min of complete coronary occlusion, MI develops, progressing from the subendocardium to the subepicardium.

The term 'acute coronary syndromes' (ACSs) describes a continuum of conditions that are associated with acute myocardial ischaemia as a result of interruption of the coronary blood supply. The syndromes range from unstable angina to full-thickness MI. ST-segment elevation MI (STEMI) exists as a distinct diagnostic entity because patients with specific ECG changes derive a unique benefit from immediate reperfusion therapy (thrombolysis or percutaneous coronary intervention [PCI]). Patients with other manifestations of ACSs are treated with low-molecular-weight heparins and antiplatelet therapy instead of fibrinolytic drugs ($\rightarrow$ later).

Every year, nearly a quarter of a million people in England and Wales have an acute MI. Up to 50% of them die in the first month. Half of these deaths occur in the first 2 h. The GRACE (Global Registry of Acute Cardiac Events) risk score is recommended (by the National Institute for Health and Clinical Excellence or NICE) as an early method of predicting 6-month mortality and thus guiding further treatment. It divides ACS patients into low-risk (<3% mortality rate), intermediate-risk (3–8%) and high-risk (>8%) groups. An online GRACE risk score calculator is available.

Diagnosis of acute coronary syndromes and evolving MI

Symptoms

The pain is classically experienced in the central chest and described as crushing or heavy. Some patients say that it feels like a tight band around their chest; others describe it as like someone sitting on them. It is common for the patient to clench his or her fist as an aid to description. The pain usually lasts longer than 15–20 min. The radiation, if any, may be to the left arm, neck or jaw. There is some suggestion that, in right coronary artery blockage, the jaw is the site of radiation whereas, in left-sided occlusions, the pain is felt in the arm.

> Chest pain that is atypical (in either site or character) can still be symptomatic of coronary ischaemia.

Accompanying symptoms such as sweating, pallor, nausea or general malaise are almost as helpful in making a diagnosis as the character of the pain. Coronary thrombosis may also present without pain ('silent MI'), with atypical pain, with complications of MI (e.g. left ventricular failure or LVF) or with an acute confusional state in elderly people.

Symptoms of 'indigestion': Be aware of the middle-aged man with 'indigestion', especially if he has no past dyspeptic history of significance. A few days of vague retrosternal pain is not a history of dyspepsia. It is much more likely to be the warning pains that often predate an MI. Recurrent belching is a sign of autonomic disturbance and as such may accompany an infarction. Even symptomatic relief from antacids should not be relied on to point away from the heart.

Some patients present with very atypical pain, in both site and character. Examples of this would be pain localised to the abdomen or to the left shoulder or arm alone.

> Many experienced doctors have sent patients home who have later proved to have an MI; sudden death may be this proof.

Signs

There are no invariable signs. Cardiogenic shock, acute pulmonary oedema or dysrhythmia makes the diagnosis much easier but physical examination of the patient is often normal. Pallor and sweating should never be ignored; they point to autonomic disturbance. The heart rate may be fast, slow or average. Likewise, the BP may be raised or low but is often normal. A slow heart rate often occurs in an inferior MI because the right coronary artery that supplies this area also supplies the conducting system. (In addition, it delivers blood to the posterior myocardium and the right ventricle, although in some patients the circumflex branch of the left coronary artery is responsible for much of this territory. The anterior and lateral myocardium is invariably supplied by the left anterior descending artery.)

Investigations in MI / ACS

- Immediate ECG (within a few minutes of arrival) is essential. Repeat ECG after 30–60 min may also be helpful.

Cardiac dysrhythmias → p. 164.
ECG changes in other acute coronary syndromes → p. 188.
ECG diagnosis of STEMI and indications for thrombolysis → below.

> A normal ECG does not exclude an MI.

- CXR is usually normal.
- Routine blood tests should be taken, especially a blood glucose to identify the need for a glucose and insulin infusion in ACS and MI.

Cardiac markers in ACS → p. 185.

- A reduction in pain after the administration of GTN may be a helpful test but unfortunately this effect also occurs in oesophageal spasm.

More advanced methods of diagnosis of myocardial ischaemia exist and some are undergoing clinical trials:

- Multi-lead 'vest' ECGs, which use over 80 chest electrodes
- High-resolution CT
- Two-dimensional echocardiography – regional motion abnormalities of the myocardium develop seconds after coronary occlusion
- Technetium scanning – a normal resting technetium-99 myocardial perfusion scintigram effectively excludes major MI. However, an abnormal scan is not diagnostic.

ECG diagnosis of coronary thrombosis and evolving infarction requiring immediate reperfusion therapy

Complete coronary occlusion causes an evolving MI that can be averted by timely reperfusion therapy. However, only when chest pain is accompanied by three specific ECG patterns has immediate reperfusion been shown to be of benefit. These three patterns are:

1 ST elevation MI (STEMI)
2 True posterior MI
3 New left BBB (LBBB).

(The term STEMI is useful in the acute situation to determine treatment and is analogous to older descriptions such as Q-wave MI and transmural infarction.)

1 ECG changes in STEMI

ST-segment elevation signifies complete occlusion of a major coronary artery and accounts for 30–40% of classic MIs. The occlusion/infarction sequence classically begins with subtle alterations in the T wave. These hyperacute T waves are tall, peaked and broadened with a loss of clear demarcation from the ST segment (→ *Figure 12.1*). Elevation of the ST segment ('convex-upwards') soon follows in leads that face the area of injury; reciprocal ST depression may also

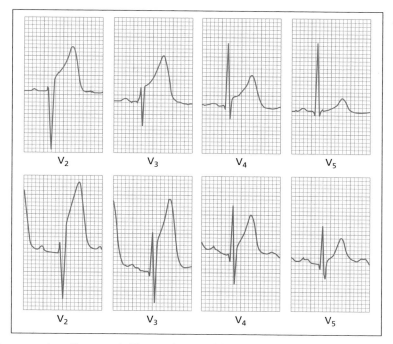

Figure 12.1 Two examples of hyperacute T waves in acute MI.

occur (→ *Figure 12.2*). Abnormal Q waves, which signify myocardial necrosis, may be present in the first ECG but in most cases do not appear for hours or even days after presentation. These pathological Q waves are wide (0.04 s – one small square – or more) and deep (4 mm or a quarter of the size of the subsequent R wave). They result from potentials that are transmitted through an electrical window of inexcitable myocardium and so suggest the presence of complete (transmural) rather than partial-thickness (subendocardial) damage (→ *later*). Severe intracellular disturbance may cause a similar picture. Finally, as the ST segment returns to the baseline, symmetrically inverted T waves appear. The timing and magnitude of all of these ECG changes vary greatly from patient to patient.

The site of a typical transmural infarction may be localised from the position of the ECG changes:

- *Anterior*: V1, V2, V3, V4
- *Lateral*: V5, V6
- *High lateral*: I, aVL
- *Inferior*: II, III, aVF (additional ST elevation in V4R [a right-sided V4] suggests infarction of the right ventricle → *Box 12.1 and p. 189*).

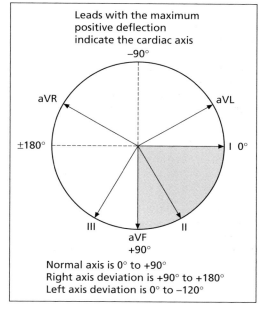

Leads with the maximum positive deflection indicate the cardiac axis

Normal axis is 0° to +90°
Right axis deviation is +90° to +180°
Left axis deviation is 0° to −120°

Figure 12.2 The ECG limb leads and the cardiac axis.

ECG changes must meet defined criteria for the diagnosis of STEMI and the initiation of reperfusion therapy:

1 ST elevation of at least 2 mm in two adjacent precordial (chest) leads (V2–V6) or
2 ST elevation of at least 1 mm in two limb leads (I, II, III, aVL or aVF).

Box 12.1 ECG signs of true posterior and right ventricular MI

Posterior infarction
• Tall R wave in the anterior leads (V1–V3)
• ST depression in the anterior leads (V1–V3), i.e. there is a mirror image of the usual Q wave and ST elevation pattern (→ *Figure 12.3*)
• ST elevation in posterior chest leads (→ *Figure 12.4*)

Right ventricular infarction
• ST elevation in V4R
• ST elevation in V1–V3 (and eventually Q waves in these leads)
• ECG changes of inferior MI

---

2 ECG changes in true posterior MI

Similar to conventional STEMI, true posterior infarction results from complete occlusion of a major coronary artery and, if untreated, leads to irreversible myocardial necrosis. The term 'true' refers to the isolation of the infarct to the posterior myocardium as opposed to being part of a posterolateral or inferoposterior picture.

ECG signs of true posterior and right ventricular MI →
  Box 12.1.
Figure 12.3 shows a 12-lead ECG of a posterior infarction.

However, although an isolated posterior infarct may be hard to diagnose on a conventional 12-lead ECG, it can be more reliably seen on a 15-lead or a 17-lead ECG. A 15-lead ECG has been described that utilises V4R and two posterior leads (→ *Figure 12.4*). This technique increases the detection of ST elevation in MI by about 10%. The extra three leads should be obtained when the standard 12-lead ECG shows either ST depression in the anterior chest leads or equivocal right-sided or inferior changes. Low-voltage ST elevation of just 0.5 mm in the posterior chest leads is sufficient to diagnose a posterior STEMI and initiate reperfusion therapy.

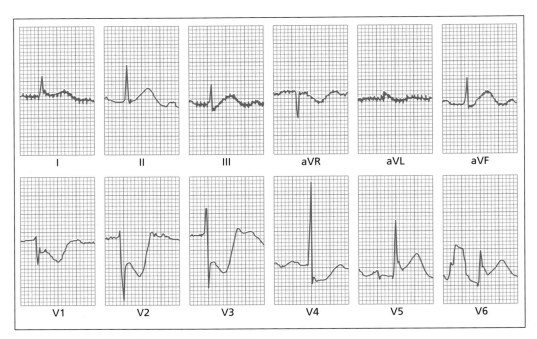

Figure 12.3 12-lead ECG of a true posterior infarction.

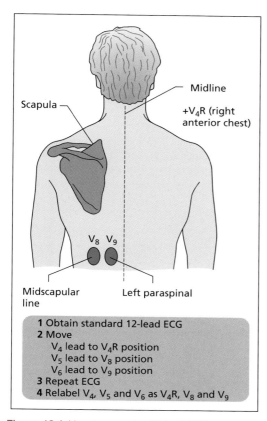

Midline

+V₄R (right anterior chest)

Scapula

V₈ V₉

Midscapular line

Left paraspinal

1 Obtain standard 12-lead ECG
2 Move
  V₄ lead to V₄R position
  V₅ lead to V₈ position
  V₆ lead to V₉ position
3 Repeat ECG
4 Relabel V₄, V₅ and V₆ as V₄R, V₈ and V₉

Figure 12.4 How to record a 15-lead ECG.

3 ECG changes in LBBB with MI

Patients with LBBB have a much worse prognosis with acute MI than patients with normal ventricular conduction, whether the LBBB is pre-existing or new. However, these patients (who account for around 0.5% of all patients with infarcts) have been shown to benefit greatly from reperfusion therapy. Consequently, in the presence of LBBB, it is essential to diagnose an MI promptly. This is difficult because the normal sequence of ventricular activation is altered and there is ST elevation because of the LBBB itself. Three ECG criteria (the Sgarbossa criteria) have been shown to have independent value in the diagnosis of MI in patients with LBBB (→ *Box 12.2*). Unfortunately, these criteria have to be scored and added to be useful and do not apply to all MIs with LBBB. Therefore, all patients with chest pain and proven or suspected new LBBB should be treated with PCI or fibrinolytic therapy without delay.

Diagnosis of LBBB → Table 11.4 and p. 167.

 Box 12.2 ECG diagnosis of MI in the presence of LBBB

Three ECG criteria have been shown to be useful in the diagnosis of MI in patients with LBBB:

1 ST-segment elevation of ≥1 mm that is concordant with (in the same direction as) a positive QRS complex
2 ST-segment depression of ≥1 mm in lead V1 or V2 or V3 (concordant change)
3 ST elevation of ≥5 mm that is discordant with (in the opposite direction from) a negative QRS complex

Treatment of ST elevation MI (STEMI)

The following section applies to new LBBB and posterior MI as well as to STEMI.

Having made the diagnosis of an evolving MI requiring immediate reperfusion therapy, the emergency treatment detailed below must not delay preparations for thrombolysis or percutaneous coronary intervention (PCI). Proceed immediately to reperfusion therapy without completing the following list:

• *Oxygen* by mask and IV access.
• *Continuous monitoring* of vital signs and ECG.
• *Analgesia* – IV morphine 5–10 mg or diamorphine 2.5–5 mg with an antiemetic (e.g. IV metoclopramide 10 mg).
• *Antiplatelet therapy* – aspirin 300 mg by mouth and oral clopidogrel. Aspirin is as effective as (and additive to) fibrinolysis in reducing death rates in STEMI. After an MI, it is continued for life at a dose of 75 mg daily. There are few contraindications to aspirin – known hypersensitivity, bleeding peptic ulcer and severe liver disease. Clopidogrel 300 mg by mouth should also be given to all patients aged <75 years with STEMI, including many of those in whom aspirin is contraindicated. However, in patients aged >75 years with STEMI, the dose of clopidogrel is omitted or reduced to 75 mg. Antiplatelet agents seem to have a synergistic effect with fibrinolytic drugs. For those patients who are having primary PCI, most centres routinely prescribe clopidogrel 600 mg or, alternatively, the newer thienopyridine antiplatelet agent prasugrel 60 mg by mouth. Prasugrel is not recommended for

patients who are aged >75 years, weigh <60 kg or have a history of transient ischaemic attack (TIA) or stroke.

- *Nitrates* – nitrates are used for persistent pain. Buccal GTN is a convenient and effective alternative to IV nitrates. The initial dose is 2 mg but this may be increased to 3–5 mg if necessary in the carefully monitored patient. A sublingual aerosol spray of GTN can be useful for a quick effect (two puffs = 800 mcg). *For GTN infusions → p. 209.*
- *Glucose and insulin infusion* – patients with diabetes and MI have double the mortality of those who do not have diabetes. In addition, there is experimental and limited clinical evidence that routine administration of glucose and insulin may improve metabolism in ischaemic myocardium. This treatment is inexpensive and should be given to all patients with either known diabetes or a blood sugar >11 mmol/L on admission. *For variable rate IV insulin regimen → Box 14.14 on p. 242.*
- *β Blockers* – if not contraindicated, early administration of a β blocker is recommended for all patients with MI. IV atenolol 5 mg is given over 5 min and the dose repeated after 10–15 min; 25 mg by mouth is an alternative. IV metoprolol is also licensed for this indication.

Inpatient treatment of MI and ACS → p. 189.
Thrombolysis → p. 183.

Reperfusion therapy for STEMI

This section applies to new LBBB and posterior MI as well as to STEMI.

There are two possible first-line reperfusion treatments:

1. *Primary PCI*: coronary angioplasty should be taking place within 90 min of arrival in hospital ('door-to-balloon' time) or within 120 min of first medical contact ('call-to-balloon' time). As a treatment standard, PCI should not be delayed for more than 60 min after the time that thrombolysis could have been given. PCI is a very effective therapy but system constraints often limit its delivery. Percutaneous transluminal coronary angioplasty (PTCA) is an older name for balloon-assisted PCI, before the common usage of stents.
2. *Immediate thrombolysis* (*→ p. 183*): thrombolysis should start within 20–30 min of arrival in hospital ('door-to-needle' time) or within 60 min of first contact with the emergency services ('call-to-needle' time). This is both effective and achievable. Even better results can be obtained with faster times or prehospital thrombolysis. Ideally, PCI should be performed during the following 24–48 h.

Local factors and protocols will control which of the above two treatments is most suitable for a particular patient. The availability of interventional cardiac catheterisation facilities is usually a major limiting factor in the UK. PCI is always the treatment of choice in cases where thrombolysis is contraindicated or has obviously failed. If the patient's chest pain started more than 3 h before arrival, (a delayed 'pain-to-needle' time), then primary PCI is much more effective than thrombolysis. PCI is contraindicated in severe thrombocytopenia. In the prehospital situation, fibrinolytic drugs offer the only possible means of reperfusion.

> There is a 'golden hour' for reperfusion therapy, which starts at the onset of pain.

PCI is better at opening closed arteries than thrombolysis. It achieves TIMI ('thrombolysis in myocardial infarction') grade 2 or 3 flow in over 95% of cases whereas fibrinolytic drugs have a maximum success rate of around 55% at completely opening up the artery responsible for the STEMI (TIMI grade 3 flow). Primary PCI is also associated with lower rates of stroke and non-fatal reinfarction than thrombolysis and goes some way to treating the underlying condition. It is much superior for patients with cardiogenic shock. When compared with tenecteplase or alteplase given within 2 h of symptom onset, very early PCI saves the lives of about 10 patients per 1000 treated. However, the added time to accomplish angioplasty often negates this advantage. Fibrinolytic drugs are most effective within 2–3 h of symptom onset. Within 6 h of the onset of chest pain, their administration prevents 30 deaths per 1000 patients treated (with aspirin increased to 50/1000 patients). Between 7 and 12 h, this reduces to 20 lives saved per 1000 patients treated. After 12 h, the risk–benefit ratio for fibrinolytic drugs is less certain. Thrombolysis increase mortality if given more than 24 h after symptom onset or to patients with ST depression or T-wave inversion without ST elevation.

> The rate of intercranial haemorrhage with thrombolysis is <1% but half of these bleeds are fatal.

Fibrinolytic drugs cause around 4 extra strokes per 1000 patients treated. These occur in the first 24 h, two patients dying and two surviving, one of whom will be disabled. The risk of stroke is predicted by advanced age, low body weight, female gender, previous cerebrovascular accident (CVA) and hypertension, especially hypertension on admission. Major non-cerebral bleeds occur in 7/1000 patients treated and are most commonly procedure related. Again advanced age, low body weight and female gender are associated factors.

> Reduction in ST elevation of >50% within 60–90 min of thrombolysis suggests a patent artery and preserved myocardium.

The resolution of chest pain and reduction in ST elevation suggest reperfusion, as does the emergence of arrhythmias. Failed reperfusion (i.e. <50% reduction in ST elevation on ECG within 90 min of starting the treatment) is an indication for rescue PCI. There is little evidence for re-thrombolysis except after the less effective drug streptokinase. Coronary artery bypass graft (CABG) surgery is becoming more common as an emergency procedure in the UK.

Thrombolytic therapy for STEMI

This section applies to new LBBB and posterior MI as well as to STEMI.

Fibrinolysis is an endogenous process whereby the insoluble fibrin that binds a blood clot together is broken down into soluble fragments (fibrin degradation products or FDPs). It is initiated by plasminogen activators such as tissue plasminogen activator (tPA), which are secreted into the circulation by the vessel wall. These substances convert plasminogen, a protein normally present in the plasma, into plasmin, which digests fibrin. Free circulating plasmin is inactivated by α_2-antiplasmin. Fibrinolytic drugs exert their effect by activating plasminogen to form plasmin, which degrades fibrin, so breaking up thrombi.

The criteria for the administration of thrombolytic therapy are as follows:

1 History compatible with MI
2 Onset of symptoms within the last 12 h
3 Diagnostic ECG changes as below (→ *also p. 178)*:
  – ST elevation of at least 2 mm in two adjacent precordial leads (V2–V6)
  – ST elevation of at least 1 mm in two limb leads (I, II, III, aVL or aVF)
  – LBBB (presumed or proven to be new)

Box 12.3 Contraindications to thrombolytic therapy

This is not an exhaustive list.

Absolute contraindications
- Known coagulation defects or bleeding diatheses
- Recent haemorrhage, significant trauma or surgery (including dental extraction)
- Haemorrhagic stroke or stroke of unknown causation at any time
- Ischaemic stroke in last 6 months
- History of central nervous system (CNS) damage, aneurysm or neoplasm
- Intracranial surgery or significant head injury within last 3 weeks
- Severe uncontrolled hypertension
- Acute pericarditis or bacterial endocarditis
- Active pulmonary disease with cavitation
- Aortic dissection
- Active peptic ulceration
- Gastrointestinal bleeding within last 4 weeks
- Acute pancreatitis
- Severe liver disease
- Oesophageal varices
- Visceral neoplasm with increased risk of bleeding
- Heavy vaginal bleeding
- Coma
- Previous allergic reaction to drug (streptokinase)

Cautions/relative contraindications *(balance risk–benefit for each patient)*
- Current oral anticoagulant therapy
- Recent non-compressible arterial or central venous puncture sites
- Traumatic resuscitation
- TIA in last 6 months
- Diabetic retinopathy (small risk of bleeding only, so not a major contraindication)
- Hypertension (systolic BP >180 mmHg)
- Abdominal aortic aneurysm
- Genitourinary (GU) bleeding in last 10 days
- Pregnant or <1 week postpartum

  – evidence of true posterior infarction (→ *Box 12.1 and Figure 12.3)*. Low-voltage ST elevation of just 0.5 mm in the posterior chest leads is sufficient to diagnose STEMI
4 No contraindications to thrombolysis (→ *Box 12.3)*.

> **Box 12.4 Thrombolytic regimens for STEMI**
>
> **Tenecteplase (TNK-tPA)**
> Single IV bolus given over 10 s + heparin for 24–48 h. Weight adjusted (500–600 mg/kg):
>
> - 30 mg if weight <60 kg
> - 35 mg if weight 60 kg to <70 kg
> - 40 mg if weight 70 kg to <80 kg
> - 45 mg if weight 80 kg to <90 kg
> - 50 mg if weight ≥90 kg
>
> **Alteplase (tPA)**
> IV bolus followed by infusion to maximum dose of 100 mg over 90 min + heparin for 24–48 h. If not using a special programmable syringe driver:
>
> - Draw up 50 mg of alteplase into each of two 50-mL syringes
> - Give an IV 15-mg bolus from the first syringe
> - Infuse 50 mg (the entire contents of the second syringe) over 30 min, using an infusion pump
> - Infuse the remainder of the first syringe (35 mg) over the next 60 min
>
> For patients <65 kg give a 15-mg IV bolus, then 0.75 mg/kg over 30 min and then 0.5 mg/kg over 60 min.
>
> **Reteplase (rPA)**
> Double IV bolus of 10 U + 10 U given 30 min apart + heparin for 24–48 h. Reteplase is not adjusted for weight.
>
> **Streptokinase**
> Infusion of 1.5 MU over 1 h. Heparin is not required (but may be given).
>
> - Dilute the contents of a 1.5-MU vial in 10 mL of 5% dextrose
> - Add this to a further 50 mL of 5% dextrose in a 60-mL infusion pump syringe
> - Run at 1 mL/min
>
> **Low-molecular-weight heparin**
> - Give 30 mg enoxaparin as an IV bolus. Omit in patients >75 years
> - Also give 1 mg/kg of enoxaparin subcutaneously. Reduce this dose to 750 mcg/kg in patients >75 years
>
> **Unfractionated heparin**
> - Give 5000 U of unfractionated heparin as an IV bolus
> - Continue with a heparin infusion for a minimum of 24 h. Infuse at 1250 U/h initially. The clotting time (activated partial thromboplastin time or APTT) should be measured within 12 h and the heparin infusion adjusted to keep the value at twice normal. These doses should be adjusted for patients with a low body weight (i.e. <60 kg)

Patients who present more than 12 h after the onset of symptoms (but not more than 24 h) may still be considered for thrombolysis if there are signs or symptoms of continuing ischaemia. Thrombolytic therapy is contraindicated in a considerable number of patients (→ Box 12.3). The contraindications are mostly those conditions that might result in severe or life-threatening bleeding. In some cases, there is a possibility of pre-existing thrombus (e.g. with aneurysms or atrial fibrillation), so there is a risk of causing an embolism by dissolution of the clot.

Heparin is given with all fibrinolytic drugs except streptokinase. It does not improve clot lysis but seems to help maintain coronary patency in the following hours and days. *For doses of thrombolytic drugs → Box 12.4.* An IV bolus of 5000 U of unfractionated heparin is followed by an IV infusion for 24–48 h.

Low-molecular-weight heparins (LMWHs) are often used in place of standard unfractionated heparin. For adults aged <75 years, an IV bolus of 30 mg enoxaparin is given together with a subcutaneous injection of 1 mg/kg. The subcutaneous dose is repeated 12-hourly for up to 8 days. The IV bolus is omitted in older patients who are given subcutaneous enoxaparin only in a dose of 750 mcg/kg. Fondaparinux (a synthetic pentasaccharide that inhibits activated factor X) is an alternative to heparins.

To be of maximum benefit, thrombolysis must be started as soon as possible and certainly within 20–30 min of hospital arrival.

Prehospital thrombolysis is a logical way of improving 'call-to-needle' times still further (often yielding time gains of up to 1 h). It has been shown to save an additional 16 lives per 1000 patients treated when

Box 12.5 Genetic modification of tPA to create TNK-tPA

Both alteplase and tenecteplase molecules are made up of 527 amino acids organised into five distinct modules. However, tenecteplase (TNK-tPA) has three modifications to specific areas of alteplase (standard tPA), which improve its pharmacokinetics:

1 Threonine (T) replaced with asparagine at position 103 (increases the half-life)
2 Asparagine (N) replaced with glutamine at position 117 (reduces plasma clearance and so increases the half-life)
3 Lysine (K), histidine and two arginines replaced with four alanines at positions 296–299 (increases fibrin specificity and gives an 80-fold greater resistance to plasminogen activator inhibitors (PAIs) such as PAI-1)

compared with conventional in-hospital thrombolysis. A recent study found that prehospital thrombolysis reduced mortality by the same amount as primary PCI.

Choice of thrombolytic drug

Contraindications to thrombolysis → Box 12.3.

Tenecteplase (TNK-tPA) is the best drug for all patients with STEMI because it combines maximum efficacy with ease of administration. It is given as a single weight-adjusted IV bolus over 10 s (→ *Box 12.4*). It is always accompanied by IV heparin to prevent re-thrombosis. An IV bolus of 5000 U unfractionated heparin is followed by an IV infusion for 24–48 h (→ *Box 12.4*). Tenecteplase is the end-result of a long research programme to find an 'ideal' fibrinolytic agent and was created by recombinant DNA modification of standard tissue-type plasminogen activator (→ *Box 12.5*). A longer half-life allows for single bolus treatment and increased fibrin specificity targets the plasminogen on the clot surface while minimising systemic plasminogen activation. This latter property leads to a decrease in non-cerebral bleeding complications and the need for blood transfusions.

The three other standard fibrinolytic drugs are alteplase, reteplase and streptokinase. Alteplase and reteplase are both plasminogen activators but streptokinase is not a naturally occurring substance in humans. Although it is cheap, it is antigenic and causes allergy and hypotension. Infusions of strep-

tokinase are often discontinued or slowed down because of these side effects – a problem that is concealed by auditing 'door-to-needle' times in isolation. Streptokinase is much less effective than tPA in patients aged <75 years with anterior infarcts and, in addition, should not be given to patients who:

1 have ever received streptokinase or anistreplase (a related drug) before
2 have had a recent, proven, streptococcal infection
3 have a systolic BP <90 mmHg
4 may need an urgent invasive procedure (e.g. pacing or PCI).

Overall, the use of tenecteplase or alteplase rather than streptokinase has been shown to save around 9 lives per 1000 patients treated.

Comparison of the four main fibrinolytic drugs → Table 12.1.
Standard regimens for all of the four main fibrinolytic drugs and heparin → Box 12.4.
Treatment of complications of thrombolytic therapy → Box 12.6.

Biochemical markers of myocardial damage

The biochemical markers of ischaemic injury include the traditional cardiac enzymes (especially creatinine kinase–myocardial band [CK-MB]) and, more recently, the cardiac proteins myoglobin and troponin. The exact use of these tests depends on local protocols; only the troponins are discussed in detail in this section. However, the use of commercial fixed combinations of cardiac markers is becoming more common in an attempt to improve the sensitivity and specificity of the biochemical diagnosis of MI in <12 h from the onset of symptoms.

Timing of the release of the three main cardiac markers into the bloodstream after ischaemic chest pain → Figure 12.5.

The cardiac specific troponins T and I (cTnT and cTnI) are proteins that are released into the bloodstream by damaged heart muscle. They are polypeptide components of the tropomyosin complex in myofibrils, which mediate actin–myosin interaction and consequent muscle contraction. The cardiac isoforms of both troponins are specific and are not found in skeletal muscle or other tissues. They are used for three main purposes:

1 To confirm or exclude the diagnosis of an ACS
2 To quantify the extent of myocardial damage and thus allow for risk stratification
3 To assess reperfusion and reinfarction.

Table 12.1 Comparison of the four main fibrinolytic drugs

	Tenecteplase	Alteplase	Reteplase	Streptokinase
Molecular weight (Daltons)	70 000	70 000	39 000	47 000
Plasma half-life (min)	20–24	4–7	15–18	23–29
Fibrin specificity	+++	++	+	−
Usual dose	0.53 mg/kg as a single bolus	100 mg over 90 min	Two 10 IU boluses 30 min apart	1.5 MIU over 60 min
Ease of use	+++	+	++	+
Reduction in mortality	++	++	+(+)?	+
Risk of haemorrhagic stroke	++	++	++	+
Antigenicity	−	−	−	++
Likelihood of hypotension	−	−	−	++

Urokinase is a direct plasminogen activator, which is produced by human kidney cells and so is non-antigenic. It is given as an IV infusion of 2 MU over 15 min but is not routinely available in the UK.

 Box 12.6 **Treatment of complications of thrombolysis**

Bleeding
Apply pressure, if possible, to any bleeding sites and, if the bleeding is severe then:

- Stop the infusion
- Start careful volume replacement
- Give cryoprecipitate 6 U or fresh frozen plasma (FFP) 2 U
- Consider antifibrinolytic drugs (tranexamic acid 10 mg/kg by slow IV injection or, exceptionally, aprotinin 500 000 U by slow IV injection)

Reperfusion arrhythmias
- Observe if transitory or minor

    Treatment of peri-arrest arrhythmias → p. 164.

Mild allergic reaction (to streptokinase)
- Give IV hydrocortisone 100–200 mg
- Give IV chlorphenamine 10–20 mg
- Continue the fibrinolytic drug with careful observation

Severe allergic reaction (to streptokinase)
- Stop the infusion
- Give hydrocortisone and chlorphenamine as above

In addition, if indicated give:
- Nebulised bronchodilators
- IM/IV adrenaline

Hypotension (following streptokinase)
- Interrupt the infusion temporarily
- Elevate the legs if necessary
- In extreme cases consider starting a low-dose noradrenaline infusion

---

Troponins have diagnostic sensitivities for acute MI, which approach 100%. The maximum sensitivity occurs 12 h after the onset of symptoms, so this is the point at which a blood sample for troponin should be taken. A normal troponin level at this time indicates a very low risk of cardiac complications in the next 30 days. However, it does not exclude the possibility of underlying CHD or that the patient's symptoms were due to myocardial ischaemia. Raised troponins (especially if elevated early in the ischaemic process) are associated with reduced ejection fractions and increased morbidity and mortality in subsequent

	Increase	Peak	Return to normal
Myoglobin	2h	6–9h	20–36h
CK-MB	3–6h	12–24h	3 days
Troponins	4–8h	12–16h	5–10 days

Figure 12.5 The release of the three main cardiac markers into the bloodstream after MI.

Box 12.7 Troponin T levels

The values given below are intended as a guide only; individual laboratories will set their own diagnostic ranges. Ranges of levels of troponin I have similar significances:

- *Troponin T <0.03mg/L*: although this does not rule out underlying CHD, a troponin T value in this category conveys no additional prognostic information. However, values between 0.01 and 0.03mg/L are abnormal and indicate either an ACS or an alternative condition
- *Troponin T 0.03–0.1mg/L*: this indicates minimal myocardial damage. Higher values are associated with greater degrees of myocardial cell loss and thus an increased likelihood of the patient developing complications
- *Troponin T 0.1–0.2mg/L*: troponin T levels >0.1mg/L suggest that significant myocardial damage has occurred. This group of patients has the greatest benefit from antiplatelet therapy
- *Troponin T >0.2mg/L*: this is the level associated with classic MI with all the attendant implications for prognosis

months. Troponin T remains elevated for 12–14 days after a large MI, troponin I for 7–10 days. *For diagnostic significance of raised levels of troponin T → Box 12.7.*

Use of troponin levels to guide safe discharge of patients from hospital: a patient who has a low clinical probability of cardiac pain, no ECG changes, a full resolution of symptoms and a normal 12-h troponin level can be safely discharged from hospital with (or sometimes without) outpatient follow-up. Use of troponins in this way has been shown to reduce the length of hospitalisation for patients with chest pain by around 33%.

False-positive troponin levels: increased troponin levels can occur in patients who do not exhibit the clinical features of an ACS. These false-positive results can lead to situations where a raised troponin is difficult to interpret. *For other clinical conditions in which raised troponins have been identified → Box 12.8.*

Acute coronary syndromes without persistent ST elevation

The ACSs without ST elevation comprise a continuum from unstable angina (UA) through to non-ST elevation MI (NSTEMI). Sensitive markers of myocardial damage (such as troponins) have revealed that there is no real qualitative difference between the various diagnostic labels. There is an underlying critical but incomplete occlusion of one or more coronary

Box 12.8 Other conditions associated with a raised troponin level

Cardiac conditions
- Myocardial contusion (raised troponin is not a sensitive indicator of trauma but has a high positive predictive value)
- Heart failure and septic shock
- Cardiac arrhythmias
- Myocarditis and cardiomyopathy
- Cardiac surgery and post-transplantation
- Cardiac electrophysiological procedures (not DC cardioversion)

Non-cardiac conditions
- Renal failure (most common reason for a false positive)
- Pulmonary embolism (associated with large emboli and right ventricular damage)
- Non-cardiac surgery

Table 12.2 Significance of T-wave inversion on a 12-lead ECG

Leads with T-wave inversion	Significance
AVR only	Normal
V1 only	Occurs in 20% of normal adults and most children
V1 and V2	Occurs in 5% of normal adults and many children
V3–V6	Always abnormal in adults
I and II	Always abnormal in adults
AVL, AVF and III	May be normal if the T-wave axis is similar to the QRS axis

Abnormal T-wave inversion may be due to ischaemia, strain or pericarditis

arteries. The ECG may show ST depression and/or T-wave inversion but is often completely normal. ST depression carries a worse prognosis. *For the significance of T-wave inversion on a 12-lead ECG → Table 12.2.* The diagnosis of myocardial necrosis may be made from the ECG alone (especially in the case of certain patterns such as subendocardial infarction (→ *below*) – but more commonly depends on the presence of raised levels of serum cardiac markers. The most commonly used cardiac markers are CK-MB, myoglobin, troponin T and troponin I (→ *p. 185*). With the aid of troponin levels, unstable angina may be somewhat arbitrarily differentiated from NSTEMI (→ *Box 12.8*). In addition, the injury may be quantified in terms of myocardial cell loss (i.e. size of infarct). Unfortunately, troponins do not reach their maximum sensitivity until 12 h after the onset of symptoms and so vigorous treatment must be initiated for all patients with suspected ACS.

Subendocardial infarction

Although the pathological and electrical findings do not correlate exactly, established MIs may be classified by ECG into two broad groups: Q-wave and non-Q-wave infarctions. Patients with ECGs in the latter group have smaller infarcts and a lower initial mortality, although they have a high risk of further (usually Q-wave) infarctions. Transmural damage to the myocardium (e.g. untreated STEMI) is usually associated with the development of Q waves and/or the loss of R-wave voltages, whereas incomplete infarction of

Box 12.9 ECG signs of subendocardial infarction

- ST-segment depression (earliest change)
- Reduction in size of R wave
- Deep symmetrical negative T wave

Unlike the more common transmural infarction, subendocardial infarction does not result in Q waves. The ECG changes are usually reflected in multiple leads but are especially frequent in the precordial leads. Exact location of the infarct site is difficult or impossible.

the ventricular wall leads to prolonged ST and T-wave changes (→ *Box 12.9*). This subendocardial infarction accounts for about 25% of all classic infarcts and represents the most severe end of the ACS spectrum, just before STEMI. It results from either diffuse three-vessel disease or a single severe stenosis.

Tx of ACS without ST elevation
- *Oxygen and IV access*
- *Continuous monitoring* of vital signs and ECG
- *Analgesia* – IV diamorphine 2.5–5.0 mg with an antiemetic (e.g. IV metoclopramide 10 mg)
- *Antiplatelet therapy* – aspirin 300 mg and clopidogrel 300 mg by mouth. *For glycoprotein(GP) IIb/IIIa inhibitors → p. 189.*

Aspirin induces a long-lasting functional defect in platelets by blocking the arachidonate metabolism (thromboxane A_2-dependent platelet aggregation). After ACS, it is continued for life in a dose of 75 mg daily. There are only a few contraindications to aspirin – known hypersensitivity, bleeding peptic ulcer and severe liver disease. Clopidogrel is a thienopyridine that inhibits ADP-induced platelet aggregation. In patients with ACS, it provides an additional 20% relative risk reduction over and above aspirin for MI, CVA and death. The loading dose is 300 mg, followed by 75 mg a day for 12 months. The onset of action of clopidogrel is delayed for 2–4 h.

- *Antithrombin therapy*
Enoxaparin 1 mg/kg subcutaneously. Low-molecular-weight heparins (LMWHs) are more effective in ACSs than standard unfractionated heparin. They have a higher plasma availability and better factor Xa inhibition. The prolonged half-life and more predictable kinetics allow them to be given subcutaneously without monitoring of clotting parameters. The best evidence is for enoxaparin – 1 mg/kg subcutaneously immediately and then twice daily for six doses or, if the pain is ongoing, until the patient has been pain free for 24 h. This dosage is reduced to 1 mg/kg once daily in severe renal impairment (i.e. creatinine clearance <30 mL/min).

- *Nitrates*
Nitrates are given for persistent pain. Buccal GTN is a convenient and effective alternative to IV nitrates. The initial dose is 2 mg but this may be increased to 3–5 mg if necessary in the carefully monitored patient. A sublingual aerosol spray of GTN can be useful for a quick effect (two puffs = 800 mcg). *For GTN infusions → p. 209.*

- *Glucose and insulin infusion*
Patients with diabetes and MI have double the mortality of those who do not have diabetes. In addition, there is experimental and limited clinical evidence that routine administration of glucose and insulin may improve metabolism in ischaemic myocardium. This treatment is inexpensive and should be given to all patients with either known diabetes or a blood sugar >11 mmol/L on admission.

Variable rate IV insulin regimen → Box 14.14 on p. 242.

- *β Blockers*
If not contraindicated, early administration of a β blocker is recommended for all patients with MI or other ACS. IV atenolol 5 mg is given over 5 min and the dose repeated after 10–15 min; 25 mg by mouth is an alternative. IV metoprolol is also licensed for this indication. β Blockers may be used for persistent or recurrent chest pain. Calcium antagonists are an alternative if β blockers are contraindicated.

Inpatient treatment: all patients with MI or a suspected ACS require admission to hospital for monitoring, 12-h troponin measurement and specialist assessment. Risk factor modification, optimisation of BP control and lipid-lowering therapy will then be considered. Ideally, an exercise ECG test and coronary angiography should be performed within 24 h.

ACE inhibitors: these drugs are of benefit to all patients with MI who have no contraindications, especially those with hypertension or poor LV function. Treatment with an angiotensin-converting enzyme (ACE) inhibitor should be started within 24 h of the acute episode and continued for at least 6 weeks. A raised troponin is strongly associated with a reduced ejection fraction and so is used in some centres as an indication for ACE inhibitor therapy.

Glycoprotein IIb/IIIa inhibitors: platelets are a key element of the thrombus formation in ACS. Their initial aggregation is caused by the formation of fibrinogen bridges between surface receptors. The glycoprotein (GP) IIb/IIIa inhibitors (abciximab, eptifibatide and tirofiban) are the most potent inhibitors of platelet aggregation available and work by blocking the binding of fibrinogen to these receptors. Abciximab is a monoclonal antibody, which binds to GP IIb/IIIa receptors, and should be used only once in an individual patient. This group of drugs is used, under specialist advice:

1 In ACSs without persistent ST elevation (usually eptifibatide or tirofiban)
2 As an adjunct to primary PCI (especially in patients with diabetes or undergoing complex procedures) (usually abciximab).

Unfortunately, GP IIb/IIIa inhibitors have been shown to cause increased bleeding when combined with fibrinolytic drugs.

Treatment of complications of MI

The outcome after acute MI is in part determined by the characteristics of the patient. Advanced age, diabetes, renal insufficiency and previous MI or CVA all contribute to a less favourable outcome.

Right ventricular infarction

This accompanies around a third of inferior MIs and causes the non-specific triad of hypotension, raised

JVP and clear lung fields. ST elevation in V4R is very suggestive of the diagnosis; ST elevation in V1–V3 is also often present ($\rightarrow$ *Box 12.1*). Echocardiography may confirm the diagnosis. Right ventricular preload must be maintained with IV fluids and vasodilators should be avoided.

Sinus bradycardia

This is common with inferior infarction because the inferior myocardium shares its blood supply with the right ventricle, posterior left heart and conducting system. (The sinoatrial [SA] node is supplied by the right coronary artery in 55% of patients and by the circumflex artery in the remaining 45%. The AV node is served by the right coronary artery in 90% of cases with just 10% of patients having a circumflex supply.) At heart rates >45 beats/min, sinus bradycardia is best just observed, but below this it starts to cause hypotension and faintness. IV atropine is effective (adult dose: 200–2000 mcg depending on the response). Tachycardia may reduce coronary perfusion while increasing oxygen demand and is thus to be avoided.

Left ventricular aneurysm

This occurs in 5% of MIs (usually large transmural anterior infarcts). Unsurprisingly, it decreases cardiac output and increases mortality by a factor of 6. Thrombus may form inside the aneurysmal sac. A CXR may show cardiomegaly and there may be persistent ST elevation on the ECG. Echocardiogram is required for a definitive diagnosis. Treatment is symptomatic together with anticoagulation.

Free wall rupture of the ventricle

This is seen after 5% of MIs, 90% of cases occurring within 14 days of infarction. Acute tearing chest pain is followed by collapse, profound shock, pulseless electrical activity (PEA) and death. Ruptured ventricle is thought to be responsible for 10–20% of post-MI deaths. Subacute free wall rupture causes a rapid-onset tamponade.

Ventricular septal rupture (acute ventricular septal defect or VSD)

This occurs in 1% of MIs, usually in the first week. The patient experiences a sudden onset of chest pain and shortness of breath. On examination, there is biventricular failure and shock. A harsh pansystolic murmur is present in 90% of cases with a systolic thrill in 50%. Echocardiogram confirms the diagnosis.

Treatment of the heart failure is aimed at keeping the patient alive while waiting for immediate surgical repair of the defect.

Acute mitral regurgitation

This occurs in 1% of MIs, usually in the first week. It is caused by LV dilatation, papillary muscle dysfunction or papillary muscle rupture. The clinical presentation ranges from tachycardia and LVF to shock and PEA. There is usually a soft pansystolic murmur. A CXR shows pulmonary oedema; echocardiogram confirms the diagnosis. Temporary medical management of the heart failure should precede immediate valve replacement surgery.

Cardiac arrest $\rightarrow$ *p. 150.*
Cardiogenic shock $\rightarrow$ *p. 238.*
Dysrhythmias $\rightarrow$ *p. 164.*
LVF and acute pulmonary oedema $\rightarrow$ *p. 208.*
Pericarditis $\rightarrow$ *p. 192.*

OTHER COMMON CAUSES OF CHEST PAIN

Pulmonary embolism

> The lung (including the visceral pleura) has no pain fibres. PE (and pneumonia) can cause chest pain only if there are peripheral parenchymal changes spreading outside the lung to the extremely sensitive parietal pleura. Thus large PEs do not cause pleuritic chest pain. Small ones sometimes do!

PE is easily missed in the following circumstances:

1 If the only symptom is breathlessness ('isolated dyspnoea') ($\rightarrow$ *p. 215*).
2 In elderly patients
3 In the presence of coexisting cardiorespiratory disease.

> A patient with increasing breathlessness, low SaO_2 and little else to find on clinical examination may be suffering from recurrent PEs. The SaO_2 can sometimes improve dramatically with oxygen therapy.

In addition to dyspnoea, PE may cause a variety of other clinical presentations:

1 Chest pain (but only rarely as an isolated symptom → *below*)
2 Haemoptysis (but again only rarely as an isolated symptom)
3 New onset of atrial fibrillation (→ *p. 171*)
4 Collapse ± hypotension
5 Shock
6 Cardiac arrest.

The diagnosis of PE is relatively unlikely in patients aged <40 years with no major risk factors who are not breathless or tachypnoeic.

> Oestrogen therapy is only a minor risk factor for venous thromboembolism.

DVT → *p. 108.*
Further details on the diagnosis and management of pulmonary embolism → p. 214.
Major risk factors for venous thromboembolism → Box 13.13 on p. 215.
Relative risks of PE and DVT for women taking combined oestrogen and progestogen contraceptive pills (and in pregnancy) → Table 7.2 on p. 109.

Isolated pleuritic chest pain as a symptom of PE

Young adults (e.g. women on oral contraception) frequently present to EDs with a single complaint of pleuritic chest pain (i.e. without breathlessness). They have a very low risk of PE if they are aged <40 years with:

- no major risk factors for thromboembolism (oestrogens are only a minor risk factor)
- no clinical features of DVT
- a respiratory rate <20/min
- a normal SaO_2 on air
- a normal CXR.

A D-dimer assay may be used to rule out PE in this situation. The test should not be requested if:

- The patient is febrile or has any evidence of inflammatory disease (febrile symptoms make the diagnosis of PE unlikely).
- There is already a clear working diagnosis.
- PE is very unlikely.
- There is a high clinical probability of PE (and so the patient will require definitive imaging).

In these circumstances, if a D-dimer assay has already been performed and is positive, it can be ignored.

Musculoskeletal chest pain → p. 195.
Pleurisy → p. 194.
Pneumothorax → p. 192.
Precordial catch/severe transitory chest pains of young adults → p. 195.

Angina pectoris (stable angina)

> Cardiac pain occurring at rest is always worrying. A couple of attacks of resting pain (i.e. unstable angina) commonly occur a few days before a fatal infarction.

The pain of angina pectoris is cardiac pain and thus is identical to that described above for MI. Even the intensity of the pain apparently overlaps that experienced in some infarctions. Angina arises from heart muscle, which is working too hard for its available blood, and hence oxygen, supply. As such it must be differentiated from the pain felt in myocardium that is losing its blood supply, i.e. infarcting.

> A patient with cardiac pain that has lasted for more than 20 min should be admitted to hospital.

To diagnose stable angina confidently the following should be confirmed.

- The patient is known to suffer from angina.
- The pain lasts only a few minutes.
- There are no atypical accompanying features, e.g. sweating.
- There is no increase in the frequency of the attacks, i.e. the patient is not developing crescendo angina.
- The pain is precipitated by the usual factors, (e.g. exercise) and it is not becoming unstable angina.
- Relief from the pain is spontaneous or by GTN.
- The ECG is unchanged.
- Everything is the same as usual.

> If this episode is so typical, why did the patient come to hospital? Resolve this question before discharge.

Tx

Treatment of unstable angina → Acute coronary syndromes on p. 187.

Box 12.10 CXR signs of thoracic aortic dissection

- Wide superior mediastinum
- Left pleural effusion
- Left pleural 'cap'
- Trachea moved to right
- Aortic outline blurred
- Left main bronchus moved down

Patients with stable angina of short duration can be allowed to go home if the above criteria are met. GP follow-up should be arranged.

Dissecting aneurysm of the thoracic aorta

This presents with severe pain radiating to the back. There may be evidence of hypertension, pregnancy, aortic coarctation or Marfan's syndrome. Pulses may be absent or unequal and acute aortic incompetence is sometimes found.

Investigations: CXR changes are often seen (→ *Box 12.10*). CT scan with contrast is diagnostic.

> A normal CXR does not exclude the diagnosis of aortic dissection.

Other (benign) causes of a widened mediastinum on CXR → p. 80.
Radiographic changes after injury to the great vessels → p. 80.

Tx Immediate consultation with a thoracic surgeon is indicated. Meanwhile, treatment should include oxygen, monitoring and IV access. The patient should be given IV analgesia and blood samples sent to the laboratory for routine tests and cross-matching. Treatment will be required for any concomitant hypertension (→ *p. 239*).

Pericarditis

Pericarditis presents as sharp, persistent midsternal chest pain, which varies in intensity with body position. The pain may be worsened by inspiration, swallowing and lying down. It is usually said that the pain is relieved by sitting and leaning forward. However, the authors have known the reverse to occur – exacerbation of the pain with flexion of the trunk.

Radiation of the pain to the area of the trapezius muscle is very suggestive of pericarditis. A rub is sometimes heard during part of the cardiac cycle and is often loudest at the left sternal border.

Investigations: The ECG may show widespread ST elevation (in all leads except aVR and V1), characteristically 'concave upwards'. There is no accompanying ST depression. Diffuse PR-segment depression is also often seen, especially in lead II. Echocardiography may detect an effusion.

Tx Treatment of viral pericarditis (the most common form) is with non-steroidal anti-inflammatory drugs (NSAIDs) and rest to avoid the development of myocarditis. Diclofenac 75 mg IM may be given in the ED.

Post-infarction pericarditis is seen in 5–20% of patients with transmural MI. The incidence is halved by the use of fibrinolytic drugs. There may be a low-grade fever and an echocardiogram may show an effusion. Post-infarction pericarditis is treated with high-dose aspirin. (NSAIDs and steroids can interfere with myocardial healing.)

Dressler's syndrome occurs in 1–5% of patients 2–3 months post-MI. It is thought to have an autoimmune origin. Pericardial effusion is rare in Dressler's syndrome. This type of pericarditis is also treated with aspirin.

Myocarditis and endocarditis → p. 239.

Pneumothorax

Spontaneous pneumothorax is most commonly seen in two groups of patients:

1 Young adults who are otherwise healthy and thus can tolerate a large air leak (primary pneumothorax)
2 Older patients with emphysema, pulmonary fibrosis or other underlying lung disease in whom even a small pneumothorax can precipitate respiratory failure (secondary pneumothorax).

> Up to 5% of people with HIV infection will develop a pneumothorax, usually with either TB or PCP (*Pneumocystis jiroveci* [formerly *P. carinii*] pneumonia) as the underlying cause.

Spontaneous pneumothorax is usually caused by rupture of a small area of abnormal lung tissue such as a bulla or subpleural bleb. This may be precipitated by increases in intra-alveolar pressure such as may occur with exertion or coughing. The patient complains of a sudden onset of pleuritic pain but this may not be severe. The degree of shortness of breath depends on the size of the pneumothorax. There may be a history of a previous episode. The signs – resonance to percussion and diminished air entry over the affected lung – also depend on the amount of pulmonary collapse.

Tension pneumothorax causes life-threatening dyspnoea. It is more common after trauma. *For the diagnosis and management of tension pneumothorax → p. 74.*

Investigations: A standard posteroanterior (PA) CXR confirms the diagnosis. Special films taken in expiration are no longer recommended. Look at the border of the lung fields, especially in the upper outer corner. Occasionally, the pneumothorax is visible only medially, in the cardiophrenic angle. If the CXR is normal despite a high degree of clinical suspicion, then a lateral chest or lateral decubitus radiograph should be requested. CT is used to differentiate a pneumothorax from complex bullous lung disease, or when the lung fields are obscured by surgical emphysema. It is also useful for the localisation of misplaced chest drain tubes!

Using the CXR, the size of a pneumothorax is described as either 'small' or 'large', depending on the distance between the lung edge and the chest wall. If this gap is <2 cm across, then the pneumothorax is classified as small; a rim of 2 cm or more defines a large pneumothorax. Other descriptions are now obsolete and percentage estimations of lung collapse are meaningless. However, a 2-cm pneumothorax has been calculated as being equivalent to a 50% loss of lung volume.

Blood gas measurements are often abnormal but are useful only in distressed patients with secondary pneumothoraces.

Tx

Aspiration of a pneumothorax → Box 12.11.
Insertion of a chest drain tube → Box 6.1 on p. 75.

Most patients with a primary pneumothorax do not have a persistent air leak. Moreover, it has been shown that the risk of recurrence is less if a chest drain tube is not inserted. For these reasons – and to minimise patient discomfort – simple aspiration is recommended as the initial treatment for primary pneumothoraces. If this fails, a second aspiration attempt is successful in a third of cases. Small-bore catheter aspiration kits with integral one-way valves are convenient and may reduce the need for repeated insertion of needles. Simple aspiration is less likely to succeed in secondary pneumothoraces (50% success rate versus 75% for primary pneumothora-

Box 12.11 Pneumothorax aspiration technique

- Locate the second intercostal space in the midclavicular line (an axillary approach is an alternative)
- Infiltrate local anaesthetic down to the pleura
- Enter the pleural cavity with a cannula and withdraw the needle (the cannula should be 16 FG or larger and at least 3 cm long)
- Connect the cannula to a 50-mL syringe via a three-way tap
- Begin aspirating air from the pleural cavity. Aspiration should be discontinued if the patient becomes distressed or coughs excessively or if >2.5 L (50 mL × 50) is aspirated
- Obtain a repeat CXR

ces). It is also less successful with increasing age of the patient (>50 years) and size of the pneumothorax (>3 L). Persistent air leak is more likely in patients with underlying lung disease and so all patients with a secondary pneumothorax should be admitted to hospital.

There is no evidence that large chest drainage tubes (20–24 Fr) are any better than smaller tubes (10–14 Fr) in the management of pneumothoraces. Therefore, smaller tubes should be used; catheter-over-guidewire (Seldinger technique) sets are now available in these sizes. The instillation of intrapleural local anaesthetic has been shown to reduce the pain caused by a chest tube *in situ*. Lidocaine 1% 20–25 mL (200–250 mg) is injected after insertion of the tube and then 8-hourly as required.

Patients with pneumothoraces that fail to expand or who have a continuing air leak after 48 h should be referred to a respiratory physician. This is an indication for suction to be applied to the drainage bottle (high volume, low pressure up to –20 cmH$_2$O). If the same problems continue for 4–5 days, then a thoracic surgeon should be consulted.

Spontaneous absorption of pneumothoraces does occur but can take several weeks as the pleura is, for obvious functional reasons, resistant to gas exchange in either direction. Around 1.5% of the volume of each pleural cavity can be absorbed per 24 h. High-flow oxygen increases this rate by a factor of 4 (but only during the period of administration).

Tx of primary pneumothorax (no underlying lung disease):

1 *Small primary pneumothorax (<2-cm rim on CXR)*: if the patient is not breathless, observation without admission is appropriate. The patient can be discharged from hospital with outpatient review and instructions to return immediately if he or she becomes short of breath.

2 *Large primary pneumothorax (≥2-cm rim on CXR) or patient breathless*: this should be treated by aspiration – *method of aspiration → Box 12.11*. If this is unsuccessful, a second aspiration should be attempted, provided that <2.5 L air was aspirated during the first attempt. After a successful aspiration, the patient may be discharged pending outpatient review, with instructions to return to hospital if he or she becomes breathless. If a second attempted aspiration is unsuccessful, then an intercostal chest drain will be required, followed by observation in hospital. The chest tube can be removed 24 h after full re-expansion of the lung and cessation of any air leakage.

Tx of secondary pneumothorax (significant underlying lung disease):

1 *Very small secondary pneumothorax (<1-cm rim on CXR or isolated apical pneumothorax) and patient asymptomatic*: observation in hospital should be arranged.

2 *Small secondary pneumothorax (<2-cm rim on CXR), patient minimally breathless and aged <50 years*: one attempt at aspiration may be made, followed by admission to hospital for 24 h. If this fails to expand the lung or there is a continuing air leak, then a chest drain will be required, followed by admission to hospital until 24 h after resolution of symptoms.

3 *Large secondary pneumothorax (≥ 2-cm rim on CXR) or patient breathless or aged >50 years*: intercostal tube drainage should be the initial treatment, followed by admission to hospital until 24 h after full re-expansion of the lung and cessation of any air leakage.

Pneumomediastinum

This is an under-recognised condition caused by the same factors as give rise to pneumothorax. The two may coexist. The most common symptom is discomfort in the neck, although chest pain is also frequently experienced. Hamman's sign, a pathognomonic crunching sound in phase with the cardiac cycle, is heard in less than 50% of cases.

Investigations: Diagnosis is by CXR. Pneumomediastinum is usually unilateral whereas air in the pericardium is seen all around the heart border.

Tx This consists of mild analgesia and observation while awaiting spontaneous resolution.

Pleurisy

Inflammation of the pleura causes a characteristic, unilateral, sharp pain, which is worse with movements of the lungs (i.e. deep breathing and coughing). Patients often describe it as being like a knife. Pyrexia is common; a pleural rub is not.

Investigations: A CXR is usually normal but may show an area of underlying pneumonia or an accompanying (small) pleural effusion.

Tx Most minor cases of pleurisy are viral in origin. Antibiotic therapy is given as for other chest infections (→ p. 209). Analgesics will be required; the addition of NSAIDs may sometimes help.

Tracheitis

In adults, tracheitis causes central chest pain of a burning nature, which is worse with deep breathing. A similar pain may be experienced after periods of hyperventilation. The patient may be pyrexial and purulent phlegm may be expectorated.

Tx This is directed at the underlying infection.

Bacterial tracheitis in children (a much more severe illness) → p. 336.

Oesophagitis

Reflex oesophagitis and oesophageal spasm cause central chest pain, which is sometimes relieved by GTN. Relief also occurs with simple antacids, suppression of acid production being the main treatment. Unfortunately, there is often no easy way to differentiate this condition from MI and thus caution is always needed (→ p. 177).

Shingles

Shingles is the infection of a peripheral sensory nerve by the chickenpox virus. It spreads from the dorsal root ganglion where it has lain dormant since primary infection.

> A patient with shingles can infect others – causing chickenpox. Shingles is the result of autoinfection and thus cannot be 'caught'.

The burning pain of herpes zoster infection always predates the characteristic vesicular rash. A thoracic nerve is often affected by shingles and initially the diagnosis can be very elusive. A vague red patch may sometimes be seen in the early stages of the disease.

Tx Treatment with aciclovir should be started as soon as possible. The adult dose is 800 mg five times daily for 7 days. Such treatment is expensive but reduces the severity of postherpetic neuralgia, a difficult and time-consuming condition to treat. There is some evidence that amitriptyline given concurrently may reduce the severity of the neuralgia still further.

Precordial catch/severe transitory chest pains of young adults

Sudden, excruciating pain in the chest is often experienced by young adults. It is usually left sided and may cause a doubled-up posture and pain with breathing. Symptoms last only for a few minutes and then disappear apart from a slight residual ache. The pain is not accompanied by nausea or sweating. The cause of the condition is unknown.

Tx Treatment consists of reasonable examination and investigation (ECG ± CXR) followed by reassurance.

Musculoskeletal chest pain

Pain in the chest wall is usually worsened by movements of the trunk such as sitting up and by deep breathing and coughing. It may also be related to movement of the arm at the shoulder joint. Sometimes the pain radiates down the arms but systemic features are usually absent. Areas of tenderness are common but by no means inevitable.

The problem may emanate from the muscles (viral myalgia or Bornholm's disease) or from the costal cartilages (Tietze's syndrome). Rib and muscle injuries can also present as unexplained chest pain. Such injuries often go unnoticed during sporting activities or periods of intoxication. Prolonged coughing is another cause of rib fractures.

Tx Treatment of musculoskeletal pain consists of analgesia and reassurance.

Rib fractures → p. 76.

Other causes of chest pain

Upper abdominal conditions such as pancreatitis, peptic ulceration, cholecystitis and renal colic can sometimes present as pain in the chest. In contrast, in communities where cocaine abuse is widespread this is one of the most common causes of chest pain (→ *p. 284*).

13

Respiratory distress

There are more emergency admissions in the UK for respiratory disease than for any other type of illness. It is responsible for 12% of urgent admissions to hospital.

THE UPPER AIRWAYS

The upper airways are very vulnerable to both infection and obstruction. Their clearance and maintenance are the primary concern in any patient with respiratory distress.

Choking and complete upper airway obstruction

Choking is the result of complete or near-complete obstruction of the upper airways by foreign or ectopic material. It is most common in children and elderly people.

> Most elderly patients who present with inhalation of foreign material have had a stroke whilst eating.

The patient may grip the throat with one hand and the wrist with the other ('the universal choking sign'). Sudden collapse with cyanosis while eating may mimic myocardial infarction (the 'café coronary').

Tx Get help. Encourage coughing in the responsive patient.

Resuscitation Council (UK) algorithms for the treatment of choking in adults and children → Figures 13.1 and 13.2.

Advanced life support entails careful judgement and an ascending hierarchy of treatment:

1 Suction and finger sweeps
2 Back blows and chest thrusts
3 The Heimlich manoeuvre
4 Direct laryngoscopic removal of foreign material
5 Surgical bypass of the obstruction.

Complete airway obstruction that does not result from foreign material (e.g. obstruction due to oedema or tumour) will always require an artificial airway – either an endotracheal tube or a surgical airway.

Notes on 1–5 above:

1 Blind probing with a finger is contraindicated in a child because it may force a foreign body further down the narrow respiratory tract and cause impaction in the conical laryngeal inlet.
2 Swift blows to the back and thrusts to the chest or abdomen may raise intrathoracic pressure sufficiently to cause foreign material to be ejected from the airway. In children, back blows can be administered with the child prone and the head lower than the trunk. In adults, the most suitable position is with the patient standing upright. Sequences of five blows or thrusts are recommended.
3 An obstructing foreign body may be expelled by means of the Heimlich manoeuvre (abdominal thrusts that work by increasing the intrathoracic pressure) (→ *Box 13.1*). The liver and spleen are less well protected by the ribs in infants, making the Heimlich manoeuvre relatively dangerous.
4 Direct laryngoscopy may allow visualisation of the obstruction and then its removal by suction or with Magill's forceps.
5 The cricothyroid membrane is the recommended site for an emergency surgical airway because a tracheotomy is difficult and time-consuming to

Emergency Medicine Lecture Notes, Fourth Edition. Chris Moulton and David Yates.
© 2012 Blackwell Publishing Ltd. Published 2012 by Blackwell Publishing Ltd.

Figure 13.1 Treatment of a choking adult. 2010 Resuscitation Guidelines. Reproduced with the kind permission of the Resuscitation Council (UK).

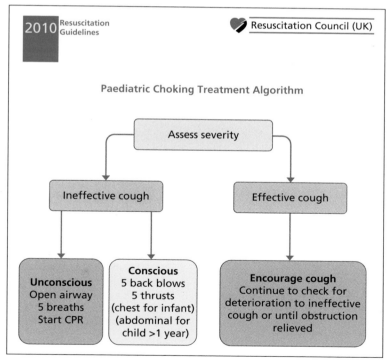

Figure 13.2 Treatment of a choking child. Reproduced with the kind permission of the Resuscitation Council (UK).

Box 13.1 The Heimlich manoeuvre

Patient standing
Place your arms around the patient's waist from behind. Grip your wrists together directly beneath the xiphisternum and then give five short, sharp 'bear hugs' up into the epigastrium.

Patient lying
Stand or kneel astride the patient's pelvis. Place the heel of one hand in the epigastrium and reinforce it with the other hand. Then give five short sharp thrusts upwards and backwards.

perform. Damage to the first tracheal ring may cause intractable stenosis. In children aged <12 years, needle cricothyroid puncture is preferable to direct surgical cricothyroidotomy. However, ventilation can then be achieved only with high-pressure oxygen and not with a bag and mask.

Cricothyroidotomy → p. 23.
Needle cricothyroid puncture → p. 23.

Postasphyxial care

All patients who have had an episode of choking should be admitted, often to the ICU. Those who remain dyspnoeic or have a depressed level of consciousness should be ventilated. Cerebral oedema is common after severe asphyxia; treatment with dexamethasone remains controversial.

Stridor and partial upper airway obstruction

Partial obstruction of the extrathoracic airways – at or above the cricoid ring – causes stridor, which is a harsh, high-pitched noise during inspiration. Intrathoracic obstruction causes wheezing. Characteristically, the patient is sat perched forward with the arms extended backward (the 'tripod position'). Other signs of partial obstruction of the upper airway are:

- drooling of saliva
- hoarseness
- rattling noises in the upper airway
- snoring (in the unresponsive patient).

Pulmonary oedema may complicate prolonged obstruction. *Also → Chapter 1, pp. 1–3.*

Absence of stridor may indicate sudden complete obstruction.

The causes of partial obstruction of the upper airway are:

- inhaled foreign body
- allergic swelling of the airway (including insect stings)
- burns to the airway
- other direct trauma to the airway (rare) (note that dislocation of the cricoid cartilage may occur in children)
- infection of the larynx (including the epiglottis) or of the trachea
- infection of the mouth, tonsils or pharynx
- infection superimposed on congenital abnormality in a small infant. Congenital abnormalities of the airway usually present in the first few weeks of life but should be considered up to the age of 6 months.

X_R Radiographs should be obtained only in a stable, calm, well-oxygenated patient with an uncertain underlying diagnosis. The only appropriate films are anteroposterior (AP) chest and lateral soft-tissue view of the neck, performed in the ED.
    A widened soft-tissue shadow on the lateral view of the neck may represent a retropharyngeal abscess or a swollen epiglottis. A coin in the trachea will have passed through the vocal folds in the sagittal plane and will thus appear end-on as a linear shadow on an AP CXR. In contrast, a coin in the oesophagus usually lies in the coronal plane.

Special problems in children

1 The flow in any tube is proportional to the fourth power of the radius. Hence, any reduction in the size of the child's small upper airway will have a much greater effect on airflow than a similar reduction in an adult.
2 Any stimulus is likely to cause increased distress, crying and consequent clinical deterioration. Therefore interventions such as venepuncture should not be undertaken until specialist help has arrived. Pulse oximetry may be useful in the interim.

T_X If there is marked stridor and cyanosis:

- Call for expert help immediately (anaesthetic and ENT specialists)

- Notify the operating theatre
- Reassure the patient and allow any position of comfort
- Give 100% oxygen or, better still, Heliox (70% helium with 30% oxygen) (helium has better flow characteristics than nitrogen or oxygen and may carry the oxygen through a small remaining passage)
- Try nebulised adrenaline (5 mg) as a temporary measure
- Consider parenteral adrenaline for allergic swelling.

> Do not examine the mouth or throat – any stimulus will increase the risk of complete obstruction.

If no help is available and the patient is about to die:

- Attempt laryngoscopy and endotracheal intubation – this is dangerous. Foreign material can be removed with suction and Magill's forceps. If the anatomy of the pharynx is distorted by oedema, ask a colleague to squeeze the chest; escaping air bubbles will help to identify the position of the upper larynx.
- Be prepared to perform cricothyroidotomy or needle cricothyroid puncture ($\rightarrow$ *pp. 22–23*).

In less urgent cases:

- Reassure the patient and allow a position of comfort
- Give 100% oxygen
- Obtain radiographs of the chest and lateral cervical spine in the resuscitation area
- Ask for ENT or paediatric advice. Be content not to make an immediate diagnosis in every case – looking for one may precipitate complete airway obstruction.

Management of specific upper airway conditions

Epiglottitis occurs in both children and adults but is often misdiagnosed in the latter. The *Haemophilus influenzae* type b (Hib) immunisation programme has led to a marked fall in the incidence in children but will have no effect on the adult disease, which is caused by different pathogens, such as staphylococci and streptococci. The clinical course can be dramatic and fatal.

Allergic swelling of the upper airways $\rightarrow$ *p. 299.*
Diphtheria $\rightarrow$ *p. 422.*
Epiglottitis in adults $\rightarrow$ *p. 422.*
Inhalational burns $\rightarrow$ *p. 136.*
Ludwig's angina $\rightarrow$ *p. 424.*
Peritonsillar infections $\rightarrow$ *p. 424.*
Retropharyngeal abscess $\rightarrow$ *p. 423.*
Stridor in children $\rightarrow$ *p. 335.*

THE LOWER AIRWAYS AND LUNGS

The restoration of adequate breathing is a priority, which is second only to the maintenance of a clear airway.

Respiratory arrest

Isolated respiratory arrest or failure of ventilation in the presence of a clear airway and a central pulse occurs in four main circumstances:

1 Poisoning with narcotic analgesics ($\rightarrow$ *p. 282*)
2 General brain-stem depression (e.g. drugs, stroke, head injury)
3 Respiratory failure with CO_2 narcosis ($\rightarrow$ *p. 217*)
4 Neuromuscular paralysis.

It may also herald cardiac arrest in conditions such as a pulmonary embolism. The treatment is artificial ventilation with 100% oxygen until the underlying cause can be remedied.

Initial assessment and management of acute breathlessness

- Ensure that airway obstruction is not the cause of the dyspnoea.
- Give oxygen by mask ($\rightarrow$ *Box 13.2*).
- Consider the need to support the ventilation:
  1 with a bag, valve and mask (a temporary measure that does not protect the airway)
  2 by intubation and ventilation, (but intubation may be extremely difficult in the patient who has not yet arrested)
  3 by requesting immediate anaesthetic support.
- Check that the circulation is adequate, otherwise the situation is that of cardiorespiratory arrest.
- Sit the patient up, loosen clothing and briefly examine the chest.
- Obtain IV access.
- Monitor SaO_2, ECG and BP.

Box 13.2 Initial oxygen therapy in a patient with respiratory distress

Is the patient known to have had previous episodes of hypercapnic respiratory failure? Is the patient drowsy?

No to both   Give 100% oxygen
Yes to either   Give 24–35% oxygen until blood gas results (and more information) are available, keeping the patient's SaO_2 around 88–92%

Box 13.3 Changes in the lung fields on a CXR

Shadows in the lung fields may be focal, multifocal or diffuse. Causes of focal and multifocal abnormalities include:

- Metastases
- Lung abscesses
- Carcinoma of the lung
- Pulmonary infarcts
- Tuberculosis
- Rheumatoid nodules
- Hydatid cysts

Diffuse changes may be of two main types: (1) alveolar or (2) interstitial. The presence of an air bronchogram indicates alveolar pathology and this may be cardiac or non-cardiac in origin. The alveoli may be filled with:

- *Blood*: lung contusion
- *Fluid*: pulmonary oedema
- *Consolidated pus*: pneumonia

Interstitial lung disease is more complex and less relevant to emergency medicine. Lung field changes caused by it may be:

- *Nodular*: small in pneumoconiosis, larger in silicosis and sometimes miliary in TB
- *Linear*: fibrosis (usually lower zone), asbestosis, connective tissue disease and cryptogenic
- *Cystic*: seen in the lower zone in bronchiectasis and cystic fibrosis and in the upper zone in histiocytosis X

- Score the level of consciousness (AVPU or GCS).
- Get a brief history.
- Obtain a CXR and ECG; check the blood gases ($\rightarrow$ below).
- Consider immediate therapy for wheezing or pulmonary oedema.

Like pain, shortness of breath must be relieved as soon as possible after initial assessment.

Investigations in respiratory distress

CXR (PA if possible)

An anteroposterior CXR taken on the trolley in the resuscitation room may be necessary in a critically ill patient but is a poor substitute for a posteroanterior erect film because:

- the mediastinum and heart size are magnified
- fluid levels are not identified
- the penetration is often inappropriate
- the film is often rotated or incomplete
- there is a potential radiation hazard to staff.

Changes in the lung fields on CXR $\rightarrow$ Box 13.3.

On a supine CXR, an effusion or haemothorax may mimic diffuse lung changes ($\rightarrow$ p. 73).

Twelve-lead ECG

A rhythm strip from a three-lead ECG is insufficient for diagnostic purposes in a patient who may have subtle changes of myocardial ischaemia or pulmonary embolism.

Pulse oximetry

Measurement of SaO_2 is extremely valuable but has some drawbacks.

- It does not assess pH and $PaCO_2$ which may both be abnormal in the presence of normal oxygen saturation.
- The steep fall of the oxyhaemoglobin curve means that SaO_2 <95% is abnormal (cf. PaO_2).
- SaO_2 is inaccurate in the presence of carboxyhaemoglobin (COHb), which is not uncommon in respiratory distress (house fires, faulty gas heaters, heavy smokers).

Box 13.4 Estimation of the expected partial pressure of oxygen in an arterial blood gas sample

With healthy lungs, the PaO_2 in (mmHg) should be approximately equal to five times the percentage of oxygen in the inspired gases (FIO_2)

i.e. expected PaO_2 (mmHg) = $5 \times FIO_2$ (%).
For example, breathing air with healthy lungs, expected $PaO_2 = 5 \times 21\% = 100\,mmHg$.

A more accurate (and more scientific) formula calculates the expected alveolar partial pressure of oxygen by subtracting the added water vapour and the alveolar carbon dioxide from the inspired oxygen tension. Using this calculation, the PaO_2 (in kPa) should be around 10 kPa less than the partial pressure of the inspired oxygen. The atmospheric pressure at sea level is 100 kPa of which 21% (21 kPa) is due to oxygen. So when breathing air with healthy lungs:

Minimum expected PaO_2 = 21 kPa − 10 kPa

$\qquad\qquad\qquad\quad$ = 11 kPa.

Thus, with healthy lungs, the minimum expected PaO_2 (in kPa) is 10 less than the inspired oxygen concentration (as a percentage).

Blood gas samples should be taken from the radial artery of the non-dominant hand.

Arterial blood gases

Estimation of the expected partial pressure of oxygen in an arterial blood gas sample → Box 13.4.

Rules of compensation in acid–base disorders → Box 14.26 on p. 252.

To convert partial pressures of gases expressed in kPa to mmHg multiply by 7.6 and vice versa.

Foreign bodies in the lower airways

Sudden onset of coughing and wheezing may accompany aspiration of a foreign body into the lower airways. Young children are especially vulnerable to this problem; a history of aspiration may be lacking. The right main, intermediate or lower bronchi are the most likely sites for obstruction to occur. Peanuts and toy fragments are the most commonly inhaled objects in children; bony food particles, broken teeth and small dental instruments predominate in adults. The presence of a unilateral wheeze, recurrent infection or other atypical symptoms and signs should always suggest the possibility of an intrathoracic foreign body.

XR The foreign body is invariably radiolucent but the obstructive emphysema or absorption collapse that it causes may often be seen. Inspiratory and expiratory CXRs should be requested to demonstrate the ball–valve effect of a partial obstruction on the lung volume.

Tx All patients with a possibility of a foreign body in the airways should be referred for bronchoscopy. This would include those with suspicious histories, signs or radiological changes.

Allergic reactions causing lower airway obstruction and respiratory distress → p. 299.
Foreign bodies in the oesophagus and gastrointestinal tract → p. 420.
Foreign bodies in the upper airways → p. 198.

Asthma in adults

Asthma continues to be a major health problem in the UK, affecting an estimated 1.4 million children and 3.7 million adults. It is responsible for the deaths of over 1500 people each year. Throughout western Europe, there is an average prevalence of asthma of 13% in children and 8.4% in adults, with a 2–4% annual increase in prevalence over the last 15–20 years. The reasons for this increase are uncertain but possible explanations include:

- a rise in the house-dust mite population
- increased diesel particulate emissions
- a decrease in exposure to bacterial pathogens in childhood
- changes in diet (more polyunsaturated fats and fewer antioxidants).

Patients with severe asthma and one or more adverse behavioural or psychosocial factors have a higher risk of death. *For risk factors for developing near fatal or fatal asthma → Box 13.5.* However, around 90% of asthma attacks that are severe enough to require admission to hospital develop relatively slowly over a period of 6 hours or more. Therefore, there is usually enough time for effective action.

Box 13.5 Patients at risk of developing fatal or near fatal asthma

Patients with a combination of one or more indicators of severe asthma:

- Previous near fatal asthma (e.g. required ventilation or had respiratory acidosis)
- Previous admission for asthma (especially if in the last year)
- Repeated attendances at ED for asthma (especially if in the last year)
- Asthma treatment requiring three or more classes of medication
- Heavy use of β_2 agonists
- Brittle asthma

And one or more adverse behavioural or psychosocial factors:

- Non-compliance with treatment, failure to attend appointments or self-discharge from hospital
- Psychiatric illness including depression and self-harm
- Current or recent major tranquilliser usage
- Alcohol or drug abuse
- Learning difficulties
- History of abuse in childhood
- Employment and income problems
- Severe domestic, marital or legal stress
- Social isolation
- Denial of illness
- Obesity

The clinical features of asthma result from a reversible inflammatory obstruction of the lower airways, which has three main components:

1 Hyperreactivity and spasm of the bronchial smooth muscle
2 Oedema of the walls of the bronchi
3 Increased production and retention of secretions.

Asthma is caused by an allergic response to a wide variety of substances but there is usually an underlying sensitivity to house-dust mite. A viral infection is a common trigger for an acute exacerbation; exercise is responsible for around 40% of attacks.

> A pneumothorax may occasionally be the cause of an acute deterioration.

Dyspnoea and wheezing are the predominant features. Bronchodilators may control these symptoms, but it is steroids that modify the underlying inflammatory processes.

Ask about

- When this attack started
- Improvement or deterioration in symptoms
- The patient's assessment of severity
- What triggers an attack and how often
- Recent hospital admissions
- Any ICU admission
- Why this time was chosen to come to hospital; this is an important discriminator when considering discharge
- Previous and current drug use, especially steroids and theophyllines
- Other conditions, including upper respiratory tract infections and pregnancy.

If nebulised drugs were given before hospital arrival by the paramedics, precise details and initial peak flow rate should be noted.

Examination begins while taking the history and setting up the nebuliser.

Look for

- Difficulty with speech – spontaneous sentences or single words?
- Reduced peak expiratory flow rate (PEFR). *For predicted values of PEFR for adults → Figure 13.3 and Box 13.6*
- Tachycardia and tachypnoea
- Indrawing of ribs, flaring of nostrils and use of accessory muscles
- Wheezing and signs of pneumothorax
- Agitation, confusion or drowsiness
- Exhaustion
- Pyrexia
- Cyanosis.

> Less wheezing than expected on auscultation may indicate less air movement, not less asthma.

Investigations in asthma

CXR is not indicated routinely in acute asthma. It should be requested only in cases of suspected pneumothorax, pneumomediastinum, pneumonic consolidation or inhaled foreign body. Patients with life-threatening asthma or failure to respond to treatment will also require a CXR as will those who have been intubated and ventilated.

Arterial blood gas analysis is required only in patients with features of life-threatening asthma and in those with an SaO_2 (on pulse oximetry) <92%. There is usually a low $PaCO_2$ as a result of hyperventilation and a low PaO_2 caused by ventilation–perfusion mismatch. A normal $PaCO_2$ is worrying and a high $PaCO_2$ (>40–45 mmHg or 5.3–6.0 kPa) indicates respiratory muscle fatigue and impending respiratory failure. Measurement of blood gas tensions should be repeated after 2 h in all patients in whom the initial PaO_2 was <60 mmHg (8 kPa) unless the SaO_2 has risen to >92% in the meantime. Electrolyte estimation is important – hypokalaemia can occur – but haematological investigation is often unnecessary. A raised white cell count is to be expected with catecholamine and steroid therapy. Theophylline levels should be measured in patients who are taking regular methylxanthines at home.

The PEFR should be measured in all patients and used as a guide to treatment. PEFR expressed as a percentage of the patient's previous best value is the most useful clinical parameter. In its absence, PEFR expressed as a percentage of the patient's predicted value is a reasonable guide. *For predicted values of PEFR for adults → Figure 13.3 and Box 13.6.*

Life-threatening asthma (PEFR 33% best or predicted)

Features include:

- unable to talk
- silent chest, cyanosis, feeble respiratory effort
- bradycardia, dysrhythmia or hypotension
- exhaustion, confusion or coma.

Pulse oximetry and arterial blood gas analysis show:

- SaO_2 <92%
- $PaCO_2$ within the normal range of 35–45 mmHg (4.6–6.0 kPa) or higher in near fatal asthma
- PaO_2 >60 mmHg (8 kPa) irrespective of oxygen therapy
- Low pH.

Tx

- Obtain anaesthetic/intensive care help immediately in life-threatening asthma.
- Give a high concentration of oxygen (at least 60%) via a well-fitting facemask. The aim is to keep the SaO_2 >92%.
- Monitor SaO_2, ECG and BP.

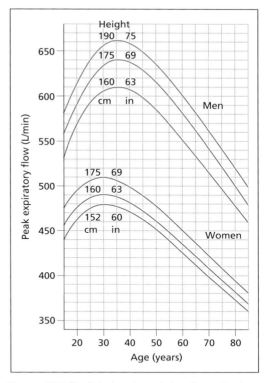

Figure 13.3 Predicted peak expiratory flow rates in adults.

Box 13.6 Predicted peak expiratory flow rates for adults of average height (in L/min)

Age (years)	15	20	30	40	50	60	70
Male	550	590	630	630	610	580	540
Female	460	480	500	480	460	430	410

The standard deviation (SD) of these values is 48 L/min for men and 42 L/min for women. Values of PEFR up to 2 SD less than predicted are within normal limits.

- Give salbutamol 5 mg (or terbutaline 10 mg) made up to 5 mL with 0.9% saline and nebulised by oxygen with a flow rate of at least 6 L/min. Add ipratropium 500 mcg to the same nebuliser. (This anticholinergic drug has been shown to produce additional bronchodilatation to that produced by

β_2 agonists alone, leading to faster recovery times and shorter durations of admission.)

- Give prednisolone 40–50 mg by mouth. If the patient cannot swallow oral medication or is vomiting, give IV hydrocortisone 100–200 mg 6-hourly. (Prednisolone 10 mg is roughly equivalent to hydrocortisone 40 mg.) Steroids should be continued for at least 5 days or until full recovery.
- Repeat the salbutamol/terbutaline and ipratropium nebulisers after 15 min. (The β_2 agonists can be administered almost continuously; the ipratropium may be repeated at 4- to 6-h intervals.)
- Commence IV fluids.
- Give a single dose of magnesium sulphate 1.2–2.0 g by IV infusion over 20 min. *For further information on magnesium → p. 250.*
- Consider continuous administration of nebulised β_2 agonists (i.e. repeated doses at 15- to 30-min intervals).
- Consider the use of IV salbutamol 200 mcg or IV terbutaline 250 mcg (given slowly over 10 min) for those patients in whom inhaled therapy cannot be used reliably.
- Consider (after consultation with senior staff) the use of IV aminophylline. This may benefit occasional patients with life-threatening asthma who are resistant to standard therapies. A loading dose of 5 mg/kg is given over 20 min under ECG control. This is followed by an infusion of aminophylline of 0.5–0.7 mg/kg per h. The loading dose (and possibly the idea of using aminophylline at all) should be abandoned in patients who are already taking oral methylxanthines. Caution is needed when giving aminophylline to patients who are hypoxic.

> Failure to recognise and act on the need for ventilation is the main preventable cause of death in asthma.

Intubation and ventilation may be required. All patients who are failing to respond to treatment should be referred to ICU specialists. This includes patients with worsening PEFR, deteriorating blood gases or acidosis, exhaustion, confusion or drowsiness.

IV adrenaline is sometimes used in a critical situation. Despite theoretical reasons for its efficacy, Heliox (helium and oxygen mixture in a 70:30 ratio) has not been shown to be of conclusive benefit in asthma. Similarly, non-invasive ventilation (NIV) is not recommended for the unstable situation of acute asthma.

Severe asthma (PEFR between 33% and 50% best or predicted)

Features include:

- inability to complete a sentence in one breath
- respiratory rate >25 breaths/min
- pulse rate >110/min.

Tx The patient should be treated as described for life-threatening asthma above, although IV magnesium should be given only if there is a poor response to inhaled bronchodilators. Aminophylline is unlikely to be considered. Admission is always required; the patient must be accompanied by a doctor or a nurse at all times.

Moderate asthma (PEF between 50% and 75% best or predicted)

The patient can finish a sentence and has no features of severe asthma.

Tx
- Give salbutamol 5 mg (or terbutaline 10 mg) made up to 5 mL with 0.9% saline and nebulised by oxygen with a flow rate of at least 6 L/min.
- Monitor SaO_2, ECG and BP.
- Wait 15–30 min after the initial nebuliser and then repeat the PEFR.
- If the patient is worse and PEFR <50% treat as severe asthma. If better and PEFR >75% consider discharge (→ *below*). If PEFR is still between 50% and 75% repeat the salbutamol or terbutaline nebuliser and give prednisolone 40–50 mg orally. Then wait a further 30 min.
- If the patient is worse and PEFR <50% treat as severe asthma. If better and PEF >75% consider discharge (→ *later*). If the same (i.e. PEFR 50–75%) wait a further 60 min while monitoring the SaO_2, heart rate and respiratory rate.
- If, at this point, the PEFR <50% treat as severe asthma. If PEFR >50% *and* the patient is stable or improving, consider discharge (→ *later*).

Mild asthma (PEFR >75% best or predicted)

- The patient can talk normally.

Tx The patient should be given his or her usual bronchodilator and then kept under observation for at least 30–60 min. If the PEFR remains >75% consider discharge (→ *later*). If the PEFR falls, treat as described in the appropriate section above.

Discharge of a patient with asthma

Most patients who are sufficiently ill to request emergency help with their chronic condition will require oral steroids (as well as inhaled steroids and bronchodilators as part of a long-term management plan). Prednisolone 40–50 mg given orally for 5 days is usually adequate. (If used within an hour of ED arrival, steroid tablets are effective at preventing admission and reducing the risk of relapse in the ensuing 21 days. Despite this, they are not always prescribed by ED staff.) There are several alternatives for high-dose inhaled steroids:

- Beclometasone 400–500 mcg twice daily
- Budesonide 400–500 mcg twice daily
- Fluticasone 250 mcg twice daily.

These doses are halved for children.

> Over 15% of patients with asthma who are discharged from an ED or hospital ward reattend within 2 weeks.

Patients who return to the ED after discharge should be automatically admitted. Referral for specialist review after ED attendance has been shown to improve outcomes significantly for most patients with asthma. The patient's GP should be informed of the attendance and arrangements made for primary care follow-up within 48 h.

Asthma in children aged <5 years → p. 336.
Predischarge checklist for moderate and mild asthma → Box 13.7.
Relative contraindications to the discharge from hospital of a patient with asthma → Box 13.8.

Acute exacerbations of chronic obstructive pulmonary disease

Chronic obstructive pulmonary disease (COPD) is the fifth biggest cause of mortality in the UK and is responsible for millions of lost working days and a huge amount of suffering. It is characterised by reduced respiratory function as a result of a combination of destruction of alveoli and obstruction of bronchioles by a chronic inflammatory process. The airflow obstruction is usually progressive, not fully reversible and relatively unchanged over a period of several months. COPD is predominately caused by smoking. Most patients have a chronic productive cough, which is worse in winter. There is no single diagnostic test for COPD but airflow obstruction is

Box 13.7 Predischarge checklist for moderate and mild asthma

Moderate asthma
- The patient is stable over at least 1 h of observation
- The PEFR is at least 75% of normal for the patient at 1 h or 50% at 2 h and improving
- The patient has both oral steroids and inhaled bronchodilators to take out
- The patient understands his or her condition and treatment and can use the inhalers satisfactorily
- Follow-up is arranged (e.g. by the GP within 48 h) and the patient has the telephone number of the ED
- There is good home support
- The patient has a letter for the GP (who must be informed within 24 h of attendance)

Mild asthma
- Oral steroids are not necessary. Otherwise as for moderate asthma

Box 13.8 Relative contraindications to discharge of a patient with asthma

- Remaining significant symptoms
- Concerns about compliance
- Psychological problems or learning difficulties
- Physical disability
- Poor social circumstances or lives alone
- Presentation at night
- Previous ICU admission for asthma
- Previous severe attacks needing hospitalisation
- Diagnosed brittle asthma
- Already on steroids
- Pregnancy
- Drug-induced attack

defined as a forced expiratory volume in 1 s (FEV_1) of <80% of the predicted value for that patient.

Acute deterioration that precipitates ED attendance is usually associated with:

- increased dyspnoea
- purulent sputum
- increased sputum volume.

This is frequently the result of superadded infection. Other causes include minor chest injury, inappropriate sedation and uncontrolled oxygen therapy. A cough fracture may also precipitate deterioration.

Patients with COPD have varying combinations of chronic bronchitis and emphysema. However, the two classic descriptions of 'blue bloaters' and 'pink puffers' are no longer thought to describe the extremes of this spectrum of lung pathologies. Instead, they represent patients with different physiological responses to abnormal blood gases – 'blue bloaters' tolerate high CO_2 levels, 'pink puffers' do not. The former is cyanosed and oedematous with signs of CO_2 retention (peripheral vasodilatation, retinal engorgement, staring eyes, confusion); the latter maintains a normal CO_2 level by hyperventilation. Most patients present with a mixture of these features, attempting to hyperventilate but failing to maintain a normal $PaCO_2$. Wheezes and rattles are heard on auscultation in bronchitis but there may be minimal chest signs with severe emphysema. Exhaustion is a common feature, with the patient sitting up using accessory muscles of respiration. Confusion and shortness of breath may make a clear history difficult to obtain.

> The risk of dying from an exacerbation of COPD is closely related to the development of a respiratory acidosis, the presence of other serious illnesses and the need for ventilatory support.

Cor pulmonale is suggested by the combination of peripheral oedema, raised venous pressure, a systolic parasternal heave and a loud pulmonary second heart sound.

Investigations:
- PFER should be measured. A PEFR <100 L/min indicates a severe exacerbation.
- Pulse oximetry will demonstrate a low oxygen saturation in most patients with COPD. Some patients may have a resting SaO_2 <90% even when stable.
- Analysis of blood gases will usually confirm hypoxia with rising hypercapnia and respiratory acidosis. The blood gas analysis should be repeated after 30–60 min of treatment.
- Full blood count, electrolytes, CXR and ECG must be obtained together with the past medical notes.
- Plasma theophylline levels should be measured in all patients who are taking regular methylxanthines.

- Sputum should be sent for microscopy and culture in patients with purulent sputum.

Tx

Immediate treatment: the patient should be sat up and given controlled oxygen by facemask to keep the SaO_2 around 90% ($\rightarrow$ Box 13.2).

Bronchodilators: Nebulised β_2-adrenoceptor agonists (salbutamol 5 mg or terbutaline 10 mg, made up to 5 mL with 0.9% saline) will treat any reversible element of the COPD. Nebulised ipratropium bromide 500 mcg is also helpful. This antimuscarinic bronchodilator has a delayed onset of action of up to 30 min but lasts for 3–6 h. The sympathomimetic nebulisers may be repeated at short intervals if they prove to be beneficial. After consultation with senior staff, IV aminophylline may be considered for patients who have a poor response to nebulised bronchodilators. A loading dose of 5 mg/kg is given over 20 min under ECG control. This is followed by an infusion of aminophylline of 500 mcg/kg per h. Aminophylline should not be used in patients who are already taking oral methylxanthines at home and great caution is required when giving it to patients who are hypoxic. (Aminophylline is a stable mixture of theophylline and ethylenediamine, which is 20 times more water soluble than theophylline alone. The plasma theophylline concentration for optimum response is 10–20 mg/L; there is a very narrow margin between the therapeutic dose and the toxic dose.)

Oxygen: the administration of a high concentration of oxygen in patients with COPD may cause increased respiratory depression, CO_2 narcosis and worsening hypoxia. It used to be said that the normal hypercapnic drive to respiration could be abolished by chronic hypercapnia and the theory ran that the patient was then reliant on the less sensitive hypoxic drive to stimulate respiratory effort. In actual fact, the clinical deterioration that may follow oxygen therapy is almost certainly due to a loss of physiological hypoxic vasoconstriction, which partially protects the patient from the effects of areas of gross alveolar hypoventilation. However, the patient has presented to an ED because of dyspnoea, so increasing hypoxia will ensure further deterioration. Immediate oxygen therapy is thus determined by the presence of drowsiness or known previous hypercapnic respiratory failure ($\rightarrow$ Box 13.2). For most patients, the target should be an SaO_2 of between 85% and 92%. The PaO_2 should certainly not fall below 50 mmHg (6.6 kPa; equivalent to an SaO_2 of approximately 80%). (A PaO_2 of <60 mmHg [8 kPa] is regarded as respiratory failure $\rightarrow$ p. 217.) The aim of controlled oxygen therapy is to raise the PaO_2 above 50 mmHg without worsening the acidosis.

Steroids: it is now recognised that almost all patients with an acute exacerbation of COPD benefit from high-dose steroids (prednisolone 30 mg daily) for 1–2 weeks. For patients who are unable to take tablets in the ED, IV hydrocortisone 200–300 mg should be given.

Antibiotics: In the presence of purulent sputum, antibacterial therapy is required. *Haemophilus influenzae, Streptococcus pneumoniae* and *Moraxella catarrhalis* are typical pathogens in COPD and so amoxicillin 500 mg three times daily or tetracycline 250–500 mg four times daily are suitable first-line antibiotics. Clarithromycin 500 mg twice daily is also often used. As a result of increasing antibiotic resistance, co-amoxiclav or quinolones (e.g. ciprofloxacin 500 mg twice daily) are given after 3 days if there is a failure to respond to first-line treatment. Patients with consolidation on CXR should be treated as pneumonia ($\rightarrow$ p. 209).

Admission to hospital: the decision to admit a patient with COPD to hospital depends on a variety of both clinical and social factors as well as the availability of a specialist home care team. *For factors that suggest that a patient with an exacerbation of COPD should be admitted to hospital $\rightarrow$ Box 13.9.* Regular physiotherapy is of great benefit to patients with retained sputum.

Respiratory support: subsequent therapy depends on the clinical findings, further history and the results of blood gas analysis. The presence of an acidosis (pH <7.35) in these often well-compensated patients is usually a bad sign and is now regarded as an indication for non-invasive ventilation (NIV). Bilevel pressure support ventilators (delivering bilevel positive airway pressure [BiPAP]) are usually used for this purpose ($\rightarrow$ *Box 13.16*). The respiratory stimulant, doxapram, is sometimes used if NIV is unavailable ($\rightarrow$ *Box 13.17*). If the pH falls to <7.25 or the $PaCO_2$ rises to >80 mmHg (10.6 kPa), or if the patient becomes drowsy or exhausted, ICU specialists should be involved with a view to instituting intubation and intermittent positive-pressure ventilation (IPPV).

Bronchiolitis in children $\rightarrow$ p. 338.
Respiratory failure $\rightarrow$ p. 217.

Acute exacerbations of bronchiectasis

Around 1 in 1000 adults in the UK has bronchiectasis, often as a result of childhood infections, cystic fibrosis, immunodeficiency or rheumatoid disease. However, in 50% of patients no cause or associated condition is found. It is believed that the bronchi are dilated and destroyed by a cycle of recurrent infection, inflammation, excessive production of mucus and reduced mucus clearance. Patients have chronic symptoms of dyspnoea and a productive cough; their sputum is mucopurulent. Some patients may present to an ED with an acute exacerbation, usually brought about by infection. Symptoms include worsening breathlessness, increased coughing and sputum production, haemoptysis (usually not severe), chest pain, fever, malaise and lethargy. Chest signs may be minimal; low-pitched crackles may be heard. In severe disease, finger clubbing and respiratory failure are seen.

Investigations: CXR shows the characteristic changes of bronchiectasis in only 50% of patients:

- Thickened bronchial walls seen as parallel 'tramlines' or ring-shaped opacities
- Cystic lesions with fluid levels
- Areas of collapse and scarring.

High-resolution CT scan or bronchoscopy may be required.

Tx Treatment includes oxygen, physiotherapy (postural drainage and percussion) and antibiotics. If likely pathogens are not known from previous sputum cultures, amoxicillin 500 mg three times daily is given for 14 days. Steroids may be used to reduce inflammation. For more severe exacerbations, blind prescription of broad-spectrum anti-pseudomonal antibiotics should be considered. Intubation and ventilation may be required. Excessive secretions

---

Box 13.9 Factors that suggest that a patient with COPD should be admitted to hospital

- Difficulty coping at home, living alone or in poor social circumstances
- Poor or deteriorating general health
- Poor activity or confined to bed
- On long-term oxygen therapy
- Significant co-morbidity (especially cardiac disease and type 1 diabetes)
- Rapid rate of onset of exacerbation
- Severe breathlessness or cyanosis
- Worsening peripheral oedema
- Acute confusion or otherwise impaired level of consciousness
- SaO_2 <90%, pH <7.35 or PaO_2 <7 kPa
- CXR changes suggestive of infection or other new pathology

tend to limit the effectiveness of non-invasive ventilation (NIV) in bronchiectasis.

Pulmonary oedema

Fluid may collect in the lung tissue for a variety of reasons, the most common being left ventricular failure (LVF). Pulmonary oedema may also be associated with the following:

1 Over-transfusion and excessive fluid therapy
2 Smoke and other noxious gas inhalation (→ p. 295)
3 Acute traumatic brain injury (neurogenic pulmonary oedema → p. 37)
4 Intracranial haemorrhage (neurogenic pulmonary oedema → p. 227)
5 Shock, from any cause (adult respiratory distress syndrome)
6 Ascents to high altitudes (→ p. 237).

Acute pulmonary oedema causes symptoms and signs of hypoxia:

- Rapidly increasing shortness of breath, which is worse on lying down
- Tachypnoea and laboured breathing (stiff water-logged lungs)
- Pallor and sweating (characteristic)
- Tachycardia
- Anxiety and distress
- Depression of consciousness (mostly caused by CO_2 narcosis).

The hypoxia leads to a vicious cycle of worsening myocardial performance and increasing oedema. On auscultation there are widespread crackles. These make the diagnostic gallop rhythm difficult to hear. Classic pink, frothy sputum is uncommon. Peripheral oedema and a raised jugular venous pressure (JVP) indicate associated right heart failure. There may be a history of ischaemic heart disease, orthopnoea or paroxysmal nocturnal dyspnoea. Chest pain results from either angina secondary to the hypoxia or from a myocardial infarction (MI) that precipitated the LVF. **'Cardiac asthma'** describes the wheeze that these patients may develop if oedema causes significant airway obstruction. The history and presentation will usually distinguish it from bronchial asthma but confusion can occur, especially in patients with both conditions.

Investigations: Arterial blood gases will show a variable degree of hypoxia, hypercapnia and acidosis.

B-type natriuretic peptide (BNP) is a cardiac hormone produced by the heart in response to ventricular stretching from volume expansion and pressure overload. It is a marker for ventricular dysfunction, the circulating BNP concentration

Box 13.10 Radiological changes in pulmonary oedema

- Widened vascular markings in the upper lung fields as a result of diversion of blood (upper lobe diversion)
- Air bronchogram
- A widened mediastinum with spreading (bat's wing) shadows
- Horizontal lines in the lower lobes (Kerley B lines)
- Small pleural effusions
- Cotton-wool shadows throughout the lung fields
- Cardiomegaly

increasing with the severity of the heart failure. BNP can also be used as a diagnostic test to help differentiate congestive cardiac failure (CCF) from COPD. A BNP level in excess of 100 picograms/mL has a high specificity for CCF.

> Over 20% of patients who are hospitalised with heart failure die within 30 days.

Radiological changes in pulmonary oedema → Box 13.10.

Tx

- Sit the patient up, with the legs dependent if possible.
- Give a high-concentration of oxygen by mask or via a continuous positive airway pressure (CPAP) circuit at $5\,cmH_2O$ pressure initially (→ below).
- Establish IV access.
- Start monitoring SaO_2, ECG and BP.
- Request a CXR and ECG. Arterial blood gases may be taken, but, unless the results are instantly available, they are unlikely to affect initial treatment.
- Give IV diamorphine 2.5–5 mg with IV prochlorperazine 12.5 mg to relieve distress and to start venodilatation.
- If the patient has a history of fluid retention (CCF), give IV furosemide 1–2 mg/kg and consider the need for a urinary catheter.
- Start nitrate therapy to further reduce venous return. Several alternative routes are effective (→ *Boxes 13.11 and 13.12*). GTN must be used with care because it may worsen hypotension and tachycardia.

Box 13.11 Alternative routes for GTN administration in LVF

1 GTN spray one to two puffs (= 400–800 mcg) or equivalent tablet sublingually, followed by a GTN 10 mg transdermal patch
2 GTN 5 mg buccal tablet, followed by a second tablet in the opposite buccal sulcus, if necessary, after 3–5 min
3 GTN infusion 10–200 mcg/min → Box 13.12

Box 13.12 Intravenous infusion of GTN

- Make 50 mg of GTN solution up to 50 mL with 0.9% saline in a large syringe in an infusion pump (i.e. mix a 1 mg/mL solution). The syringe and the giving-set should be made of polyethylene because PVC (polyvinyl chloride) absorbs GTN
- The IV dose of GTN is from 0.6 mg/h to 12 mg/h (equivalent to 10–200 mcg/min)
- Start the infusion at 1.5–3.0 mL (1.5–3 mg)/h and adjust this dose by a factor of two every 15–30 min according to the patient's clinical condition

Inotropes such as dobutamine are indicated in low output states (forward failure) (→ p. 238). When the clinical picture is dominated by wheezing (cardiac asthma), nebulised salbutamol may be given (aminophylline is no longer used in LVF). Conventional positive-pressure ventilation (IPPV) may be required in a rapidly deteriorating patient.

CPAP and BiPAP: in LVF, CPAP and BiPAP may help to alleviate respiratory distress and improve some metabolic parameters to a limited extent (they have been shown to be equivalent in this respect). However, neither treatment modality has a beneficial effect on either short-term or long-term survival and so both CPAP and BiPAP are best used very selectively in acute cardiogenic pulmonary oedema.

BiPAP → Box 13.16 on p. 217.

Pneumonia

This is the most common serious infection seen in adults in the ED and may be fatal even in people who have been previously healthy. The outcome is greatly improved by very early treatment with appropriate antibiotics. The patient with pneumonia presents with a short history of fever and productive cough ('rusty' sputum with *Streptococcus pneumoniae* infection). There may be tachycardia, shortness of breath and pleuritic chest pain. Findings on examination vary from obvious lobar consolidation to minimal crepitations. Lethargy and confusion are often the first signs in elderly people. Children may present with abdominal pain (→ p. 339). Pneumonia is defined as severe (with a mortality rate in excess of 10%) if two or more of the following criteria are present:

- PaO_2 <60 mmHg (8 kPa)
- C: new confusion
- U: urea >7 mmol/L.
- R: respiratory rate >30 breaths/min
- B: systolic BP <90 mmHg or diastolic BP <60 mmHg
- 65: age >65 years.

The last five of these criteria are the basis of the CURB-65 scoring system. This is used to predict mortality and thus suggest the need for admission. It can also be used to guide the prescription of antibiotics. One point is allocated for each of the CURB-65 criteria, giving a score from 0 to 5. Patients with a score of 0 or 1 have a relatively low risk of death (<5%) and can be treated as outpatients. Those with a score of 2 or 3 have an intermediate mortality rate of around 15% whereas the risk of death rises to 40–60% in patients with scores of 4 or 5. Delay in obtaining a plasma urea concentration can be a problem in the ED with the use of the CURB-65 scoring system.

> Patients with diffuse and severe changes on CXR should be admitted and treated aggressively even if their CURB-65 score is 0 – such patients always get worse!

Community-acquired pneumonia

Previously fit people are most likely to have been infected by pneumococci although previously esoteric causes of pneumonia are becoming more common. Pneumonia caused by *Mycoplasma pneumoniae* occurs in epidemics every 3–4 years. Extrapulmonary manifestations of mycoplasma infection include skin rashes, musculoskeletal pain, gastrointestinal upset, haemolytic anaemia and neurological disease. TB and AIDS may both present as an acute community-acquired pneumonia.

Acute infection complicating COPD → p. 205.
Bacterial causes of community-acquired pneumonia in adults in the UK → Figure 13.4.

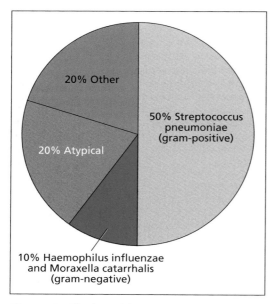

50% Streptococcus
pneumoniae
(gram-positive)

20% Other

20% Atypical

10% Haemophilus influenzae
and Moraxella catarrhalis
(gram-negative)

Figure 13.4 The bacterial causes of community-acquired pneumonia in adults in the UK.

HIV infection/AIDS → p. 261.
Legionnaires' disease → p. 211.
Pneumonia in children → p. 339.
Q fever → p. 212.
TB → p. 213.

Hospital-acquired pneumonia

This is defined as a pneumonia that occurs after at least 3 days in hospital and so should be of no direct relevance to an ED. However, patients may present themselves from institutions such as nursing homes where hospital-type opportunistic organisms abound. Pathogens gain access by inhalation or aspiration, directly via the bloodstream or by local spread.

Every sick or badly injured patient who passes through the ED is at risk of subsequent nosocomial (i.e. hospital-acquired) infection. This can be reduced by the following:

1 Using sterile techniques when siting IV lines and catheters
2 Ensuring that all airway equipment, including suction, is completely clean
3 Maintaining good tissue perfusion (i.e. promptly treating shock)
4 Humidifying inspired gases (dry gases damage the airways, thereby impairing normal respiratory defence mechanisms).

Patients at an increased risk of pneumococcal infection

Patients who have had a splenectomy, no matter how long ago, are at a high risk of developing overwhelming pneumococcal infection. Similarly, some other conditions may cause a functional hyposplenism:

• Sickle cell disease and thalassaemia
• Coeliac disease
• Systemic lupus erythematosus
• Lymphoma and leukaemia
• Other immunodeficiencies.

Such patients should have received pneumococcal vaccine and must be regarded with a high level of suspicion whenever they develop a pyrexia or acute respiratory symptoms.

Investigations: A CXR may show a variable picture; a classic lobar atelectasis is unusual. *For the appearances of lobar collapse-consolidation on CXR → Figure 13.5.* The distinction between pneumonia and an exacerbation of COPD depends on the presence or absence of the radiological signs of pneumonia; patients with consolidation on a CXR should be treated for pneumonia. Identification of the causative organism will be aided by the cultures of blood (taken before the administration of antibiotics), sputum, pleural aspirate and bronchial lavage fluid. Blood specimens should also be taken for a full blood count, blood chemistry and arterial blood gases. A urine sample may be obtained to look for pneumococcal antigen in patients with severe pneumonia.

Tx

• Sit the patient up and give a high concentration of humidified oxygen.
• Start IV rehydration.
• Monitor SaO_2, ECG and BP.
• Consider immediate transfer to the ICU if the PaO_2 cannot be maintained above 60 mmHg (8 kPa). (This level of desaturation is regarded as respiratory failure → p. 217.)

Almost all patients who present to hospital with pneumonia will require admission. Intravenous antibiotics should be started in the ED for those patients who have severe infections (→ p. 209 for the definition of severe pneumonia) or who are obviously frail. Physiotherapy is contraindicated in pneumonia unless the patient is producing large amounts of sputum (usually because of underlying COPD).

Community-acquired pneumonia is often caused by *Streptococcus pneumoniae* or *Mycoplasma pneumoniae* although a variety of atypical pathogens may also be responsible. If the infection is not severe (→

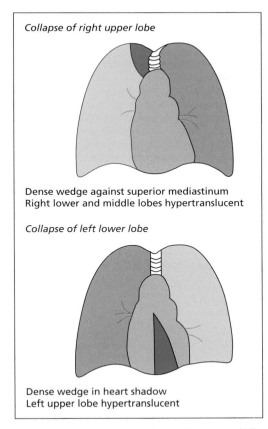

Collapse of right upper lobe

Dense wedge against superior mediastinum
Right lower and middle lobes hypertranslucent

Collapse of left lower lobe

Dense wedge in heart shadow
Left upper lobe hypertranslucent

Figure 13.5 Appearance of lobar collapse on a CXR.

before) and the patient has not been previously treated in the community, amoxicillin 500 mg–1 g three times daily by mouth (for at least 7 days) is an appropriate antibiotic. For patients who are allergic to penicillins, clarithromycin 500 mg twice daily or doxycycline 200 mg daily can be used. If there is no response to amoxicillin after 2 days, or if atypical pathogens are suspected, then clarithromycin should be added. For patients who have already been treated in the community, or those with more severe features, the combination of amoxicillin and clarithromycin (or doxycycline alone) is used immediately. All patients with a severe community-acquired pneumonia (→ *p. 209 for definition of severe*) should be given IV co-amoxiclav 1.2 g three times daily with IV clarithromycin 1 g twice daily from first presentation for 7–10 days. Cefuroxime and cefotaxime are alternatives to co-amoxiclav in this situation.

Hospital-acquired pneumonia may be caused by a wide variety of pathogens including Gram-negative bacilli and *Streptococcus pneumoniae*. Early onset hospital-acquired pneumonia (i.e. occurring within 5 days of admission) can be treated with co-amoxiclav. Late-onset infection requires an anti-pseudomonal penicillin combination (e.g. piperacillin with tazobactam) or a quinolone (e.g. ciprofloxacin).

Post-influenza pneumonia is caused by secondary bacterial infection of inflamed lung tissue. The same situation may occur after measles. The mortality associated with staphylococcal superinfection is particularly high and, if it is suspected, flucloxacillin should be added to the above antibiotics. Vancomycin (or teicoplanin) is used in cases caused by meticillin-resistant *Staphylococcus aureus* (MRSA).

***Pneumocystis jiroveci* pneumonia** (formerly known as *Pneumocystis carinii* pneumonia or PCP – this acronym is still in use) is invariably associated with AIDS (→ *p. 261*). The CXR shows diffuse interstitial changes. The diagnosis may be confirmed by culture of sputum or broncho-alveolar lavage specimens. PCP is treated with co-trimoxazole 120 mg/kg per day in two to four divided doses either by mouth or intravenously.

Aspiration pneumonia may occur in emergency patients with impaired airway reflexes from a wide variety of causes including depressed consciousness, neurological disease and general debilitation. Radiographic changes are often inconclusive or delayed for several hours after aspiration. Consolidation appears most usually in the right upper or middle zones. Pathogens in this situation include *Streptococcus pneumoniae*, *Klebsiella pneumoniae* and anaerobic bacteria. IV co-amoxiclav 1.2 g three times daily is given together with IV metronidazole 500 mg three times daily. For less serious cases, ciprofloxacin 500 mg orally twice daily can be used. There is little evidence for the efficacy of steroids in aspiration pneumonia.

Clearance and protection of the airway → *pp. 2 and 196.*
Prophylaxis of gastric acid aspiration in pregnant patients with major trauma → *p. 32.*
Respiratory failure → *p. 217.*

Legionnaires' disease

This atypical pneumonia is caused by infection with the Gram-negative organism *Legionella pneumophila*, which is harboured in institutional water systems. The disease is spread by airborne droplets, most commonly to middle-aged men in warm conditions. There may be a history of a recent stay in a hotel, hospital or other large building. Legionnaires' disease starts with a flu-like illness and then develops into a severe chest infection, often with accompanying gastrointestinal features. Symptoms and signs include:

- fever and rigors
- pleurisy and haemoptysis
- abdominal pain, diarrhoea and vomiting
- a relative bradycardia.

Investigations: These may reveal:

- raised WCC with neutrophilia and lymphopenia
- low plasma sodium (<130 mmol/L)
- proteinuria and haematuria
- unilateral patchy shadowing (often confined to a lower lobe) and pleural effusions on CXR.

The specific urinary antigen test is diagnostic (although the result is not available immediately).

Tx Patients in whom the diagnosis of legionellosis is suspected should be admitted to hospital. Clarithromycin 500 mg twice daily by mouth is the first-line antibiotic; ciprofloxacin 500 mg twice daily is an alternative. Severe infections may require the addition of rifampicin 600 mg twice daily by mouth. Ten or more days' treatment may be required. Legionnaires' disease is notifiable in the UK (except in Scotland).

Further treatment of pneumonias → p. 209.

Q fever

This highly infectious zoonosis occurs throughout the world and is caused by the bacterium *Coxiella burnetti*. Humans become infected by inhaling or ingesting infected dust. (A single organism can cause disease if inhaled by a susceptible individual.) The primary vector of *Coxiella burnetti* is the tick that infests large, domesticated animals, so there is usually a history of recent contact with cattle, sheep or goats. Abattoir workers, meat packers and farmers are mostly affected; the peak incidence in the UK is associated with the spring lambing season. The incubation period of Q fever is 7–30 days. Most infections are asymptomatic but there are two main acute presentations:

1 Pyrexia, sweating, fatigue, headache and malaise (an influenza-like illness); retro-orbital pain is very suggestive of Q fever.
2 Chest pain and cough (atypical pneumonia with patchy basal consolidation on CXR; hepatitis may occur).

The most common manifestation of chronic Q fever is endocarditis in those with underlying cardiac structural abnormalities. Q fever in pregnancy, whether symptomatic or asymptomatic, may result in abortion or adverse pregnancy outcomes.

Q fever is treated with doxycycline 200 mg daily or tetracycline 250–500 mg four times daily for 10–14 days.

Further treatment of pneumonias → p. 209.

Influenza

Every winter in the UK, during a 6- to 8-week period, influenza is associated with a sharp increase in both mortality and requests for medical attention. At this time, consultations for respiratory illness may increase up to 10-fold. In an average year, an estimated 2000–3000 people die in the UK from influenza-related causes; in years with major epidemics there have been over 20 000 excess deaths. People at an increased risk from influenza (and who should be immunised against it) include those who are aged ≥65 years, residents in long-term care and people with certain chronic illnesses including:

- respiratory disease (especially COPD and asthma)
- heart disease
- renal disease
- immunosuppression (from any cause and including asplenia)
- diabetes.

The symptoms of influenza are relatively non-specific – pyrexia, malaise, anorexia, myalgia, nausea and unproductive coughing. The incubation period is only 2 days and viral shedding lasts for 48 h on average.

Tx The treatment of influenza is mostly symptomatic – fluids and antipyretic analgesics. However, during an epidemic, high-risk patients in the groups listed above who present within 36 h of the onset of symptoms should be considered for antiviral therapy. For adults and children >40 kg, oseltamivir 75 mg is given by mouth twice daily for 5 days. An alternative for patients >12 years is zanamivir 10 mg by inhalation twice daily for 5 days. These antiviral compounds (neuraminidase inhibitors) are licensed for the treatment of both influenza A and B but are not suitable for pregnant or breast-feeding women.

Avian influenza (bird flu) is a disease of birds caused by influenza viruses that are closely related to human influenza viruses. It is an important disease economically for farmers because of losses in poultry flocks. Transmission to humans in close contact with poultry or other birds occurs rarely and only with some strains of avian influenza (e.g. subtype H5N1) (→ *Figure 13.6*). The potential for transformation of avian influenza into a form that both causes severe disease

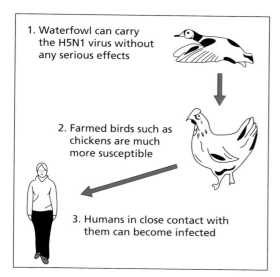

1. Waterfowl can carry the H5N1 virus without any serious effects

2. Farmed birds such as chickens are much more susceptible

3. Humans in close contact with them can become infected

Figure 13.6 The transmission of avian influenza.

in humans and spreads easily from person to person is a great concern for world health. During a pandemic, it is estimated that one in four of the population could become ill and that the deaths could number over 50 000 in the UK alone.

Swine influenza A (swine flu) is another form of zoonotic influenza that is usually caused by an H1N1subtype. This influenza A virus is sensitive to oseltamivir and zanamivir but resistant to amantadine and rimantadine.

Infection control principles in respiratory epidemics →
  SARS below.
Treatment of post-influenza pneumonia → p. 211.

Severe acute respiratory syndrome

SARS (severe acute respiratory syndrome) is the term used to describe an emerging disease that first appeared in southern China at the end of 2002 and has since been described in many countries around the world. It is a serious respiratory infection, which may lead to pneumonia and respiratory distress syndrome (RDS). The causative organism is the SARS coronavirus (SARS-CoV), a newly discovered member of the coronavirus family. (Coronaviruses are the second most common cause of a cold – after rhinoviruses.) The SARS-CoV has been isolated from wild animals native to the Guangdong Province and other parts of China. It appears to be less infectious than the influenza viruses, with a short

incubation period of 2–10 days (usually less than a week). Transmission occurs through close contact with an infected person, probably by droplet spread. Many of the outbreaks have been in hospital workers or close family members of known cases. The reported death rate for probable cases of SARS is 4–10%. The main features of the disease are similar to severe influenza – high fever, sore throat, headache, myalgia, dry cough and dyspnoea. CXR changes suggestive of pneumonia may occur. The WHO clinical case definition of SARS has been developed for public health purposes:

1 Respiratory illness severe enough to warrant hospitalisation
2 Fever of ≥38°C (documented or reported)
3 One or more symptoms of lower respiratory tract illness (cough, difficulty breathing, shortness of breath)
4 Radiological evidence of lung infiltrates consistent with pneumonia or RDS or postmortem findings consistent with the pathology of pneumonia or RDS without an identifiable cause
5 No alternative diagnosis to fully explain the illness.

Investigations:
• Routine blood tests and CXR
• Blood (30–40 mL) for serology (ELISA [enzyme-linked immunosorbent assay] antibody test and PCR [polymerase chain reaction] for SARS-CoV)
• Nasopharyngeal and throat swabs
• Urine and stool specimens.

Tx There is no specific treatment or vaccine against SARS-CoV. Control of SARS (and similar infective pathogens) depends on the following:

1 Early recognition of the symptoms and signs of the disease
2 Immediate isolation of suspected cases
3 Effective means to reduce cross-infection, by means of exceptional standards of environmental hygiene
4 No inappropriate reuse of equipment that has been used on or near a suspected case
5 Early involvement of infection control staff.

Respiratory failure → p. 217.

Tuberculosis

TB was known as the 'white plague' in Europe during the industrial revolution and has continued to ravage developing countries ever since. For the major part of the twentieth century, it was well controlled in the developed world but 25 years ago (in

1986) it began to increase in the USA and Europe. The reasons for the increase are complex but include social changes, immigration, new diseases (AIDS) and changing antimicrobial resistance in mycobacteria. The causative organism of TB, *Mycobacterium tuberculosis*, is an obligate parasite with no free-living saprophytic forms. It is capable of both intracellular and extracellular existence. Other mycobacteria (e.g. *Mycobacterium avium-intracellulare*) are increasingly recognised as human pathogens, which cause both pulmonary and systemic disease. High-risk groups for TB (and some other mycobacterial infections) include the following:

- Children and young adults
- Immigrants from the developing world
- People with poor socioeconomic status
- Residents of prisons, nursing homes and other institutions
- Individuals who are alcohol and IV drug abusers
- People with AIDS and other causes of immunodeficiency
- People with some chronic illnesses (e.g. diabetes)
- People on long-term steroid therapy
- Health-care providers.

Patients with pulmonary TB may present to an ED with chronic respiratory symptoms, general illness and weight loss, complications of TB or superadded infection. Sometimes TB may be an incidental finding on a CXR.

> A person with undiagnosed smear-positive pulmonary TB infects around 10 other people each year.

Investigations: The CXR in primary TB is likely to show changes in the lower lobes with mediastinal or hilar lymphadenopathy and, sometimes, a pleural effusion. Post-primary TB is caused by either reinfection or reactivation of a primary lesion (tubercle bacilli can remain dormant but viable in the body for many years). The altered immune response of the host results in a different radiographic picture:

- Disease in the upper lobe or superior segments of the lower lobes
- Pleural effusions and cavitating lesions
- Pneumonic consolidation, nodules or miliary spread.

In immunodeficient patients (e.g. those with AIDS) mycobacterial infection causes lymphadenopathy or minimal changes on a CXR. In almost all patients, a tuberculin skin test will confirm the diagnosis. However, tuberculin skin testing (TST) is being replaced by interferon-γ-release assay (IGRA), in the form of a single blood test. IGRA is both more specific and more sensitive than a Mantoux skin test and is not affected by previous BCG (bacille Calmette–Guérin) immunisation. It can be used at all ages (including in babies) and is safe for immunosuppressed patients. Like TST, IGRA does not differentiate between latent and active TB. Microbiology, in the form of a positive sputum sample, remains the gold standard!

Tx Patients with suspected TB should be referred to a respiratory physician for specialist treatment. In the UK, antimicrobial therapy with three drugs (rifampicin, isoniazid and pyrazinamide) is recommended, with the addition of a fourth drug (ethambutol) if there is a risk of isoniazid resistance. After 2 months, rifampicin and isoniazid are given alone for another 4 months – 'four drugs for 2 months, then two drugs for 4 months'. TB is a notifiable disease throughout the UK.

Collapse of the lung (atelectasis)

Segmental collapse is generally a result of sputum retention or infection. Lobar collapse occurs with pneumonia, TB, malignancy and foreign body aspiration. The treatment of collapse is that of the primary condition. *For the radiological appearances of lobar collapse → Figure 13.5 on p. 211.*

Pulmonary embolism

The overall incidence of PE in the UK is 60–70/100 000 people per year with an in-hospital mortality rate of around 10%. The incidence of venous thromboembolism (VTE) rises exponentially with increasing age above 40 years but age may not be an independent risk factor. *For recognised risk factors for VTE → Box 13.13.* A positive family history causes a variable increase in risk of VTE; the risk associated with cigarette smoking is still uncertain. About 50% of PEs occur in patients in hospital or long-term care, 25% in patients with other recognised risk factors and the final 25% are idiopathic. Without prophylaxis, up to 50% of patients undergoing major orthopaedic surgery, around 25% of general surgical patients and almost 20% of general medical patients will have a VTE. Thromboprophylaxis with heparin reduces these figures by around 50%.

DVT → p. 108.
Relative risks of PE and DVT for women taking combined oestrogen and progestogen contraceptive pills (and in pregnancy) → Table 7.2 on p. 109.

Box 13.13 The risk factors for venous thromboembolism

Major risk factors (relative risk = 5 to 20 fold):
- Late pregnancy or puerperium
- Caesarean section
- Major abdominal or pelvic surgery (usually procedures lasting >30 min)
- Major orthopaedic surgery (e.g. hip or knee replacement)
- Postoperative intensive care
- Malignancy (especially advanced or metastatic or in the abdomen/pelvis)
- Lower limb fracture (especially with cast)
- Previous proven VTE
- Varicose veins
- Reduced mobility (hospitalisation or other institutional care and especially critical care admission)

Minor risk factors (relative risk = 2 to 4 fold):
- Age >60 years
- Oral contraceptives and hormone replacement therapy (*also → Table 7.2 on p. 109*)
- Heart disease (congenital disease, cardiac failure, acute MI)
- Hypertension
- Other chronic diseases (e.g. COPD, infection, metabolic diseases, renal dialysis and neurological disability)
- Thrombotic disorders including known thrombophilias
- Central venous catheter *in situ*
- Previous superficial venous thrombosis or phlebitis
- History of VTE in a first-degree relative
- Dehydration
- Obesity (body mass index [BMI] >30 kg/m²)
- Long-distance sedentary travel (both by air and by road).

crepitus or a pleural rub is sometimes heard, as is a pulmonary flow murmur. Thrombosis of the deep veins may be present but is usually occult.

PE is present in less than 10% of patients with a low clinical probability of the condition. The clinical features compatible with PE are breathlessness and tachypnoea ± chest pain ± haemoptysis. In the presence of these symptoms, two further features help to determine the patient's clinical probability of having a PE:

1 There is no other likely explanation for the patient's symptoms.
2 The patient has a major risk factor. (*For major risk factors for VTE → Box 13.13.*)

Both 1 and 2 = high clinical probability.
Either 1 or 2 = intermediate clinical probability.
Neither 1 nor 2 = low clinical probability.

Isolated dyspnoea: the diagnosis of PE may be overlooked in patients with shortness of breath as their only symptom ('isolated dyspnoea'). In addition, recurrent small PEs are very often forgotten as a cause of a stepwise increase in dyspnoea. PEs in elderly patients or in those with pre-existing cardiorespiratory disease are similarly misdiagnosed.

Pleuritic chest pain as an isolated symptom of PE →
p. 191.

Massive pulmonary embolism: sometimes, the presenting symptoms of PE are collapse, syncope, hypotension, shock or even cardiac arrest. A diagnosis of massive PE is likely in the presence of unexplained hypoxia, engorged neck veins and a right ventricular gallop rhythm. An overwhelming urge to defecate may herald the onset of the illness. Urgent treatment is vital (*→ later*).

Massive PE accounts for 10% of patients arriving at an ED in cardiac arrest and up to 50% of those arriving with pulseless electrical activity or asystole. The prognosis in these cases is very poor.

Over 90% of patients with PE are breathless or have a raised respiratory rate (>20 breaths/min). Only 3% will not have dyspnoea, tachypnoea or pleuritic chest pain. Haemoptysis occurs in around 10% of cases of PE but, in the absence of respiratory symptoms, a patient's pleuritic chest pain or haemoptysis is usually due to another cause. A fifth of patients with a PE have a cough. Tachycardia is also fairly common but other symptoms and signs are very variable. Areas of

Investigations:
- Routine FBC/WCC (to look for infection) and blood chemistry should be requested.
- A negative D-dimer assay may be used to exclude PE in patients with low or intermediate clinical probability. (D-dimer is a breakdown product of cross-linked fibrin.)

Box 13.14 ECG signs of PE

- Sinus tachycardia (most common positive finding)
- New atrial fibrillation
- S1, Q3, T3 (an S wave in lead I and a Q wave with T-wave inversion in lead III)
- ST depression and T-wave inversion in the right chest leads

Box 13.15 CXR signs of PE

- Segmental collapse
- Pleural effusion
- Area of peripheral infarction ('sail' shadow)
- Raised hemidiaphragm
- Prominent pulmonary artery
- Localised absence of vascular markings

In a breathless, hypoxic patient, the more abnormal the CXR, the less likely the diagnosis of PE. Conversely, a normal CXR increases the likelihood of PE.

- Blood gases and SaO_2 may show hypoxia on air but this is not invariable with small pulmonary emboli. Measurement of the blood gases is not indicated if there is a normal SaO_2 on air.
- Around a third of patients with a moderate or large pulmonary embolus have a raised troponin level. This is associated with right ventricular damage and may in the future be used as an indication for thrombolysis in PE.
- Investigations for occult cancer in idiopathic VTE (present in 7–12% of such patients) are indicated only if the presence of malignancy is clinically suspected or suggested by a CXR or blood tests. Tests for thrombophilia are indicated in patients aged <50 years with recurrent PEs or a strong family history of thromboembolic disease.
- ECG may be normal; any changes are the result of right heart strain (→ *Box 13.14*).
- CXR is often unremarkable – *for possible changes in PE → Box 13.15*. After upper abdominal surgery, PE may be confused on a CXR with segmental collapse of the lung or pulmonary infection.
- Identification of a deep vein thrombosis (DVT) will help in the diagnosis of PE (→ *p. 108*). Venography will identify twice as many thromboses as ultrasonography in this situation. Ultrasonography

is obviously adequate if a DVT is clinically identified.
- Definitive imaging should take place within an hour in massive PE and within 24 h in all other cases. A ventilation–perfusion scan of the lungs is the classic investigation for suspected PE but is often unavailable in the acute situation. Moreover, although a normal isotope scan can reliably exclude PE, a significant proportion of results are false positives. Isotope scanning is even less reliable in the presence of an abnormal CXR or concurrent cardiorespiratory disease. CTPA (computed tomographic pulmonary angiography) is rapidly replacing it as the first-line investigation in PE. Patients with a good-quality negative CTPA do not require further investigation or treatment for PE. Echocardiography may be diagnostic in massive PE where the patient cannot be safely moved to a CT scanner.

Tx

Initial treatment: includes high-concentration oxygen, monitoring and analgesia.

Anticoagulation with heparin: should be started before imaging in patients with anything more than a low clinical probability of PE. Enoxaparin 1.5 mg/kg is given subcutaneously immediately and then daily for at least 5 days (and until oral anticoagulation is established). In pregnancy, a regimen of 1 mg/kg stat and then 1 mg/kg twice daily is used (based on weight in early pregnancy). The dose of enoxaparin should be reduced to 1 mg/kg once daily in patients with severe renal impairment (i.e. creatinine clearance <30 mL/min). Standard unfractionated heparin is a less convenient and less effective alternative to low-molecular-weight heparins (LMWHs) with more unwanted effects. An initial IV loading dose of 80 U/kg is followed by a continuous IV infusion of 15–25 U/kg per h (1000–2000 U/h). An IV bolus dose of unfractionated heparin (80 U/kg) should also be given (instead of LMWH) to unstable patients, to those with massive PE or in situations where rapid reversal of anticoagulation may be required. Fondaparinux (a synthetic pentasaccharide that inhibits activated factor X) is an alternative to heparins.

Thrombolysis: may be considered for massive life-threatening emboli. IV alteplase 10 mg is given over 1–2 min followed by an IV infusion of 90 mg over 2 h (maximum dose 1.5 mg/kg in patients <65 kg). The accelerated MI regimen for alteplase (→ *Box 12.4 on p. 184*) can also be used. Streptokinase is a less effective alternative to alteplase; urokinase may also be used. Thrombolysis is followed by unfractionated heparin after 3 h. An IV bolus of alteplase 50 mg can be administered during cardiac arrest, which is most probably due to PE or if cardiac arrest is thought to be imminent. A few units have the facility for clot fragmentation via a pulmonary artery catheter. Elsewhere, contraindications to thrombolysis should be ignored in life-threatening PE.

Oral anticoagulation (e.g. warfarin): commenced once the diagnosis of PE is confirmed. The target international normalised ratio (INR) is 2.0–3.0 and, when this is achieved, heparin can be discontinued. Warfarin is given for 4–6 weeks to patients with temporary risk factors, for 3 months to patients with a first idiopathic thrombosis and for at least 6 months to most other patients. Oral anticoagulants are teratogenic and so should not be given to pregnant patients (although they are not contraindicated during breast-feeding). Pregnant patients must be anticoagulated with heparin, which should be reduced a few hours before expected delivery and then restarted after the baby has been born.

Admission to hospital: this is required for the majority of patients with PE. A proportion of patients can be managed in the community but this depends on local protocols and services.

Respiratory failure

This is developing when the patient's conscious level begins to fall and the PaO_2 cannot be maintained above 60 mmHg (8 kPa). A normal $PaCO_2$ in the presence of tachypnoea, which should reduce it, is a worrying feature. Anaesthetic/ICU help should be requested at once.

Type I respiratory failure

Low PaO_2 (<60 mmHg or 8 kPa) with a normal or low $PaCO_2$ may result from any of the many pathological causes of maldistribution of ventilation and perfusion in the lungs. The definitive management is intubation and mechanical ventilation (IPPV) while treating the underlying cause. Continuous Positive Airway Pressure (CPAP) is a technique that uses a tight-fitting facemask to deliver oxygen at pressure throughout the ventilatory cycle and thus improve oxygen delivery to underventilated areas.

Type II (ventilatory) respiratory failure

Low PaO_2 (<60 mmHg or 8 kPa) with a raised $PaCO_2$ (>45 mmHg or 6 kPa) most commonly results from COPD ($\rightarrow$ p. 205). Other causes include:

- paralysis of the respiratory muscles
- chest deformity, especially with superadded infection

> **Box 13.16 Use of BiPAP**
>
> *Absolute exclusion criteria*
> - Tracheostomy *in situ*
> - Inability to protect airway/manage secretions
> - Pneumothorax confirmed by CXR with no chest drain *in situ*
>
> *Relative exclusion criteria*
> - Confusion and agitation
> - Systolic BP <90 mmHg
> - Head and facial trauma or burns
> - Recent facial, oesophageal or gastric surgery
> - Uncontrolled vomiting
> - Respiratory arrest
>
> Commence BiPAP starting with 4 cmH$_2$O expiratory PAP and 10 cmH$_2$O inspiratory PAP Increase inspiratory PAP in 2 cmH$_2$O increments (up to a maximum of 25 cmH$_2$O) to obtain inspiratory time <33% of total respiratory time (*Ti TOT*)
> Ensure that rise time is optimised
> Ensure that leak is no more than 20 L

- depression of the respiratory centre by sedative or narcotic/opiate drugs.

Non-invasive ventilation (NIV) can be very effective in ventilatory failure. It is indicated when the pH is <7.35. NIV is also known as non-invasive positive pressure ventilation (NIPPV). Bilevel pressure support ventilators are the most common machines to be used for NIV. They deliver two levels of positive airway pressure over the respiratory cycle (BiPAP). *For the use of BiPAP $\rightarrow$ Box 13.16.*

> A hypercapnic patient who is receiving BiPAP with a 10–15 cmH$_2$O inspiratory : expiratory (*I/E*) pressure difference, and who is not triggering or synchronising with the machine's flow, is being ventilated albeit with low pressures, a mask and no ventilator!

The analeptic and respiratory stimulant drug, doxapram, is sometimes used if NIV is unavailable. Its main functions are the following:

1 To reduce oxygen-induced CO$_2$ retention
2 To treat a patient who is not thought to be suitable for assisted ventilation

Box 13.17 Doxapram and oxygen therapy for ventilatory failure

PaO_2 >45 mmHg (6 kPa) give 28% oxygen and observe.
PaO_2 <45 mmHg (6 kPa) give 24% oxygen and if:

- the PaO_2 fails to improve or
- the $PaCO_2$ is rising more than 10 mmHg or 1.5 kPa in less than 1 h,

then doxapram should be commenced as follows:

    4.0 mg/min × 15 min
    3.0 mg/min × 15 min
    2.0 mg/min × 30 min
    1.5 mg/min thereafter

Control of the CO_2 rise may enable a change to 28% oxygen

3 As a holding measure while awaiting anaesthetic help.

Controlled oxygen therapy with doxapram in type II respiratory failure → Box 13.17.

Intubation and conventional IPPV remain the definitive treatment of both types of respiratory failure.

Hyperventilation syndrome

Although some people are prone to attacks of hyperventilation, it is rare for significant psychiatric disease to be the cause. There is usually underlying anxiety and social stress.

The patient becomes increasingly frightened by an apparent inability to breathe adequately. Attempts to breathe rapidly result in dizziness and further anxiety. Tachypnoea blows off CO_2 and the resultant respiratory alkalosis causes a fall in ionised calcium. Paraesthesiae in the fingers and around the mouth are common consequences but tetany with carpopedal spasm is relatively unusual (→ *p. 249*).

Tx Investigation should accompany treatment; the confirmation of normality with warm reassurance is essential. Organic respiratory problems, such as spontaneous pneumothorax, PE or salicylate poisoning must be ruled out. This will certainly entail physical examination and pulse oximetry; ECG, CXR and blood gas analysis may also be needed in some cases.

If no organic cause can be found, then re-breathing into a closed bag-and-mask system without oxygen supplement may be helpful. Requests for tranquillisers should be resisted. The patient should either be discharged home with relatives and a note sent to the GP or else, in severe cases, be admitted for further assessment. Outpatient psychiatric review, via the GP, may be required for patients who suffer from frequent attacks.

Other causes of respiratory distress

A wide range of other conditions may lead to respiratory distress, including shock from any cause, trauma, poisoning and metabolic upset.

Diabetic ketoacidosis → p. 241.
Inhalation of fumes, smoke and other gases → pp. 136 and 295.
Myocardial infarction → p. 177.
Salicylate poisoning → p. 277.
Spontaneous pneumothorax → p. 192.

Haemoptysis

Patients may present with haemoptysis as an isolated symptom. The blood is usually coughed up in a small quantity mixed with sputum. History and examination must aim to exclude serious illnesses such as chest infection, LVF, PE, TB or malignancy. FBC, ECG and CXR should be performed on all such patients with the same aim. Patients who are then found to have no other apparent abnormalities or stable conditions can be referred back to their GP for further management. Most haemoptysis in young people is idiopathic.

Pulmonary embolism → pp. 190 and 214.

Collapse and sudden illness

COLLAPSE

The term 'collapse' is generally used to describe a sudden deterioration in health and thus it covers a wide spectrum of disease. To collapse implies a change of such magnitude that an upright posture cannot be maintained; it does not necessarily refer to a depression in the level of consciousness. However, some collapsed patients will be comatose and many will have a history of having been unresponsive at some time. The priorities in patients who present with a sudden onset of illness or who have collapsed are to:

- start resuscitation
- seek out easily reversible conditions and treat them
- begin a structured assessment.

Assessment and management of the collapsed patient

Details of immediate assessment and management applicable to all emergency patients are given in *Chapter 1*. The same structured system can be used for the collapsed patient.

A – Airway

- Clear the airway with suction or other physical means.
- Maintain the airway by positioning or using airway adjuncts.
- Protect the airway by positioning the patient in the recovery position and having suction available.

- Consider the need for endotracheal intubation.
- Protect the cervical spine at all times if the history is unknown, vague or suggests the possibility of trauma.
- Consider specific treatment for foreign body obstruction ($\rightarrow$ *p. 196*) or anaphylaxis ($\rightarrow$ *p. 299*).

B – Breathing

- Give a high concentration of oxygen by mask if the arterial O_2 saturation (SaO_2) is <94% on air.
- Briefly look at the adequacy of respiration.
- Consider the need for immediate ventilation.
- Establish monitoring (SaO_2, BP [blood pressure] and ECG).
- If the SaO_2 is low or if there is a suggestion of CO_2 narcosis, check the blood gases.
- Commence therapy to relieve hypoxia and dyspnoea; consider specific treatment for:
  - cardiorespiratory problems (severe left ventricular failure, chronic obstructive pulmonary disease [COPD], asthma, pneumonia, pulmonary embolism and spontaneous pneumothorax $\rightarrow$ *Chapter 13*)
  - CO_2 narcosis $\rightarrow$ *p. 217*
  - anaphylaxis $\rightarrow$ *p. 299*.

C – Circulation

- Establish venous access and give intravenous (IV) fluids as necessary.
- Examine the cardiovascular system.
- Consider the possibility of bleeding into the abdomen or the gut (abdominal + rectal examination).

Emergency Medicine Lecture Notes, Fourth Edition. Chris Moulton and David Yates.
© 2012 Blackwell Publishing Ltd. Published 2012 by Blackwell Publishing Ltd.

Look for melaena or coffee-ground vomit and vaginal or rectal bleeding.

- Consider specific treatment for:
  - cardiothoracic problems (myocardial infarction [MI], pulmonary embolism → *Chapter 12*; dysrhythmia → *Chapter 11*)
  - abdominal problems (gastrointestinal bleed, intra-abdominal bleeding or sepsis → *Chapter 16*)
  - anaphylaxis → *p. 299*.

D – Disability

- Record the level of consciousness.
- Look at the pupils, muscle tone and reflexes and record any localising signs.
- Run your hands over the scalp to discover any swelling or bleeding.
- Look in the ears for signs of base of skull fracture.
- Look in the fundi for preretinal haemorrhage (from a subarachnoid bleed).
- Look for photophobia, neck stiffness, Kernig's sign and purpura.
- Listen for neck bruits (cerebral ischaemia).

A decreased level of consciousness indicates that something is wrong with the brain or its fuel supply. It may be:

1 Poisoning or gross metabolic disturbance (including CO_2 narcosis and hypothermia)

2 Cerebral injury or pathology (head injury, intracranial bleeding, thrombosis, embolism, infection, swelling, tumour, fitting, etc.)

3 Failure of the brain's fuel supply (hypoxia, hypovolaemia, cerebral ischaemia or hypoglycaemia)

Common causes of sudden collapse with coma → Box 14.1.

 Box 14.1 Common causes of sudden collapse with coma

- Subarachnoid haemorrhage
- Brain-stem cerebral vascular accident (CVA)
- Hypoglycaemia
- Poisoning (e.g. tricyclic antidepressants)
- Head injury

E – Environment and exposure

- Take the temperature (tympanic or rectal).
- Remove clothing (but keep warm), and examine the whole patient – front and back. Search the clothing for treatment cards, drugs, suicide notes and identification. Consider forensic needs.
- Protect the eyes.
- Consider specific treatment for:
  - hypothermia → *p. 243*
  - infection
  - hyperpyrexia → *pp. 245 and 271*.

F – Fits

- Control any tonic–clonic activity with benzodiazepines (→ *p. 231*).
- Protect the tongue from the teeth with a Guedel airway.

G – Glucose

Check the blood sugar in any patient who is unresponsive or behaving strangely and administer IV glucose if necessary.

H – History

- Get as much detail as possible from bystanders, ambulance crew and relatives. The essentials are AMPLE (→ *p. 12*).
- Obtain hospital records or details from the GP by telephone.

I – Immediate analgesia and investigations

- Give analgesia, if required, and look for the cause of any pain.
- Request a chest radiograph (CXR).
- Obtain an ECG.
- Take blood for full blood count (FBC), urea and electrolytes (U&Es), sugar and C-reactive protein (CRP). Consider also requesting a serum osmolality. The osmolar gap is a useful and easily available indicator of toxic and metabolic disorders → *Boxes 14.2 and 14.3*.
- Consider the need for a nasogastric tube and/or a urinary catheter in all unresponsive patients.
- Consider the need for radiographs of the hips and pelvis in any older person who has collapsed or been found on the floor.

Box 14.2 The osmolar gap

This is useful as a screening test for osmotically active poisons in the bloodstream and in the search for a cause for a metabolic acidosis.

Osmolar gap is the difference between measured serum osmolality and calculated serum osmolality.

Measured serum osmolality is normally 280–300 mosmol/L (easily measured by freezing point osmometry).

Calculated serum osmolality is twice the serum sodium concentration plus the glucose and the urea levels (in mmol/L).

$$\text{Calculated osmolality} = (2 \times Na^+)$$
$$+ \text{glucose} + \text{urea}$$

This is a simplification of a more accurate formula:

$$\text{Calculated osmolality} = (1.86 \times Na^+)$$
$$+ \text{glucose} + \text{urea}/0.93$$

If the osmolar gap is >10 mosmol/L then there are probably abnormal osmotically active substances in the bloodstream such as:

- ethanol
- methanol
- ethylene glycol
- mannitol.

These are all substances with a small molecular weight. Even in poisoned patients, most other drugs do not achieve a high enough molar concentration to contribute to osmolality, which depends purely on the number of molecules present.

The osmolar (or more correctly osmolal) gap should be interpreted cautiously in the critically ill patient because circulatory failure may cause it to increase. Hyperosmolar IV infusions, ketoacidosis and chronic (but not acute) renal failure may do the same.

 Box 14.3 The anion gap

The anion gap refers to the concentration difference between the measured serum cation (sodium) and the measured serum anions (chloride and bicarbonate). It is normally 12 mmol/L (±2). An anion gap of >20 is definitely abnormal.

$$\text{Anion gap} = Na^+ - (Cl^- + HCO_3^-)$$
$$= 10 - 14 \text{ mmol/L}$$

An increased anion gap suggests an underlying metabolic acidosis – usually as a result of poisoning, renal failure or excess production of lactate or ketones. This is because, in metabolic acidosis, excess acids are titrated by bicarbonate, the level of which then falls – resulting in an increase in the calculated anion gap. *Metabolic acidosis → p. 251.*

Collapse in children

Collapse in children usually accompanies overwhelming pathology such as shock, respiratory failure or intracranial infection.

Meningococcal septicaemia → p. 341.
Miscellaneous paediatric conditions → Chapter 18.
Paediatric resuscitation → p. 151.

Collapse in elderly people

Collapse in elderly people is common because of the following:

1 Homeostatic mechanisms and physiological reserves are impaired – a relatively small change in health can cause sudden decompensation of an already failing system.
2 Lack of social support and delayed access to carers may prevent timely interventions that could have avoided gross deterioration.
3 Elderly patients are often taking a multiplicity of drugs.
4 Symptoms and signs tend to be less focused, so that the patient presents with global vague problems rather than specific and localised abnormalities.

The cause of a sudden deterioration in an elderly patient may not be immediately apparent from the history or clinical examination. For this reason,

Poisoning

Treatment of poisoned patients → Chapter 15.

Unexplained collapse with generalised or bizarre signs must always raise the possibility of poisoning, even if this is strenuously denied. In unresponsive patients, a gastric lavage may yield useful information and remove toxic substances from the stomach.

most collapsed older patients will need investigation before discharge to exclude diagnoses such as the following:

- MI or pulmonary embolism
- Heart block or other dysrhythmia
- Pneumonia, pyelonephritis or other infection
- Gastrointestinal bleeding or other blood loss
- Anaemia or renal failure
- Chronic subdural haemorrhage or CVA
- Fractured neck of femur.

FBC, standard blood chemistry, glucose, ECG and CXR are essential. CRP, plasma calcium and osmolality are useful in non-specific illness.

Patients who have been found lying on the floor are often cold, dehydrated and frightened; they must be admitted for further assessment and stabilisation. The plasma creatinine kinase should be measured and the urine tested for myoglobin (*For crush injuries → p. 265 and hypothermia → p. 243*).

Prevention of pressure sores

Pressure sores cause a great deal of morbidity among hospitalised patients and are difficult and expensive to treat. They will begin to form or worsen during a period of immobility on an emergency department (ED) trolley, especially if the time is >2 h. Thus all patients who are recumbent should be assessed for risk factors using a predetermined scoring system.

There are general risk factors including the following:

- Obesity or low body weight
- Thin, oedematous, sweaty or damaged skin
- Reduced or restricted mobility, including that caused by pain or splintage
- Incontinence of urine or faeces
- Low intake of food and drink
- Increasing age (>50 years)
- Female gender.

Problems that carry a special and very high risk of skin breakdown include the following:

- Cachexia
- Cardiovascular disease
- Neurological disease
- Major trauma
- History of lying on the floor
- Hypothermia
- Treatment with steroids and cytotoxics.

Patients who are found to be at risk of developing pressure sores should receive pressure area care from trained nursing staff and be moved to a suitable ward bed as soon as possible.

Prevention of venous thromboembolism

Venous thromboembolism (VTE) usually starts as a deep vein thrombosis (DVT) and is not just a problem in surgical patients. Sick patients of all types are susceptible, especially if their mobility is reduced for 3 days or more. Moreover, the risk of DVT doubles with serious infections. Up to 20% of general medical patients are believed to have VTE that is very often undiagnosed. The incidence of VTE has been found to be 100 times greater in hospital patients than in similar populations in the community. It is the most common cause of preventable death in British hospitals and is responsible for 25 times more deaths than meticillin-resistant *Staphylococcus aureus* (MRSA)! For this reason, prophylaxis against DVT is recommended for almost all medical patients. Exceptions include those who present with a condition that might be haemorrhagic in origin or who:

- are aged <40 years and fully mobile
- have a congenital or acquired bleeding disorder (including severe liver disease)
- have thrombocytopenia (platelets $<75 \times 10^9/L$)
- are already on anticoagulants (with an international normalised ratio or INR >2)
- have a history of haemorrhagic stroke or subarachnoid haemorrhage
- have uncontrolled systolic hypertension (>230/120 mmHg)
- have a recent history of GI bleeding
- are known to have pericarditis or diabetic retinopathy
- have had a lumbar puncture or epidural injection in the previous 4 h or are expected to require one of these procedures in the next 12 h.

A suitable regimen is enoxaparin 40 mg daily by subcutaneous injection, started in the ED. Alternative anticoagulants for this purpose include other low-molecular-weight heparins, unfractionated heparin and fondaparinux. Mechanical DVT prophylaxis with stockings or pneumatic devices is also possible. Aspirin and other antiplatelet agents do not provide adequate protection against VTE.

Diagnosis and treatment of DVT → p. 108.
Risk factors for VTE → Box 13.13 on p. 215.

Driving after a collapse or sudden illness

Patients who have conditions that may result in a sudden and dramatic change in health are not fit to drive or operate dangerous machinery → p. 376. An escort home should be arranged for all such patients and they should be warned of the possible dangers to themselves and others. *For advice on driving after a CVA or transient ischaemic attack (TIA) → p. 230.*

NEUROLOGICAL PROBLEMS

Acute confusional states → p. 358.

Syncope (transient loss of consciousness)

Transient loss of consciousness ('blackout') is a common presentation to an ED, particularly in teenagers, young adults and elderly people. It affects almost half the population at some point in their lives. A careful history is essential to ascertain the following:

- What the patient was doing at the time of the syncope
- What posture he or she was in
- What warning signs were experienced
- Whether the person feels that he or she has fully recovered
- The past medical history and medications.

'Red flag' symptoms include:

- Collapse and loss of consciousness during exertion
- Dyspnoea, chest pain or headache
- Tongue-biting, incontinence or post-ictal drowsiness/confusion
- Family history of sudden cardiac death before age 40.

Information from observers and paramedics can be extremely useful in this respect.

Subsequent examination and investigations can be tailored to the likely causes of the syncope as suggested by the history. Older people will require an ECG and possibly routine blood tests and measurement of lying and standing BPs. Possible diagnoses at all ages include epilepsy, cardiac causes and psychogenic syncope.

Vasovagal syncope (the common faint) often occurs in pregnancy or during the prodromal phase of a viral illness. There should be a history of some warning symptoms before the faint, a full recovery and no features to suggest alternative diagnoses. A mild degree of bradycardia is a common finding even when the patient appears to have fully recovered. Sudden arising to an upright posture, prolonged standing, excessive heat and anticipated medical procedures may all induce this type of syncope. Occasionally, a vasovagal faint will be followed by a brief convulsion – an 'anoxic' fit. The patient can be reassured if there is a good history of a simple faint, no previous similar episodes, and a full and rapid recovery.

Situational syncope may occur during micturition or coughing. There should be a clear history, a full recovery and no features to suggest alternative diagnoses.

Orthostatic syncope is caused by postural hypotension and can be diagnosed when there is a drop in systolic blood pressure upon standing of >20 mmHg (or a drop in diastolic BP >10 mmHg). The first BP reading should be taken after the patient has been lying supine for 5 min and then the second reading is taken 1 min later after standing. Postural hypotension is usually associated with medications such as vasodilators, antihypertensives and antidepressants. Dehydration, arteriosclerosis, diabetes and some other metabolic diseases are also implicated in orthostatic drops in BP. A change of drug therapy should be considered in liaison with the GP.

Some patients with transient loss of consciousness can be safely discharged whereas others will require admission. Those who have fully recovered but have some worrying features, a history of a possible fit or abnormal investigations should be sent to an appropriate specialist clinic. Patients aged >65 years with no prodromal symptoms should always be considered for further investigation. All patients who are waiting for specialist assessment should be warned not to drive and to take appropriate precautions at home and at work.

Headache

The discomfort described as a headache may result from the following:

- Muscular tension (tension headache)
- Arterial dilatation (hypertension, nitrates)
- Traction on arteries (raised intracranial pressure)
- Traction on venous sinuses (low pressure headache after cerebrospinal fluid leak or dehydration)
- Inflammation (meningitis, arteritis)
- Referred pain (sinusitis, glaucoma).

Common pathological causes of a headache → Box 14.4.

Worrying features in the history of a patient with a headache include:

- sudden onset of symptoms
- neck stiffness
- loss of consciousness, however transient
- fit or other collapse
- visual loss or other visual change
- other neurological symptoms

Box 14.4 Causes of a headache

- Tension headache
- Migraine/cluster headache
- Subarachnoid haemorrhage (SAH)
- Other intracranial bleed
- Post head injury headache
- Intracranial infection
- Systemic febrile illnesses
- Space-occupying lesion
- Temporal arteritis
- Malignant hypertension
- Paget's disease
- Hypercapnia/hypoxia
- Poisoning (CO_2, nitrates)
- Glaucoma
- ENT infection and nasal trauma
- Dental problems
- Neck problems
- Cerebrospinal (CSF) fluid leakage
- Dehydration
- Psychogenic factors, including anxiety and depression

Consider the possibility of SAH in all patients with a headache:

- 50% of patients with SAH have a warning headache in the week before a big bleed
- 50% have a warning headache without major physical signs
- nearly 50% have seen a doctor about the headache
- 50% with missed initial bleeds die

- change in personality, memory or mental ability
- pain worse on waking or straining
- worst-ever headache
- first severe headache in a patient aged >35 years.

The minimum examination of an ambulant patient with a headache should record the following:

- Cortical functioning/Glasgow Coma Scale (GCS)
- Gross neurological state
- Pupillary signs
- Fundoscopy
- The presence or absence of meningism or neck tenderness
- Temperature
- The presence or absence of rashes
- Otoscopy
- BP
- Palpation of the scalp and sinuses for tenderness.

XR CT is the most useful first-line investigation of a headache unless lumbar puncture is needed to exclude meningitis. A negative scan does not rule out SAH.

TX Patients with a headache who have symptoms or signs suggestive of serious pathology should be referred to the physician on call. Even with no neurological signs and a GCS score of 15/15, more than 1 in 20 patients with a 'thunderclap' headache will be found to have an SAH.

Head injury

Chronic subdural haematoma → p. 45.
Management of patients with head injuries → Chapter 3 on p. 33.

Head injury must always be considered as a cause of collapse and may often coexist with it. Where there is doubt as to the relative influences of intracranial injury and other conditions, then a CT scan should be performed.

Subarachnoid haemorrhage

Primary SAH occurs in 1 in 1000 adults. Most (80–85%) of these bleeds are caused by the rupture of saccular ('berry') aneurysms, usually situated around the circle of Willis or one of its major branches. In the remaining 15–20% of cases, no aneurysm is detected and about half of these bleeds are attributed to non-aneurysmal perimesencephalic haemorrhage, in which the blood is limited to the subarachnoid spaces around the midbrain (i.e. the mesencephalon) and its exact origin is uncertain. Another group of spontaneous SAHs are due to other disorders affecting the blood vessels (such as arteriovenous malformations). If untreated, saccular aneurysms have a 20–40% chance of re-bleeding in the following month with an 80% chance of death or residual disability. Perimesencephalic haemorrhages have a very good prognosis and can be treated conservatively. Overall, 10% of patients with primary SAH die in the first few hours and this rises to 50% in the first few weeks. Bleeding recurs in one in five patients, usually at the end of the first week. Secondary SAH may occur from extension of an intracerebral bleed or after trauma.

SAH usually presents as one of the following:

1 Sudden collapse with a depressed level of consciousness with or without convulsions and/or vomiting

2 Sudden onset of severe occipital headache ('thunderclap' headache) with or without other neurological features. There may be a history of recent 'warning' episodes of sudden headache. The patient may be feeling much better at the time of ED examination.

Meningism is often present even in the comatose patient although neck pain and photophobia are not essential for the diagnosis. Lateralising signs are usually 'soft' or absent.

Fundoscopy of comatose patients with SAH may reveal preretinal (subhyaloid) haemorrhages; this sign is pathognomonic. Tropicamide mydriatic drops may be used to dilate the pupils; pupillary signs must be recorded first.

> Beware of the patient who collapses with SAH but sustains a coincidental traumatic brain injury.

Investigations: Non-contrast CT scan of the brain is more than 95% sensitive at detecting subarachnoid blood. It also shows the amount and distribution of the blood and complications such as surrounding oedema, hydrocephalus or ischaemic damage. Larger bleeds or those with extension into the brain parenchyma almost always yield a positive result. However, the sensitivity of CT falls to less than 50% after a week and the blood may have been completely reabsorbed by 10 days.

> A negative CT scan of the brain does not completely exclude SAH.

When the history is suggestive of SAH and the CT scan is negative, lumbar puncture will be required. This should not be performed until at least 6 h (and preferably 12 h) have elapsed since the onset of symptoms. A bloody tap can be distinguished from true SAH by levels of red cells that remain constant in successive collection tubes and by the presence of breakdown products of haemoglobin. MRI, conventional catheter angiography and MR or CT with angiography are all used as further investigations for SAH.

Tx
- ABCs
- Terminate convulsions
- Check the blood sugar
- Refer the patient to the general physicians/neurosurgeons as appropriate.

The calcium antagonist nimodipine (60 mg every 4 h) is used to prevent the development of secondary cerebral ischaemia. This occurs in 50% of patients, usually in the first 5–10 days after the bleed.

Intracranial infection

Impaired consciousness and pyrexia suggest intracranial infection. Meningitis is the most common cause and may be associated with infection elsewhere. Encephalitis (usually herpetic) may present as confusion, disorientation, drowsiness or bizarre behaviour.

Encephalitis → p. 340.
Features and treatment of both bacterial and viral meningitis → pp. 339 and 340.
Prophylaxis of meningitis contacts → p. 343.

> Neck stiffness is absent in up to 30% of cases of bacterial meningitis.

Meningococcal disease is especially important for ED personnel to recognise because very early treatment (with IV antibiotics, fluids and ventilation) improves the prognosis. In the UK, cases of meningococcal infection, both meningitic and septicaemic, usually rise in the autumn and reach a peak early in the New Year. This annual rise in cases starts in students in colleges of higher education, although the highest incidence rates are in children aged <2 years. Muslim visitors to Saudi Arabia for the Hajj or Umrah pilgrimages are also at a high risk of meningococcal infection.

Meningococcal disease → p. 341.

Temporal arteritis

Cranial or giant cell arteritis is a panarteritis of unknown aetiology, which affects medium-sized vessels, particularly those of the scalp. Affected arteries are thickened and tender and thrombosis may occur. The condition is related to polymyalgia rheumatica and is predominantly seen in patients aged >60 years (and hardly ever in people aged <50). The incidence of giant cell arteritis continues to rise with increasing age.

Temporal arteritis – the most common manifestation – starts with an acute onset of headache. There is a sharp, burning pain over the temporal artery, which may be locally tender or even pulseless.

Neurological signs are caused by ischaemia in the territory of other inflamed arteries:

- *Visual impairment*: which may progress to blindness caused by ischaemia of the optic nerve and retina
- *Ophthalmoplegia*: due to ischaemia of the ocular motor nerves
- *Pain on eating*: due to masseter claudication
- *TIA/stroke*: caused by involvement of branches of the vertebral or carotid arteries.

Systemic malaise and weight loss may sometimes occur. In many cases, the features are atypical.

Investigations: A raised erythrocyte sedimentation rate (ESR) may confirm the diagnosis but a normal ESR does not exclude it. Plasma CRP is also elevated in most cases. Serial ESRs and biopsy of the superficial temporal artery may be required.

 Tx As soon as the diagnosis is suspected, parenteral methylprednisolone should be given (up to 500 mg by slow IV injection). Oral prednisolone (40 mg) is an alternative (60 mg if there are visual symptoms). Soluble aspirin (300 mg) should also be administered. Prompt treatment with high-dose systemic steroids does not usually improve vision but prevents further deterioration, especially in an eye that has not already been affected. Analgesia and admission for observation are also required. Recovery can take several months and recurrence is always a possibility.

> The primary aim of treatment in temporal arteritis is to prevent the occurrence of permanent neurological damage, especially blindness.

Migraine

The first severe attack of migraine usually occurs in the teenage years or early 20s. There may be an isolated unilateral throbbing headache (common migraine) or a more complicated syndrome preceded by some form of aura (classic migraine). In the latter case, the headache may be accompanied by:

- gross malaise
- pallor and tremor
- nausea and vomiting with gastric stasis
- visual disturbance
- abdominal pain
- focal neurological signs such as paraesthesia and numbness or even hemiparesis.

Over half of all patients with migraine have a family history of the condition and many have suffered from travel sickness as children.

Episodes of migraine may last for hours or even days. Those attacks that are atypical in severity or duration should be given special consideration.

 Tx A severe headache can often be avoided if simple analgesics are taken early enough in the course of an attack. Unfortunately, by the time most patients present to an ED, the opportunity for this has passed and vomiting then makes oral drugs useless. A parenteral non-steroidal anti-inflammatory drug (NSAID) (e.g. diclofenac 75 mg IM) can be given together with an antiemetic injection. Sumatriptan is a specific treatment for migraine (→ *Boxes 14.5 and 14.6*) but it is only effective in about 75% of patients.

Box 14.5 Use of sumatriptan

Oral dose = 100 mg, can be repeated if symptoms return (maximum oral dose = 300 mg in 24 h)
Subcutaneous dose = 6 mg, can be repeated after an hour if symptoms recur (maximum subcutaneous dose = 12 mg in 24 h)
Sumatriptan may cause:

- lethargy
- dizziness or vertigo
- sensations of warmth
- feelings of pressure or heaviness in any part of the body

Box 14.6 Contraindications to sumatriptan

- Known hypersensitivity to the drug
- Ischaemic heart disease
- Conditions predisposing to ischaemic heart disease
- Prinzmetal's angina
- Poorly controlled hypertension
- Renal or hepatic impairment
- Hemiplegic migraine
- Patients taking monoamine oxidase inhibitors, selective serotonin reuptake inhibitors (SSRIs) or lithium
- Pregnancy or lactation
- Children
- Age >65 years

Neurological symptoms should be treated by oral aspirin and admission for observation. Most severe attacks finally terminate when the sufferer falls asleep. Not surprisingly, a feeling of euphoria may accompany the subsequent relief.

Cluster headache (migrainous neuralgia)

This is a related condition that is more common in men and is often misdiagnosed. There is severe unilateral facial pain (orbital, supraorbital or temporal) with lacrimation and rhinorrhoea. Each attack starts abruptly and lasts from 15 min up to 3 hours. In over 80% of patients, the headaches 'cluster' into episodes over a period of a few weeks before there is a time of remission. This unpleasant neuralgic headache is treated in a similar way to migraine in the acute phase although specialist assessment should be arranged.

Cluster headache is a member of a group of comparatively rare conditions called trigeminal autonomic cephalalgias. They are characterised by severe unilateral pain in a trigeminal distribution and are associated with ipsilateral cranial autonomic features. Paroxysmal hemicrania is another member of the group with similar features to cluster headache although attacks are shorter, more frequent and more common in women.

Tension headache

This is the most common cause of a headache, occurring more often in females than in males. Symptoms may persist for several days and occur up to 14 days/month. The pain is usually described as a tight cap or band pressing around the head. The distribution of the sensation is that of the occipitofrontalis muscle and tension in this muscle is probably the cause of the pain. Nausea and difficulty getting to sleep may also be experienced. The muscular tension may be precipitated and maintained by:

- personal worries and difficulties
- constant unremitting stress (e.g. mother with young children)
- depression
- a minor injury (e.g. whiplash type).

Tx The patient has often found that simple analgesics have not relieved the pain. Non-steroidal anti-inflammatory drugs (NSAIDs) may help, as may psycho- and physiotherapy. Tricyclic antidepressants are sometimes prescribed in relatively low doses (e.g. amitriptyline 50–100 mg at night). Referral should be made to the GP. SAH must be excluded → p. 224.

Other headaches: Most other patients with headaches should also be referred back to the GP but those with neurological signs should be admitted for investigation.

Brain-stem CVA

Sudden catastrophic collapse may be caused by haemorrhage into or infarction of the brain stem. There will be:

- coma
- small fixed pupils (exclude narcotic/opiate poisoning)
- few, if any, lateralising signs.

Respiration continues but other brain-stem functions and reflexes are attenuated. The prognosis is grave.

XR It is important to make an accurate diagnosis as soon as possible to avoid inappropriate and distressing life support measures. A CT scan will be needed for this purpose.

Tx As soon as the prognosis is assured, the relatives must be gently informed. The patient should be admitted to a bed and kept comfortable while nature takes its course.

Bereavement counselling → p. 163.
Diagnosis of brain-stem death → p. 386.

Cerebrovascular events

Cerebrovascular disease is the third most common cause of death in the UK and the single most common cause of severe disability. After a stroke, approximately 23% of people die within 30 days and, of the initial survivors, only 30–40% are alive after 3 years and 25–30% remain permanently disabled. In Europe, people of West Indian origin have a particularly high risk of CVA.

> Collapse associated with unilateral abnormal neurological signs is most commonly caused by a stroke or a TIA (→ *later*). The distinction between the two overlapping conditions is impossible in patients who are not already recovering when seen.

Most CVAs (80%) are a result of thrombotic or embolic cerebral infarction rather than haemorrhage. The most common causes of cardiac emboli are atrial fibrillation (AF), mural thrombosis and valvular heart disease, and these emboli lodge in the large cerebral arteries, particularly the middle cerebral arteries. Atherosclerosis causes both intracerebral thrombosis and thromboembolism from the extracranial internal carotid arteries. It also affects the vertebral and basilar arteries. The Oxford system of stroke classification defines a total anterior circulation stroke as having three components: contralateral motor or sensory deficit, homonymous hemianopia and higher cortical dysfunction such as dysphasia and visuospatial disturbance. The combination of any two of these features is called a partial anterior circulation stroke. A posterior circulation stroke may manifest itself as cerebellar ataxia or brain-stem signs or isolated homonymous hemianopia. Occlusion of deep perforating arteries (which arise from both the anterior and posterior circulation and supply the white matter of the cerebral hemispheres and brain stem) causes a lacunar stroke. This leads to pure motor, pure sensory or mixed sensorimotor deficit.

Cerebral infarction leads to a progressive neurological deficit. Signs may be minimal at first with subjective weakness or paraesthesia only. The CVAs that result from intracerebral haemorrhage (the remaining 20%) are more sudden in onset with headache and rapidly established signs.

> A patient who complains of vague unilateral symptoms must be taken seriously.

A stroke causes loss or disturbance of motor and sensory function. The exact clinical picture depends on the territory of the blood vessel involved (→ *Box 14.7*). Posterior lesions may affect conscious level (→ *p. 227*) or more rarely there may be cerebellar signs. In the very early stages, spinal reflexes are usually

---

Box 14.7 **Symptoms of a TIA**

TIA in the carotid territory (80% of TIAs):

- Unilateral paresis
- Unilateral sensory loss
- Aphasia
- Monocular visual loss

Vertebrobasilar TIA:

- Bilateral or alternating weakness or sensory loss
- Bilateral visual loss/hemianopia
- Two or more of the following: vertigo, diplopia, dysphagia, dysarthria, ataxia

---

depressed although the plantar response may be extensor. Severe hypertension may be present but intervention to lower it in the ED is contraindicated because this may precipitate further cerebrovascular damage.

Investigations: Routine blood tests, CXR and ECG should be performed. Coincidental hip fracture must be considered and excluded. Brain imaging should be undertaken as soon as possible in all patients, certainly within 24 h of the onset of symptoms unless there are good clinical reasons for not doing so. The brain scan must be performed urgently if the patient has:

- a known bleeding tendency or is taking anticoagulants
- a depressed level of consciousness
- a severe headache at the onset
- an uncertain diagnosis or atypical features (most doctors would consider age <60 years as atypical)
- unexplained, progressive or fluctuating signs
- papilloedema, neck stiffness or fever
- indications for thrombolysis or early anticoagulation (→ *later*).

> Non-contrast CT is most useful for excluding intracerebral haemorrhage and conditions such as brain metastases. It should be performed as soon as possible. However, it has a low sensitivity (around 26%) for detecting early ischaemia when compared with MRI (83%).

Elderly people often fall at the onset of a stroke, but this history may be lacking. Traumatic intracranial blood (acute or chronic subdural or even extradural) may mimic a CVA. Sudden deterioration, in particular with a fixed, dilated pupil, raises the suspicion of an expanding lesion. A CT scan is indicated to confirm the suspected sequence of events.

Tx

- Give oxygen, if required, to maintain the SaO_2 >94%.
- Monitor vital signs. Current guidelines do not recommend routine lowering of BP in the acute phase of a stroke unless there are specific circumstances such as hypertensive encephalopathy or aortic dissection.
- Check the blood sugar. In the absence of diabetes, there is no evidence to support treating hyperglycaemia in the acute phase of a stroke.
- Establish IV access and give maintenance IV fluids. The patient should be kept nil by mouth until there

has been a proper assessment of the airway and swallowing reflexes.

- Treat complications (e.g. fits).
- Treat pyrexia with standard drugs. It is associated with a poor outcome, possibly because of its effects on free radical production or cerebral metabolism.
- Admit the patient to hospital for assessment and rehabilitation – usually in a specialist stroke unit.

Patients have a risk of a further stroke within 5 years of between 30% and 43%, and also an increased risk of other cardiovascular events. Therefore, consideration needs to be given to lifestyle factors (smoking, diet and exercise), BP and cholesterol reduction. Stroke patients should have an annual immunisation against influenza.

Anticoagulants are usually prescribed for all patients with persistent or paroxysmal AF. There is a 68% reduction in the risk of stroke for patients with AF on warfarin compared with a 25–30% risk reduction with aspirin. Other patients with an ischaemic stroke require antiplatelet therapy such as low-dose aspirin (75 mg a day), clopidogrel (75 mg a day), or a combination of low-dose aspirin and modified-release dipyridamole (200 mg twice daily). Dipyridamole has both antiplatelet and vasodilating properties and is thought to inhibit the uptake of adenosine (a potent inhibitor of platelet activation and aggregation) into platelets and vascular cells. Dipyridamole may also inhibit the breakdown of cyclic guanosine monophosphate. *For the mechanism of action of other antiplatelet drugs → p. 181.*

Thrombolysis for CVA

Thombolysis with alteplase is proven to be beneficial if given within 4.5 h of an ischaemic stroke in selected patients. However, in Europe, alteplase is licensed to be given only in ischaemic stroke within 3 h of symptom onset. The aim is to limit the size of the cerebral infarct and thus improve the functional outcome. Alteplase (tPA) is given intravenously over 60 min in a dose of 900 mcg/kg (to a maximum of 90 mg). The initial 10% of the dose should be given by bolus injection and the remaining 90% by infusion. Thrombolysis is not yet proven to be of value for patients aged >80 years. A CT brain scan must be performed before thrombolysis to exclude intracerebral haemorrhage.

General contraindications to thrombolysis → Box 12.3 on p. 183.

Specific contraindications to the use of thrombolysis in ischaemic stroke → Box 14.8.

Box 14.8 Specific contraindications to the use of thrombolysis in ischaemic stroke

Also → Box 12.3 on p. 183 for the general contraindications to thrombolysis.

- Onset of symptoms more than 4.5 h previously or unclear time of onset
- Age <18 or >80 years
- Previous stroke within the past 3 months
- Previous stroke with concomitant diabetes
- Evidence of intracranial or subarachnoid haemorrhage
- Mild stroke or rapid improvement
- Very severe stroke
- Seizure at onset of stroke
- Systolic BP >185 mmHg or diastolic BP >110 mmHg
- Platelet count below 100 × 10⁹/L
- Heparin within the last 48 h with raised PTT (prothrombin time)

By 6 months after their stroke, 50% of all patients will need some help with daily living, 15% will have communication problems and >50% will have some residual weakness. Many will also have mood or cognitive problems. Their carers also suffer.

Transient ischaemic attack

A TIA is defined as an abrupt loss of focal cerebral or monocular function with symptoms lasting <24 h which, after adequate investigation, is presumed to be caused by embolic or thrombotic vascular disease.

There is no qualitative difference between a TIA and an ischaemic stroke. Truly transient cerebrovascular events last for only a matter of minutes!

The risk of having a stroke after a hemispheric TIA is over 5% in the first 7 days, with the greatest risk occurring in the first 72 h. In addition, a TIA is a marker for general vascular disease (→ *Box 14.9*). Half

Box 14.9 Risk of cardiovascular diseases after a TIA

- The average annual risk of stroke is about 7% (seven times the risk in the normal population)
- The greatest risk of a stroke is in the first year (half will occur in the 2 days after a TIA)
- The annual risk of MI is 2–3%
- The annual death rate from CVA, MI or other vascular death is about 9%

Box 14.10 The ABCD2 score

The ABCD2 score can be used to predict the risk of stroke in the period immediately after a TIA. The following risk factors are added to give a total score out of a maximum of 7. A score >5 equates to high risk, 4 or 5 indicates moderate risk and <4 signifies a lower degree of risk (although still a 1% chance of a stroke in the next 2 days).

Risk factor	Score
Age ≥60 years	1
Diabetes	1
Raised blood pressure (>140/90 mmHg)	1
Unilateral weakness	2
Speech impairment without weakness	1
Duration ≥60 min	2
Duration 1–59 min	1

of all TIAs are caused by the thromboembolic complications of arteriosclerosis in the arteries that supply the brain; emboli from the heart account for a further 20%.

The diagnosis of TIA is based on the history. Symptoms – usually loss of function – are of sudden onset and are maximal from the start (→ *Box 14.7*). As TIAs are focal events, global symptoms such as light-headedness, dizziness and syncope are rarely consistent with the diagnosis. The following predisposing factors should be sought:

- AF or other source of cardiac embolism
- Hypertension
- Carotid disease (bruits)
- History of smoking
- Hypercholesterolaemia.

Investigations: All patients should have a routine screen (FBC, ESR, U&Es, LFTs [liver function tests], glucose, random cholesterol, ECG and CXR). An urgent CT scan of the brain should be considered for patients aged <60 years and for those with atypical features, reasons for bleeding or an uncertain diagnosis. Carotid duplex scan is usually requested from the clinic by investigating physicians.

Tx Once the symptoms are clearly resolving, oral aspirin (300 mg) should be given to all patients in whom it is not contraindicated. Patients should be risk-assessed using the ABCD2 score (→ *Box 14.10*) and admitted to hospital if they have any of the following:

1 Residual symptoms or signs (i.e. not a TIA!)
2 A history of more than one TIA in a week
3 An ABCD2 score ≥5 (→ *Box 14.10*).

Other patients (i.e. ABCD2 score ≤4) may go home, provided that there are arrangements for assessment by a specialist service within 7 days of the TIA at the latest. The GP must be notified and aspirin (300 mg daily for 2 weeks and then 75 mg a day) prescribed for all patients (aspirin therapy reduces the incidence of CVA in patients who have had a TIA by around 3%/annum). Patients who are intolerant of aspirin (hypersensitivity or severe dyspepsia induced by low-dose aspirin) should be prescribed modified-release dipyridamole 200 mg twice daily. In the specialist clinic, the patient will be prescribed modified-release dipyridamole 200 mg twice daily in addition to aspirin or be changed to treatment with clopidogrel. If a patient is found to be in AF (and not anticoagulated), he or she should be prescribed aspirin 300 mg/day as above until seen in clinic.

Driving after a CVA or TIA

The UK Driver and Vehicle Licensing Agency (DVLA) rules on fitness to drive state that a patient with a diagnosis of CVA or TIA must not drive for at least 1 month. He or she may resume driving after this time if his or her clinical recovery is judged to be satisfactory and he or she has not had any fits. There is no need to notify the licensing authority (DVLA) unless there is a residual neurological deficit 1 month after the episode. A patient with multiple TIAs will require an attack-free period of 3 months before resuming driving and must notify the DVLA. This advice has obvious implications for patients discharged from an ED with a diagnosis of TIA.

Transient global amnesia

Transient global amnesia (TGA) describes a sudden and temporary loss of memory in an otherwise well patient who is fully conscious throughout the episode. Distant memories are preserved, as is immediate recall of current events. There is complete recovery within 24h (and usually much sooner). TGA is of unknown aetiology and carries no increased risk of CVA or other illness although there is a small risk of recurrence. Intracranial venous congestion has been implicated in its causation but the main known risk factor is a history of migraine. Treatment centres around excluding other conditions and reassuring the patient.

Labyrinthitis (vestibular neuronitis)

Presumed viral infection of the inner ear or its nerve supply may cause an unpleasant condition closely related to motion sickness. The symptoms are the same:

- Profound nausea and vomiting
- Vertigo and ataxia
- Pallor, sweating and gross malaise.

The vertigo is positional and usually worsened by movements of the head and reduced by keeping still. Nystagmus may be present (fast component towards the affected side) but there is no hearing loss.

Tx Other conditions must be excluded before treatment is initiated. Bed rest is essential and affected patients cannot go home alone. The symptoms may persist for several days or even weeks, during which time the patient must not drive. (In its duration and dubious aetiology, vestibular neuronitis resembles another common cranial mononeuropathy, Bell's palsy.)

If not contraindicated, the most effective drugs are:

1 The sedative anticholinergic hyoscine hydrobromide. This is known as scopolamine in some countries and differs from the antispasmodic hyoscine butylbromide (Buscopan). It is given in an initial IV or IM dose of 0.4 mg but may also be administered as a tablet or a transdermal patch.
2 The phenothiazine-derived antihistamine promethazine, given in an IM or oral dose of 25–50 mg.

This drug also (and uniquely) seems to help 'reset' the labyrinthine mechanisms to their new state.
3 Sedative antihistamine tablets such as meclozine (marketed for motion sickness).

Standard phenothiazines (e.g. prochlorperazine) and the serotonin $5HT_3$-receptor antagonists (e.g. metoclopramide) are relatively ineffective for vestibular conditions.

Other vestibular or cerebellar signs

Sudden onset of ataxia must generally be referred to the physicians for investigation. Sometimes people with chronic alcohol problems and known cerebral degeneration present with an apparent disproportionate worsening of the cerebellar component of this disease. They should be admitted because the combination of alcohol, ataxia and the environment is often fatal.

Also → CVA and TIA on pp. 227 and 229.

Convulsions (seizures)

Treatment of fits in children → p. 343.

Fits occur when there is one of the following:

- *Deprivation of cerebral fuel supply (anoxic convulsion):*
  - hypoglycaemia or hypoxia
  - transient dysrhythmia or cardiac arrest
  - syncope
- *Cerebral irritation:*
  - head injury
  - cerebral tumour or infection
  - poisoning
  - fever (viraemia) in children
  - primary epilepsy
- *Withdrawal of sedatives:* alcohol or drug withdrawal.

A fit causes a dramatic increase in the cerebral metabolic demand for oxygen and also partial airway obstruction and decreased ventilation. Hypoxia must be prevented by urgent airway control and rapid treatment of the fit before elucidation of the underlying cause can be undertaken.

Tx
- Protect or remove the patient from harm.
- Give high-concentration oxygen by facemask. Never attempt to force open the airway by inserting a wedge in the mouth – use a Guedel airway once the jaw has relaxed.

- Obtain venous access.
- Give IV diazepam emulsion (initially 5–20 mg for adults in incremental doses). If IV access cannot be obtained, then diazepam can be given rectally. Midazolam or lorazepam, at approximately a third of the dose recommended for diazepam, are useful alternatives.

When the fit has stopped:

- place the patient in the recovery position
- monitor vital signs
- check the blood sugar
- start investigating the circumstances that led to the fit and perform a full physical examination.

If the fit is not terminated within 30 min, the patient has status epilepticus (permanent damage is common, 10% mortality rate). Call for urgent help – an anaesthetist may be needed – and then consider the therapies below:

- Paraldehyde – 5–10 mL (up to 5 mL by deep IM injection into each buttock). This is useful if IV access is problematic.
- Phenytoin – immediate loading dose of 15 mg/kg by IV infusion at a rate of no more than 50 mg/min (or 1 mg/kg per min). Fosphenytoin sodium is a prodrug, which is converted to phenytoin immediately after administration. It is prescribed in milligram PE (phenytoin equivalents). Unlike phenytoin sodium, it dissolves freely in aqueous solutions and can be infused intravenously at rates up to three times faster than the parent drug (i.e. 100–150 mg PE/min). In the case of both drugs, the ECG must be monitored throughout the infusion and for at least 30 min afterwards.
- Phenobarbital – 15 mg/kg by IV infusion at a rate of not more than 100 mg/min.

As soon as it becomes apparent that more than one drug is required, consideration should be given to the need for general anaesthetic techniques. This usually entails either sedation with thiopental (up to 5 mg/kg) and then a thiopental infusion (1–3 mg/kg per h) accompanied by intensive care unit (ICU) monitoring or full anaesthesia, paralysis and ventilation.

Status epilepticus must be distinguished from serial seizures without full recovery. If the patient stops tonic–clonic seizures but does not regain full consciousness consider 'absence' or complex partial seizures. These are difficult to detect but important to stop because ongoing cerebral ischaemia is a strong possibility.

A fully recovered patient with known epilepsy may go home under the following circumstances:

- There are no unusual features in this episode.
- He or she remains well after 2 h observation.
- There is continuous social support both en route and at home.
- The GP is informed of the discharge.
- The usual drug supply is available.

Pseudo-fits

The possibility of pseudo-fits must be considered. These are an attention-seeking device, often manifest in a public arena. They can be distinguished from genuine convulsions because:

- the patient is rarely injured
- there is no incontinence or tongue biting
- the plantar response remains flexor
- pulse oximetry remains normal, as opposed to the marked fall in saturation seen in a genuine fit.

Nevertheless, these patients cannot simply be dismissed. The pseudo-fit represents abnormal behaviour, often prompted by chronic and complex social problems. Discharge and follow-up should be discussed with the GP over the telephone.

Peripheral neuropathies and similar conditions

There are many causes of failure of conduction of the peripheral nerves including drugs, diabetes, infections, vitamin deficiencies and alcoholism. Many cases are idiopathic. Guillain–Barré syndrome is the most common type of acute polyneuropathy in the UK → *later*.

Isolated peripheral neuropathies may follow stretching or compression of nerves while intoxicated with alcohol or drugs. Radial nerve palsy (wrist drop) often occurs in these circumstances. Patients with foot drop sometimes present to an ED. Both of these conditions should be treated by splintage and referral for investigation.

Acute (transverse) myelitis may look similar to a polyneuritis. It causes a specific sensory level with bilateral leg weakness and bladder and bowel dysfunction.

Multiple sclerosis (MS) is not a peripheral neuropathy but may be mistaken for one because the multiple central nervous system (CNS) lesions responsible are scattered in both time and place. MS may present with a vast array of different neurological features including loss of vision, diplopia, spastic weakness of the legs, numbness and paraesthesia, sphincter disturbance, painful flexor spasms and cerebellar signs (vertigo, tremor and nystagmus).

Botulism → p. 234.
Myasthenia gravis → below.
Poliomyelitis → p. 254.
Tetanus → pp. below and 396.

Guillain–Barré syndrome (acute polyneuritis)

Guillain–Barré syndrome is an ascending polyneuritis of unknown aetiology, which has an annual incidence of 1–2 cases per 100 000 throughout the world. It is the most common form of acute peripheral neuropathy in the UK and also the most common cause of acute neuromuscular paralysis. There are at least four clinicopathological subtypes. Most cases (90%) are described as 'acute inflammatory demyelinating polyradiculoneuropathy'. Between 25 and 30% of patients require artificial ventilation. Mortality rates range from 3% to 6% overall but rise to around 20% in ventilated patients.

The features of Guillain–Barré syndrome develop over the course of a few days or sometimes several weeks. There may be a history of a preceding infection and then severe backache before the development of neurological symptoms and signs as below:

- Progressive, symmetrical, ascending weakness, which may include ocular, bulbar and respiratory muscles
- Diminished or absent tendon reflexes
- Variable sensory loss and pain (in up to 90% of patients)
- Autonomic disturbances such as tachycardia, cardiac dysrhythmias and labile blood pressure.

Motor involvement (which may be either proximal or distal) usually predominates over sensory loss (often distal). Of the cranial nerves, the facial nerve is the most commonly affected. Measurement of peak expiratory flow rate is useful to assess the degree of respiratory impairment. Very few investigations are helpful in the diagnosis of acute polyneuritis. The cerebrospinal fluid (CSF) usually contains an increased amount of protein.

Hyperacute cases of Guillain–Barré syndrome may resemble a stroke, cases with pain may masquerade as spinal cord (or cauda equina) lesions and pure motor cases may be confused with poliomyelitis, acute transverse myelitis, myasthenia or acute muscle disease.

Tx If the condition is clinically suspected, then the patient must be admitted to hospital. Intensive care is appropriate if there is bulbar or respiratory weakness or autonomic signs. Most cases of Guillain–Barré

syndrome recover spontaneously over several weeks. Immunotherapy with intravenous immunoglobulin or plasma exchange has been shown to hasten recovery but corticosteroids do not help. Residual disability is found in 20% of those patients who survive the illness.

Cholinergic and myasthenic crises

In myasthenia gravis, too high a dose of anticholinesterase drugs may make the weakness worse (cholinergic crisis). This is easily mistaken for exacerbation of the primary disease (myasthenic crisis). Differentiation can be achieved by IV injection of edrophonium 2 mg (the 'Tensilon' test), which will induce a transient improvement in myasthenic crisis only.

> This test may precipitate ventilatory failure, so should be carried out only by those who can deal with this eventuality.

Tx In both conditions, artificial ventilation may be required from the outset. For myasthenic crisis, IM neostigmine 0.5 mg should be given and repeated every 20 min as necessary. For cholinergic crisis, the treatment is pralidoxime 1–2 g by slow IV injection, again repeated every 20 min as required. The muscarinic effects of anticholinesterases must be controlled with IV atropine.

Tetanus

Gas gangrene (Clostridium perfringens infection) → p. 266.
Prophylaxis against tetanus infection in wounds → p. 394.

Cases of tetanus have increased in the UK during the past decade. Infection is caused by contamination of a wound with the spores of the bacillus *Clostridium tetani*. Days or even weeks after infection, local multiplication of the organism occurs with release of its neurotoxin. Even the most trivial of wounds can introduce tetanus into the body, but some wounds carry a particularly high risk of infection. *Factors that help to identify tetanus-prone wounds → Box 21.6 on p. 396.* The incubation period of tetanus is between 4 and 21 days (usually about 10 days) and the case fatality rate is almost 30%. Tetanus is a notifiable disease.

Active immunisation against tetanus was introduced into some areas of the UK as part of the primary immunisation of infants from the mid-1950s and was adopted nationally from 1961. As a result, tetanus virtually disappeared in children aged <15 years by the 1970s. Until recently, the majority of cases of tetanus in the UK were in people aged >65 years who had not been previously immunised. Two-thirds of the victims were women who, unlike most older men, had not been immunised during military service (immunisation against tetanus was provided by the British armed forces from 1938 onwards). However, in the last few years, men and women seem to be equally at risk from the disease. More recently still, tetanus has been seen in young adults who abuse IV drugs. (In the USA, 20% of tetanus cases are associated with IV drug abuse.) IM and subcutaneous injections are particularly likely to result in a suitable environment for spore germination because citric acid (which is used to dissolve heroin) may damage muscle tissue. Neonatal tetanus is still a major public health problem in many developing countries but there have been no cases in the UK for over 30 years. It is usually caused by infection of the umbilical stump as a result of poor hygiene.

It is important to understand the mechanism of action of tetanus toxin. In the ventral horn of the spinal cord, negative feedback loop neurons (Renshaw cells) limit the activity of the α-motoneurons. Tetanus toxin prevents the release of the inhibitory neurotransmitter glycine from these cells, which allows uncontrolled spasms of skeletal muscle. Strychnine (and brucine) compete with glycine for its receptors on the α-motoneurons and thus cause a very similar clinical picture. Acute dystonic reactions ('oculogyric crises') may also mimic tetanus → p. 300.

For the role of the Renshaw cell in tetanus and strychnine poisoning → Figure 14.1.

The clinical features of tetanus can progress slowly over as much as 2 weeks. In the usual order of appearance they are as follows:

- Stiff muscles near the wound (or injection site)
- Jaw stiffness and trismus ('lock-jaw')
- Abdominal rigidity
- Progressive painful muscle spasms (the fixed mocking grin caused by facial muscle tightening is known as the 'risus sardonicus' and extensor spasms of the back, neck and limbs are called opisthotonus)
- Dysphagia and respiratory difficulty
- Autonomic dysfunction.

Consider the diagnosis of tetanus in IV drug abusers presenting with muscle stiffness or muscle spasms.

Tx Supportive therapy is essential with special attention given to the airway, respiration and autonomic activities. IV benzodiazepines or even general anaesthesia may be required to control spasms. The tetanus bacillus is sensitive to both benzylpenicillin and metronidazole. Immunoglobulin against tetanus toxin (HTIg) 150 IU/kg is given intramuscularly in multiple sites (a range of doses from 30 IU/kg to 300 IU/kg has been suggested.) Tetanus immunoglobulin for IV use is also available on a named-patient basis. The dose is 5000–10 000 IU by IV infusion. Surgical debridement of wounds may help to reduce the toxin load. Suspicion of tetanus infection should provoke a discussion with a specialist in infectious diseases. Strychnine poisoning is treated with similar supportive and relaxant therapy.

Botulism

Botulinum toxin is one of the most poisonous substances known to humans. Several countries are known to have attempted weaponisation of the toxin for airborne dispersal leading to inhalation.

Food-borne botulism: the features of botulism typically begin between 12 and 36h after ingestion of contaminated food but may start after as few as 6h. The earliest symptoms are usually gastrointestinal (nausea, vomiting and abdominal pain) and neurological (dysfunction of the cranial nerves).

Wound botulism: this variant of botulism has recently been seen in IV drug abusers, probably as a result of contaminated drugs and citric acid damage to muscle. Unlike the classic food-borne disease (which is caused by the ingestion of preformed toxin), wound botulism occurs when the spores of the anaerobic bacterium *Clostridium botulinum* contaminate a wound, germinate and produce toxin in vivo.

Botulinum toxin blocks the release of acetylcholine from the neuromuscular junction and characteristically causes a descending flaccid paralysis:

- Dysphonia, dysarthria and dysphagia (in >95% of cases)
- Blurred or double vision and ptosis (in >90% of cases)
- Dizziness and general muscle weakness (in >70% of cases)
- Immobility and respiratory distress.

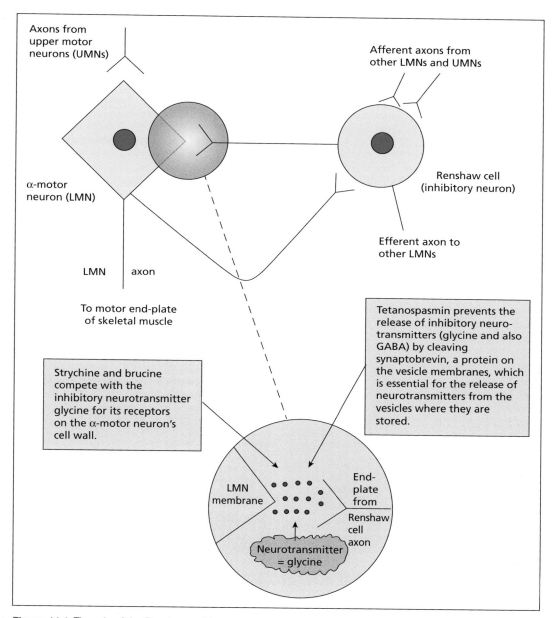

Figure 14.1 The role of the Renshaw cell in tetanus and in strychnine poisoning. Strychnine and brucine are alkaloids from plants of the genus *Strychnos*. Tetanospasmin is the neurotoxic component of the exotoxin produced by the tetanus bacillus. LMN, lower motor neuron; UMN, upper motor neuron.

Patients are afebrile with no sensory loss and no confusion. Autonomic signs include dry mouth, dilated pupils, constipation and urinary dysfunction; postural hypotension may also occur. Surprisingly, deep tendon reflexes are preserved. Diagnosis is confirmed in a reference laboratory using serum samples and wound swabs. Botulism is fatal in 10% of victims and those who recover are usually debilitated for many months.

Tx Ventilatory support may be required, as may surgical debridement of wounds. *Clostridium botulinum* is sensitive to benzylpenicillin and metronidazole. Botulinum antitoxin should always be given because it is effective in reducing both the severity and the duration of symptoms.

Conditions caused by diving

Decompression sickness

Decompression sickness or caisson disease may occur up to 48 h after diving. It is caused by nitrogen (which has been dissolved in the blood under pressure) coming out of solution and forming bubbles in the bloodstream and tissues. The patient may present as a collapse without giving a history of recreational diving because many people do not appreciate the potential for delayed onset of symptoms. There is:

- malaise
- joint pains (the 'bends')
- itching and rashes
- lymphadenopathy and oedema.

In severe cases there are signs and symptoms of cardiopulmonary, vestibular and CNS involvement such as:

- chest pain
- dyspnoea
- coughing and haemoptysis
- hypertension or hypotension
- tinnitus or deafness
- nausea
- vertigo and nystagmus
- headache
- behavioural changes
- altered consciousness
- convulsions
- motor and sensory deficits, including hemiplegia, paraplegia and urinary retention.

Tx
- Give oxygen
- Commence IV fluid resuscitation

- Control fits and agitation
- Discuss the patient with a specialist in diving and hyperbaric medicine. Recompression in a hyperbaric chamber may be required.

Nitrogen narcosis and oxygen toxicity in divers ('rapture of the deep')

Nitrogen toxicity: When breathed under pressure (at depths in excess of 100 feet or 30 m), nitrogen has an intoxicating effect. There is light-headedness, impairment of judgement and loss of coordination. Hallucinations, coma and death may occur at extreme depths. The narcosis reverses spontaneously on ascent to normal air pressures.

Oxygen toxicity: Breathing oxygen at high partial pressures (at depths over 200 feet or 60 m) causes CNS toxicity. Dizziness, nausea, disorientation, visual abnormalities and facial twitching occur; convulsions and coma can prove fatal. Treatment is supportive. Recompression requires careful oxygen monitoring because high inspired concentrations of oxygen may worsen the condition.

Barotrauma from diving

The pressure changes associated with diving may also cause the following:

- Pneumothorax and surgical emphysema
- Air embolism (neurological signs may mimic decompression sickness)
- Rupture of the tympanic membrane (pain, bleeding, hearing loss)
- Disturbance of the inner ear (nausea, vomiting, vertigo, tinnitus and deafness may also look like decompression sickness)
- Pain around the sinuses and in the mouth (from air trapped in cavities beneath fillings or caries)
- GI pain, colic and flatulence.

If the clinical picture suggests a possibility of decompression sickness then the patient must be discussed with a hyperbaric specialist.

Altitude-related illness

Altitude, hypoxia and acclimatisation: barometric pressure falls logarithmically with increasing altitude. The partial pressure of oxygen (21% of barometric pressure) falls at the same rate. At 19 000 feet (5800 m), these pressures are 50% of their values at sea level, falling to 28% at the summit of Mount Everest. The ambient temperature also drops by 6.5°C with every additional 3300 feet (1000 m) in altitude. The complex physiological changes of acclimatisation include increased minute ventilation, increased sympathetic tone, increased pulmonary vascular resistance and, after several weeks, an increased haematocrit.

Acute mountain sickness: This affects around 75% of people who ascend rapidly to heights of more than 10 000 feet (3000 m) above sea level and even troubles 20% of people at just 7500 feet (2300 m). It is usually defined as a headache accompanied by any of the following symptoms: nausea, vomiting, malaise, fatigue, lethargy, anorexia and insomnia. Sleep may be disturbed by periodic breathing or even apnoea. Acute mountain sickness (AMS) usually resolves within 3 days of arriving at altitude but sometimes leads to life-threatening cerebral or pulmonary oedema. The causes of these altitude-related illnesses are poorly understood. There is some genetic predisposition associated with capillary leakage, fluid retention and stimulation of chemoreceptors in the presence of hypoxaemia. The risk is increased with rapid ascents and failure to acclimatise. All patients will have a low SaO_2. It is said that AMS can be minimised by 'climbing high and sleeping low'.

High-altitude cerebral oedema: the most severe manifestation of altitude sickness is acute cerebral oedema, which can be overwhelming if untreated. It is thought to have the same pathophysiology as AMS and may represent the extreme form of the condition. In addition to the usual symptoms of mountain sickness, there is a progressive deterioration in mental status with ataxia and, in some cases, focal neurological deficits. Eventually coma supervenes.

High-altitude pulmonary oedema: this is seen in 2–4% of climbers once 14 000 feet (4300 m) is reached and is the most common medical cause of death at altitude. Atmospheric hypoxia is thought to cause pulmonary hypertension, uneven perfusion and capillary leakage. The first symptoms are cough and tachypnoea, followed by increasing dyspnoea and cyanosis.

Tx Sufferers must be advised to stop and rest immediately before the condition worsens. Oxygen, analgesics and antiemetics should be given and descent arranged. A reduction in altitude of as little as 1500–3000 feet (450–900 m) may be all that is required. Acetazolamide 125–250 mg twice daily may be given to increase the rate of acclimatisation. High-altitude cerebral oedema is treated with dexamethasone 4 mg (by any route) every 6 h and hyperbaric therapy (in a portable unit such as a Gamow bag) if available. Patients with high-altitude pulmonary oedema should be given nifedipine 10 mg by mouth 4-hourly and hyperbaric therapy, in addition to standard treatments for the oedema.

Prophylaxis for AMS

Acetazolamide is a sulfonamide that inhibits carbonic anhydrase. It decreases renal bicarbonate reabsorption, causing a mild metabolic acidosis and also decreases the formation of CSF. Acetazolamide 125 mg twice daily is an effective prophylaxis for AMS that increases the rate of acclimatisation and reduces the severity of symptoms. Treatment should be started 2 days before ascent and continued for up to 5 days at altitude. The main side effects are diuresis and paraesthesiae. Chemoprophylaxis does not reduce the risk of altitude sickness; gradual ascent and physiological acclimatisation are still essential.

Other risks in climbers

These include hypothermia, frostbite, UV keratitis, exacerbation of pre-existing diseases and, of course, trauma.

> British expeditions to peaks higher than 23 000 feet (7000 m) have experienced death rates of 4.3 per 100 climbers.

CARDIOVASCULAR PROBLEMS

Anaphylaxis → p. 299.
Cardiac dysrhythmias → p. 164.
Dyspnoea → Chapter 13 on p. 196.
Myocardial infarction → p. 177.
Pneumonia → p. 209.
Pulmonary embolism → pp. 190 and 214.

Shock

Shock is a state of inadequate perfusion of vital tissues. This may be caused by inadequacies in the pump (heart), the delivery system (blood vessels) or the perfusing fluid (blood). There are therefore three basic types of shock:

1 Central shock – pump failure
2 Hypovolaemic shock – decreased blood volume
3 Distributive shock – leaky or dilated blood vessels.

The effects of septic, anaphylactic and neurogenic shock are mostly attributable to maldistribution of fluid but there may also be elements of cardiac depression and true hypovolaemia.

Table 14.1 Blood loss and signs of shock

Blood loss (% total)	<15	15–30	30–40	40
Blood pressure	Normal	Normal	Decreased	Decreased
Heart rate	Normal	Raised	Rapid	Very rapid
Respiratory rate	Normal	Raised	Rapid	Very rapid

Anaphylactic shock → p. 299.
Hypovolaemic and cardiogenic shock → below.
Neurogenic shock → p. 51.
Septic shock → p. 260.

Hypovolaemic shock

Loss of blood or other body fluid may result in hypovolaemic shock. The classic signs may become obvious only as sudden decompensation occurs (→ *Table 14.1*).

Tx
- Manage the airway and breathing. Give high-concentration oxygen.
- Keep the patient supine.
- Insert two large IV lines. Large (Seldinger-type) peripheral lines are better than central lines. Short thick lines are the best.
- Cross-match blood.
- Give IV fluids in boluses of 10–20 mL/kg for an adult (20 mL/kg for a child).
- Institute full monitoring.
- Look for the cause of the shock (→ *appropriate section of book for specific treatment*).
- Refer to the appropriate specialty, usually surgical.
- Insert a urinary catheter and record the fluid balance.

Cardiogenic shock

Collapse with hypotension may occur secondary to asymptomatic MI or overt causes of cardiac depression. Cardiogenic shock is 'forward failure' of the heart as opposed to the 'backward failure' of congestive cardiac failure. In the absence of external factors, it is caused by insufficiency in the muscles that power the pump and thus primary pulseless electrical activity or electromechanical dissociation (PEA/EMD) is the final phase (→ *p. 151*).
Investigations: There may be ECG changes but these cannot be guaranteed.

Box 14.11 Intravenous infusion of dobutamine

- Mix 500 mg dobutamine in 500 mL 5% glucose or 0.9% saline to give a solution of 1 mg (1000 mg)/mL
- This infusion can be given into a peripheral vein in the short term. In contrast, dopamine must always be given into a central vein
- A reasonable starting dose is 5 mcg/kg per min. The infusion rate in mL/h needed to give this dose can be calculated by multiplying the patient's body weight in kilograms by 0.3 e.g. to give 5 mcg/kg per min to a 70-kg man: 70 kg × 0.3 = 21 mL/h of the above mixture

Tx
- Ensure that the airway and breathing are satisfactory. Give high-concentration oxygen. Intubation and ventilation may become necessary.
- Allow the patient to adopt whatever posture is most comfortable; this will usually be partially sitting up.
- Correct any bradycardia with IV atropine to a rate >60 beats/min, but avoid tachycardia because this impairs coronary perfusion.
- Consider the need for IV fluids. The failing heart needs a high filling pressure, hence LVF causes pulmonary oedema.
- Institute full monitoring.
- Refer to the ICU.
- Look for the secondary causes of pump (heart) failure. These are identical to the causes of PEA (→ *p. 151*).
- Insert a central venous line.
- Insert a urinary catheter.
- Request a CXR, ECG, FBC and U&Es.
- Begin inotropic support – an IV infusion of dobutamine or dopamine. (*For a method of setting up an IV infusion of dobutamine → Box 14.11*).

Cardiac tamponade

This causes:

- hypotension
- raised jugular venous pressure (JVP) unless hypovolaemic
- muffled heart sounds
- pulsus paradoxus
- breathlessness.

If the signs suggest a diagnosis of tamponade, then look for an underlying reason for a pericardial effusion or haemorrhage such as:

- MI
- trauma ($\rightarrow$ *p. 78*)
- neoplasia
- renal failure.

Tx In a collapsed patient with a tamponade, attempt pericardiocentesis ($\rightarrow$ *p. 78*). This procedure may buy time but is not a definitive treatment so seek help immediately.

Accelerated or very severe hypertension

Accelerated or very severe hypertension (diastolic blood pressure >140 mmHg) requires urgent treatment in hospital but is not usually an indication for parenteral antihypertensive therapy.

Tx Oral therapy should be instituted with a β blocker (atenolol or labetalol) or a long-acting calcium channel blocker (modified-release nifedipine or amlodipine). The aim should be to reduce diastolic BP to 100–110 mmHg within the first 24 h. Then, over the next 2 or 3 days, BP can be normalised with additional drugs such as diuretics and angiotensin-converting enzyme (ACE) inhibitors. Very rapid reduction in BP can reduce organ perfusion leading to cerebral infarction, myocardial ischaemia and renal failure. Parenteral antihypertensive drugs are only rarely necessary; sodium nitroprusside by infusion is the best drug in these exceptional circumstances.

Malignant hypertension refers to the syndrome of:

- severe diastolic hypertension
- papilloedema
- retinal exudates and haemorrhages
- renal failure.

It occurs mainly in men in their third and fourth decades and pursues a rapidly downhill course to death from uraemia within a year unless properly treated.

Hypertensive encephalopathy is a rare condition in which transient neurological symptoms occur in the presence of a very high BP. The underlying acute focal cerebral ischaemia is caused by a mixture of cerebrovascular spasm, oedema and thrombosis. Treatment is as described above for accelerated hypertension.

Myocarditis

Although it can be subclinical, inflammation of the myocardium can lead to debilitating cardiomyopathy. The damage to the muscle tissue is thought to be caused by either toxins or an immunological reaction. A vast array of organisms and diseases have been associated with myocarditis. Enteroviruses (especially Coxsackie B virus) are the most common pathogens in the developed world. Diphtheria toxin, HIV infection, Lyme disease ($\rightarrow$ *p. 256*), rheumatoid arthritis and Kawasaki's disease ($\rightarrow$ *p. 348*) are less common causes of myocarditis. Ethanol can cause cardiomyopathy and AF. The heart failure that follows Chagas' disease (caused by *Trypanosoma cruzi*) is an enormous problem in Central and South America. Clinical presentations of myocarditis range from a mild flu-like illness to overwhelming congestive cardiac failure. ECG and CXR changes are variable; echocardiography typically shows a globally dilated left ventricle. ESR, CRP, CK-MB and troponin may be raised. Treatment is supportive and symptomatic.

Endocarditis

Infective endocarditis is a serious condition with a mortality rate of 20% or more. Although it is primarily a disease of older people and those with congenital or acquired structural heart disease ($\rightarrow$ *Box 14.12*), IV drug abusers have a 30-fold higher incidence of endocarditis than the general population. HIV infection and diabetes are also risk factors. Infected vegetations occur on the endothelium of the heart usually, but not always, on areas of previous abnormality or damage. Left-sided infections are mostly found in patients with acquired valvular heart disease (e.g. rheumatic heart disease), but either side of the heart may be affected in those with congenital heart disease or prosthetic valves. The most common pathogens are *Streptococcus viridans*, *Staphylococcus aureus* and *Staphylococcus epidermis*. Most cases of right-sided

Box 14.12 Cardiac conditions that cause an increased risk of developing infective endocarditis

- Acquired valvular heart disease with stenosis or regurgitation
- Valve replacement
- Structural congenital heart disease (including surgically corrected conditions, but excluding isolated atrial septal defect, fully repaired ventricular septal defect or fully repaired patent ductus arteriosus)
- Hypertrophic cardiomyopathy
- Previous episode of infective endocarditis

endocarditis occur in IV drug abusers as a result of *Staphylococcus aureus* infection of the tricuspid valve.

The symptoms of infective endocarditis are vague and may be the result of valvular emboli. There is fatigue, weight loss and fever (above 38°C). Nausea, back pain and arthralgia may also occur. Cardiac murmurs are usually pre-existing. Septic emboli cause pulmonary, cerebral or systemic symptoms (e.g. pneumonia, headache, renal or splenic infarcts). Splinter haemorrhages and petechiae are classic signs of the disease.

> Endocarditis should be considered in all patients with malaise and fever of uncertain origin.

Investigations: FBC, ESR, CRP and blood cultures may all yield useful information. Mild anaemia is often found. CXR and ECG are usually non-specific. Echocardiography is used to detect predisposing heart disease.

Tx Initial 'blind' antibiotic therapy is IV flucloxacillin and gentamicin. The flucloxacillin should be replaced with vancomycin and rifampicin if the patient has cardiac prostheses *in situ* or is allergic to penicillins or if MRSA is thought to be a likely pathogen.

Prophylaxis against infective endocarditis

Antibiotics to prevent infective endocarditis are no longer recommended for adults and children with structural cardiac defects who are undergoing dental and non-dental interventional procedures. This is because there is no consistent association between having such a procedure and the development of infective endocarditis. Everyday activities such as tooth brushing can cause repetitive bacteraemias that almost certainly pose a greater risk for developing infective endocarditis than a single interventional procedure. In addition, the clinical effectiveness of antibiotic prophylaxis is not proven. Good oral health is more important, as is the avoidance of non-medical procedures such as body piercing and tattooing.

Palpitations

Palpitations are a common presentation to an ED. The underlying causes include the following:

- Sinus tachycardia
- Ectopic beats (→ *p. 174*)
- Paroxysmal dysrhythmias (→ *Chapter 11*)
- Chronic dysrhythmias (→ *Chapter 11*).

Sinus tachycardia may result from:

- anxiety or other emotion
- pyrexia
- anaemia
- drugs including excessive caffeine intake
- hyperthyroidism.

A rapid onset and cessation of palpitations with polyuria in an otherwise normal individual are extremely suggestive of a paroxysmal dysrhythmia.

Investigations: FBC, electrolytes, glucose and thyroid function tests should be performed. An ECG is essential to demonstrate:

- the exact rhythm and rate
- congenital abnormalities of the cardiac conducting tissue
- unsuspected myocardial ischaemia and infarction.

Tx

Treatment of patients with a frank cardiac dysrhythmia → *Chapter 11.*

Patients with an abnormal ECG should be discussed with a physician. Excessive and unexplained sinus tachycardia should also be investigated. Those with normal physical findings and a normal ECG can be referred to their GP for further assessment.

METABOLIC DISORDERS

Hypoglycaemia

The symptoms of low blood sugar are the most common presentation of diabetes to an ED. Hypoglycaemia results from:

- too much insulin or oral hypoglycaemic by either accident or intent
- insufficient food
- change of routine, e.g. site of injection, type of insulin, new syringe size.

Initially, a hypoglycaemic patient is restless and agitated but, if untreated, rapidly becomes unresponsive. There is pallor, profuse sweating and a bounding pulse. Aggression can be such that the patient arrives in police custody and may be thought to be intoxicated. False localising neurological signs are sometimes seen.

Investigations: Venous blood should be taken for measurement of baseline glucose before treatment is instituted. In cases of unexplained hypoglycaemia samples should also be sent for LFTs, insulin, C-peptide and paracetamol assay.

Tx Like hypoxia, hypoglycaemia rapidly leads to permanent brain damage. This can be avoided by prompt treatment with IV glucose into a large vein (50 mL of 50% solution for an adult). In a child, the dose is 0.2–0.5 mg/kg of glucose, which should be given as 10% dextrose (i.e. 2–5 mL/kg of 10% dextrose).

IM glucagon 1 mg (equal to 1 U) is an alternative treatment if venous access is delayed, although it is rather slow to work. The dose for children is 20 mcg/kg.

When the patient has fully recovered, the reasons for the low blood sugar must be explored. The patient should be allowed home only if:

- he or she has been fully awake for a couple of hours and has had some food
- continuous supervision is available
- there has been an attempt to prevent a recurrence of the problem
- follow-up arrangements have been made.

Diabetic ketoacidosis

DKA in children → p. 344.

Diabetic ketoacidosis (DKA) is a life-threatening metabolic condition with three main components: hyperglycaemia, acidosis and ketonaemia. In the UK, it still has a mortality of 1 in 150. Most of the cells of the body need insulin to allow them to take up glucose from the bloodstream. Ketoacidosis starts when this process is critically interrupted by absolute or relative deficiency of insulin. This is accompanied by an increase in counter-regulatory hormones (glucagon, cortisol, growth hormone and adrenaline) that stimulate hepatic gluconeogenesis and glycogenolysis. Two main problems result:

1 The body cells have no glucose to metabolise and so are starving. They burn fat and then produce an excess of the ketoacids.
2 Gross hyperglycaemia causes an osmotic diuresis, decreased tissue perfusion and circulatory collapse. There is dehydration and gross metabolic upset, failure of all body systems, and eventually coma and death.

The patient looks ill and may have a decreased level of consciousness. The skin is dry, not sweaty and there is tachycardia and hypotension. Kussmaul's respiration describes the characteristic deep, sighing breathing. Some patients present with only modest elevation of blood glucose, but with acidosis secondary to ketonaemia ('euglycaemic diabetic ketoacidosis'). The resolution of DKA in all cases depends on the suppression of ketogenesis.

Near patient testing for 3β-hydroxybutyrate (the predominant ketone in DKA) is now readily available. This means that the level of ketonaemia can be used to guide treatment rather than just the plasma glucose readings.

Tx Hyperglycaemia is of less importance than the hyponatraemic dehydration and the cellular ketogenesis.

- The airway must be protected and oxygen given.
- Resuscitation should be commenced with 0.9% saline (at least 15 mL/kg in the first hour and similar amounts in each of the next 2-hour intervals) (→ *Box 14.13*). Hartmann's solution is an alternative to saline that provides less of a chloride load. Colloids should not be used. Fluid resuscitation should be slower and more cautious in children and adults aged <25 years because of the risk of cerebral oedema (→ *Box 18.12 on p. 345*).
- Full monitoring is essential.
- Plasma sugar, bicarbonate, U&Es, haematocrit and blood gases should be measured. Plasma ketones (3β-hydroxybutyrate) can also be measured (>2–3 mmol/L is significant).
- Hyperglycaemia is initially treated by rehydration. Soluble insulin is then given in an IV bolus of 6–10 U (for an adult). The use of an initial bolus of insulin has been questioned in adults and is not now recommended in children. Traditionally, the rate of the subsequent insulin infusion has been governed by the patient's clinical condition and biochemical results, using a sliding scale (→ *Box 14.14*). However, a fixed rate soluble insulin infusion of 0.1 U/kg is now recommended as the best

> **Box 14.13 Typical water and electrolyte deficits in DKA**
>
> | | |
> |---|---|
> | Water | 100 mL/kg |
> | Sodium | 7–10 mmol/kg |
> | Chloride | 3–5 mmol/kg |
> | Potassium | 3–5 mmol/kg |
> | Phosphate | 1 mmol/kg |

Box 14.14 Insulin infusion

- Soluble insulin binds to plastic; this can be prevented by mixing the insulin with Haemaccel or a similar modified gelatin solution
- Human soluble insulin 50 U added to 50 mL gelatin solution gives a 1 U/mL mixture, which is easy to administer via an infusion pump
- The usual rate for an adult is 2–3 U insulin/h. A typical variable rate IV insulin regimen ('sliding scale') is shown below:

Blood glucose (mmol/L)	Insulin (U/h)
0–4.0	0.5
4.1–8.0	1
8.1–10.0	2
10.1–14.0	3
14.1–22.0	4
>22.0	6

When restarting subcutaneous insulin, the IV insulin infusion must be continued for 30 min after the administration of the first subcutaneous dose.

It is usually recommended that the long-acting recombinant human insulin analogues, insulin glargine and insulin detemir, are continued as a baseline therapy to ensure stabilisation despite the addition of a variable IV infusion.

 Box 14.15 Treatment targets in DKA

- Reduction of the blood ketone concentration by 0.5 mmol/L per h
- Increase of the venous bicarbonate by 3 mmol/L per h
- Reduction of the (capillary) blood glucose by 3 mmol/L per h
- Maintenance of the plasma potassium between 4.0 and 5.0 mmol/L

If these rates are not achieved then the fixed rate insulin infusion should be increased (by 1 U/h increments hourly).

- Catheterisation allows a careful check on fluid balance. A strict recording of fluid input and output must be maintained in any case.
- The administration of prophylactic low-molecular-weight heparin (LMWH) should be considered → p. 184.
- A cause for the development of the ketoacidosis must be sought. The condition usually develops over several days and is often precipitated by infection or other coexisting illness. Samples of blood, sputum and urine should be collected for culture and sensitivity. CXR and ECG should also be requested.
- The patient should be discussed as soon as possible with a physician who specialises in diabetes. Patients with heart failure, renal failure and other co-morbidities need special attention, as do those who are elderly, pregnant or aged <25 years.

way of suppressing ketogenesis → *Box 14.15*. An infusion of 10% glucose is introduced when the blood glucose falls to <14 mmol/L. The initial rate should be around 125 mL/h. The saline infusion should be continued as required.

- Metabolic acidosis is best treated by 'switching off' ketogenesis and restoring blood volume and renal function as above. Bicarbonate should not be given.
- Serum potassium may be normal or high initially as a result of haemoconcentration. It will fall rapidly when the hypovolaemia and acidosis are corrected and will follow the glucose into the cells. For this reason, plasma potassium should be measured regularly and replacement initiated early on (usually after 1–2 h of resuscitation). (*For potassium therapy → p. 249.*)

Recent evidence has shown that the difference between venous and arterial pH is between 0.02 and 0.15 pH units only and the difference between arterial and venous bicarbonate is 1.88 mmol/L. This is not significant in the management of DKA and thus it is not necessary to use arterial blood to measure acid–base status.

Hyperosmolar (non-ketotic) diabetic coma

A hyperosmolar state is usually seen in older patients who are not insulin dependent. In fact, most have no history of diabetes although there may have been polyuria and polydipsia for up to 2 weeks before presentation. As there is some insulin available to the body, ketoacidosis is not a feature of this condition. It is precipitated by infection or other illness in just the same way as DKA but drugs, especially diuretics, may also play a part. Hyperosmolar coma has a very high mortality because of coexisting disease and late diagnosis.

There is profound dehydration with depression of consciousness (not necessarily coma) and other neurological signs. There may be symptoms and signs of the precipitating disease.

Investigations:

- Blood glucose, U&Es, haemoglobin, white cell count and haematocrit should be checked together with blood gases. Haemoconcentration and infection are likely findings. Potassium depletion is common. *For potassium therapy → p. 249.*
- Serum osmolality is, of course, very high (>350 mmol/L) as a result of hyperglycaemia (>30 mmol/L) and hypernatraemia.
- Investigations for infection and other illness are as detailed above for ketoacidosis.

Tx This is similar to that for DKA. Vigorous fluid resuscitation is essential. Hypotonic solutions may precipitate cerebral oedema and so should be withheld until monitored parameters have stabilised; 0.45% saline is then used. Insulin requirements are low, so insulin therapy should again await fluid resuscitation.

Patients with hyperosmolar coma are at great risk of thromboembolism, so they should be given prophylactic subcutaneous LMWH.

Hypothermia

Hypothermia is defined as a core temperature <35°C:

- Mild hypothermia – <35°C
- Moderate hypothermia – <32°C
- Severe hypothermia – <30°C.

Core temperature must be measured with a suitably low reading and accurate device.

There are three main types of accidental hypothermia:

1 Acute (immersion) hypothermia: heat production is overwhelmed by sudden cold stress (immersion, lying injured in snow or drunk on a very cold, wet day)
2 Acute (exhaustion) hypothermia: cooling occurs only as energy reserves are exhausted (endurance sports, outdoor pursuits and immersion in relatively warm water)
3 Subacute (urban) hypothermia: the victim has been exposed to moderate cold for days, often with several predisposing factors (elderly or other → *later*).

> Up to 3% of medical patients admitted to UK hospitals during winter months have core temperatures <35°C.

The factors predisposing to hypothermia include the following:

- Relatively large surface area, large head and immature thermoregulatory mechanism in babies and young children
- Impairment of thermoregulatory mechanisms in old age. This may be potentiated by immobility after a minor accident, poor personal and environmental insulation, and inadequate heating in the home
- Altered behaviour patterns in patients taking drugs or alcohol; alcohol also causes peripheral vasodilatation
- Direct metabolic effect of certain drugs (e.g. chlorpromazine) and endocrine disorders (e.g. myxoedema).

There are several important haemodynamic changes in hypothermia:

- Profound vasoconstriction occurs. This is accompanied by a diuresis.
- Fluid moves into the extracellular compartment and cells.
- Immersion in water causes hydrostatic compression of the body – an effect similar to vasoconstriction and hence removal from water may cause 'rescue collapse'.
- As the core temperature decreases, the risk of VF increases.

The reversal of these effects during re-warming creates a danger of fluid overload. *For causes of death in hypothermia → Box 14.16.*

Hypothermia also induces metabolic upset:

- There is both respiratory and metabolic acidosis. Serum potassium levels rise.
- As the body temperature falls, carbohydrate is progressively replaced by fat as the metabolic fuel.
- Insulin resistance develops but the blood sugar level may be high or low.
- Cortisol levels are uniformly high.
- Pancreatitis may occur.

- Hypothyroidism is only rarely the cause of hypothermia presenting to an ED but cold, elderly patients may look myxoedematous. Consider taking a blood sample for subsequent estimation of thyroid-stimulating hormone, triiodothyronine (T_3) and thyroxine (T_4). T_3 (or T_4) must not be given except on the instructions of an endocrinologist – it may precipitate cardiac failure.

Tx Hypothermia is a reversible condition. Recovery has been reported from core temperatures as low as 13.7°C. Cardiovascular complications may make re-warming hazardous, but if normothermia can be regained patients rarely show any residual stigmata in the CNS or elsewhere. The 'afterdrop' phenomenon – whereby cooling of the patient continues after removal from the cold – is of little clinical significance.

- Seek advice.
- Treat the patient gently – the most common precipitant of VF in hypothermia is mechanical irritation of the body.
- Give oxygen.
- Institute careful monitoring – the key to success.
- Start passive re-warming:
- Remove clothing, especially if wet.

Box 14.16 Causes of death in hypothermia

- Hypovolaemia and circulatory collapse
- Fluid overload leading to cardiac failure and pulmonary or cerebral oedema
- Ventricular fibrillation
- Hypoxia
- Continued cooling and cardiac standstill
- Underlying pathology that predisposed patient to hypothermia (e.g. poisoning or CVA)

- Gently dry the skin.
- Wrap the patient in woollen blankets. Space blankets are no better than a comparable sheet of plastic.
- Dry and cover the scalp.
- Establish an IV line, although fluid therapy must be carefully monitored.
- Take blood for baseline Hb, white blood cells, glucose, U&Es and amylase.
- Obtain an ECG. It may show bradycardia and a characteristic notching of the S wave (usually seen best in V4) referred to as a J wave (present in 80% of patients with severe hypothermia) → *Figure 14.2*.
- Consider coincidental injury. Request radiographs of the chest and skull and any areas that may have been injured. Bruising and swelling are slow to appear in hypothermia and examination may be deceptively normal. The skin is abnormally susceptible to burns and pressure effects because of its poor blood supply.
- Consider active methods of re-warming (→ *Box 14.17*) in elderly patients with a core temperature <32°C and in younger patients with a temperature <30°C. ICU level monitoring and facilities for IPPV (intermittent positive pressure ventilation) must be available for these groups. Patients with the slow-onset (subacute) type of hypothermia (invariably elderly people) should probably be re-warmed at a rate no faster than 0.5°C/h to avoid the risk of pulmonary and cerebral oedema.
- Admit the patient to a suitable ward or to the ICU.

Hypothermic patients with no detectable cardiac output

- Diagnosis of arrest (feeling for a central pulse) should take place over about 60 s. The depressed circulation is difficult to assess; inappropriate cardiopulmonary resuscitation may precipitate VF.
- Ventilation and compression for cardiopulmonary resuscitation should then probably follow the same guidelines as in normothermia, although some authorities advocate slower rates. The compliance

Figure 14.2 J waves on the ECG in hypothermia.

Box 14.17 Re-warming in hypothermia

Re-warming may be of two main types:

1 Passive re-warming: insulation and other measures to prevent further heat loss
2 Active re-warming: heat supplied to the surface or the core of the body

Cold is a slow killer but inappropriate warming treatment can be fatal in a matter of minutes. Aim for safe, rather than rapid, re-warming.

Active re-warming of the surface of the body
Radiant surface heat can be dangerous because it may:

- reduce vasoconstriction leading to hypotension and collapse and the release of acidotic blood
- cause burns even at low temperatures if the circulation is sufficiently impaired
- inhibit shivering and reduce heat production

However, when applied to the trunk only, radiant heat is useful in patients with mild-to-moderate hypothermia. A warm bath (40°C) is effective but makes other management difficult. Hot water bottles around the neck, axillae and groins are probably the best compromise.

Active re-warming of the core of the body
This is more effective and logical than surface warming and should be employed in severe hypothermia. Techniques include the following:

- Airway warming: warm, moist air is supplied from a humidifier. This is effective as the entire cardiac output passes through the lungs. However, the energy that can be supplied is limited (only 10–15 kcal/h) and the main value is to prevent heat loss from the lungs
- Gastric or peritoneal lavage with warm saline
- Extracorporeal blood warming: this requires specialised facilities
- Irrigation of other body cavities and orifices with warm saline: this is usually impractical

The administration of warm (40°C) IV fluids is attractive but technically difficult to achieve because the high flows and volumes required may lead to fluid overload.

of the lungs, heart and chest wall is decreased in hypothermia.

- Defibrillation for VF is increasingly ineffective as the core temperature falls – especially to <28°C. Thus it is usually recommended that, if there is no response to the initial three shocks, subsequent attempts at defibrillation are delayed until the core temperature rises to >30°C. If the deep body temperature is <25°C, consider opening the chest through the fourth left interspace, assessing cardiac activity directly and, if necessary, performing internal cardiac massage. Warm saline packs can be applied to the heart and internal defibrillation is an option (→ p. 80).
- Metabolism of drugs is impaired in hypothermia and toxic accumulation of drugs may thus occur. For this reason, it is usually recommended that adrenaline and other drugs are withheld until the patient's core temperature reaches 30°C. At this point, the interval between drug doses is doubled (adrenaline is given every 6–10 min) until at least 32°C has been reached.
- Apparently dead patients may be hypothermic but recoverable ('never dead until warm and dead'). The heart can still be working even if this is clinically undetectable. Patients who may have suffered from hypothermia must therefore be re-warmed before assessing viability. This is particularly important in children. However, hypothermia and collapse may be agonal features of a terminal illness. If the prognosis is known to attending relatives discuss the management with them; re-warming is usually inappropriate.

Cardiac arrest → Chapter 11.

Hyperpyrexia and hyperthermia

Normal basal metabolism creates a heat load of around 65–90 kcal/h for an adult. This is enough to raise the body temperature by about 1°C/h in the absence of normal thermoregulation. Moderate exercise increases the generation of heat by a factor of five (300–500 kcal/h). A third of basal heat production is the result of cellular membrane ion pumps.

Hyperpyrexia is defined as a core temperature in excess of 41°C. This can result from two main causes:

1 Febrile illnesses
2 Hyperthermic conditions.

In a fever, the thermoregulatory set point of the hypothalamus is raised. This usually causes temperatures of between 38 and 41°C, and rarely up to 42°C – a response that may be protective against some infectious diseases. The most effective treatment is antipyretics such as paracetamol, which reset the temperature control mechanism. Cooling measures alone are relatively ineffective and short-lived.

Hyperthermia is a condition in which there is an imbalance between heat production and heat loss. Unlike hypothermia, this is not an inherently benign state. Urgent treatment is required to lower the temperature. Brain damage continues throughout the period of hyperpyrexia.

Causes of hyperthermia include the following:

- The extreme effects of drugs (e.g. levothyroxine and atropine; amphetamines, cocaine, PCP [phencyclidine] and other stimulants)
- Idiosyncratic reactions to drugs (e.g. neuroleptic malignant syndrome and malignant hyperthermia → *p. 300*; ecstasy and other stimulant drugs → *pp. 282 and 283*)
- Tetanus and other severe tonic–clonic conditions (→ *p. 233*)
- Excessive exercise, exhaustion and dehydration (heat exhaustion → *below*)
- Combinations of the above (e.g. febrile illnesses accompanied by convulsions or profound dehydration; stimulant drugs and prolonged dancing with an inadequate fluid intake).

> If the patient's temperature is >42°C, then hyperthermia is the likely diagnosis rather than fever.

Treatment of hyperthermia → p. 271.

Heat exhaustion

Heat exhaustion or heat stroke results from a combination of excessive exercise, exhaustion of energy stores and dehydration. Symptoms include headache, malaise, nausea, vomiting, faintness and muscle cramps. Core temperature is usually <41°C and mental status is unaffected. Treatment is rest, cooling, fluids and glucose. In most cases, the condition runs a benign course and does not lead to a hyperpyrexic emergency.

Addison's disease

Adrenocortical deficiency may be a consequence of autoimmune disease, TB or, most commonly, the cessation of long-term steroid therapy. In the last case, the deficiency may become obvious only several months after the therapy has stopped.

An Addisonian 'crisis' is often precipitated by infection. It presents with hypotension, collapse and vomiting. Pigmentation and weight loss are features of the underlying disease.

Investigations: The plasma potassium and urea are high and the sodium is low (due to aldosterone deficiency). Blood glucose may be normal or low. A plain abdominal radiograph may show calcification in tuberculous adrenal glands and the CXR may also reveal TB.

Tx

- Give a high concentration of oxygen as required to maintain the SaO_2 >94%.
- Take blood for routine tests and plasma cortisol level.
- Start fluid resuscitation with 0.9% saline.
- Give IV hydrocortisone 200 mg.
- Refer the patient to the general physicians on call.

Hepatic coma

Acute hepatic failure is usually caused by alcoholic cirrhosis or hepatitis (→ *p. 306*) but can also be caused by other diseases and drugs. There are three main problems:

1 Impaired gluconeogenesis
2 Coagulopathy
3 Failure to break down toxic metabolites.

Clinical features include:

- hypoglycaemia
- hypothermia
- neurological changes and coma as a result of underlying cerebral oedema or encephalopathy
- renal failure and metabolic disturbance
- hypotension and pulmonary oedema
- bleeding
- infection
- jaundice and hepatic fetor.

Paracetamol poisoning – a common cause of hepatic failure in emergency medicine – may present late with:

- a vague, non-specific history
- a few days of malaise, anorexia, nausea and vomiting

- hypoglycaemic coma
- low levels of paracetamol detectable in the plasma.

> Hepatic coma can be partially reversed by the benzodiazepine antagonist flumazenil; this can be misleading in coma of unknown causation.

Tx
- Oxygen and fluids
- Treatment of complications (e.g. hypoglycaemia, bleeding)
- Admission.

Renal failure

Shock from any cause may result in a temporary 'pre-renal failure' with anuria. Sustained hypotension leads to acute tubular necrosis and, in extreme cases, to acute cortical necrosis also → *Box 14.18.*

Acute renal failure is also seen in the following:

- Acute-on-chronic failure – precipitated by renal infection or dehydration
- Primary renal disease – acute glomerulonephritis or collagen vascular disease
- Hepatorenal syndromes – including Weil's disease (→ *p. 306*)
- Postrenal obstruction.

Oliguria is the cardinal sign (<300 mL in 24 h) because the clinical features of severe uraemia are variable and non-specific:

- *Cardiovascular:* hypertension, heart failure, pericarditis
- *Neurological:* lethargy, weakness, confusion and eventually coma
- *Gastrointestinal:* anorexia, nausea, vomiting and hiccoughs

- *Dermatological:* pruritus, pallor, petechiae
- *Haematological:* anaemia, bleeding tendency, immunosuppression.

Other changes seen in acute renal failure are caused by hyperkalaemia and acidosis (→ *pp. 248 and 251*). **Investigations:** The diagnosis is confirmed by the high blood urea and creatinine. Hyperkalaemia is common. Other investigations that should be performed are:

- FBC – low platelets
- Blood gases – acidosis
- CXR – pulmonary oedema
- ECG – *For changes in hyperkalaemia* → *Box 14.19*
- Blood sugar
- Calcium studies
- Urine microscopy and culture – haematuria, casts and infection.

The urinary sodium concentration is a useful investigation if there is any doubt about whether the oliguria is prerenal and amenable to fluid therapy or a result of acute tubular necrosis → *Box 14.20.*

Tx
- Record fluid balance carefully.
- Restore intravascular volume in prerenal failure.
- Perform an aseptic catheterisation.
- Treat complications (e.g. LVF or hypokalaemia).
- Discuss the patient with a physician and arrange admission.

Nephrotic syndrome: this may present with oedema. There is heavy proteinuria and hypoalbuminaemia. Various types of glomerulonephritis account for 80% of cases in adults whereas there is usually minimal change glomerulonephritis in children.

> **Box 14.18 Causes of acute tubular necrosis**
>
> - Sustained hypotension
> - Massive haemorrhage
> - Septicaemia, especially when caused by Gram-negative organisms
> - Free circulating haemoglobin or myoglobin (→ *crush injuries on p. 265*)
> - Poisoning

> **Box 14.19 ECG changes in hyperkalaemia**
>
> - Tall, peaked (tented) T waves (early change)
> - Shortened Q–T interval (early change)
> - Widened QRS complex
> - Small or absent P waves
> - Increased P–R interval
> - Depressed ST segment
> - Ventricular dysrhythmias (fibrillation and asystole)
>
> Note that tall peaked T waves are higher than they are wide.

> **Box 14.20 Distinction between prerenal and renal uraemia**
>
> In volume depletion or hypoperfusion with a healthy kidney the intact tubules are able to conserve sodium and concentrate the urine by the tubular reabsorption of sodium and water. In contrast, in acute tubular necrosis (renal uraemia) the tubular function is impaired and the urinary sodium concentration rises.
>
> - Prerenal problem: urinary sodium ≤20 mmol/L
> - Acute tubular necrosis: urinary sodium ≥40 mmol/L

Hyperkalaemia

High plasma potassium (>5.5 mmol/L) may be caused by the following:

- *Release from damaged cells*: burns, crush injury and rhabdomyolysis, transfusion
- *Abnormal movement out of cells*: acidosis, transfusion, hyperkalaemic periodic paralysis
- *Decreased excretion*: renal failure, Addison's disease, drugs such as potassium-sparing diuretics and NSAIDs
- *Poisoning*
- *Excessive intake*: rarely.

The effects of hyperkalaemia are:

- paraesthesia
- muscle weakness (flaccid paralysis)
- ventricular dysrhythmias (eventually asystole).

Dangerous effects are to be anticipated when the plasma potassium exceeds 6.5 mmol/L.

Investigations: The plasma potassium may be spuriously raised by haemolysis in the specimen tube. Blood gases should be taken to check for acidosis and the plasma potassium should be measured before commencing treatment. There are characteristic ECG changes in hyperkalaemia → Box 14.19.

Tx

Patients with severe elevation of the plasma potassium concentration (i.e. plasma potassium ≥6.5 mmol/L) and with toxic ECG changes: the first priority is to protect the patient from life-threatening cardiac dysrhythmias by giving:

- *Calcium*: under ECG control, give 10 mL of 10% calcium chloride by slow IV injection over 2–5 min (10 mL of 10% calcium chloride contains 6.8 mmol calcium ions). This has an immediate effect that lasts for up to 1 h. Up to 20 mL of 10% calcium gluconate (equivalent to 4.5 mmol calcium ions) is an alternative. Calcium stabilises the myocardial cell membrane but does not affect the plasma potassium.

Then proceed as below to redistribute potassium and remove it from the body.

Patients with severe elevation of the plasma potassium concentration (i.e. plasma potassium ≥6.5 mmol/L) but without toxic ECG changes: potassium can be redistributed out of the plasma into the cells by the administration of the following:

- *Bicarbonate*: if the patient has a metabolic acidosis (pH <7.20), give IV sodium bicarbonate (1 mmol/kg) over 5–15 min (→ Box 14.24 on p. 252). This acts within 15–30 min but has a limited effect on potassium levels when used alone.
- *Salbutamol*: give salbutamol 10 mg by nebuliser (2.5–5.0 mg in children). Up to 20 mg may be required. IV salbutamol 0.5 mg (4 mcg/kg in children) is an alternative. Patients with known ischaemic heart disease may be safer with inhaled salbutamol. Via β_2 receptors in liver and muscle, salbutamol stimulates the Na^+/K^+ ATP pump to move potassium into cells. Within 30 min, the plasma potassium begins to fall (by up to 1.5 mmol/L after IV salbutamol and up to 1.0 mmol/L after the nebulised drug). The effect of salbutamol is additional to that of insulin and reduces unwanted hypoglycaemia.
- *Insulin*: give 10 U soluble insulin in 50 g glucose intravenously over 15–30 min. Insulin stimulates the Na^+/K^+ ATP pump to increase the intracellular uptake of potassium. This effect is independent of its hypoglycaemic action. Reduction in plasma potassium starts within 15 min and is maintained for 1–2 h; a drop of around 1 mmol/L is to be expected. In children (who increase their insulin production more rapidly than adults) IV glucose 0.5 g/kg may be given alone.

Then proceed as below to remove excess potassium from the body.

Patients with mild or moderate elevation of the plasma potassium concentration: the ECG should be monitored in all patients. If the plasma potassium concentration is moderately elevated (i.e. 6.0–6.4 mmol/L) insulin and glucose should be given as described above before instituting treatment to remove excess potassium from the body. In patients who have only a mild elevation of the plasma potassium concentration (i.e. 5.5–5.9 mmol/L), therapies to remove potassium from the body are adequate alone.

All patients with hyperkalaemia: remove potassium from the body with an ion exchange resin such as calcium (or sodium) polystyrene sulphonate 15 g four times daily by mouth. Administration of 30 g by retention enema is an alternative. If renal function is normal, increase potassium excretion with furosemide 0.5–1.0 mg/kg orally or intravenously. Sufficient oral or IV fluid must be given in addition. Referral to a physician for further investigation is essential; dialysis may be required.

Hypokalaemia

Low plasma potassium (<3.5 mmol/L) results from the following:

- *Abnormal movement into cells*: alkalosis, insulin, hypokalaemic periodic paralysis
- *Excessive loss from the GI tract*: diarrhoea or vomiting
- *Excessive renal loss*: Cushing's disease, diuretics, renal tubular acidosis.

The most common symptoms of hypokalaemia are tiredness and weakness. These may be the only symptoms and examination may be unremarkable. However, there may also be:

- paraesthesia
- metabolic alkalosis
- polyuria
- paralytic ileus.

Investigations: The blood gases should be checked. The ECG may show characteristic changes → *Box 14.21*.

Tx Under ECG control, IV potassium replacement can be commenced in symptomatic or at-risk patients. The rate can be up to 0.5 mmol/kg per h (no more than 30–40 mmol/h for an adult). Many patients

---

> **Box 14.21 ECG changes in hypokalaemia**
>
> - Flattening or inversion of the T wave
> - Depression of the ST segment
> - Prolongation of the Q–T interval
> - Ventricular dysrhythmias including VF

---

with no symptoms and normal ECGs will respond to oral supplements. All patients should be referred to a physician.

Hypercalcaemia

Older people may present with non-specific symptoms that are attributable to hypercalcaemia:

- Weakness and lethargy
- Confusion and other mental changes
- Anorexia, nausea and vomiting
- Constipation
- Polyuria and dehydration.

The most common causes are malignancy (lung, breast and kidney) and primary hyperparathyroidism.

Tx
- Monitoring, especially of the ECG
- Forced saline diuresis
- IV furosemide 0.5 mg/kg
- Admission for investigation and specific calcium-reducing therapy (steroids, calcitonin, etc.).

Hypocalcaemia and tetany

Hypocalcaemia gives rise to the state of increased neuromuscular excitability known as tetany. The features are:

- paraesthesia
- carpopedal spasm and muscular cramps
- stridor, caused by laryngospasm
- other signs of neuromuscular irritability (twitching, hyperreflexia, Trousseau's and Chvostek's signs)
- convulsions.

Tetany most commonly accompanies the calcium changes of hyperventilation (→ *p. 218*) but may also be seen in hypoparathyroidism and a variety of other diseases. A similar state is seen in hypomagnesaemia → *p. 250*. Hypocalcaemia and hypomagnesaemia may coexist.

Tx
Hyperventilation syndrome → p. 218.

Other patients with tetany should be carefully monitored, given appropriate therapy and discussed with a physician. The initial dose of calcium in hypocalcaemic tetany is 2.25 mmol, which is present in 1 g calcium gluconate (i.e. 10 mL calcium gluconate 10% solution). This is given slowly intravenously and may be doubled if the response is unsatisfactory. It should be followed by an IV infusion of around 9 mmol/day.

Volume for volume, a solution of calcium chloride contains three times as much ionised calcium as a similar strength solution of calcium gluconate, e.g. 10 mL calcium chloride 10% contains 6.8 mmol calcium ions; 10 mL calcium gluconate 10% yields 2.25 mmol calcium.

Hypomagnesaemia and magnesium therapy

Magnesium is an essential constituent of many enzyme systems, particularly those involved in energy generation. Its salts are not well absorbed from the GI tract – hence their use as osmotic laxatives. As magnesium is present in large amounts in the GI secretions, excessive losses in diarrhoea, stoma or fistula fluids are the most common causes of hypomagnesaemia; deficiency may also occur in people who abuse alcohol and patients on diuretics. Hypomagnesaemia often causes secondary hypocalcaemia – with which it may be easily confused ($\rightarrow$ p. 249). Resistant tetany may result from a combination of the two. Symptomatic patients should be treated with a starting dose of 8 mmol (2 g) magnesium, diluted to 20 mL with saline and given intravenously over 15 min.

Other indications for treatment with magnesium in emergency medicine $\rightarrow$ *Box 14.23.*
Serum levels of magnesium $\rightarrow$ *Box 14.22.*

Hyponatraemia

Hyponatraemia is a relatively common electrolyte disorder, especially in hospitalised elderly patients.

It may occur in hypervolaemic, hypovolaemic and euvolaemic states. Low sodium levels lead to extracellular hypo-osmolarity and consequent movement of free water into the intracellular spaces. Causes of hyponatraemia include the following:

- Loss of body fluids (diarrhoea, vomiting, sweating, heat exhaustion, burns)
- Congestive heart failure
- Liver and kidney disease (including acute alcohol poisoning)
- Pulmonary and mediastinal disease
- CNS disease (including head injury)
- Endocrine disease (especially hypoadrenalism and hypothyroidism)
- Malignancies
- Polydipsia (including psychogenic polydipsia and beer 'potomania')
- Iatrogenic (too much IV dextrose)
- Feeding tap water or diluted milk to infants
- SIADH (syndrome of inappropriate antidiuretic hormone secretion)
- Antidepressant drugs, especially SSRIs (hyponatraemia with antidepressant therapy usually occurs in elderly people and may be due to SIADH)

 Box 14.22 Serum levels of magnesium

Normal range	0.7–1.1 mmol/L
Therapeutic range	1.5–2.5 mmol/L
Toxic range	>4 mmol/L

A bolus dose of 8 mmol of magnesium will approximately double the serum concentration; this will return to normal levels within 20 min. Toxic levels of magnesium cause neuromuscular blockade and muscle weakness. Calcium is a specific antagonist and will reverse these effects.

 Box 14.23 Indications for magnesium therapy in emergency medicine

1 Control of some resistant ventricular dysrhythmias:
  – VT secondary to hypokalaemia
  – VT that is resistant to DC shock
  – torsade de pointes ($\rightarrow$ p. 173)
  – some tachycardias that are secondary to the effects of drugs including digitalis, antiarrhythmics and occasionally tricyclics
2 Treatment of eclamptic fits ($\rightarrow$ p. 317)
3 Treatment of asthma ($\rightarrow$ p. 204)
4 Treatment of hypomagnesaemic tetany ($\rightarrow$ above)

The recommended starting dose of IV magnesium varies with the condition being treated. The total dose may be up to 16 mmol, followed by an infusion of 2.5 mmol/h; 1 g magnesium sulphate contains approximately 4 mmol magnesium ions; a 50% solution contains approximately 2 mmol/mL. Transient flushing – sometimes accompanied by hypotension – is to be expected in almost all patients.

- Diuretic drugs
- Many other drugs (including MDMA [3,4-methylenedioxymethamfetamine]/'ecstasy').

The symptoms of low plasma sodium are vague and non-specific and mostly due to cerebral oedema. They include fatigue, irritability, anorexia, nausea, headache, weakness, cramps, confusion, hallucinations and convulsions. Hyponatraemia that develops over a short period (<48h) is more dangerous than a more chronic fall in sodium levels. Rhabdomyolysis may occasionally occur (→ p. 265) and herniation of the brain stem is a risk with very low sodium levels.

Investigations: Plasma sodium and osmolality should be measured. An acute drop in plasma sodium to <120mmol/L is likely to be symptomatic with fits occurring at levels <110mmol/L. Urinary sodium and osmolality should also be measured. The avid reabsorption of sodium in most cases of hyponatraemia leads to a urinary sodium concentration <20mmol/L whereas, with renal causes and SIADH, the urinary sodium is >20mmol/L. SIADH causes inappropriately concentrated urine with an osmolality in excess of 100mosmol/L. In most other cases of hyponatraemia, the urinary osmolality is <100mosmol/kg.

A CT scan of the brain may be required to exclude other causes of cerebral swelling.

Tx Sodium levels must be increased slowly to prevent the development of osmotic demyelination syndrome (→ below). The plasma sodium concentration should not increase by >10mmol/L in 24h and should not normalise (or increase by >15–20mmol/L) for at least 48h.

If the plasma sodium is <115mmol/L, hypertonic saline (i.e. triple strength = 2.7% saline containing sodium 450mmol/L) should be given in an amount dependent on the patient's weight. The aim is to increase the plasma sodium concentration by just 5mmol/L in the first couple of hours. A bolus of 2.7% saline of 1.5–2.0mL/kg will usually raise the patient's plasma sodium by around 1–2mmol/L and, after measuring the biochemical effect (or if the patient continues to fit), a second bolus of 1.5–2.0mL/kg may be given. Isotonic saline (i.e. normal strength = 0.9% saline containing sodium 150mmol/L) should then be infused as a maintenance fluid; 0.9% saline should also be the initial IV fluid for patients with plasma levels of sodium >115mmol/L. IV furosemide 20–40mg is given to help excrete water and to block the ADH secretion that follows the administration of hypertonic saline.

SIADH is treated initially by water restriction. If this does not raise sodium levels sufficiently (or is not tolerated), then demeclocycline (a tetracycline antibiotic) may be given to block the renal tubular effects of ADH. Tolvaptan (a vasopressin V_2-receptor antagonist) may also be used for this purpose.

Osmotic demyelination syndrome (also known as cerebral pontine myelinolysis) may actually be a form of hypoxic encephalopathy, rather than an iatrogenic disorder. It is more common after chronic hyponatraemic states and people who abuse alcohol seem to be particularly at risk from it. Symptoms start 1–3 days after treatment and include dysarthria, dysphagia, paresis, fits and reduced level of consciousness. Unilateral signs may occur.

Metabolic acidosis

In emergency medicine, metabolic acidosis is most commonly a result of hypoxia and increased lactate production. This accompanies poor tissue perfusion or fitting. Other causes of metabolic acidosis include:

- poisoning (e.g. salicylic acid, methanol, carbon monoxide or cyanide)
- renal failure
- diabetic ketoacidosis
- rapid saline infusion (dilutional acidaemia).

Correction of hypoxia and restoration of tissue perfusion is the mainstay of emergency treatment. Bicarbonate therapy should be used with caution only in the patient with adequate ventilation (→ Box 14.24). It is not indicated for DKA. *For use of bicarbonate in tricyclic poisoning → p. 279.*

> In a simple metabolic acidosis, the $PaCO_2$ in mmHg will be approximately the same as the last two digits of the arterial pH.

Metabolic alkalosis

Diagnosis and treatment of metabolic alkalosis → Box 14.25.
Respiratory causes of acid–base disorders → p. 205.
The rules of compensation in acid–base disorders → Box 14.26. (These rules predict the expected compensation that results from a given primary change in acid–base status.)

> The direction of the pH change (acidosis or alkalosis) indicates the primary disorder; overcompensation does not occur.

Box 14.24 Bicarbonate therapy

Correction of an acidosis with IV sodium bicarbonate generates CO_2, which must be eliminated via the lungs:

$$HCO_3^- + H^+ = H_2O + CO_2$$

Thus adequate ventilation is a prerequisite for treatment.

Listed below are the two main solutions of bicarbonate:

1 Sodium bicarbonate 8.4% contains 1 mmol bicarbonate and 1 mmol sodium/mL. It is thus easy to calculate the required dosage but the concentrated solution is caustic to veins and should be given through a central venous line
2 Sodium bicarbonate 1.26% is isotonic. It contains 150 mmol bicarbonate and 150 mmol sodium/L. It is thus similar in composition to 0.9% saline (150 mmol chloride and 150 mmol sodium/L). This dilute solution can be given into a peripheral vein and provides fluid in addition to bicarbonate and sodium

Box 14.25 Differential diagnosis of metabolic alkalosis

Saline responsive (urinary chloride <10 mmol/L)
If the urinary chloride concentration is <10 mmol/L, the metabolic alkalosis is likely to be responsive to therapy with IV 0.9% saline. The condition is characterised by sodium chloride and volume depletion, so both sodium and chloride are avidly reabsorbed by the kidney. This type of alkalosis usually results from:

- loss of gastric secretions (e.g. vomiting)
- diuretic therapy
- chloride diarrhoea

Saline resistant (urinary chloride ≥20 mmol/L)
If the urinary chloride concentration exceeds 20 mmol/L, the metabolic alkalosis is probably resistant to simple infusion of saline. The underlying metabolic disturbance is excessive hydrogen ion secretion by the kidney. This occurs in hyperadrenal states and severe hypokalaemia. Chloride excretion remains unaffected. Causes include the following:

- Primary aldosteronism
- Cushing's disease
- ACTH-producing tumours
- Steroid therapy
- Severe potassium depletion

Box 14.26 Rules of compensation in acid–base disorders

Primary disturbance	Normal compensatory response
Metabolic acidosis	The $PaCO_2$ (mmHg) is equal to 1.5 times the plasma bicarbonate concentration +8 (±2)
Metabolic alkalosis	The $PaCO_2$ (mmHg) is equal to 0.9 times the plasma bicarbonate concentration +9 (±2)
Acute respiratory acidosis	For each mmHg rise in $PaCO_2$, the bicarbonate concentration increases by 0.1 mmol/L
Chronic respiratory acidosis	For each mmHg rise in $PaCO_2$, the bicarbonate concentration increases by 0.4 mmol/L
Acute respiratory alkalosis	For each mmHg fall in $PaCO_2$, the bicarbonate concentration decreases by 0.2 mmol/L
Chronic respiratory alkalosis	For each mmHg fall in $PaCO_2$, the bicarbonate concentration decreases by 0.4 mmol/L

ZOONOSES AND DISEASES RELATED TO TRAVEL

Travel to exotic places is now commonplace, so patients with a large variety of tropical and other unusual diseases may present to an ED. In addition, many of the infections described below (especially the zoonoses) have been included because of their potential for 'weaponisation', i.e. use in a biowarfare or bioterrorist incident. The UK's Health Protection Agency lists 10 such types of infective organism → p. 293.

> Meningococcal infection has recently occurred in outbreaks among travellers making pilgrimages to holy shrines in the Islamic world.

Malaria

> Malaria is commonly misdiagnosed as flu or viral hepatitis. A history of chemoprophylaxis does not exclude the diagnosis because patients may fail to take the right dose for the right period.

Malaria is the world's most important parasitic disease. It is a protozoal infection that is transmitted to humans by the bite of an infected female anopheline mosquito. Four species of the parasite are infectious to humans: *Plasmodium falciparum*, *P. vivax*, *P. ovale* and *P. malariae*. Half the world's population live in areas where malaria is endemic; 400 million people contract the disease each year and 2 million die from it, invariably from *P. falciparum* malaria.

Even the most fleeting visit to an area where malaria is endemic may result in infection. The time that it takes for an aeroplane to refuel is longer than the time that it takes for a mosquito to bite.

For predisposing factors → Box 14.27.

The initial features last for 2–3 days – malaise, anorexia, fever and headache. There is then an abrupt onset of rigors and sweating without specific clinical findings. There may also be:

- nausea, vomiting and diarrhoea
- tachycardia
- splenomegaly and occasionally splenic rupture
- jaundice.

The fever may become periodic as the erythrocytic phases of the parasite's life cycle become synchro-

 Box 14.27 Factors predisposing to malaria

- Travel – occasionally just a visit to an airport – within the last 2 months
- Inadequate prophylaxis – but there is no chemoprophylaxis that is 100% effective
- Age <5 years or >65 years
- Pregnancy
- Previous splenectomy

nous; every 48 h or 'tertian' for *P. vivax* and *P. ovale* infection and every 72 h or 'quartan' for infection with *P. malariae*.

The addition of acute neurological findings (disorientation, fits or coma) indicates cerebral malaria, a complication of *P. falciparum* infection. Blackwater fever, where malaria causes haemoglobinuria and renal failure, is another potentially fatal variant of this infection.

Investigations: The diagnosis is confirmed by microscopic examination of blood films (fresh or EDTA samples if stained within 3 h) but this may require up to six films. Nevertheless, in the vast majority of patients with a final diagnosis of malaria, the first blood film gives a positive result. A negative blood film suggests that the risk of developing an overwhelming disease in the next 24 h is very small because the level of parasitaemia correlates well with the severity of the infection.

Tx In patients who are very unwell start an IV infusion. Measure the blood sugar and correct any hypoglycaemia. A specialist in infectious diseases should be contacted for advice in all cases. Quinine is still the first-line drug in severe (invariably *P. falciparum*) infection, although there is increasing evidence that artesunate may be more effective. Quinine is given orally unless the patient is vomiting or deteriorating rapidly. Admission is usually required only for infection with *P. falciparum*; other forms of malaria can be treated in the community (with chloroquine). The disease is not contagious and so the patient does not have to be isolated.

Rabies

Any bite from an animal outside the UK carries a potential risk of rabies. Within the UK, bats can transmit EBLV2 (European bat Lyssavirus type 2), which is closely related to the classic rabies virus. Most cases of rabies occur within a few days of the bite but occasionally symptoms are delayed for weeks or even months.

It is said that, the more peripheral the wound, the longer the incubation period is likely to be because it takes time for the virus to migrate to the CNS.

> An unprovoked attack may suggest a rabid animal, but an animal that is known to be alive and well several days after the bite is unlikely to be rabid.

Rabies flourishes in dirty, contused wounds. The earliest signs are a failure of wound healing and paraesthesia or anaesthesia at the site of the injury. Eventually, florid CNS signs, including hydrophobia, develop. If untreated, symptomatic rabies has a 100% case fatality rate!

*For features that suggest the development of rabies →
Box 14.28.*

Tx
- Clean, debride and dress the wound.
- Give antitetanus therapy.
- Discuss the patient with a specialist in infectious diseases. Human diploid cell rabies vaccine should be given as soon as possible. Induction of a deep coma is often advised to protect the brain.

Box 14.28 Features of an animal bite that are suggestive of rabies infection

- Bite occurred outside the UK or from a bat within the UK
- Animal dead or whereabouts unknown
- Dirty wound; wound not healing well; paraesthesia
- Accompanying CNS symptoms or signs

Poliomyelitis

This highly infectious disease is still prevalent in many parts of the world, although the last 'non-imported' case in the UK was in 1982. The polio virus is spread by droplet infection and faecal–oral contamination with an incubation period of 3–21 days. An initial flu-like illness is followed by a pre-paralytic phase. This is essentially a meningitis (pyrexia, headache, vomiting and neck stiffness) accompanied by muscle pain and tenderness. Symptoms may subside after 48 h but in susceptible patients (around 1 in 75 adults and 1 in 1000 children) a paralytic phase will ensue as the muscle pain continues and weakness

develops. This is a result of the involvement of the anterior horn cells and the onset of an irreversible motor neuropathy. Signs are asymmetrical and may include the brain stem and bladder as well as the limbs.

Tx Patients must be isolated and discussed with a specialist immediately.

Haemorrhagic fevers

These deadly viral diseases have short incubation periods and are unlikely diagnoses if the patient has been out of an endemic area for more than 3 weeks.

- *Lassa fever:* Nigeria and other west African countries
- *Marburg fever:* northern Zaire and southern Sudan
- *Ebola fever:* Zaire.

The haemorrhagic fever starts abruptly as a flu-like illness with malaise, shivering and pyrexia. Other features that quickly develop are:

- severe headache, backache and other myalgia
- pharyngitis
- anorexia, nausea and vomiting
- abdominal pain and diarrhoea (watery stools often containing blood and mucus)
- maculopapular rash
- chest pain and pleural effusions
- spontaneous bleeding.

Tx Seek advice from a consultant specialising in infectious diseases before taking blood samples. Barrier nurse the patient in the interim. Patients are not infectious until they become very ill but transmission may occur through contact with infected body fluids.

Travellers' diarrhoea and vomiting

This has many different infectious causes:

- Viral infections, especially Noro (Norwalk) virus
- Coliform infections.
- Staphylococcal toxins: abrupt onset of violent symptoms within a few hours of a meal
- *Bacillus cereus* toxins: diarrhoea 12–24 h after eating recooked rice
- *Shigella sonnei* and *Shigella shigae*: bacillary dysentery with pyrexia, abdominal pain and bloody diarrhoea
- *Entamoeba histolytica*: amoebic dysentery (chronic diarrhoea)

- *Salmonella* spp. (including *paratyphi* A and C): abdominal pain and pyrexia
- *Salmonella paratyphi* B: paratyphoid fever

Tx

- Commence rehydration.
- Take blood for FBC, U&Es and glucose.
- Send stools for microscopy, including ova, cysts and parasites, and culture.
- Prevent spread of infection – wash hands and advise the patient accordingly.

The duration of travellers' diarrhoea can be halved by a 3-day course of either co-trimoxazole or ciprofloxacin. Single doses have also been shown to be effective. Food poisoning, infectious bloody diarrhoea and suspected *Escherichia coli* O157 infection are all notifiable diseases.

'Chinese restaurant syndrome' → *p. 291.*
Diarrhoea and vomiting in children → *p. 348.*
Gastroenteritis → *p. 311.*
Notifiable diseases → *p. 388.*
Scombroid fish poisoning → *p. 291.*

Other infections in travellers

Cholera

Infection with the causative organism of cholera – *Vibrio cholerae* – causes profound diarrhoea ('rice-water' stools) and the rapid development of life-threatening dehydration. This is accompanied by hyponatraemia and hypokalaemia. Rehydration is essential.

Typhoid fever

Infection with *Salmonella typhi* causes a non-specific fever for the first week of the illness. During the second week more specific signs develop:

- Abdominal pain and diarrhoea
- Relative bradycardia, considering the high pyrexia
- 'Rose spots'
- Splenomegaly.

Typhoid fever is treated with ciprofloxacin, chloramphenicol or cefotaxime. Infections from India and south-east Asia may be resistant to antibiotics.

Sandfly fever

This disease is a viral infection, transmitted by the bite of the sandfly. There is sudden onset of:

- pyrexia
- frontal headache

- neck stiffness
- ocular pain
- muscle pain
- red face, neck and conjunctivae.

Dengue fever

This is a mosquito-born viral infection with clinical features almost identical to sandfly fever.

Yellow fever

Yellow fever is a dangerous viral infection, which is also transmitted by mosquitoes. Three to six days' incubation is followed by profound illness:

- Pyrexia
- Headache, nausea, vomiting and photophobia
- Jaundice
- Hypotension
- Purpura and bleeding.

Chikungunya fever

Chikungunya is a relatively rare form of viral fever that, although regarded as a tropical illness, is now established in Europe. It is caused by an alphavirus that is spread by bites from *Aedes aegypti* mosquitoes and also by the Tiger mosquito (*Aedes albopictus*), which is common in southern Europe. Infection with the virus causes fever, headache, photophobia, muscle and joint pains, conjunctivitis, and bleeding from the nose and ears. Severe symptoms usually last less than 7 days and most patients recover fully after a few weeks. However, up to 1 in 10 people is left with chronic joint pain, stiffness and swelling. There is no vaccine against Chikungunya virus and no specific treatment for it.

Typhus fever

Louse-borne or epidemic typhus is caused by *Rickettsia prowazeki* and is transmitted by the infected faeces from a human louse, usually inoculated by scratching. After 2 weeks' incubation, there is a sudden onset of rigors, frontal headaches, and pain in the back and limbs. Chest infection and confusion develop, with a rash appearing on days 4–6. At first, this rash is morbilliform but it soon becomes petechial and mottled. During the second week, symptoms may increase in severity and overwhelming septicaemia, pneumonia or renal failure may lead to death. Tetracycline antibiotics are effective against rickettsial infections and additional treatment is mainly supportive.

Plague

Bubonic plague presents with pyrexia, malaise and discharging 'buboes'. These are purulent lymph nodes in the groin or axilla. *Yersinia pestis* is transmitted by flea bites but, if inhaled, causes a very contagious pneumonia (pneumonic plague).

Smallpox

Smallpox starts with an initial febrile episode, followed by severe prostration. The characteristic vesicular rash then develops in a single eruption with a dense distribution on the face and limbs. The palms and soles are particularly badly affected. (Chickenpox begins with a mild prodromal period. The vesicles appear at different times in several crops, mostly on the trunk. The palms and soles are spared and the lesions are relatively superficial.)

Infectious hepatitis → p. 306.
Influenza and SARS see → pp. 212 and 213.
Weil's disease (leptospirosis) → p. 306.

Zoonoses (human infections of animal origin)

Lyme disease

Visits to parks or woods where there may have been deer, or sometimes other animals, may lead to infection by *Borrelia burgdorferi*, a tick-born spirochaete. There is:

- a papule at the site of the bite
- fever, headache and fatigue
- polyarthritis and lymphadenopathy.

Lyme disease is on the increase in the UK.

Brucellosis (undulant or Mediterranean fever)

Brucellosis is a highly transmissible zoonosis, which is caused by bacteria of the genus *Brucella*. It affects a wide variety of mammals; human infections arise through direct contact with infected animals or their milk, by either ingestion or inhalation. After an incubation period of 5–30 days, there is fever, malaise, headache and joint pains. The disease is rarely fatal but causes debilitation for many weeks. Brucellosis is treated with a combination of doxycycline and rifampicin for at least 6 weeks.

West Nile fever

Despite its name, West Nile fever is endemic in southern Europe, the USA and Canada. The causative flavivirus (WNV) is transmitted to humans from its primary hosts, birds and horses, by mosquitoes and the incubation period is usually 3–15 days. Around 80% of those infected with WNV have no symptoms at all but 20% have a mild flu-like illness (fever, headache and muscle pains), sometimes with swollen lymph glands or a rash on the trunk. However, a small proportion (about 1 in 150 people infected) develop more severe disease – usually an encephalitis, meningitis or meningoencephalitis. These people may have headaches, fever, stiff neck, sore eyes, disorientation, muscle weakness, convulsions and coma; numbness and paralysis may also occur. People over the age of 50 are more likely to develop this serious form of West Nile fever.

Rocky mountain spotted fever

This tick-borne typhus fever is caused by *Rickettsia rickettsi* and is usually confined to dogs and rodents. It occurs in the western and southern states of the USA and also in South America. After an incubation period of 7 days, there may be an eschar at the site of the tick bite with enlargement of regional lymph nodes. Symptoms closely resemble those of louse-borne typhus (→ p. 255). A blotchy rash appears on day 3 or 4 and gradually becomes petechial. Untreated, the course of the disease may be mild or rapidly fatal. Tetracyclines remain the most effective antibiotics against rickettsiae.

Glanders

This zoonosis is caused by the bacterium *Burkholderia mallei* and is primarily a disease of donkeys, mules and horses. Human infection is rare but may be rapidly fatal. Glanders is spread to humans by inhalation or directly into wounds and has an incubation period of 10–14 days before symptoms appear. There is a high fever, malaise and muscle pains. Abscesses of the skin, nasal passages or lungs may be followed by septicaemia. Cases should be isolated.

Melioidosis

The causative organism of melioidosis, *Burkholderia pseudomallei*, is found in the soil and water of tropical regions such as Thailand, India and northern Australia. It may enter the body through wounds or by inhalation. Features include fever, headache, muscle pains, pneumonia and septicaemia. Untreated severe disease is nearly always fatal. Cases should be isolated.

Anthrax

Infection by the organism *Bacillus anthracis* occurs most often in wild and domestic animals in Asia, Africa and parts of Europe; humans are rarely infected. The organism can exist as spores that allow survival in the environment for many years. (*Cutaneous form of anthrax → p. 408*). Inhalational anthrax presents with a flu-like illness that progresses to severe respiratory difficulties and shock. Signs on CXR include pleural effusions, mediastinal widening, paratracheal/hilar fullness and parenchymal infiltrates. Progressively enlarging, haemorrhagic pleural effusions are a consistent feature. The disease is often biphasic, with a prodrome of general malaise for 2–3 days, followed by a day or two of apparent remission before the full-blown picture develops. Swabs, sputum samples, blood cultures and EDTA blood for polymerase chain reaction (PCR) should be taken before starting treatment for *Bacillus anthracis* with ciprofloxacin, clindamycin and a penicillin. Anthrax is a notifiable disease and should be considered in IV drug users with any severe soft-tissue or systemic sepsis. The source, in these cases, is presumed to be contaminated heroin.

Cutaneous anthrax → p. 408.
Q fever → p. 212.
Tularaemia → p. 408.

HAEMATOLOGICAL AND OTHER IMPORTANT DISEASES

Indications for transfusion of different blood components → Box 14.29 on p. 258.
Use of prothrombin complex concentrate → Box 14.30 on p. 259.

Sickle cell disease

Sickle cell disease is hereditary and occurs predominantly in African and African–Caribbean patients. It is also seen to a lesser extent in those from the Middle East, India and Mediterranean countries.

Polymerisation of abnormal haemoglobin S leads to deformity of the red cells, with a consequent increase in blood viscosity and blockage of capillaries. This 'sickling' is usually precipitated by hypoxia, dehydration or infection, although there are many other causes. Induction of anaesthesia can provide just such a stimulus. Attacks start in infancy.

Clinical presentations of sickling include the following 'crises':

- *Severe bone pain* (ischaemic): this may be in the spine
- *Abdominal pain and vomiting*: splenic infarction causes pain in the left upper quadrant of the abdomen
- *Pleuritic chest pain*: pulmonary infarction
- *Convulsions and strokes*: cerebral ischaemia
- *Visual loss*: retinal infarction
- *Infection*: the leading cause of death – note that loss of splenic function predisposes to pneumococcal infection
- *Hypotension*: visceral sequestration of blood; enlarged, tender liver and spleen
- *Priapism*
- *Rhabdomyolysis* (→ p. 265)
- *Haemolytic and anaemic crises.*

Investigations: A full screen should be carried out. Haemoglobin is normally low in patients with sickle cell disease and will be very low in a crisis.

CT brain scan is indicated in the presence of neurological signs.

Before general anaesthesia, patients at genetic risk of sickle cell disease need a simple laboratory test to screen for HbS (sickle cell haemoglobin). Application of a tourniquet (e.g. for Bier's block) is contraindicated in sickle cell disease.

Tx

- Give a high-concentration of oxygen.
- Commence rehydration with IV fluids. Blood transfusion dilutes HbS but may increase blood viscosity.
- Give adequate analgesia, usually morphine.
- Arrange admission.

Penicillin prophylaxis against pneumococcal septicaemia is advisable in at-risk children. If in doubt, seek advice from the nearest NHS Sickle Cell and Thalassaemia Counselling Centre.

Acquired haemophilia

Acquired haemophilia is a rare condition caused by an autoimmune depletion of clotting factor VIII. It is most commonly seen in elderly patients without any underlying disease but also occurs:

- as a feature of autoimmune diseases
- as a drug reaction
- in some malignancies and lymphoproliferative disorders
- in young women up to 12 months postpartum.

Box 14.29 Indications for transfusion of blood components in emergency medicine

The codes given are those assigned to the indication by the National Blood Service of the UK.

Red cell concentrates

R1 Acute blood loss – to maintain circulating blood volume and haemoglobin >7 g/dL in otherwise fit patients and >9 g/dL in older patients or those with known cardiovascular disease. Usually required only when there is 30–40% loss of blood volume (1500–2000 mL for an adult)

R7 Anaemia – to maintain the Hb above the symptomatic level (usually around 8 g/dL)

Cryoprecipitate
Dose = 1 U/5 kg body weight (equivalent to 10 U for an adult)

C1 DIC (disseminated intravascular coagulation) with bleeding and a fibrinogen level <1 g/L

C2 Advanced liver disease with bleeding and a fibrinogen level <1 g/L

C3 Bleeding associated with thrombolytic therapy and hypofibrinogenaemia

C4 Hypofibrinogenaemia (<1 g/L) secondary to massive transfusion

C5 Renal or hepatic failure associated with bleeding where DDAVP (desmopressin) is ineffective

Fresh frozen plasma (FFP)
Dose = 12–15 mL/kg (equivalent to 4 U for an adult)

F1 Single coagulation factor deficiency where a specific or combined factor concentrate is unavailable (e.g. factor V)

F2 Bleeding due to warfarin if prothrombin complex concentrate is unavailable (→ *Box 14.30 on p. 259 for the use of prothrombin complex concentrate*)

F3 DIC with bleeding and abnormal coagulation results

F5 Massive blood transfusion – coagulation testing should be performed before administration, if possible. If this is impractical in massive haemorrhage, use the formula: 4 U FFP for every 8 U red cell concentrate. Alternatively, empirical administration: coagulation factor deficiency can be expected after blood loss of 1.5 times blood volume or if >8 U red cells have been given

F6 Liver disease with bleeding

Platelet concentrates
Dose = 15 mL/kg (equivalent to one therapeutic dose for an adult)

P1 Thombocytopenia – to prevent spontaneous bleeding when the platelet count is <10 × 10⁹/L

P2 Thombocytopenia – to prevent spontaneous bleeding when the platelet count is <20 × 10⁹/L in the presence of additional risk factors for bleeding such as sepsis

P3 Thombocytopenia – to prevent bleeding associated with invasive procedures (such as central line insertion) when the platelet count is <50 × 10⁹/L

P4 Massive blood transfusion – the platelet count will usually be <50 × 10⁹/L after replacement of 1.5–2 times the blood volume. Aim to keep the platelet count >75 × 10⁹/L or >100 × 10⁹/L in cases of multiple, eye or CNS trauma

P6 DIC with bleeding and thrombocytopenia

P8 Autoimmune thrombocytopenia with a major haemorrhage

The haemophilia may present with a rapid onset of bleeding into the muscles, soft tissues or retroperitoneum or may complicate a situation in which there is already severe bleeding. Sometimes, prolongation of the activated partial thromboplastin time (APTT) is the first sign of abnormal clotting. Diagnosis depends on finding a reduced level of factor VIII in the plasma together with factor VIII inhibitors. Acquired haemophilia is treated by intravenous administration of activated recombinant human coagulation factor VIIa (rFVIIa, also called eptacog alfa), which directly activates the conversion of factor X to factor Xa.

Children with congenital haemophilias should be given factor VIII (or IX) concentrate after even very minor injuries.

Box 14.30 Prothrombin complex concentrate

Prothrombin complex concentrate (PCC) is a human activated coagulation factor concentrate containing the vitamin K-dependent factors, II, VII, XI and X, and also protein S and protein C. It is indicated for the treatment of bleeding and for perioperative prophylaxis in acquired deficiency of PCC factors due to vitamin K antagonists or autoantibodies. In emergency medicine, it is used primarily for patients who require rapid reversal of warfarin therapy, especially in cases of intracranial haemorrhage or other major haemorrhage (instead of the less effective FFP). It is issued as Octaplex from the blood transfusion laboratory. The concomitant administration of IV vitamin K (5 mg) should always be considered because warfarin activity can last longer than the effect of PCC. The dose is prescribed in mL/kg, according to the patient's INR and weight in kilograms:

Initial INR	2.0–2.5	2.5–3.0	3.0–3.5	>3.5
Approximate dose (PCC in mL/kg body weight)	0.9–1.3	1.3–1.6	1.6–1.9	>1.9

The single dose should not exceed 3000 IU (120 mL or six vials of PCC) in 24 h. The main risk is that of thromboembolic complications but allergic reactions may also infrequently occur.

Low platelets

There are many causes of thrombocytopenia (a platelet count $<150 \times 10^9$/L):

1 *Decreased production*: bone-marrow failure due to disease, cytotoxic therapy or irradiation; acute leukaemias; uraemia
2 *Decreased survival*: usually immunological causation such as idiopathic thrombocytopenic purpura (ITP) or drugs
3 *Increased consumption:* DIC; thrombotic thrombocytopenic purpura (TTP); large haemangiomas; some infections
4 *Sequestration*: hypersplenism and hypothermia
5 *Excessive loss*: massive haemorrhage and consumption coagulopathy
6 *Dilution*: massive transfusion of stored blood.

There are also congenital causes of low platelets and conditions where platelets exist in sufficient numbers but are dysfunctional. The diagnosis and specific treatment of all these conditions are beyond the scope of this book. However, severe bleeding and the indications for platelet transfusion are discussed below.

Platelet transfusions are used for the prevention and treatment of bleeding associated with thrombocytopenia or platelet function defects. Serious spontaneous haemorrhage due to thrombocytopenia alone is unlikely to occur at platelet counts $>10 \times 10^9$/L. Massive haemorrhage, DIC, bone marrow failure and acute leukaemias are all indications for platelet therapy, as is post-transfusion purpura (PTP). In ITP, TTP and heparin-induced thrombocytopenia (HIT) platelets are contraindicated unless there is life-threatening bleeding.

Platelet concentrates from donors of the identical ABO group to the patient should be used. Rhesus D-negative women of child-bearing age should receive RhD-negative platelets. The initial transfusion should be one adult therapeutic dose over 30 min. This may be expected to increase the patient's platelet level by at least 20×10^9/L. To treat massive bleeding, much larger doses may be required (four bags or more). Small children should be given 10–15 mL/kg of platelet concentrate at a rate of 20–30 mL/kg per h.

Adverse effects from oral anticoagulant drugs

The main adverse effect of drugs such as warfarin and acenocoumarol is haemorrhage. Bruising and bleeding increase significantly with INRs >5 (therapeutic INRs are between 2 and 4). Vitamin K_1 (phytomenadione) can be used to reverse the effects caused by over-anticoagulation, the dose being dependent on the INR result and the presence of bleeding. Oral administration of vitamin K is nearly as effective as IV administration; it is almost completely absorbed from the gut and the onset of action is not significantly delayed. The solution for injection can be taken by mouth. If given IV, vitamin K_1 should be injected slowly at a rate of 1 mg/min.

INR 6.0–8.0 with minor or no bleeding: stop oral anticoagulants and recheck the INR every 2 days to ensure that it is falling. Recommence anticoagulants when the INR is <5. There is no indication for vitamin K.

INR >8.0 with minor or no bleeding: stop oral anticoagulants and recheck the INR every 2 days to ensure that it is falling. Recommence anticoagulants when the INR is <5. If the patient has risk factors for bleeding (age >70 years, previous history of bleeding including epistaxis), give oral vitamin K 0.5–2.5 mg stat. Recheck the INR after 24 h and repeat the vitamin K if necessary.

Major bleeding: stop oral anticoagulant drugs. The anticoagulation can be rapidly and effectively reversed with prothrombin complex concentrate (→ *Box 14.30)* and IV vitamin K_1 5 mg stat. Partial reversal can be achieved using FFP 15 mL/kg and IV vitamin K_1 5 mg stat. Complete reversal of anticoagulation with higher doses (6–10 mg) of vitamin K results in prolonged resistance to oral anticoagulants with the risk of thrombosis. The INR should be rechecked daily.

Neutropenic sepsis

Certain categories of patients are at a high risk of developing neutropenia (a neutrophil count <1.0 × 10^9/L) and consequent life-threatening sepsis:

- Patients who have received recent cytotoxic chemotherapy
- Patients who have an acute haematological malignancy (such as acute lymphoblastic or myelobastic leukaemia)
- Patients with an absolute neutrophil count of ≤0.5 × 10^9/L for any reason.

In such patients, all febrile episodes must be taken very seriously and treated urgently with antibiotics. For this purpose, fever is defined as a temperature of 38.5°C or more on one occasion or 38°C or more on two occasions (separated at least by an hour during a 12-hour period). However, fever may not be present and the possibility of infection should be considered in all neutropenic patients who are unwell. Shock, acute respiratory distress and multiple organ failure are possible extreme presentations of neutropenic sepsis.

> There is a particularly high risk of neutropenia around one week after receiving chemotherapy.

Over 50% of febrile neutropenic patients prove to have an infection and many have a bacteraemia. This is usually due to Gram-positive cocci or Gram-negative bacilli such as *Escherichia coli, Klebsiella* spp. or *Pseudomonas aeruginosa.* Acute respiratory viral infections may also be associated with severe illness in the immunocompromised host. Infections in neutropenic patients typically take between 2 and 7 days to respond to antimicrobial therapy.

Chemotherapy patients with central venous catheter infections will not necessarily be neutropenic. In these cases, all IV antibiotics should be administered through the catheter and not through a peripheral cannula.

Investigations:
- Blood cultures and also cultures from any indwelling lines
- FBC, blood chemistry, LFTs, glucose, CRP, plasma lactate and coagulation screen
- CXR and MSU (midstream urine).

Tx
- A broad-spectrum carbapenem antibacterial (such as IV meropenem 1 g three times daily) should be given as soon as cultures have been obtained. (The dose must be reduced for patients with a creatinine clearance <50 mL/min.)
- IV teicoplanin 400 mg 12-hourly should be added for catheter-related infections or if meticillin-resistant *Staphylococcus aureus* (MRSA) is likely. Vancomycin is an alternative.
- A stat dose of recombinant human granulocyte colony-stimulating factor (lenograstim or filgrastim) should also be given subcutaneously to stimulate the production of neutrophils.
- Antipyretic drugs should not be given because the level of fever is a guide to further treatment.
- Admission should be arranged to a clean, spacious, enclosed area. The advice of a haematologist can be invaluable.
- If the patient is stable with a neutrophil count that is >1.0 × 10^9/L, then it may be appropriate to discharge them with a 5-day course of oral ciprofloxacin 500 mg twice daily and co-amoxiclav 625 mg three times daily.

Sepsis and septic shock

Sepsis is a systemic inflammatory response syndrome (SIRS) triggered by an infection. SIRS is defined as two or more of the following:

- Temperature >38.3°C or <36°C
- Heart rate >90 beats/min
- Respiratory rate >20 breaths/min or $PaCO_2$ <32 mmHg (4.23 kPa)
- White cell count >12 or <4 × 10^9/L
- Acute change in mental state
- Hyperglycaemia in the absence of diabetes.

Severe sepsis = sepsis with at least one organ failure or dysfunction:

- New requirement for oxygen to maintain SaO_2 >90%
- Systolic BP <90 mmHg

- Urine output <0.5 mL/kg per h (for 2 h or more)
- Lactate >2 mmol/L
- Creatinine >177 mcmol/L
- Bilirubin >34 mcmol/L
- INR >1.5 or APTT >60 s
- Platelets <100 × 10⁹/L.

Septic shock = severe sepsis with hypotension that is unresponsive to fluid resuscitation (i.e. systolic BP <90 mmHg and/or serum lactate >4 mmol/L after 60 mL/kg of IV fluid).

Potentially overwhelming sepsis with multiplying bacteria (and their toxins) in the bloodstream is called septicaemia.

Severe sepsis and septic shock are common causes of collapse, especially in elderly people and children. Sepsis is often overlooked as a cause for severe illness because:

- the temperature may not be raised
- the white blood cell count may be normal or low
- blood cultures may be negative.

The hallmark is impaired tissue perfusion.

Tx The resuscitation of a patient with severe sepsis or sepsis-induced hypoperfusion (hypotension or lactic acidosis) should begin as soon as the syndrome is recognised. The severe sepsis care pathway describes six key interventions (the 'Sepsis Six'):

1 Oxygen (to keep SaO_2 >94%)
2 Blood cultures and other routine blood tests (the haemoglobin must be maintained >7 g/dL)
3 IV antibiotics (septicaemia is treated with the antibiotics that are appropriate for its most likely source; in the absence of an obvious cause, a broad-spectrum anti-pseudomonal β-lactam antibacterial should be given (e.g. piperacillin enhanced with tazobactam) or a carbapenem (e.g. meropenem)
4 IV fluids (20 mL/kg boluses of 0.9% saline, up to 60 ml/kg)
5 Lactate measurement (a serum lactate >4 mmol/L [36 mg/dL] denotes very poor tissue perfusion)
6 Fluid balance monitoring (this may require a catheter).

Senior review and an ICU opinion should be arranged as soon as possible. Careful and continuous monitoring and recording of physiological parameters are essential. The immediate aim of treatment is to achieve a systolic BP >90 mmHg, a urinary output of at least 0.5 mL/kg per h and a serum lactate <4 mmol/L.

Meningococcal septicaemia in both children and adults → p. 341.

Acquired immune deficiency syndrome

The causative organism of AIDS – human immunodeficiency virus (HIV) – is transmitted by the following:

1 Unprotected sexual intercourse with an infected person
2 Injection of infected blood, usually the result of drug abusers sharing equipment
3 An infected mother to her baby before or during birth or by breast-feeding.

Infected blood and other body fluids that are splashed on to body surfaces in the normal course of resuscitation have not been shown to transmit HIV. Current evidence indicates that a significant volume of infected material has to be injected in order to transmit infection. HIV is easily neutralised by the common disinfecting agents.

HIV infection can be encountered in any patient although it is most common in:

- homosexual men
- IV drug abusers
- people from sub-Saharan Africa (or sexual contacts of people from sub-Saharan Africa).

The most common presentation of a patient with AIDS to an ED is with fever and malaise caused by an opportunistic infection (→ *Box 14.31*). Unexplained coma may occur. It is important to consider the possibility of HIV infection, because late diagnosis remains a common cause of avoidable death.

 Box 14.31 Opportunistic infections in AIDS

- Pneumonia, classically caused by *Pneumocystis jiroveci* (formerly called *Pneumocystis carinii*)
- Tuberculosis
- Meningitis and encephalitis (headache, fever, fits and coma – toxoplasmosis and sometimes herpes viruses)
- Gastrointestinal upset (anorexia, weight loss and diarrhoea – cytomegalovirus, salmonellae or atypical mycobacteria)
- Hepatitis
- Fungal infections
- Skin infections

Before an HIV test, lengthy counselling is not required (unless a patient requests or needs it). The minimum requirement is just to ensure informed patient consent to the test.

Moist primary and secondary syphilitic lesions are highly infectious!

Investigations: A full screen should be performed. CXR shows diffuse interstitial changes in pneumocystis pneumonia. TB should also be considered when looking at the CXR.

Tx All HIV-positive patients with unexplained fever, neurological signs or any suggestion of significant infection should be admitted for investigation. *Pneumocystis jiroveci* pneumonia (= PCP or *Pneumocystis carinii* pneumonia) is very suggestive of AIDS and is treated with high-dose co-trimoxazole. TB is also increasing in the HIV-positive population.

Pneumonia → *p. 209.*
Post-exposure prophylaxis against HIV infection in health-care workers → *Box 21.10 on p. 404.*
TB → *p. 213.*

Syphilis

Syphilis is on the increase in the UK. Men account for over 90% of the cases, most of whom are either homosexual or bisexual. Acquired syphilis is divided into early (primary, secondary and early latent infection) and late (>2 years after infection) stages:

- *Primary syphilis* presents as a painless ulcer usually (but not always) in the anogenital area with regional lymphadenopathy. This ulcer heals in a few weeks and may go unnoticed. The incubation period of the underlying treponemal infection is usually 3–4 weeks (range 9–90 days).
- *Secondary syphilis* causes a widespread, polymorphic rash on the trunk (typically with involvement of the palms and soles as well). There is lymphadenopathy, mucocutaneous ulcers (especially in the mouth), headache and vague malaise.
- *Early latent syphilis* is characterised by positive treponemal serology with no symptoms.

Around a third of diagnosed patients are found to have primary syphilis, another third secondary syphilis and the remainder early latent syphilis. The incidence of late syphilis (latent, cardiovascular, neurological or gummatous disease) has not increased in the UK.

Investigations: Patients from high-risk groups presenting with genital or oral ulceration, non-itchy rashes or lymphadenopathy should be tested for syphilis. The diagnosis is confirmed by positive serology (send 10 mL of clotted blood marked '?syphilis'), although serology may be negative in very early infection.

Tx Patients with positive serological tests or with suspicious ulcers on their genitalia should be referred urgently to a genitourinary (GU) clinic.

Pelvic inflammatory disease (gonococcal or chlamydial infection) → *p. 314.*

Haemolytic uraemic syndrome

Haemolytic uraemic syndrome (HUS) is a systemic disease with three main components:

1 Haemolytic anaemia
2 Acute renal failure
3 Thrombocytopenia.

HUS is caused by the effects of a circulating toxin that binds to endothelium, particularly in the renal, gastro-intestinal and central nervous systems. Thrombin and fibrin are deposited in the damaged microvasculature and erythrocytes are then injured (and subsequently haemolysed) as they pass through the partially occluded blood vessels. Platelets are sequestered but coagulation is relatively unaffected.

Typical (infection-induced) HUS is caused by a toxin from *Escherichia coli* O157:H7 (i.e. somatic [O] antigen 157 and flagellar [H] antigen 7) called verocytotoxin (or Shiga toxin). Other bacteria and some viruses (including HIV) may also be associated with HUS and the atypical form of the disease (10% of cases) may be induced by certain drugs, systemic lupus, cancer and pregnancy. Verotoxin (or Shiga toxin)-producing *Escherichia coli* (STEC or VTEC) are found in the gut of cattle and other farm animals. Contaminated food products (e.g. beef and milk) are therefore the usual source of infection but fruit and vegetables may be contaminated by infected manure. Water and direct contact with farm animals or infected people are other possible routes of transmission. The disease (which is notifiable) occurs as both sporadic cases and larger outbreaks. It is most common at the extremes of age, in summer months and in rural communities.

VTEC may cause a haemorrhagic colitis but only around 15% of cases progress to HUS (after 5–14 days) and many infected adults remain asymptomatic. Initial profuse diarrhoea becomes bloody after a couple of days with fever, vomiting and abdominal pain. In the UK, HUS is the most common cause of acute renal failure in children. Other causes of abdominal pain and diarrhoea, TTP and HELLP syndrome (**h**aemolysis, **e**levated **l**iver enzymes and **l**ow **p**latelet count) may all mimic HUS.

Investigations:
- FBC and blood film (looking for anaemia, haemolysis and a low platelet count)
- Blood chemistry (to show renal involvement)
- Stool sample (for culture and phage typing of *Escherichia coli*).

Tx The treatment of VTEC-induced bloody diarrhoea and HUS is supportive, with no evidence for specific treatments. Antibiotics are not beneficial and anti-diarrhoeal drugs should be avoided. Fluid and electrolyte losses may be high due to both diarrhoea and capillary leakage. The case fatality rate is 2–5% with most deaths occurring in children and elderly people.

Hereditary and other non-allergic angio-oedemas

Allergic angio-oedema and anaphylaxis → p. 299.

There are several types of angio-oedema that do not respond to treatment with antihistamines, corticosteroids or epinephrine. These include:

- Hereditary angio-oedema (HAE): this affects 1 in 50 000 people. There is an inherited mutation in the C1-inhibitor gene, leading to a reduced level of C1 esterase inhibitor or a C1 inhibitor protein that does not work properly. The lack of this physiological regulator results in an overproduction of bradykinin and consequent leaky blood vessels (→ *Figure 14.3*). The absence of a family history does not rule out the diagnosis of HAE; in up to 25% of cases a spontaneous mutation is responsible. The frequency, severity and duration of attacks are very variable but most patients have a first attack before the age of 20. There are many possible triggers including concurrent illnesses, surgery, emotional stress, hormonal changes and specific foods. Many patients experience prodromal symptoms of some sort.

- Drug-induced angio-oedema: ACE inhibitors may often be responsible (→ *Figure 14.3*).
- Acquired angio-oedema: this can develop during serious illnesses such as malignancies or autoimmune disorders.
- Pseudoallergic angio-oedema: drugs such as NSAIDs may affect the production and regulation of inflammatory mediators.
- Idiopathic angio-oedema.

At least the first three of these angio-oedemas are mediated by excess bradykinin production (→ *Figure 14.3*). There may be swelling of the face, lips, tongue, pharynx and larynx. The extremities of the limbs and the genitalia may also be involved and around 25% of patients have an erythematous, non-pruritic rash. The oedema may cause airway obstruction and shock (due to fluid redistribution). In HAE, recurrent colicky abdominal pain (sometimes with vomiting and diarrhoea) may be repeatedly misdiagnosed.

Tx Oxygen and fluids. Advanced airway care may be required. Any precipitating factor must be withdrawn.

Icatibant, a synthetic decapeptide, is a specific and selective competitive bradykinin B_2-receptor antagonist that is indicated for the emergency treatment of HAE. It displaces bradykinin from its receptor and thus reduces the oedema and shortens the duration of attacks. It is given subcutaneously in a dose of 30 mg (up to three times in 24 h). Symptoms usually improve in less than an hour.

C1 inhibitor concentrate may be administered intravenously in an acute attack (500–1500 U, with an additional infusion if symptoms persist for more than 2 h). Two units of FFP can be used if C1 inhibitor concentrate is not available. Conestat alfa, a recombinant C1 esterase inhibitor, is now available as an alternative to the plasma-derived concentrate. The dose is 50 U/kg (up to a maximum of 420 U) and a response is anticipated within 4 h. It contains traces of rabbit protein, so it is recommended that recipients are tested for the presence of IgE antibodies against rabbit allergens.

Attenuated androgens (such as danazol or stanazolol) are used to activate liver enzymes to produce more C1 inhibitor and thus shorten the duration of an attack. Antifibrinolytics (such as tranexamic acid 1 g four times daily for 48 h) affect the complement cascade and are sometimes recommended. A kallikrein inhibitor may be available in the UK in the near future. In the absence of type 1 hypersensitivity, adrenaline is not particularly effective.

Figure 14.3 The role of the kallikrein–kinin system in the pathogenesis and treatment of non-allergic angio-oedemas. ACE, angiotensin-converting enzyme.

Acute porphyrias

Acute hepatic porphyrias are rare diseases, which are often under-diagnosed or mistaken for NSAP (non-specific abdominal pain). Drugs that are prescribed to alleviate symptoms may exacerbate the attack.
A list of potentially unsafe drugs is available on the European Porphyria Initiative website.

Porphyrias are uncommon inherited disorders of haem biosynthesis, each of which is related to a specific enzyme deficiency. Transmission is usually autosomal dominant. The defective synthetic pathway results in accumulation and increased excretion of porphyrins and their precursors. Of the seven types of porphyria, three are described as 'acute' and all produce similar clinical pictures:

1 Acute intermittent porphyria (the most common form)
2 Hereditary coproporphyria (there may be skin lesions).
3 Variegate porphyria or mixed porphyria (skin lesions are present).

Around 80% of sufferers are women aged 15–45 years. Drugs, alcohol, infections, fasting or hormonal changes may trigger an attack. There is persistent and intense abdominal pain, often accompanied by low back pain, vomiting and constipation. Tachycardia, fever and sweating may be present. On examination, there is tenderness and guarding over the liver. Psychiatric symptoms are present in over a quarter of patients and neurological features include fits, local paresis and generalised paralysis.

Investigations: Radiological examination of the abdomen is normal. There may be hyponatraemia. With exposure to light for 10–30 min, the urine turns from reddish brown to black. The urinary levels of ALA (δ-aminolevulinic acid) and PBG (porphobilinogen) are elevated.

Tx Attacks of acute porphyria require hospitalisation and urgent treatment to avoid life-threatening complications. Any neurological symptoms should provoke an ICU admission to anticipate possible respiratory paralysis. Immediate treatment includes the following:

- Analgesia with morphine or pethidine
- Prochlorperazine for nausea (not metoclopramide)
- Rapid IV fluids
- Oral or IV carbohydrates as soon as possible: 500 g in 24 h (this prevents the induction of ALA synthase)
- Chlorpromazine for psychiatric disturbance
- Specific therapy with human hemin (an infusion of 3 mg/kg is given immediately and then daily for a further 3 days. This infusion is run over an hour through a central or large peripheral vein. The vein should be thoroughly flushed with a saline infusion after administration. A glass bottle is recommended for the diluted hemin solution but a PVC bag is adequate in the emergency situation. An inline filter and shielding of the hemin infusion from light are also required). The administered hemin corrects the haem deficiency and thus restores negative feedback control to its metabolic pathway to reduce the production of toxic precursors.

Dermatological emergencies

Acute generalised pustular psoriasis (of von Zumbusch) is an explosive, eruptive form of psoriasis accompanied by fever and toxicity. The patient (who is often middle-aged) initially has red, tender skin and feels ill. Clusters of superficial, sterile pustules (2–3 mm in diameter) appear within hours. They are widely distributed over the body but concentrated in the flexures, genital regions and fingertips. Within 24 h, the pustules coalesce, dry and desquamate. The underlying skin is smooth and erythematous but new crops of pustules may appear over a period of days or weeks. There is a neutrophilia and a raised ESR. Albumin, calcium and zinc levels are low and renal tubular necrosis may occur. This is a life-threatening condition and the patient must be admitted to hospital for skin care and IV rehydration.

Acute erythrodermic psoriasis refers to a very extensive or whole body eruption of red, thickened and often scaly skin. There may be fluid imbalance and pyrexia. Admission is required for skin care and IV fluids.

Bullous pemphigoid is a blistering skin disease that usually affects older people. The blisters are due to an immune reaction within the skin and cause intense itching. Crops of tense, fluid-filled bullae develop which are filled with clear, cloudy or blood-stained fluid. The eruption may be very widespread and, in severe episodes, there may be blisters over the entire skin surface and in the mouth. In such cases, hospital admission may be required so that the blisters and raw areas can be carefully dressed. IV fluids and steroids are usually given and antibiotics may be required for secondary bacterial infection.

Rhabdomyolysis and myoglobinuria

Extensive contusion to muscle resulting in rhabdomyolysis and myoglobinuria may occur in several ways:

1 As a consequence of an acute crushing injury (e.g. trapped in a pit or under a lorry) (also → traumatic asphyxia syndrome on p. 78)
2 From other direct muscle injury, e.g. deep burns or severe and untreated compartment syndrome
3 After lying immobile for a long time on a hard surface. This is seen in:
   – elderly or debilitated people after a collapse (found on the floor)
   – alcohol-intoxicated patients
   – those who are drug abusers
   – those who have been in prolonged coma from an overdose
4 Following the excessive muscle activity caused by prolonged seizures, extreme exercise and some stimulant drugs (e.g. phencyclidine, cocaine and ecstasy)
5 In some severe infections and metabolic disorders. In addition, drugs of the statin class may sometimes cause a dose-related myositis, which in rare cases leads to rhabdomyolysis.

The diagnosis should be suspected in any patient in the above categories. Muscle pain and tenderness may be absent.

The main consequences of the damaged and necrotic muscle are:

- metabolic and volume disturbance
- acute renal failure from myoglobinuria
- local tissue destruction
- compartment syndrome in the limbs ($\rightarrow$ *p. 87*).

Investigations: The urine usually tests positive for blood and the laboratory may find granular casts in it. A raised plasma creatinine kinase is also strongly suggestive of the diagnosis of rhabdomyolysis. Concentrations of creatinine kinase >5000 U/L are associated with a high incidence of acute renal failure. The serum myoglobin peaks at 4 h and returns to normal within 12 h of injury. As a result of this rapid clearance, myoglobin in the urine may easily be missed. Arterial blood gases, plasma electrolytes and calcium should also be measured.

Tx Initial resuscitation with IV fluids should be followed by a continuous infusion of sodium bicarbonate 1.26% solution in order to:

1 maintain normovolaemia (large quantities of fluid can be sequestered in damaged muscle)
2 ensure a steady urine output of >100 mL/h
3 create an alkaline urine, aiming for a urinary pH of >7 (alkalisation of the urine increases the solubility of the myoglobin-derived tubular protein casts).

Catheterisation is mandatory. There must be careful monitoring of clinical and biochemical parameters. Hyperkalaemia occurs in most cases and may need treatment. Bicarbonate is of use for hyperkalaemia but IV calcium may increase the destruction of the muscle tissue. Mannitol 0.5–1.0 g/kg or furosemide 1–2 mg/kg is sometimes used to achieve a forced diuresis. Dialysis may be required.

Early amputation of extensively crushed limbs has been advocated to remove the source of toxic metabolites and infection but is of unproven value. In contrast, rapid fluid replacement and electrolyte control increase the chances of survival. Fortunately, the prognosis for renal failure induced by myoglobinuria is excellent, with most survivors recovering fully within 3 months.

Necrotising soft tissue infections

There is a large spectrum of clinical conditions in which there is a spreading necrosis of soft tissue ranging from relatively localised pyodermas to fulminating gas gangrene. Anaerobic streptococci, staphy-lococci, *Bacteroides* spp., enterococci and clostridia are the most commonly implicated organisms, but many other bacteria are also sometimes involved. Intravenous drug users have an above-average risk of such infections, especially those who inject subcutaneously ('skin-popping') or use large amounts of citric acid to dissolve their drugs (citric acid causes local tissue necrosis). The possibility of anthrax infection ($\rightarrow$ *pp. 257 and 408*) should be also considered in any IV drug user with a necrotising soft-tissue infection.

Necrotising fasciitis

Spreading necrosis of the fascial plane is usually polymicrobial in nature with cultures yielding a mixture of four or more species of both anaerobic and aerobic bacteria. Exotoxin-producing anaerobic streptococci are the most common single organism isolates at present but 'clostridial cellulitis' was well recognised in the past. Although rare, the condition has a mortality rate of around 25%. It is more common in males and in people aged >60 years. Victims often have an underlying condition that predisposes to infection such as diabetes, peripheral vascular disease, alcoholism or IV drug abuse. Fournier's gangrene of the scrotum (which tracks abdominally via Scarpa's fascia) is an eponymous variant of the same condition.

Necrotising fasciitis can affect any part of the body. It usually follows a trivial injury such as an insect bite or a small abrasion. An initial cellulitis is followed by necrosis of the fascia and subcutaneous tissue with relative sparing of the underlying muscle. Symptoms develop over a period of hours or even days and presentations vary greatly. The patient is pyrexic, tachycardic and unwell with a seemingly disproportionate amount of pain. A diffuse erythema of the whole body (similar to toxic shock syndrome) may occur. The necrosing skin is erythematous and oedematous at first but, as the infection develops, it becomes dusky and haemorrhagic with bullae formation. Overwhelming sepsis can progress rapidly to shock and multiorgan failure.

Gas gangrene (necrotising myositis)

Fulminating necrosis of muscle occurs when damaged or devitalised tissue becomes contaminated with anaerobic bacteria from soil or the intestines of humans and animals. The Gram-positive anaerobe *Clostridium perfringens* (formerly called *Clostridium welchii*) is the classic cause of gas gangrene but other clostridial species (e.g. *Clostridium novyi* and *Clostridium septicum*) and anaerobic streptococci are also sometimes implicated, especially in IV drug users. As the bacteria multiply, they produce toxins (such as lecithinase), which digest muscle and subcutaneous tissues. The destructive processes liberate free gas and an assortment of noxious metabolites.

In this situation, clostridia have a short incubation period; contaminated wounds begin to putrefy around 1–3 days after injury. The surrounding tissues crepitate because of the free gas and emit a foul odour. The patient has a high fever, hypotension and usually a toxic delirium. The condition progresses rapidly to systemic sepsis and organ failure. First World War surgeons noted jaundice as a preterminal feature of gas gangrene.

Investigations: Diagnosis of soft-tissue necrosis is almost entirely clinical. However, around 50% of patients with necrotising fasciitis (and many more with gas gangrene) have air in the soft tissues on plain radiography. Almost all patients have an elevated white cell count and urea. In the later stages, there is metabolic acidosis and coagulopathy.

Tx Resuscitation with IV fluids and administration of broad-spectrum IV antibiotics (e.g. co-amoxiclav and metronidazole or piperacillin/tazobactam and clindamycin) is required (clindamycin and ciprofloxacin can be given to patients who are allergic to penicillins). Extensive surgical debridement of affected wounds must not be delayed.

15

Poisoning

GENERAL PRINCIPLES IN POISONING

Poisoning may be the result of:

1 accidents
2 social drug abuse
3 deliberate self-harm
4 attempts to harm others.

> Bizarre symptoms and signs or unusual combinations of clinical features should always suggest the possibility of poisoning.

Initial assessment and management

ABCs → Chapter 1.

In all cases, approach the patient without condemnation. If the patient has a reduced level of consciousness or immediately appears unwell:

- Protect the airway.
- Administer a high concentration of oxygen by mask.
- Obtain venous access.
- Control fits with intravenous (IV) diazepam.
- Connect the patient to monitoring devices – ECG, BP (blood pressure) and SaO_2 (arterial O_2 saturation); measurement of core temperature is also important.
- Measure the blood glucose.
- Request an urgent ECG.
- Seek senior/anaesthetic advice.

> Narcotic (opiate) and sedative drugs may depress the protective reflexes of the airway more than might normally be expected for a given level of consciousness.

Further assessment and management

Ask about

- Nature of substance taken
- Type of preparation taken.

> Slow-release preparations may cause delayed or protracted poisoning.

- Other substances (e.g. alcohol) also taken. Ask specifically about paracetamol and aspirin. Poisoning with these two drugs is common, dangerous and treatable
- Route of poisoning (e.g. oral, IV)
- Time taken
- Intended result of poisoning
- Previous episodes of poisoning.

> Over half of all self-poisoned patients present within 4 h of ingestion.

Look for

- Dyspnoea, bronchospasm and pulmonary oedema
- Tachycardia and hypotension

Emergency Medicine Lecture Notes, Fourth Edition. Chris Moulton and David Yates.
© 2012 Blackwell Publishing Ltd. Published 2012 by Blackwell Publishing Ltd.

- Dysrhythmias and widening of the QRS complex
- Depressed level of consciousness
- Agitation, restlessness and hallucinations
- Pupillary changes
- Extensor plantar reflexes
- Lowered or raised core temperature.

Specific actions

- Measure the plasma urea and electrolytes (U&ES) and glucose.
- Consider the need to measure the blood gases, plasma osmolality and plasma chloride. The osmolar gap and the anion gap can then be calculated → p. 221.
- Measure or screen for plasma aspirin and paracetamol levels 4 h after the estimated time of ingestion.
- Obtain a 12-lead ECG.
- Seek specific poisons advice *(Sources of advice →* p. 271).
- Consider the need for gastric decontamination *(→ later)*.
- Consider the need for specific supportive measures *(→ p. 271)*.
- Consider requesting toxicology levels (e.g. lithium, iron, theophylline, methanol, ethylene glycol, digoxin, paraquat and carboxyhaemoglobin).
- Consider the need for specific therapies *(→ below)*.

> Most patients should be screened for aspirin and paracetamol 4 h from time of ingestion, irrespective of the history of substances taken.

In patients with a reduced level of consciousness, consider the need to:

- give IV saline (at least 10 mL/kg) unless there is a specific contraindication
- catheterise the bladder and measure the urine output.

Metabolic acidosis, anion gap and osmolar gap in poisoning

A metabolic acidosis with an increased anion gap (and a normal chloride concentration) indicates retention of non-volatile organic acids such as may be present in renal failure, ketoacidosis and lactic acidosis, or following the ingestion of substances such as methanol, ethylene glycol, salicylate and iron. In the absence of circulatory failure, diabetes, alcoholism or uraemia, an increased anion gap clearly indicates poisoning with one or more of these substances.

An increased osmolar gap indicates that one or more substances are present in high molar concentrations. Most drugs, including salicylates, are not identified this way because they are dissociated or do not attain high enough serum concentrations on a molar basis. The ingested substances best able to increase the osmolar gap are those that have a low molecular weight and are present in high mass units – such as the lower alcohols and glycols. Poisoning with methanol or ethylene glycol commonly causes severe metabolic acidosis and elevation of both the anion and osmolar gaps → p. 221.

Calculation of the anion gap → p. 221.
Calculation of the osmolar gap → p. 221.
Metabolic acidosis → p. 251.

Gastric decontamination

Controversy still surrounds the efficacy of the different modes of gastric decontamination although none is a mainstay of modern treatment. All methods aim to reduce the absorption of residual toxins from the gastrointestinal (GI) tract. The risks must be carefully weighed against the likely benefits. Any form of gastric decontamination is of doubtful value if more than 1 hour has passed since the ingestion of poisons, except in specific cases:

1. Modified-release preparations of drugs
2. Drugs that possess anticholinergic (antimuscarinic) properties (e.g. tricyclic antidepressants)
3. Drugs that directly delay gastric emptying (e.g. salicylates)
4. Drugs, the elimination of which may be increased by active charcoal after they have been absorbed → p. 270.

Gastric lavage

Gastric lavage is effective only if the substance ingested is still in the stomach → *above*. It should be reserved for intubated patients with a depressed level of consciousness from unknown substances or specific indications such as highly toxic drugs. It may be useful to remove large quantities of alcohol in patients with acute poisoning. A general anaesthetic may sometimes be necessary, especially in children. Gastric lavage is contraindicated in the following circumstances:

- There are not adequate facilities and skills available to protect the airway or deal with any complications that might arise.

Box 15.1 Procedure for gastric lavage

- Move the patient to the resuscitation area
- Secure the airway; request anaesthetic help if required
- Put the patient in the recovery position on a tiltable trolley The stomach is easier to drain in the right lateral position
- Monitor the patient's SaO_2 throughout the procedure
- Have a high-volume suction pump switched on
- Carefully insert a lubricated lavage tube
- Siphon the gastric contents into a bucket, checking for tablet material; gentle pressure over the stomach may facilitate drainage
- Lavage the stomach with warm water or saline until the drainage fluid is clear; in small children isotonic fluids in aliquots of 10 mL/kg should be used
- Instil activated charcoal if indicated → *later*
- Remove the lavage tube

- The substance taken is relatively safe (e.g. benzodiazepines).
- The substance ingested is safer in the stomach than anywhere else. This applies to the following:
  - *Oily or petroleum-based substances*: relatively harmless in the stomach, but accidental spillage into the lungs during lavage will cause a life-threatening pneumonitis.
  - *Corrosives and caustics*: may cause oesophageal perforation, especially with the help of a lavage tube.

Technique of gastric lavage → *Box 15.1*.

Emesis and whole bowel irrigation

Emesis removes at least as much material from the stomach as gastric lavage. It also has the same contraindications as lavage → *before*. It is possible to vomit up tablets, which would not fit through the small Murphy's eye of a lavage tube. However, emesis is dangerous in obtunded patients and activated charcoal cannot be subsequently given. For this reason, emesis is no longer routinely recommended in the UK. For those situations or in places where there is no alternative, syrup of ipecacuanha is usually used to induce vomiting (30 mL in an adult and 15 mL in a child). It should be followed by a reasonable volume of fluid and can be repeated after 20 min if necessary.

Whole bowel irrigation is also of doubtful value and has not been shown to improve outcomes.

Milk

Milk is often advocated to assuage the effects of ingested substances that are:

- irritant
- of low toxicity
- dangerous to remove by lavage or emesis.

Activated charcoal

Heating of charcoal with chemical activators increases its surface area to between 1000 and 2000 m^2/g and thus enhances its ability to reversibly absorb small molecules. (A standard 50-g dose has an internal surface area that is larger than 20 football pitches!)

> Charcoal is extremely dangerous if aspirated; airway protection must therefore be ensured whenever it is used.

Activated charcoal will not absorb:

- iron, lithium and other metallic compounds
- cyanides
- strong acids and alkalis
- alcohols
- petroleum distillates
- malathion and DDT.

Repeated administration of charcoal absorbs drugs re-excreted into the bowel via the enteroenteral and enterohepatic circulations. This 'gastrointestinal dialysis' is indicated for:

- theophyllines
- carbamazepine
- phenobarbital
- quinine
- dapsone

and may be useful for:

- tricyclic and related antidepressants
- barbiturates
- salicylates
- sotalol
- phenytoin
- paraquat
- digoxin and other cardiac glycosides
- ciclosporin.

Activated charcoal should be administered in a dose equal to 10 times that of the poison to be absorbed. An initial dose of 50–100 g (or 1 g/kg for children) will usually ensure that this ratio is met. Paracetamol and aspirin are taken in gram rather than milligram quantities and so a second dose of charcoal may be needed after a few hours. For repeated dosing 50 g (1 g/kg) should be given every 4 h or smaller doses more frequently. Large doses of charcoal may form concretions in the bowel and so lactulose (or sorbitol) should be given with each repeated dose.

Treatment of respiratory depression

There are four main factors:

1 Airway protection – positioning and suctioning
2 Airway maintenance – positioning and adjuncts
3 Support of breathing – assisted ventilation
4 Reversal of specific opioid-induced respiratory depression – naloxone.

Specific respiratory stimulants (e.g. doxapram) have little place in the treatment of drug-induced respiratory depression.

Treatment of circulatory depression

This involves the following:

- Maintenance of adequate oxygen supply to the heart → *before*
- Maintenance of normovolaemia – IV fluids; vasoconstrictors (e.g. ephedrine) are sometimes used in specific treatment situations
- Correction of cardiac dysrhythmias – may need specialist advice to avoid dangerous interactions (e.g. prolongation of the Q–T interval → *p. 174*)
- Correction of bradycardia – atropine initially; may need an adrenaline infusion or cardiac pacing (→ *p. 164*)
- Maintenance of cardiac contractility – inotropes such as dobutamine (→ *p. 238*). Specialist monitoring is necessary to optimise cardiac output in this situation.

Treatment of hyperthermia

Hyperthermia may result from the following:

1 Stimulant drugs (e.g. amphetamines)
2 Excessive exercise and dehydration
3 Idiopathic reactions to drugs (e.g. neuroleptic malignant syndrome (→ *p. 300*) and malignant hyperthermia)
4 A combination of the above (e.g. ecstasy and prolonged dancing; amphetamines and convulsions → *p. 282*).

Treatment must be promptly instituted to prevent the development of multiorgan failure. Cooling measures include:

- removal of clothing
- cool sponging and promotion of evaporation with an electric fan
- placement of ice-packs in the axillae and groins
- infusion of cooled IV fluids
- gastric lavage with cool fluids in the unresponsive (intubated) patient
- administration of oral or rectal paracetamol.

Exotic lavages of cool fluids into the peritoneal and pleural cavities, colon and bladder are often advocated but are usually impractical in the ED. Drugs that may be used in some situations by the specialist to promote cooling include the following:

- Chlorpromazine: vasodilator, sedative, hypothermic effect
- Diazepam: muscle relaxant and sedative
- Dantrolene: muscle relaxant. Dantrolene is used for the treatment of malignant hyperthermia and as such is kept in all operating theatres. Its use should usually be discussed with an intensivist. An initial dose of 1 mg/kg is given intravenously over 10 min, repeated if necessary every 15 min to a maximum of 10 mg/kg in 24 h.

Convulsions → p. 231.
Hyperpyrexia and hyperthermia → p. 245.
Sedative drugs that may cause hypothermia → p. 243.

Poisons information services

Specific poisons information may be obtained from the following:

1 The internet (TOXBASE, the primary clinical toxicology database of the UK National Poisons Information Service is available on the internet to registered users)
2 Telephone enquiries to the UK National Poisons Information Service
3 Textbooks, including the front of the *British National Formulary*
4 Databases (e.g. tablet, plant and fungi identification charts).

Management of poisoning with unknown substance(s)

- Obtain as much history and background information as possible; consider alternative diagnoses.
- Examine the patient and his or her clothing and possessions for further clues. Beware of needles in the pockets.
- Consider trauma or coexistent disease.
- Monitor the patient.
- Check the blood sugar.

- Send off blood for full blood count (FBC), blood chemistry, and aspirin and paracetamol screen.
- Consider the need for ECG and blood gases. Plasma osmolality can be a useful test to establish the presence of extraneous substances in the blood ($\rightarrow$ *p. 221*).
- Consider the administration of activated charcoal.
- Administer IV fluids and measure urine output.
- Admit for observation.

POISONING WITH COMMON MEDICINES

The frequency with which poisoning with a drug occurs usually reflects its availability in a society.

Treatment of toxicity caused by local anaesthetic agents $\rightarrow$ *p. 393*.

Paracetamol (acetaminophen)

> Paracetamol 150 mg/kg or 12 g (24 standard tablets) for an adult (whichever is the smaller amount) constitutes a significant ingestion of the drug.

Paracetamol is the most common drug involved in self-poisoning in the UK. This reflects its widespread usage and over-the-counter availability. It is also a common ingredient in compound tablets, combined with opiates, caffeine and many other drugs. The only early features of isolated paracetamol poisoning are nausea and vomiting, which usually settle within 24 h. Malaise beyond this time, especially if accompanied by right subcostal pain and tenderness, usually indicates the development of hepatocellular necrosis, the major toxic effect of paracetamol poisoning. There may also sometimes be delayed renal tubular necrosis, usually in association with liver damage. These serious problems occur 3–4 days after ingestion, although patients may sometimes present even later with:

- hypoglycaemia
- bleeding
- encephalopathy and cerebral oedema.

The fatal dose of paracetamol may be as low as 10–15 g (20–30 tablets). Fortunately, the specific antidotes, *N*-acetylcysteine and methionine, are very effective if given early enough. Children rarely ingest large quantities of paracetamol and so deaths attributable to this drug before the teenage years (and especially age <6 years) are extremely unusual.

> Patients who present 15 h or longer after ingestion tend to be more severely poisoned and at a greater risk of serious liver damage.

Tx

> Be aware of the units used by the laboratory to measure paracetamol concentration. At least two different units are commonly used in the UK.

All patients should have their plasma paracetamol concentration measured as soon as 4 h have passed since the ingestion (measurements before 4 h have passed are unreliable because of continuing absorption and distribution). The plasma salicylate should be simultaneously measured because patients are not always able to differentiate between the two drugs. The need for specific treatment can usually be determined from this single measurement when it is plotted on a reference treatment curve ($\rightarrow$ *Figure 15.1*). If the time of ingestion is in doubt, the worst case option should be assumed to have occurred. After 15 h, the estimates of risk are less reliable and clinical judgement is more important.

> Accurate timing of the overdosage is critical when interpreting plasma paracetamol levels on a treatment nomogram. The recommended graph for use in the UK and Ireland starts at 4 h post-ingestion with a plasma concentration of 200 mg/L (the '200' line) ($\rightarrow$ *Figure 15.1*). However, in Australia, New Zealand and the USA, a similar semi-logarithmic plot is used that starts with paracetamol levels that are 25% lower at 4 h (the '150' line) in order to allow for a wider margin of error. For the same reason, the UK will use the high risk treatment line (the '100' line) for all patients in the very near future.

The usual antidote is IV *N*-acetylcysteine (NAC) ($\rightarrow$ *Box 15.2*), but up to 10% of patients treated with this drug may have an allergic response to it, with 3–6% having a severe reaction ($\rightarrow$ *Box 15.3*). Patients who are given IV NAC despite having plasma paracetamol levels that are not in the toxic range are more likely to have these reactions. Oral methionine is an alternative to IV NAC that is widely used in some countries ($\rightarrow$ *Box 15.4*). Some patients have an increased risk of liver damage after paracetamol ingestion ($\rightarrow$ *Box 15.5*). Antidote treatment should be instituted for

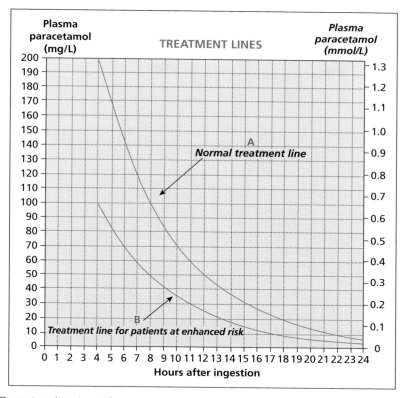

Figure 15.1 Paracetamol treatment lines.

 Box 15.2 **Treatment with *N*-acetylcysteine**

For adults, infuse NAC in three aliquots:

1 150 mg/kg in 200 mL of 5% glucose over 15 min
2 50 mg/kg in 500 mL of 5% glucose over 4 h
3 100 mg/kg in 1000 mL of 5% glucose over 16 h

- For very obese patients (i.e. body weight >110 kg), the dose of NAC should be calculated on a maximum weight of 110 kg.
- For children >20 kg, use the same dose of NAC in half the volume of 5% glucose. For children <20 kg, the same dose can be used in a still

smaller volume of fluid (e.g. aliquot 1 = 3 mL/kg, aliquot 2 = 7 mL/kg and aliquot 3 = 14 mL/kg).
- Physiological (0.9%) saline may be substituted for 5% glucose.
- In exceptional circumstances without IV access, NAC may be administered by mouth. (But it is poorly tolerated because of the high doses required due to its low oral bioavailability. It also has a very unpleasant taste and odour and causes nausea and vomiting.)

---

these patients if their plasma paracetamol concentration is 50% or more of the normal reference treatment value (→ *Figure 15.1*).

Mechanism of action of antidotes in paracetamol toxicity → Figure 15.2.

Patients who have received NAC or methionine will subsequently require measurements of clotting time (international normalised ratio or INR), glucose, U&Es and creatinine. Vitamin K should be given if the INR is increased (>2) with fresh frozen plasma (FFP) and clotting factors reserved for active bleeding.

Box 15.3 Adverse reactions to N-acetylcysteine

Reactions usually occur during the first 30 min of treatment (when large amounts of NAC are being given rapidly) and consist of:

- nausea
- flushing
- itching, urticaria and other erythematous rashes
- angio-oedema
- bronchospasm
- hypotension or (rarely) hypertension

Most reactions are mild and will resolve if the infusion is stopped and IV chlorphenamine is given. The infusion can then be restarted at the rate of 50 mg/kg over 4 h. Severe reactions require urgent treatment; methionine can then be given as an alternative.

Box 15.4 Treatment with oral methionine

Oral dose of methionine: 2.5 g initially followed by three further doses of 2.5 g every 4 h.

Useful if:

- past or present allergic reaction to N-acetylcysteine
- difficulty obtaining, or maintaining, IV access
- patient refuses other treatment
- patient is going to take own discharge
- awaiting plasma paracetamol concentration

Unsuitable if:

- patient is nauseous or vomiting
- activated charcoal has been given (it will absorb methionine)

Patients with signs of liver damage should be discussed early on with a specialised liver unit. This would include those with:

- INR >3.0
- elevated plasma creatinine (>300 mcmol/L)
- hypoglycaemia
- severe acidosis (arterial pH <7.3 or lactate >3.5 mmol/L)
- encephalopathy
- hypotension (mean arterial pressure <60 mmHg)
- pre-existing liver disease.

Box 15.5 Patients at special risk of liver damage (treated according to the 'high risk' line on the graph in Figure 15.1)

- Has a condition that causes glutathione depletion (i.e. malnutrition, cachexia, failure to thrive, anorexia nervosa and other eating disorders, malabsorption states and chronic debilitating illnesses, including cystic fibrosis, malignancies, alcoholism, hepatitis C, HIV infection and AIDS)
- Is taking hepatic enzyme-inducing drugs such as carbamazepine, phenytoin, phenobarbital, primadone, rifampicin, rifabutin, efavirenz, nevirapine or St John's wort
- Drinks excessive amounts of alcohol (>21 units/week in males and >14 units/week in females)

High risk is suggested by the history, abnormal liver function tests (LFTs), raised INR, low urea and urinary ketones.

Severe liver damage after paracetamol poisoning has been defined as a peak plasma alanine aminotransferase (ALT) activity exceeding 1000 IU/L. An aspartate aminotransferase (AST) level >1000 IU/L is similarly diagnostic. Most patients who are clinically unwell have peak ALT and AST levels of several thousand units per litre. In clinical practice, the prothrombin time (PT) or INR is a more accurate test for assessing prognosis.

Children: paracetamol poisoning with paediatric preparations is rarely serious as toxic amounts are not usually ingested. In addition, young children may metabolise the drug differently from adults. However, children poisoned with adult preparations may be at risk of liver damage and so assessment and treatment are virtually identical to those for adults. Nausea and vomiting are very common in children who have ingested excessive amounts of paracetamol. If there is a certainty of an accidental ingestion of a single dose of paracetamol of <150 mg/kg (or 75 mg/kg in children at enhanced risk → Box 15.5), then measurement of paracetamol levels is unnecessary and the child can be discharged. However, all children with deliberate self-poisoning, including those who have taken insignificant amounts, should be admitted for child psychiatric assessment → *p. 365*.

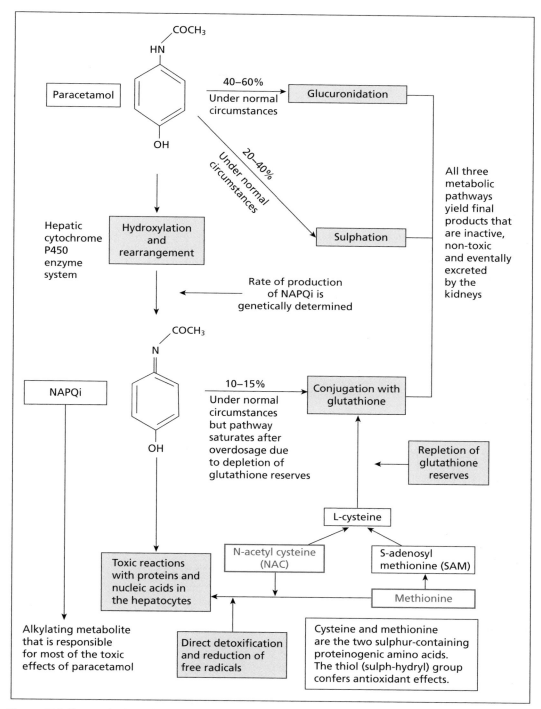

Figure 15.2 The mechanism of action of antidotes in paracetamol toxicity.
NAPQi, *N*-acetyl-*p*-benzoquinoneimine.

Management of patients who present within 8h of ingestion

- For patients who present within 1 h of a significant ingestion, give activated charcoal 50 g, although it is of unproven benefit in this situation.
- Assess whether the patient is at an enhanced risk of severe liver damage (→ Box 15.5).
- Measure the plasma paracetamol concentration as soon as 4 h or more have elapsed since the ingestion.
- Start treatment with NAC if the plasma paracetamol level is on or above the relevant treatment line (→ Figure 15.1) (for normal patients, this is 200 mg/L at 4 h and 110 mg/L at 8 h, and for high-risk patients 100 mg/L at 4 h and 55 mg/L at 8 h). If the paracetamol concentration is unavailable within 8 h of ingestion and if >150 mg/kg (or 12 g) of paracetamol has been taken, then the antidote should be started anyway and treatment stopped if the result subsequently indicates that it was not required.
- Arrange admission to a medical ward or psychiatric referral as appropriate. Patients who have received NAC within 8 h of a paracetamol overdose can be expected to be fit for discharge on completion of its administration. However, INR, ALT and plasma creatinine should be measured before discharge in everyone who has received NAC. Patients should be advised to return to hospital if vomiting or abdominal pain develops or recurs.

Management of patients who present 8–15h after ingestion

- Measure the plasma paracetamol concentration immediately. Also take blood for INR, plasma creatinine and ALT.
- Start IV NAC, without delay, while waiting for the paracetamol concentration result if a significant amount (>150 mg/kg or total 12 g) is thought to have been taken. The efficacy of the antidote declines progressively from 8 h after ingestion.
- Assess whether the patient is at special risk of severe liver damage (→ Box 15.5).
- Discontinue NAC only if the paracetamol level is below the relevant treatment line (→ Figure 15.1) (for normal patients, 110 mg/L at 8 h and 35 mg/L at 15 h; for high-risk patients, 55 mg/L at 8 h and 15 mg/L at 15 h) and the patient is asymptomatic with a normal INR, plasma creatinine and ALT. If there is any doubt about the timing of the overdose, then continue the infusion of NAC.
- Arrange medical admission or psychiatric referral as appropriate. INR, ALT and plasma creatinine should be measured before discharge in all patients who have received a full course of NAC. Patients

should be advised to return to hospital if vomiting or abdominal pain develop or recur.

Management of patients who present 15–24h after ingestion

- Measure the plasma paracetamol concentration immediately, together with the INR, ALT, glucose, U&Es, creatinine, LFTs and venous bicarbonate.
- Start IV NAC, without delay, while waiting for the paracetamol concentration result in all patients unless convinced that a significant amount (>150 mg/kg or total 12 g) has not been ingested. Urgent action is required because the efficacy of NAC is limited when more than 15 h have passed since the ingestion.
- Assess whether the patient is at special risk of severe liver damage (→ Box 15.5).
- Discontinue NAC only if the paracetamol level is below the relevant treatment line (→ Figure 15.1) and the patient is asymptomatic with a normal INR, plasma creatinine and ALT. If there is any doubt about the timing of the overdose, then continue the infusion of NAC. The prognostic accuracy of the treatment lines after 15 h is uncertain but a plasma paracetamol concentration above the applicable treatment line should be regarded as indicative of a serious risk of severe live damage.
- Arrange admission for patients with abnormal clotting, renal function or liver enzymes or whose paracetamol level exceeds the relevant treatment line.

Patients can be discharged 24 h after paracetamol ingestion if all of the following criteria are met:

- No symptoms
- Normal INR, ALT and creatinine
- Plasma paracetamol concentration <10 mg/L
- Normal mental state (confirmed by psychiatric review) and adequate social circumstances.

Management of patients who present more than 24h after ingestion

- Measure the plasma paracetamol concentration together with the INR, ALT, glucose, U&Es, creatinine, LFTs and venous bicarbonate.
- Start IV NAC immediately in all patients who have taken an overdose of paracetamol within the last 36 h (as recommended by the British National Formulary), unless convinced that a significant amount (>150 mg/kg or total 12 g) has not been ingested.

- Arrange admission or referral if a significant ingestion is thought to have occurred. All patients with abnormal clotting or liver enzymes or renal function require admission and monitoring and should be discussed with a specialist liver unit or the National Poisons Information Service. An infusion of NAC may still be recommended for some of these patients.

Management of patients who ingest a significant amount of paracetamol over a short period of time, as opposed to a single ingestion (staggered overdose)

Staggered overdose of paracetamol is particularly difficult to assess and treat. The paracetamol treatment graph relates to a single acute ingestion rather than ingestion over a period of time.

- Measure the plasma paracetamol concentration, but accept that it is very difficult to interpret.
- These high-risk patients should all be considered for treatment with NAC. They should be discharged only if they are asymptomatic and the INR, ALT and creatinine are normal at 24h after the last dose of paracetamol.
- In patients who have ingested the paracetamol over <12h, the plasma paracetamol concentration should be measured again 4h later. If the second level is more than half the first level, then a significant overdose is likely to have occurred.

Aspirin

Aspirin poisoning is now relatively uncommon. The main features of salicylate toxicity are:

- hyperventilation
- tinnitus and deafness
- vasodilatation
- sweating
- hypoglycaemia (especially in children).

In severe poisoning, convulsions and coma may occur and complex acid–base disturbances are inevitable. Initial stimulation of the respiratory centre causes a respiratory alkalosis. As more of the drug is absorbed, a metabolic acidosis supervenes. In between these two phases there may be a transitory period with a relatively normal blood gas picture.

Tx
- Plasma salicylate concentration must be measured in all patients in whom analgesic poisoning is suspected. It is usually measured with the plasma

paracetamol level 4h after ingestion. Peak levels may not be reached, however, for at least 6h. U&Es, glucose and blood gases must also be measured.
- It is worth attempting to decontaminate the stomach with charcoal for up to 8h after ingestion as salicylates markedly delay gastric emptying.

> 'It is never too late for salicylate.'

- Repeated doses of charcoal may also be useful.
- Intravenous fluid should be administered.
- Forced alkaline diuresis (with sodium bicarbonate 1.26% → *p. 252*) should be considered in cases of significant poisoning, i.e. when the plasma salicylate concentration is:
  >500 mg/L (3.6 mmol/L) in adults
  >350 mg/L (2.5 mmol/L) in children.
- Haemodialysis may be required if the plasma salicylate concentration is >700 mg/L (5.1 mmol/L) or in the presence of a severe metabolic acidosis.

Ibuprofen, mefenamic acid and other NSAIDs

Ibuprofen is of low toxicity; poisoning with <100 mg/kg does not require any treatment. Ingestions in excess of 400 mg/kg will cause symptoms including nausea, vomiting and epigastric pain. Diarrhoea, GI bleeding, headache and tinnitus may also occur, but more severe toxicity (convulsions, central nervous system [CNS] depression and metabolic acidosis) is very uncommon. The half-life of ibuprofen in overdosage is 2–3h.

Mefenamic acid is the most dangerous non-steroidal anti-inflammatory drug (NSAID) when taken in overdosage. It may cause convulsions.

Tx
Ibuprofen and mefenamic acid: treatment with activated charcoal is indicated if ibuprofen >100 mg/kg has been taken within the preceding hour (or longer for sustained-release preparations). All patients who have ingested in excess of this amount will require observation for at least 4h and monitoring of plasma electrolytes. A good urine output must be maintained.

Activated charcoal effectively absorbs mefenamic acid and should be considered for all patients, even when only small amounts of the drug have been ingested. Observation and monitoring of plasma electrolytes should be arranged.

Other NSAIDs:
- Ascertain the time and amount of the ingestion.
- Seek specific information concerning the toxicity and treatment of poisoning with that drug.
- Consider the need for gastric decontamination.
- Consider admission for observation and supportive therapy.

Salbutamol

This β_2-receptor agonist causes predictable adrenergic side effects:

- Tremor
- Tachycardia
- Agitation and headache
- Hypokalaemia.

Tx
- Consider activated charcoal for all patients, especially if a controlled-release preparation has been taken.
- Monitor the heart rate, BP and ECG continuously.
- Measure the U&Es and glucose.
- Consider specific therapy with a cardioselective β blocker. This would probably be contraindicated in patients with a history of bronchospasm.
- Admit for observation and monitoring.

β Blockers

The effects of poisoning vary considerably according to the specific drug. Sotalol in particular, may cause bizarre dysrhythmias (*For torsade de pointes and prolongation of the Q–T interval by sotalol → p. 173*). In overdosage, most β blockers can cause:

- severe bronchospasm
- bradycardia, hypotension and syncope
- heart failure
- coma and convulsions (especially with propranolol).

Tx
- Apply supportive measures.
- Consider activated charcoal in recent ingestions and for modified-release preparations (repeated doses for sotalol in particular).
- Give nebulised salbutamol for wheezing.
- Administer IV atropine for bradycardia and hypotension (up to 3 mg for an adult and 40 mg/kg for a child).
- Give IV glucagon for hypotension refractory to atropine (boluses of 2 mg, up to a maximum of 10 mg for an adult; 50–150 mcg/kg for a child).
- Give IV dobutamine for severe cardiac depression or an infusion of isoprenaline for resistant bradycardia.

- Establish transvenous pacing for intractable bradycardia.

Calcium channel blockers

Poisoning with calcium channel blockers causes nausea, vomiting, dizziness, confusion and coma. Metabolic acidosis and hypoglycaemia can occur. Depending on the exact drug, hypotension may be primarily due to cardiac depression (verapamil and diltiazem) or profound vasodilatation (nifedipine), although the selectivity of calcium antagonists tends to disappear on overdosage.

Tx Activated charcoal is effective if given within 1 h of ingestion or after modified-release preparations (when repeated doses may also be considered). IV calcium may be used in severe poisoning → *p. 249*. For symptomatic bradycardias and hypotension, atropine and inotropes are indicated. An insulin and glucose infusion may be used in the management of severe hypotension and myocardial failure.

Tricyclic and related antidepressants

Poisoning with tricyclic antidepressants (TCAs) is dangerous and common, being implicated in over a fifth of all fatal ingestions. Dosulepin is the most common drug involved. Some of the newer cyclic antidepressants – with different ring structures – seem less toxic. Ingested amounts are usually significant because the patient who needs TCAs will often have a mental state compatible with suicide. One in 40 patients who overdoses on TCAs will die. An ingestion of 35 mg/kg is the median lethal dose for an adult.

The effects of TCAs are largely related to their anticholinergic activity and so include peripheral effects such as:

- blurred vision and dry mouth
- dilated pupils
- urinary retention
- diverse GI symptoms
- tachycardia and dysrhythmias

and central effects such as:

- agitation and anxiety
- hyperactivity
- disorientation and confusion
- drowsiness and lethargy
- hallucinations
- nystagmus, dysarthria, ataxia and movement disorders

- hyperreflexia and extensor plantar response
- hyperthermia or hypothermia.

However, the most serious features are probably unrelated to anticholinergic activity:

1 *Coma*: a Glasgow Coma Scale (GCS) score of ≤8 occurs in about a third of cases but rarely lasts more than 24 h. Comatose patients are likely to develop complications.
2 *Convulsions*: these are associated with severe toxicity, hypoxia and metabolic acidosis. They occur in up to 20% of patients.
3 *Cardiorespiratory collapse*: hypotension or cardiac dysrhythmias may occur. The latter are the most common cause of death. Tachycardia (rate >120 beats/min) is worrying, especially with ECG change. Prolongation of the QRS complex >100 ms suggests cardiotoxicity. A QRS duration of >160 ms (four small squares) is associated with a very high risk of life-threatening dysrhythmia.

Tx This depends very much on the time of ingestion and the condition of the patient. Serious complications occur within 12 h of ingestion. Rapid deterioration may occur. Most patients will require the following:

- Gastric decontamination (worthwhile for up to 8 h after ingestion – little absorption of TCAs takes place in the stomach). The administration of activated charcoal may be repeated because charcoal prevents absorption in the small intestine
- A 12-lead ECG
- Referral for monitoring and observation.

Agitation or convulsions should be controlled with IV benzodiazepines.

Patients with a significantly depressed level of consciousness or fitting also require:

- airway protection
- high-concentration oxygen
- blood gas analysis
- monitoring
- anaesthetic advice and a consideration of the need for paralysis and ventilation (this may need to be accompanied by an infusion of thiopental to control fits)
- intensive care unit (ICU) admission.

Cardiovascular complications should be treated by alkalisation (→ *later*). Antidysrhythmic drugs are best avoided in TCA poisoning because conduction deficits may make the ECG difficult to interpret. Moreover, some of these drugs will produce a synergistic cardiotoxicity. Torsade de pointes should be treated with magnesium (→ *p. 250*). Mild hypotension usually responds to IV fluids; for more severe hypotension alkalisation is appropriate.

Alkali therapy for TCA poisoning: induction of an alkalosis with IV sodium bicarbonate reduces mortality in TCA poisoning. The mechanism of action is not fully understood but is related to protein binding of the TCA and the movements of ions into the heart. The benefits of alkalisation are seen not only in patients who are acidotic – those with a minimal or absent base deficit also show improvement. Suggested indications for bicarbonate in TCA-poisoned patients are:

- systemic acidosis
- QRS duration of >120 ms
- ventricular dysrhythmia
- hypotension
- cardiac arrest.

The aim of therapy is to maintain a pH of between 7.50 and 7.55. The initial dose of bicarbonate can be up to 1–2 mmol/kg; further doses will depend on the clinical picture. Hyperventilation can be used as an adjunct to the bicarbonate to help achieve the desired pH.

Bicarbonate therapy (general information) → *p. 252*.

Selective serotonin reuptake inhibitors

Selective serotonin reuptake inhibitor (SSRI)-type drugs inhibit the reuptake of serotonin (5-hydroxytryptamine or 5HT). Some related compounds (serotonin–noradrenaline reuptake inhibitors or SNRIs) also inhibit the reuptake of noradrenaline. These drugs are widely prescribed for the treatment of depression and consequently self-poisoning with them is common. SSRIs in overdose cause:

- sweating and dizziness
- drowsiness, convulsions and coma
- tachycardia, hypotension or hypertension (prolongation of the Q–T interval and the QRS complex may also occur with consequent ventricular dysrhythmias; torsade de pointes is a particular risk → *p. 173*).

Tx Activated charcoal may be given if a significant amount of an SSRI has been ingested within the previous hour. Observation for at least 6 h is indicated. Otherwise, treatment is supportive.

Serotonin syndrome (which may be a feature of SSRI poisoning) → *p. 301*.

Table 15.1 Therapeutic and toxic levels of common drugs

Drug	Lower level (mg/L)	Upper level (mg/L)	Possible toxicity (mg/L)	Severe toxicity (mg/L)
Theophylline	10	20	20	60
Phenytoin	8	15	20	40
Carbamazepine	4	10	25	40

Theophylline

Large doses of slow-release theophylline preparations may be taken intentionally. They cause:

- severe and intractable vomiting
- agitation and restlessness
- dilated pupils
- tachycardia and tachydysrhythmias
- convulsions
- haematemesis
- hyperglycaemia and hypokalaemia.

Tx
- Consider gastric lavage within 2 h of ingestion and give repeated doses of activated charcoal.
- Administer potassium, anticonvulsants, sedatives and other supportive treatment as indicated.
- Intravenous propranolol may be considered in patients who are not asthmatic to reverse tachycardia, hypokalaemia and hyperglycaemia.
- Large clumps of drug in matrix may require endoscopic removal.

Plasma levels → Table 15.1

Lithium

Lithium toxicity may occur as a complication of long-term therapy or after a deliberate ingestion. Dehydration and infection may precipitate a crisis by reducing renal excretion of the drug. The symptoms of acute overdosage of lithium may be delayed for 12 h or more. Initially, there is lethargy and restlessness and later the patient may have:

- diarrhoea and vomiting
- thirst and polyuria
- ataxia and dysarthria
- muscle weakness, twitching and tremor
- convulsions and coma
- dehydration and hypotension
- renal failure and electrolyte imbalance.

Tx The serum lithium should be measured. Therapeutic concentrations are within the range 0.4–1.0 mmol/L; concentrations in excess of 2.0 mmol/L may be associated with serious toxicity. Forced diuresis is often advocated. Haemodialysis is required in the presence of renal failure. Otherwise, treatment is supportive with special regard to electrolyte imbalance and renal function. Activated charcoal is ineffective.

Phenytoin

The average lethal dose for adults is between 2 and 5 g but there is a marked variation among individuals with respect to the toxic effects of a given serum level of phenytoin. The initial symptoms are nystagmus, ataxia and dysarthria but later on there may be:

- coma
- fixed pupils
- hypotension
- respiratory depression.

Tx Activated charcoal should be given; repeated doses are sometimes advised. Subsequent treatment is supportive and symptomatic.

Plasma levels → Table 15.1

Carbamazepine

Overdose may cause:

- tremor and excitation
- convulsions
- impairment of consciousness and coma
- hypotension or sometimes hypertension
- cardiac dysrhythmias.

Tx Activated charcoal should be given; repeated doses are indicated, especially if a slow-release preparation has been taken. Subsequent treatment is supportive and symptomatic.

Plasma levels → Table 15.1

Benzodiazepines and related minor tranquillisers

Self-poisoning with prescribed (or illicit) minor tranquillisers is common but hardly ever fatal. They are often taken together with alcohol, which leads to a synergistic effect. Benzodiazepines exert their action on specific BZ receptors, which are closely associated with γ-aminobutyric acid (GABA) receptors. GABA is an inhibitory neurotransmitter that is widely distributed throughout the brain and spinal cord. Potentiation of GABA transmission thus causes a generalised depression of CNS activity and results in:

- reduced level of consciousness
- flaccidity
- ataxia and dysarthria
- hypotension
- hypothermia.

Poisoning with non-benzodiazepine hypnotics such as zopiclone, which also act at the benzodiazepine receptor, is similar in both effects and treatment.

Tx Supportive therapy and observation.

Comparative doses and half-lives of benzodiazepines → Table 15.2.

Flumazenil: This is a specific benzodiazepine antagonist that:

- wears off sooner than most oral ingestions of benzodiazepines
- may precipitate fitting if TCAs have also been taken and so should never be used in poisoning with unknown or mixed substances

- may partially reverse hepatic coma
- can occasionally be useful as a diagnostic tool.

It is given as a bolus of 200 mg (2 mL) by slow IV injection and then repeated doses of 100 mg (1 mL) after 1-min intervals, depending on effect. Infusion of 100–400 mg/h may sometimes be required.

Barbiturates

Barbiturates are now infrequently prescribed, so poisoning with them is much less common than in the past. Findings include:

- depressed level of consciousness
- respiratory depression
- hypotension
- hypothermia
- palmar and plantar blistering.

Tx Supportive therapy and administration of activated charcoal are appropriate. Repeated doses of charcoal may increase drug elimination, especially of phenobarbital. Forced alkaline diuresis and charcoal haemoperfusion may be necessary.

Phenothiazines and other major tranquillisers

These drugs cause:

- drowsiness and confusion
- hypotension
- hypothermia
- sinus tachycardia and cardiac dysrhythmias, (especially with thioridazine)
- convulsions and coma (with large doses).

There is often less depression of consciousness and respiration than is seen with other sedatives. Extrapyramidal effects including acute dystonic reactions may occur but are not dose related. Neuroleptic malignant syndrome, although related to long-term use of major tranquillisers, is not usually a feature of poisoning → p. 300.

Tx Activated charcoal should be given to all patients who present within 1 h of ingestion of a potentially toxic amount. Otherwise treatment is supportive. Fluids and dobutamine can be used to treat severe hypotension. Convulsions respond to lorazepam. Symptomatic patients should be monitored (including ECG) for at least 4 h.

Table 15.2 Comparison of different benzodiazepines

Drug	Half-life (h)	Equivalent dose (mg)
Diazepam	20–50	5
Chlordiazepoxide	6–30	15
Nitrazepam	24	5
Lorazepam	12	0.5
Temazepam	8	10
Oxazepam	6–8	15

POISONING WITH DRUGS OF ABUSE

Misuse of Drugs Act 1971 and the Misuse of Drugs Regulations 2001 → p. 374.
Poisoning with barbiturates → p. 281.
Poisoning with minor tranquillisers → p. 281.

Narcotic analgesics (opioids)

Opioid poisoning occurs by both oral and parenteral routes. If a combination analgesic has been taken, narcotic effects may accompany paracetamol poisoning (→ p. 272). Signs of acute poisoning with opioids include:

- a depressed level of consciousness
- respiratory depression (usually the respiratory rate is most affected)
- pinpoint pupils.

Methadone and dextropropoxyphene have particularly long durations of action. Codeine (methylmorphine) and dihydrocodeine are changed in the body to their active metabolite morphine and thus may also have a prolonged course in overdosage. The effect of naloxone can be used as a diagnostic test in cases of suspected acute opioid poisoning.

Tx Emergency treatment involves naloxone therapy in variable amounts (and sometimes by IV infusion), support of vital functions and close observation. The initial dose of IV naloxone for adults is 400–2000 mcg, repeated at 2- to 3-min intervals as required. For children 10 mcg/kg should be given, increased to 100 mcg/kg if the desired improvement is not seen with the first dose. *For a suggested approach to a patient with an overdose of IV opioids → Box 15.6.*
Withdrawal from opioid drugs is rarely as traumatic as is popularly believed. Most patients should be referred to a specialised treatment and counselling facility. Prescription of substitute opioids is best left to such agencies.

Withdrawal from opioid drugs → p. 366.

> If a vein cannot be found, naloxone may be given via the intraosseous route.

Stimulant drugs

The abuse of stimulant drugs is on the increase (for supposed enhancement of academic performance as

Box 15.6 Management of heroin overdose

- Attend to the ABCs; assisted ventilation with a bag and mask is often required
- Draw up two ampoules of naloxone (800 mcg) in a 2-mL syringe
- Insert an IV cannula; this may be difficult. Often only a tiny spidery vein is available. Enter this vein with an orange (25 G) needle attached to the syringe of naloxone
- Inject the naloxone, ensuring that it is not extravasated
- Inject a further 800 mcg naloxone intramuscularly to sustain the blood levels. This is very important
- Continue ventilatory support until recovery occurs
- Once the patient is alert and oriented, discuss the further management options with him or her

Do not forget to check the blood sugar as hypoglycaemia is a good mimic of this condition.

well as recreational usage). Amfetamine is used as the basis for several more potent variants (e.g. ecstasy → p. 283). Patients present with varying degrees of:

- wakefulness and hyperactivity
- agitation and confusion
- paranoia and hallucinations
- hypertension and dysrhythmias
- convulsions
- exhaustion and coma
- sweating and hyperthermia.

Later on, in extreme cases, gross electrolyte disturbance, rhabdomyolysis, disseminated intravascular coagulation (DIC) and multisystem failure may occur. Sometimes, just one tablet can provoke an idiosyncratic life-threatening hyperthermia.

Tx This mainly consists of supportive therapy:

- Give oxygen.
- Start vigorous IV rehydration.
- Consider giving activated charcoal in recent ingestions.
- Give sedatives and anticonvulsants (e.g. lorazepam or diazepam) as necessary.
- Summon anaesthetic help early on.
- Measure the core temperature continuously.

- Start active cooling if indicated ($\rightarrow$ *p. 271*).
- Consider the need for paralysis and ventilation and/or ICU care.
- Measure the U&Es, glucose and blood gases.
- Consider giving bicarbonate for metabolic acidosis.
- Monitor the urine output.
- Consider the use of nifedipine (5–10 mg by mouth) for hypertension and β blockers for tachycardias (do not use β blockers if cocaine may be involved).
- Consider the need for dantrolene therapy $\rightarrow$ *p. 271*.
- Consider forced acid diuresis to increase excretion.

Extreme mental disturbance secondary to stimulant drugs: The diagnosis is not usually difficult – the patient is violent, agitated and confused. The patient should be restrained and sedated for the safety of both him- or herself and others and can then be examined properly. This kind of immediate sedation presents no special legal problems ($\rightarrow$ *p. 377*).

MDMA ('ecstasy')

> At least 16 compounds related to MDMA are available on the illicit market. These include its 'sister' drug MDEA (methylenedioxyethamfetamine or 'Eve') and their common metabolite MDA (methylenedioxyamfetamine or 'Ice').

Methylenedioxymethamfetamine (MDMA, 'ecstasy', 'Adam') is a semi-synthetic drug that is sold in single tablets containing 30–150 mg of active substance. It causes increased levels of serotonin, dopamine and noradrenaline in the CNS. Effects occur within 1 h and last for 4–6 h after 75 mg and up to 48 h with higher doses. The half-life of MDMA is 7.6 h. *For clinical features that are suggestive of MDMA usage $\rightarrow$ Box 15.7.* Ecstasy gives the user a tremendous feeling of energy and vitality, is mildly hallucinogenic, and can engender feelings of peace, love and sensuality. Unfortunately, it is much more dangerous than cannabis, its 1960s' predecessor. At moderate doses (75–100 mg) it causes the following:

- Mild mental changes as described above
- Variable autonomic upset (dilated pupils, dry mouth, tachycardia and hypertension); these may be influenced by the degree of dehydration
- An increase in muscle tone, sometimes with myalgia
- A partial failure of temperature homeostasis; when this is combined with excessive dancing in a hot,

> **Box 15.7 Features suggestive of MDMA poisoning ('ecstasy' usage)**
>
> - History of ingestion or likely circumstances from user and friends
> - Fever, sometimes with absence of perspiration
> - Mydriasis (dilated pupils)
> - Dry mouth and throat
> - Bruxism (tightening of the jaw muscles)
> - Tachycardia and hypertension (hypotension in some cases)
> - Fits, confusion, mania, headaches, ataxia or nystagmus
> - Unexplained pains
> - Coma or sudden collapse

dry atmosphere with a low fluid intake, simple heat-stroke-type collapse may occur ($\rightarrow$ *p. 246*).

At higher doses, panic attacks and psychosis may appear. Severe and even fatal idiopathic reactions can follow the ingestion of amounts that were previously tolerated. These dramatic, but rare, events seem to be an idiosyncratic reaction related to the neuroleptic malignant syndrome ($\rightarrow$ *p. 300*). There is hyperpyrexia, coma, convulsions and circulatory collapse. Rhabdomyolysis, renal failure and DIC may occur. MDMA may also trigger the serotonin syndrome ($\rightarrow$ *p. 301*). It must be remembered that similar, unidentified or impure drugs may corrupt the clinical picture described above, as may self-induced water intoxication.

Tx Rehydration and observation is the mainstay of treatment for mild cases. Activated charcoal may be given for recent ingestions. *For severe features, $\rightarrow$ treatment of poisoning with stimulant drugs on p. 282.* 5HT agonists (e.g. cyproheptadine) may be useful.

Mephedrone and other cathinones

A new generation of stimulant drugs has recently been synthesised by underground chemists in order to capitalise on the internet market for 'legal highs'. Cathinones are ketoamfetamines and have very similar effects to standard amfetamines and MDMA: they cause the same overstimulation of the CNS and sympathetic nervous system. Cathinone itself is a naturally occurring alkaloid found in the leaves of the khat plant. Mephedrone (4-methylmethcathinone), the most readily available of these new substances, is sold as a whitish powder and is usually snorted or swallowed. It is now classified as a class B drug (→ p. 374). Its euphoric effects last for only 1 or 2 h, so there is a tendency for users to take repeated doses. Mild cases of mephedrone poisoning can be treated with fluids and observation.

MDMA (ecstasy) poisoning → p. 283.
Severe poisoning with stimulant drugs → p. 282.

Cocaine and 'crack'

The plant alkaloid cocaine and its more potent, free base form, 'crack', are increasingly abused by smoking, sniffing or injection. They are reuptake inhibitors of dopamine, noradrenaline and serotonin. The resulting CNS stimulation causes:

- agitation and hallucinations
- dilated pupils
- tachycardia and hypertension
- hyperthermia
- hypertonia and hyperreflexia
- convulsions and coma.

There may be a metabolic acidosis and chest pain (caused by coronary vasospasm) often occurs. It may lead to dysrhythmias and even myocardial infarction.

Tx
- Give supportive therapy (oxygen, rehydration and cooling measures).
- Consider sedation with IV benzodiazepines.
- Treat chest pain with analgesia and nitrates. Calcium antagonists may be helpful.
- In the presence of ECG changes, initiate appropriate therapy for an acute coronary syndrome → p. 177.

> Do not use β blockers as they may cause worsening of the hypertension because of unopposed α-receptor stimulation.

Cocaethylene

This substance is produced by the liver when cocaine and alcohol have been taken simultaneously – a transesterification process that is catalysed by carboxyl esterases. Cocaine (or cocamethylene) is the methyl ester of benzoylecgonine and cocaethylene is

the corresponding ethyl ester. Cocaethylene is not found in coca leaves but causes a more euphoric and longer-lasting stimulation than its naturally occurring relative. It is also more toxic to the cardiovascular system. Treatment of cocaethylene poisoning is identical to that of cocaine toxicity; it should be suspected when there is evidence of both alcohol and cocaine usage.

Gamma-hydroxybutyrate

Gamma-hydroxybutyrate (GHB) is a potent CNS sedative that is easily synthesised and then sold in clubs. Several precursor drugs (such as 1,4-butanediol or pine needle oil) are metabolised in the body to GHB and so may also be used for the same effect. GHB may cause a rapid onset of coma and respiratory depression such that 10% of patients presenting to an ED after its ingestion require endotracheal intubation. Concurrent ethanol usage exacerbates its effects. Treatment is largely supportive. One of the hallmarks of GHB intoxication is a rapid recovery to full consciousness after profound coma.

Ketamine and phencyclidine

Ketamine ('Special K') and phencyclidine (PCP) are also encountered as drugs of abuse. They cause a variable depression of consciousness and dissociative behaviour. Trance-like staring may occur with hallucinations and agitation. The diagnostic ocular finding is rotatory nystagmus. Treatment is supportive.

Lysergic acid diethylamide (LSD)

The potent hallucinogen lysergic acid diethylamide (LSD) causes excitement and euphoria before agitation, tachycardia and vivid visual hallucinations. Extreme dysphoria and bizarre behaviour may require sedation. A similar condition may be seen in people who have eaten bread made with grain (principally rye) contaminated with the fungus *Claviceps purpurea* (which produces ergot alkaloids related to LSD). Outbreaks of collective madness (known in the Middle Ages as 'St Anthony's fire') have occurred in villages and on cruise ships where contaminated bread has been distributed. Treatment is symptomatic.

Cannabis (marijuana or Indian hemp)

Patients may present to an ED who are intoxicated with tetrahydrocannabinols, the active substances in cannabis resin. They are usually mildly disoriented; on rare occasions a frank psychosis is seen. No specific therapy is indicated.

Mushroom poisoning

Patients may accidentally or deliberately eat poisonous fungi.

Death cap mushrooms (*Amanita phalloides*) are the most dangerous fungi in the British Isles. They contain phallotoxins and amatoxins. Several hours after ingestion there is abdominal pain, vomiting and continuous diarrhoea. Renal and hepatic failure may follow in 2–3 days with death within a week.

'Magic mushrooms' contain the hallucinogens psilocybin and psilocin which can cause an organic psychosis. Disturbed patients may require sedation with diazepam or lorazepam followed by close observation.

Solvent abuse

This was originally described as 'glue sniffing' in teenagers; toluene is the usual solvent in glue but benzene and xylene are found in plastic cement. However, the sensations of early anaesthesia can be obtained from most inhalable organic materials and so many products have abuse potential. Lighter fuel (butane) appears to be one of the most dangerous because sudden death may result from a cardiac dysrhythmia. Solvent abuse usually causes no symptoms or signs after the initial effects but should always be considered in young people with bizarre behaviour or collapse. There may sometimes be:

- euphoria and 'drunkenness'
- headache
- nausea and vomiting
- dizziness and ataxia
- fits
- cardiac dysrhythmias, which are precipitated by a mixture of cardiac irritation, hypoxia and hypercapnia.

Chronic abusers may also have:

- sores around the nose and mouth
- signs of bone marrow suppression
- encephalopathy.

Tx
- Give high-concentration oxygen.
- Establish ECG monitoring.
- Obtain blood gas analysis.
- Request an FBC.
- Refer for observation and follow-up.

It is tempting to ask why people seek the disordered sensations of cerebral poisoning. The questioner should remember that there are whole industries, both legal and illegal, devoted to providing human beings with strange sensations – the fairground and distilling industries, for example. Every civilisation sets its own standards of acceptable behaviour. The emergency physician must not let these social and legal codes influence management or attitudes to care.

Alcohol (ethanol)

The world's favourite poison is freely available in most societies and is associated with many social problems (→ *Chapter 20*). It is frequently taken as a component of self-poisoning. In acute ingestions there may be a combination of signs such as:

- a smell of alcoholic beverage on the breath
- red, injected conjunctivae
- loss of inhibition and judgement
- aggression and excitability
- ataxia and slurred speech
- depression of consciousness.

There may also be:

- hypoglycaemia – seen in children and adult patients with poor liver glycogen reserves
- fluid depletion – in severe poisoning
- a loss of airway protection – with a risk of aspiration
- coexisting head injuries – especially subdural haematoma (→ *p. 44*).

Ethyl alcohol is metabolised in the liver to carbon dioxide and water via acetaldehyde and acetate. This breakdown normally occurs at a constant rate (about 10–15 g/h) irrespective of the amount of alcohol present in the body (zero-order kinetics). Above a level of about 100 mg/dL, liver metabolism is unable to cope and further alcohol intake may cause a very rapid increase in blood concentrations. Similarly, at very high blood levels (probably >300 mg/dL) alcohol concentration decreases more quickly than can be explained by zero-order kinetics alone.

Tx Several substances have been shown to hasten the recovery from alcohol intoxication:

- *Insulin*: speeds up the catabolic process
- *Fructose (laevulose), galactose and sorbitol*: these substances may precipitate lactic acidosis, especially in the presence of hypovolaemia
- *Naloxone*: inconclusive
- *IV fluids*.

The risk is greater than the benefit with all these therapies, except in the case of IV fluids. Isotonic saline should therefore be given (at least 10–20 mL/kg in the first hour if not contraindicated). Further treatment consists of supportive measures and a consideration of other injuries. The blood sugar should be measured routinely in all patients thought to be drunk.

> In a patient with a depressed level of consciousness thought to be caused by alcohol, a CT scan of the brain is indicated if a GCS score of 15 is not reached within about 6–8 h of arrival.

Box 15.8 Management of the aggressive drunk patient

- Observe the patient carefully
- Enquire about the possibility of trauma from the patient and any bystanders
- Examine the patient as fully as possible but without risk to yourself. Try especially to feel the head for cuts or swellings
- Measure blood sugar
- Get senior help. Options for further management include:
  - sedate the patient and observe in hospital
  - let the patient go home with friends or relatives, to whom are given verbal and written head injury instructions
  - let the patient go to a police cell, verbal and written head injury instructions being given to the police

Measurement of blood alcohol: Level of consciousness bears little relationship to initial blood alcohol level. However, it is unusual for a blood alcohol concentration <200 mg/dL to cause depression of consciousness. Coma generally occurs with alcohol levels >300 mg/dL. Serial measurements of blood alcohol show that the concentration of alcohol in the blood often increases for the first 2 h after presentation. The explanation for this phenomenon is that alcohol is continuing to be absorbed from the gastrointestinal (GI) tract at a rate that exceeds its metabolism in the body. Gastric lavage may be useful in unresponsive patients to prevent this continuing absorption of alcohol.

Alcohol withdrawal states → p. 360.
Management of the aggressive, intoxicated patient → Box 15.8.
Medicolegal aspects of alcohol abuse (including driving) → p. 374.

POISONING WITH SUBSTANCES FOUND AT HOME AND AT WORK

Iron

Iron poisoning is most common in children aged <5 years and so is usually accidental. The toxicity of iron may be underestimated by both parents and medical staff.

In normal circumstances, iron is absorbed by the mucosal cells of the duodenum and jejunum and transported in the blood bound to transferrin. After an acute overdose, the intestinal barrier is overwhelmed and the transferrin is saturated. Unbound iron then causes cardiovascular, hepatic, CNS and metabolic damage.

Oral iron preparations are ferrous salts and contain differing amounts of elemental iron (e.g. 200 mg ferrous sulphate contains 60 mg pure iron). Toxicity is dependent on the amount of elemental iron ingested:

- <30 mg/kg causes mild toxicity
- >30 mg/kg causes moderate toxicity
- >60 mg/kg causes severe toxicity
- >150 mg/kg is potentially lethal.

The early features of iron poisoning, which occur at 1–6 h post-ingestion, result from corrosive damage and haemodynamic effects (vascular dilatation and capillary leakage). There may be:

- nausea and vomiting (vomitus may have a metallic odour)
- abdominal pain and diarrhoea
- haematemesis and rectal bleeding
- hypovolaemia, hypoxia, acidosis and collapse.

Drowsiness, coma and convulsions may also occur; signs of gastric and jejunal perforation are a possibility.

A relatively quiescent phase then follows. This lasts for 6–12 h, after which there is either a recovery or a further exacerbation of symptoms. These later effects are mostly the result of intracellular poisoning and include:

- coma and convulsions
- circulatory collapse and pulmonary oedema
- profound metabolic acidosis
- liver failure with hypoglycaemia and coagulopathy
- renal failure
- further GI haemorrhage.

Delayed sequelae, after at least 2 weeks, include stricture formation, pyloric stenosis and small bowel obstruction.

Investigations: Patients who have ingested <30 mg/kg of elemental iron will not require either investigations or active treatment. In those who have taken in excess of this amount:

- An abdominal radiograph should be obtained in order to determine the need for GI decontamination and the site to target.
- The serum iron must be measured to determine the need for chelation therapy → *later*.
- FBC, electrolytes and glucose should be requested.

Patients with severe symptoms will also require LFTs, clotting studies, blood gases and ECG. Measurement of total iron-binding capacity (TIBC) is of little value. Raised white cell count and blood sugar are typical findings.

The serum iron should be measured 4 h post-ingestion or immediately before desferrioxamine administration. Levels taken later than 6 h post-ingestion may underestimate the amount of free iron because of tissue uptake. If slow-release tablets have been taken, the serum iron should be rechecked after 4 h. Patients who present late and have low iron levels must be regarded as at high risk of toxicity.

The anticipated effect of the measured serum iron concentration must be interpreted in conjunction with the history and clinical findings:

- >20 mcmol/L (>110 mcg/dL) – mild toxicity
- >55 mcmol/L (>300 mcg/dL) – moderate toxicity
- >90 mcmol/L (>500 mcg/dL) – severe toxicity
- >180 mcmol/L (>1000 mcg/dL) – extreme toxicity.

The advice of a chemical pathologist should be sought as soon as possible.

Tx Patients who have ingested <30 mg/kg of elemental iron do not require either investigations or active treatment.

Tablets that are visible on a radiograph must be removed from the stomach by lavage or endoscopy.

Iron tablets beyond the pylorus are an indication for whole-bowel irrigation or even surgical removal. Whole-bowel cleansing may be performed with polyethylene glycol electrolyte solution (Klean-Prep). The dose is 15–40 mL/kg per h given orally until the rectal effluent runs clear (maximum 6–8 h). Repeat radiographs must be obtained in all cases requiring decontamination to confirm a satisfactory result.

Dissolved tablets are not radio-opaque. Patients who have ingested a significant amount of iron, which is not visible on radiograph, should be treated with emesis or lavage (with 1% sodium bicarbonate solution, if possible). Activated charcoal is not indicated because it does not bind iron.

Subsequent management depends on the clinical findings and serum concentrations of iron. All patients should be rehydrated with care; fluid balance must be recorded. Patients with serum iron levels <55 mcmol/L can be managed at home. Those with serum iron concentrations of 55–90 mcmol/L and minimal symptoms should be observed in hospital for 48 h.

Parenteral desferrioxamine chelates free iron and the resulting complex is excreted in the urine, which then turns pink. It should be given to all patients with:

- serum iron concentrations in excess of 90 mcmol/L
- cardiovascular symptoms
- CNS symptoms
- significant GI haemorrhage.

The dose of IV desferrioxamine is 15 mg/kg per h up to a maximum of 80 mg/kg in 24 h. It may cause hypotension. A successful outcome is heralded by cessation of symptoms, return of normal urine colour and low serum iron (<18 mcmol/L). Oral or intramuscular (IM) desferrioxamine is no longer recommended.

All patients with significant iron poisoning must be followed up for 6 weeks because of the risk of stricture formation.

Vitamins

These are not harmful in an isolated acute ingestion but the estimated amount taken should be checked against known poisons information. Some compound preparations may contain iron and other substances.

Oral contraceptives

These are not harmful although nausea and vomiting may occur. Female patients should be warned about the slight possibility of withdrawal bleeding.

Methanol and glycols

Substances such as methanol (methyl alcohol or wood alcohol) and ethylene glycol (antifreeze) cause drunkenness in the early stages followed by a severe metabolic acidosis as toxic metabolites are formed in the liver.

> Methylated spirits and surgical spirits contain 95% ethanol; car antifreeze contains 95% ethylene glycol.

Although comparatively rare, this type of poisoning should be suspected in the following circumstances:

- There is a distinct latent period between ingestion and the development of toxic features.
- There is an unexplained metabolic acidosis (or hyperventilation).
- There is an inexplicably raised anion or osmolar gap (with a normal serum chloride).

Ethylene glycol

Ethylene glycol (also known as 1,2-ethanediol or glycol alcohol) is a dihydroxy-alcohol derivative of the aliphatic hydrocarbons that is essentially non-toxic. However, its hepatic metabolites, glycolate and oxalate, cause extensive cellular damage to various tissues, especially the kidneys. The lethal dose of ethylene glycol is around 1.5 mL/kg (about 100 mL in an average adult) but as little as 30 mL may sometimes prove fatal. It is rapidly absorbed from the GI tract, reaching peak blood concentrations between 1 and 4 h after ingestion. Approximately 80% of ethylene glycol is metabolised in the liver and 20% is excreted unchanged by the kidneys. The elimination half-life of ethylene glycol is approximately 3 h but this is prolonged to around 18 h after inhibition of alcohol dehydrogenase.

Three stages of ethylene glycol poisoning are classically described: a neurological stage, followed by a cardiopulmonary stage and, finally, a renal stage. In many cases, however, there is a considerable overlap between these three phases:

1 *Neurological features (1–12 h after ingestion):* symptoms similar to those of ethanol intoxication may be observed. Nausea and vomiting can occur. As metabolism progresses, acidosis and CNS features are seen. The latter include hypotonia, hyporeflexia, nystagmus, ataxia, ophthalmoplegia, myoclonic jerks, seizures, meningism and coma. In most cases of ethylene glycol poisoning, the optic fundus is normal; however, in some situations, the presence of papilloedema may mimic methanol poisoning.

2 *Cardiopulmonary features (12–24 h after ingestion):* tachycardia and mild hypertension frequently occur. In serious cases, severe metabolic acidosis with compensatory hyperventilation can develop, accompanied by multiple organ failure. Most deaths occur in this stage.

3 *Renal features (24–72 h after ingestion):* the symptoms of the third stage can include oliguria, flank pain, acute tubular necrosis, renal failure and, rarely, bone marrow suppression. Recovery of renal function is often complete but may require several months of haemodialysis. Serious damage to the liver is rare.

Methanol

Although methanol itself is only mildly intoxicating, it is converted in the liver to highly toxic metabolites. The lethal dose of pure methanol is estimated to be around 1–2 mL/kg but both permanent blindness and death have been reported with as little as 0.1 mL/kg (i.e. 6–10 mL in adults). Methanol is rapidly absorbed from the gut, skin and lungs with peak serum concentrations occurring within 30–60 min after oral ingestion. It distributes throughout the body water and is then slowly metabolised by the liver, following zero-order kinetics. First, methanol is slowly oxidised by the enzyme alcohol dehydrogenase to yield formaldehyde. This is then further oxidised by formaldehyde dehydrogenase to create formic acid (this second step occurs rapidly so that little formaldehyde accumulates in the serum). Finally, the formic acid is metabolised to carbon dioxide and water. It is the accumulation of formic acid that is responsible for metabolic acidosis. Formic acid also inhibits cellular respiration with consequent lactic acidosis and directly damages the retina and the optic nerve.

Initial symptoms of methanol poisoning may appear as soon as 12 h post-ingestion but usually develop after 24 h. There is drowsiness, confusion and ataxia, as well as weakness, headache, nausea, vomiting and abdominal pain. Collectively, these symptoms may mimic those of ethanol. As methanol metabolism proceeds, a severe anion gap metabolic acidosis will develop. This acidosis, in association with visual symptoms, is the hallmark of methanol poisoning. Patients usually describe blurred or double vision or changes in colour perception. There may be visual field loss and partial blindness with pupillary dilatation and loss of pupillary reflexes.

Further features include respiratory changes, amnesia, confusion, agitation, coma, seizures, electrolyte disturbances and profound hypotension. Poor outcomes are associated with coma, seizures or pH <7 on presentation.

Tx

Ethylene glycol: rapid diagnosis of poisoning with ethylene glycol is critical because therapy can be very effective when administered within a reasonable period of time after ingestion. The most conclusive method of diagnosis is direct measurement of serum or urine ethylene glycol concentration. However, because this substance induces toxicity after conversion to its metabolites, there is little correlation between blood concentrations and the harmfulness of the poisoning. The severity of the acidosis is a better guide to treatment. There are three primary aims: correction of the patient's metabolic acidosis, prevention of metabolism of the compound to its toxic metabolites, and removal of ethylene glycol and these metabolites. Gastric lavage may be indicated if performed soon after ingestion or in patients who are comatose or at risk of convulsions. Activated charcoal is of no real benefit.

Supportive measures include airway care, IV fluids and careful measurement of urine output. Early and aggressive treatment with sodium bicarbonate is essential to correct the initial acidosis; >500–1000 mmol bicarbonate may be needed within the first few hours. Pyridoxine and thiamine may be administered in order to promote alternative metabolism or formation of the non-toxic metabolites glycine and α-hydroxy-β-ketoadipate. Calcium should not be given for hypocalcaemia (unless there is tetany or seizures) because it may increase precipitation of calcium oxalate crystals in the tissues. Haemodialysis is effective at removing ethylene glycol and its major metabolite glycolate; it should be considered in cases with a serum ethylene glycol concentration >500 mg/L. Peritoneal dialysis is less efficient and haemoperfusion is ineffective for this purpose.

Methanol: as with ethylene glycol above, the three primary goals of therapy include treatment of metabolic acidosis, inhibition of methanol metabolism, and enhanced elimination of the unmetabolised compound and its toxic metabolites. Gastric decontamination is unlikely to be beneficial because methanol is rapidly and completely absorbed from the gut. Stabilisation of the critical patient must be attempted before other therapies can be instituted – airway care, IV fluids, treatment of fits and arterial blood gas analysis. Sodium bicarbonate should be given to correct acidosis. The elimination of methanol may be enhanced by administering folic acid, a co-factor in the conversion of formic acid to carbon dioxide and also by haemodialysis.

Specific therapy with fomepizole: fomepizole (also known as 4-methylpyrazole or 4-MP) is a competitive inhibitor of alcohol dehydrogenase, the enzyme that catalyses the oxidation of ethanol to acetaldehyde and is responsible for the preliminary step in the metabolism of methanol and ethylene glycol to their toxic metabolites. A loading dose of 15 mg/kg should be given, followed by four doses of 10 mg/kg at 12-h intervals and then 15 mg/kg every 12 h until the plasma concentration of the poison has reduced to a non-toxic level. All doses are given as a slow IV infusion over 30 min. The most frequent adverse effects of fomepizole are headache, nausea, dizziness and minor allergic reactions. Ethyl alcohol may be given in an attempt to saturate the alcohol dehydrogenase-binding sites if fomepizole is not available.

Mechanism of action of antidotes in poisoning with methanol and ethylene glycol → Figure 15.3.

Household substances

Children may be suspected of ingesting an enormous variety of domestic substances. Most of these are harmless but some are not and so caution is always advisable. Many household substances are caustic or contain petroleum distillates. Thus, in almost all cases, emetics are contraindicated. Treatment consists of milk and the recommendations of a poisons information service.

Cleaning materials

Most are harmless. Two notable exceptions are bleach and dishwasher products for machines. These can burn the mouth and damage the oesophagus. Emesis is therefore contraindicated. Patients should be given milk and observed in hospital.

Turpentine

This can be lethal. Its abbreviated name, 'turps', usually refers to a white spirit substitute that is not very dangerous. Check the bottle.

Cosmetics

These are usually harmless but may contain a large amount of alcohol (→ p. 285). Perfume oil ingestions (which may sometimes be dangerous) should be treated with milk and observation.

Chronic poisoning with heavy metals in cosmetics → p. 298.

Figure 15.3 The mechanism of action of antidotes in poisoning with methanol and ethylene glycol.

Pet foods

Not surprisingly, most pet foods are completely safe to eat.

Mercury and lead

Mercury from a broken thermometer has a very low risk of toxicity. Most 'lead' shot/pellets and 'lead' fishing weights no longer contain lead.

Mercury and lead poisoning → p. 298.

Plants and garden substances

Earth, faecal material, insects and worms generally present little risk. The possibility of ingesting ova, cysts and parasites is probably quite small.

Berries and seeds are commonly ingested. Some such as laburnum seeds may cause GI upset and drowsiness. Deadly nightshade may be mistaken for elderberry and lead to atropine poisoning. If the ingested plant material is presented, it may be identified with the aid of a guidebook.

Tx Most ingestions of this type, including those where the material is unidentified, should be treated by observation for around 6 h.

Paraquat

The industrial liquid (e.g. Gramoxone) contains 10–20% paraquat and is deadly. Granular preparations for the garden contain only 2.5% paraquat and have caused few deaths. The chemical is highly irritant to the skin, eyes and other membranes. Inhalation of paraquat spray causes a sore throat and epistaxis but not systemic toxicity. Ingestion causes:

- nausea, vomiting and diarrhoea (after a few hours)
- painful ulceration of the lips, tongue and throat (36 h)
- renal failure (48 h)
- dyspnoea (after a few days). There is pulmonary fibrosis with proliferative alveolitis and bronchiolitis.

Tx
- Expert advice should be sought as soon as possible. The Central Toxicology Laboratory at Imperial Chemical Industries Ltd can help with plasma estimations of paraquat in the UK.
- Activated charcoal should be administered immediately (with an IV antiemetic if required). Fuller's earth and magnesium sulphate are no longer recommended.
- Oxygen therapy should be avoided in the early stages of treatment because it may exacerbate damage to the lungs. All patients should have blood gas analysis performed.
- Local irritation of mucous membranes, eyes and skin should be treated by irrigation.
- Mannitol (200 mL 20%) can be given orally as a purgative but is of doubtful value.
- ICU admission must be arranged.

Toxic effects from foods
Scombroid fish

If not completely fresh, fish of the family *Scombridae* (which includes mackerel and tuna) may be decomposed by bacteria such as *Proteus morgani* to form heat-stable substances that are unaffected by cooking. Similar processes may occur in both tinned and fresh fish of other non-scombroid species such as herring. Histamine is produced from histidine and levels are very high in affected fish. However, there are other (as yet unidentified) toxins also involved.

Around 30 min to several hours after eating the fish, the seafood lover experiences widespread erythema and blotchy urticaria of the skin with headache, colic, diarrhoea and vomiting. Bronchospasm, tachycardia and hypotension may also occur. This combination of features is easily mistaken for an allergic reaction or even bacterial food poisoning. The illness is treated with IV antihistamines (both H_1- and H_2-receptor blockers), IV fluids and nebulised bronchodilators. Symptoms resolve within 24 h.

Chinese restaurant syndrome

Monosodium glutamate (MSG) is used as a flavour enhancer in a variety of foods. It is sold as a fine white crystalline powder, which does not have a distinct taste of its own. The mechanism by which MSG adds flavour to other foods is not fully understood. However, the human body uses the amino acid glutamate as a neurotransmitter and it may be that MSG stimulates glutamic acid receptors in the tongue to augment meat-like flavours.

Excessive quantities ($\geq$3 g) of MSG cause a toxic reaction in susceptible individuals around 1 h after ingestion. There is flushing and paraesthesia of the skin with nausea, headache, a sensation of facial pressure and chest discomfort. Bronchospasm may occur in people with asthma. The syndrome is rarely seen nowadays as restaurant cooking practices seem to have changed.

> Food poisoning is a notifiable disease throughout the UK.

Allergic reactions to foods (and other substances) →
p. 299.
Bacterial and viral food poisoning → *p. 254.*

Envenoming

Exotic pets may inflict exotic bites and stings. In addition, unlucky world travellers may encounter poisonous insects, spiders, snakes, fish, corals, hydroids, anemones, jellyfish and octopuses.

Tx All such wounds must be cleaned thoroughly and then dressed. Tetanus prophylaxis must be ensured. It may occasionally be necessary to give antivenom and it is important that each ED knows where the nearest supply is kept. (The *British National Formulary* contains up-to-date telephone numbers of regional depots). Twenty-four-hour help and advice can be obtained from the following centres in the UK:

- The Liverpool School of Tropical Medicine
- The Hospital for Tropical Diseases in London.

In the case of travellers, expert local advice is essential for both diagnosis and treatment.

Jellyfish, weever fish, caterpillar, wasp and bee stings in the British Isles → p. 400.

> Worldwide, around two-thirds of snake bites are from non-venomous varieties. Of the remaining third, half are dry bites where the snake does not inject sufficient venom to be toxic. Therefore, over 80% of people bitten by a snake have nothing to worry about!

Adder bites

The European Viper or adder (*Vipera berus*) is the only poisonous snake that is native to the British Isles. It is not found in Ireland.

Adder bites are occasionally seen in EDs, especially in the south of England. The viper venom causes three main groups of effects:

1 *Local effects*: pain, swelling and bruising at the site of envenoming with tender enlargement of regional lymph nodes
2 *Early anaphylactoid effects*: angio-oedema, urticaria, transient hypotension and syncope; diarrhoea and vomiting with colic
3 *Severe systemic toxic effects*: hypotension, ECG abnormalities, coagulopathy, acute renal failure and adult respiratory distress syndrome.

Tx Anaphylactoid symptoms should be treated with adrenaline (→ p. 299). Systemic effects or persistent and worsening local swelling are indications for treatment with European viper venom antiserum. The dose for both adults and children is 10 mL (diluted in saline) by IV infusion over 30 min. If there is little improvement, this may be repeated after 1–2 h. The antivenom itself may cause an anaphylactic reaction.

Carbon monoxide

This under-recognised condition hospitalises more than 200 people and causes about 50 deaths every year in the UK. Carbon monoxide is a colourless, tasteless, non-irritating gas produced by incomplete combustion of any carbon-containing material (including gas, oil, wood and coal) and so is a sinister and insidious enemy. The main causes of poisoning with carbon monoxide in the UK are as follows:

1 *Deliberate self-harm* (45%)
2 *Faulty domestic heating and cooking apparatus* (33%)
3 *Smoke inhalation in fires* (20%) (note that cyanide and other toxic fumes may be released during the combustion of common materials such as polyurethane foam in furniture → p. 296).

Think of carbon monoxide poisoning if a patient has:

• a history of smoke inhalation (→ p. 136)
• unexplained neurological symptoms, including headache
• an unexplained metabolic acidosis

and if:

• more than one patient presents from the same site
• there are known to be animals that are also unwell
• the patient gets better when away from home
• the patient comes from a community that uses traditional, ethnic cooking methods
• the patient reports that there are black, sooty marks on the walls around stoves, boilers or fires or that their gas appliances burn with yellow rather than blue flames.

Carbon monoxide causes tissue hypoxia by the following methods:

1 Binding to haemoglobin (to form carboxyhaemoglobin or COHb) and thus preventing the carriage of oxygen (its affinity for haemoglobin is 240 times greater than that of oxygen)
2 Moving the oxyhaemoglobin dissociation curve to the left
3 Binding to cellular proteins (such as cytochrome oxidases) which are essential for oxidation.

Tissues with a high requirement for oxygen, such as nervous tissue and myocardium, are most severely affected. The atmospheric level of carbon monoxide considered to be immediately dangerous is 1500 parts per million or ppm (0.15%) but exposure to 1000 ppm (0.1%) may result in 50% saturation of haemoglobin with the gas.

Symptoms and signs: Symptoms vary widely and include malaise, headache, nausea and myalgia (→ *Table 15.3*). A collection of these vague symptoms may mimic influenza or food poisoning. However, there may also be overt neurological, cardiovascular and biochemical findings such as:

• confusion, coma and psychological changes
• dysphasia, dyskinesia, paresis and cortical blindness
• angina, dysrhythmias and left ventricular failure

Table 15.3 Common symptoms of carbon monoxide poisoning

Symptom	Approximate frequency (%)
Headache	90
Nausea and vomiting	50
Vertigo	50
Alteration in mental state	30
Subjective weakness	20

- hypotension
- metabolic acidosis, hypokalaemia and leukocytosis
- rhabdomyolysis (very rarely).

These problems may persist or reoccur and are not well related to the COHb level. This is probably because the half-life of carbon monoxide bound to intracellular myoglobin and respiratory enzymes is up to 48 h, as opposed to 5 h (300 min) in the blood as COHb. Binding to mitochondrial cytochrome A_3 is thought to be particularly important in the causation of carbon monoxide toxicity. Neurological damage seems to be the result of free radical generation and lipid peroxidation.

Patients with coexisting medical problems (heart disease, respiratory disease and anaemia) and children are usually the worst affected and may experience symptoms at lower levels of COHb. Carbon monoxide has a special affinity for fetal haemoglobin and so babies and pregnant women present a special risk.

The severity of poisoning is related to:

1 the concentration of carbon monoxide inhaled
2 the length of exposure
3 the level of activity during the exposure.

> A cherry-red skin colour occurs only when COHb concentrations exceed about 20% and is rarely seen in living patients.

Investigations: Investigations may include:

- *blood gases* – metabolic acidosis with normal oxygen tension
- *ECG* – ischaemia
- *fetal cardiotocograph (FCTG)* – fetal hypoxia

 Box 15.9 The effects of increasing carboxyhaemoglobin levels

- COHb should be <5% of total haemoglobin in a non-smoker and <10–13% in a smoker
- COHb >10% causes mild headache and dyspnoea on vigorous exertion
- COHb >20% causes severe headache, dyspnoea on mild exertion and sometimes early neurological symptoms and signs
- COHb >30% causes severe headache, irritability, fatigue, dimness of vision and other neurological symptoms and signs
- COHb >40% causes severe headache, tachycardia, lethargy, confusion, collapse and sometimes coma
- COHb >60% causes coma, convulsions and cardiovascular collapse
- COHb >70% is very rapidly fatal

- *plasma electrolytes, glucose and osmolality* – to exclude other causes of poisoning
- *COHb levels* ($\rightarrow$ Box 15.9).

> Laboratory measurement of arterial blood gases looks at oxygen dissolved in the plasma rather than oxygen bound to haemoglobin and so the PaO_2 level in CO poisoning may be surprisingly near to normal. Traditional pulse oximeters will also give a false normal value because they cannot differentiate between oxyhaemoglobin and carboxyhaemoglobin. However, pulse CO-oximeters are now available.

Tx This should include the following:

- High-concentration oxygen therapy for 120 min, given via an endotracheal tube or tight-fitting mask (the half-life of COHb is reduced to around 1 h (80 min) when breathing 100% oxygen).
- Close observation and monitoring.
- A consideration of the need for hyperbaric oxygen therapy ($\rightarrow$ Box 15.10) (the half-life of COHb is reduced to 23 min when breathing oxygen at twice atmospheric pressure although there is very little evidence of a beneficial effect from this expensive and inconvenient treatment). The telephone number of the nearest hyperbaric unit should

> **Box 15.10 Indications for hyperbaric oxygen therapy in CO poisoning**
>
> - Symptoms of poisoning and COHb >40%
> - Last trimester of pregnancy with FCTG changes and COHb >20%
> - Comatose at any time
> - Neurological signs after 2 h treatment with high-concentration oxygen
> - Severe cardiovascular problems (e.g. continuing myocardial ischaemia on ECG)

Chemical agents

> Intentional spread of a chemical or biological agent might occur in a biowarfare or bioterrorist incident anywhere in the world. A deliberate release could be overt and clearly identifiable. In this case, there might be a prior warning or an obvious distribution of a toxic substance by an explosive device. However, covert release is also a possibility, in which circumstances the release would not be apparent until the first cases of disease presented – probably to an ED!

be available in the ED; suitable patients can usually be discussed with an expert at the hyperbaric facility.
- All unresponsive patients should be intubated and ventilated. Acidosis will resolve with oxygenation and should not be treated with bicarbonate.

Cyanide → p. 296.
Methaemoglobinaemia → p. 295.
Noxious fumes, vapours and gases → p. 295.

POISONING WITH HARMFUL AGENTS THAT HAVE BEEN RELEASED INTO THE ENVIRONMENT

Incapacitating sprays and aerosols

Patients may present who have been assaulted with a variety of irritant powder aerosols, e.g. pepper spray, CS (tear gas) or CN (mace). There is profound irritation of the eyes, skin and respiratory tract. Water 'activates' the powder and may temporarily increase symptoms but it is usually impractical to avoid irrigation during treatment.

Tx The effects of these agents are usually self-limiting (within 30 min). Most patients require irrigation to the face and eyes only; a weak alkaline solution (or soap and water) can be used for the skin. Continuing discomfort of the eyes merits examination with fluorescein to exclude chemical damage. Severe dermatitis can be treated with topical steroids. Good ventilation of treatment areas is essential to protect staff and other patients.

Chemical warfare has not gone away. With modern aeromedical evacuation patients suffering from its effects may present to distant hospitals. In addition, the threat of terrorist attack has necessitated a knowledge of substances that might be deliberately released into the environment. There are five main types of agents used for such purposes:

1 Irritants and asphyxiants such as chlorine, phosgene, ammonia and ammonium nitrate
2 Vesicants (blistering agents) such as mustard gas and the arsenical vesicants (e.g. Lewisite)
3 Blood agents such as the compounds of cyanide – hydrogen cyanide (AC) and cyanogen chloride (CK)
4 Nerve gases – the G agents (e.g. tabun, sarin, cyclosarin and soman), the GV agents and the V agents (e.g. VX)
5 Miscellaneous substances such as ricin, abrin and botulinum toxin and Kolokol-1 (an extremely potent opioid-based incapacitating agent containing carfentanil).

Tx All cases should be discussed with a specialist, initially a public health consultant or a poisons unit adviser.

Ammonium nitrate → p. 295.
Botulinum toxin → p. 234.
Chemical accidents and decontamination → p. 146.
Chlorine, phosgene, ammonia and sulphur dioxide → p. 295.
Cyanide → p. 296.
Mustard gas → p. 295.
Organophosphate and carbamate insecticides and nerve gases → p. 296.
Ricin and abrin → p. 297.
Strychnine and brucine → p. 235.

In the UK, the National Blood Service can supply multi-dose antidote pods containing botulinum antitoxin, cyanide antidotes and nerve agent antidotes.

Methaemoglobinaemia

Exposure to toxic fumes or drugs may oxidise the iron of haem to its ferric (Fe^{3+}) form. The resulting methaemoglobin (met-Hb) cannot carry oxygen. This leads to acute dyspnoea with headache, lethargy, dizziness, nausea and other symptoms of hypoxia. There is a variable degree of cyanosis. Met-Hb causes cyanosis at a third of the level of deoxygenated haemoglobin (deoxy-Hb) (i.e. $1.5 \, g/dL$ of met-Hb causes equivalent cyanosis to $5 \, g/dL$ of deoxy-Hb). The presence of met-Hb is suggested by characteristic chocolate-coloured blood but laboratory confirmation of the diagnosis must be obtained. High doses of the local anaesthetic prilocaine may sometimes cause methaemoglobinaemia.

Tx
- Give oxygen
- Administer IV methylthioninium chloride (methylene blue) 1% at a dose of $1 \, mg/kg$.

Noxious vapours and gases

Occupational poisoning may occur with gases such as sulphur dioxide, chlorine, ammonia and phosgene. In most cases, there is immediate dyspnoea, choking, coughing, watering eyes and incapacity. However, pulmonary oedema may develop up to 36h after a severe exposure, especially following exertion.

Both chlorine (Cl_2 – a greenish-yellow gas) and phosgene ($COCl_2$ – a colourless gas) react with water in the lungs to form hydrochloric acid. This causes extensive cellular damage to both terminal airways and the alveolar–capillary membrane.

Tx Most patients will require inpatient observation. Symptomatic treatment may include:

- oxygen therapy
- nebulised steroids (e.g. budesonide $2 \, mg$ repeated as necessary)
- cough suppressants

- continuous positive airway pressure (CPAP)
- ventilation with positive end-expiratory pressure (PEEP).
- correction of methaemoglobinaemia ($\rightarrow$ *above*).

Ammonium nitrate (which releases ammonia and other substances) $\rightarrow$ below.
Carbon monoxide $\rightarrow$ p. 292.
Cyanide $\rightarrow$ p. 296.

Hydrogen sulphide

'Detergent suicide' is a recently recognised phenomenon whereby a person uses common household chemicals to make a lethal gaseous combination. The method has been able to gain popularity due to precise instructions on the internet. A domestic cleaning fluid (an acid source) is mixed with a sulphur-containing substance. This combination of ingredients yields hydrogen sulphide (H_2S), a colourless gas that may cause immediate death after just a few breaths. Emergency responders should be aware that these suicides typically take place in a confined space such as a vehicle, cupboard, small room or toilet. The person usually places the chemicals in a bucket and then mixes them together.

Ammonium nitrate

Ammonium nitrate appears as either a colourless, crystalline, solid substance or a white granular powder that is used to make matches, explosives and fertilisers. It is one of the substances that is considered by the Health Protection Agency (UK) to have a high potential for deliberate release. When mixed with other substances, it is highly explosive and can self-ignite to produce ammonia and toxic oxides of nitrogen. Exposure to these fumes causes severe irritation of the eyes, nose, throat and skin; inhalation inflames the respiratory tract and lungs. Absorption may occur through either the skin or lungs and leads to nausea, vomiting, headache and collapse. It may cause methaemoglobinaemia ($\rightarrow$ *above*).

Treatment is symptomatic; nebulised steroids may be of benefit (e.g. budesonide $2 \, mg$ repeated as necessary).

Mustard gas

The toxic effect of the vesicant agent mustard gas is primarily due to its alkylating ability. It can penetrate clothing (including leather) and even the 'off-gassing' from casualties may be sufficient to cause symptoms in emergency personnel. There is usually no pain at the time of exposure; symptoms may be delayed for up to 4–6h. Higher environmental concentrations shorten the time for effects to develop but a typical progression is as follows:

- <1 h: irritation of the eyes, nausea and vomiting are the first signs (if any); facial erythema may start to appear.
- 2–6 h: there is nausea, fatigue, headache, inflamed eyes, lacrimation, photophobia, rhinorrhoea, sore throat, hoarse voice, erythema of exposed skin (usually face and neck) and tachycardia.
- 8–12 h: the erythema worsens and oedema of the skin develops.
- 12–24 h: there is severe inflammation in areas where there was tight clothing and of the axillae, inner thighs, genitalia, perineum and buttocks; pendulous blisters appear, which are filled with clear, yellow fluid; death at this stage is uncommon.
- 48–72 h: this is the stage of maximum blistering; there is intense itching of the skin with an increase in pigmentation. Coughing leads to expectoration of mucus, pus and necrotic debris from the airways.

Skin changes continue until 7–10 days when healing begins to occur. Recovery is usually complete by 21–28 days.

Tx Treatment is symptomatic and depends on the level of exposure. Patients with minimal symptoms and signs can be discharged after 4–6 h of observation. Those with respiratory distress may require intensive care.

Cyanide

Cyanide ions block the electron transport chain between the carrier proteins (the mitochondrial cytochromes) and oxygen. This results in a reversible inhibition of oxidative phosphorylation that is the endpoint of cellular respiration. As rapid measurement of blood cyanide levels is not usually available, the diagnosis must be suspected from circumstantial evidence:

- Fire brigade suspicion (materials involved, etc.)
- Coma/convulsions
- Cardiovascular collapse/dysrhythmias
- Metabolic acidosis/reduced arteriovenous oxygen content difference
- Other signs of inhalation of smoke and fumes (→ p. 136; *carbon monoxide* → p. 292)
- Possibility of deliberate release.

Ingestion of cyanide salts may cause delayed poisoning and is an indication for gastric lavage.

Tx Initial treatment includes administration of 100% oxygen using a non-re-breathing system.

Clothing should be removed, skin decontaminated and the eyes irrigated. Cyanide is rapidly detoxified by the human body. Any casualty who is fully conscious and breathing normally more than 5 min after removal from cyanide exposure will recover spontaneously and does not require treatment with an antidote. Blood for cyanide levels (10 mL in a lithium heparin tube) should be taken before antidotes are given because they interfere with the interpretation of cyanide concentrations.

There are several possible antidote regimens for the treatment of severe, life-threatening cyanide poisoning:

1 Hydroxocobalamin (70 mg/kg [5 g for an adult] by IV infusion over 15 min; repeated, if necessary, over 15–120 min according to the severity of the poisoning). (In this situation, vitamin B_{12} acts as a chelating agent.) This is the safest first-line treatment, especially after smoke inhalation.
2 Combination therapy with sodium nitrite – given intravenously over 5–20 min (adult dose 300 mg or 10 mL of 3% solution; child 4–10 mg/kg) – and sodium thiosulphate – given intravenously over 10 min (adult dose 12.5 g or 25 mL of 50% solution; child 400 mg/kg). Sodium nitrite exerts its therapeutic effect by inducing methaemoglobinaemia; methaemoglobin binds cyanide ions. An excess of this process will impair oxygen delivery.
3 If the patient is severely ill (with coma or respiratory depression) and cyanide poisoning is thought most likely to be responsible and sodium nitrite has not been given already, treatment is with dicobalt edetate – given intravenously over 1 min (adult dose 300 mg or 20 mL of 1.5% solution) – followed immediately by 50 mL of 50% IV glucose. This can be repeated once or even twice as necessary. Dicobalt edetate is extremely toxic in the absence of cyanide ions. It can cause laryngeal and pulmonary oedema.

Cholinesterase inhibitors (nerve agents)

This form of poisoning has occurred following the deliberate release of chemical warfare agents and in workers exposed to the related organophosphate and carbamate insecticides. The principal weaponised substances in this group are tabun (GA), sarin (GB), soman (GD), GF and VX. Nerve agents are absorbed through intact skin as well as through the lungs and the gut. Off-gassing from casualties may cause symptoms in emergency personnel. The mechanism of toxicity is inhibition of cholinesterase enzymes (both acetylcholinesterase and pseudocholinesterase) and thus the effects are those of endogenous acetylcholine in massive excess:

1 *Muscarinic (parasympathetic) effects*: miosis, lacrimation and rhinorrhoea; hypersalivation and sweating; bronchospasm, bronchial hypersecretion and pulmonary oedema; colic and diarrhoea; bradycardia and dysrhythmias

2 *Nicotinic (motor and postganglionic sympathetic) effects*: muscle weakness, fasciculation and flaccid paralysis; hypertension and hyperglycaemia

3 *CNS effects*: headache, nausea and vomiting; anxiety and restlessness; dizziness, ataxia, confusion, convulsions and coma; central respiratory depression.

Death is usually due to respiratory arrest.

Tx Further absorption must be prevented by emptying the stomach, giving oxygen by mask, and removing clothing and washing the skin. Supportive therapy includes oxygen and bronchial suctioning. There are three types of antidote for organophosphorus poisoning:

1 Atropine antagonises the muscarinic effects of acetylcholine (especially hypersecretion and bradycardia). The IV dose of 2 mg (20 mcg/kg for a child) can be repeated every 10 min until the pupils dilate and a tachycardia develops.

2 Oximes reactivate inhibited enzyme and thereby decrease the amount of excess acetylcholine. Pralidoxime mesylate (P2S) 30 mg/kg is diluted and given slowly intravenously over 5–10 min. It improves muscle tone within 30 min and lasts for 4 h. Oximes must be given within 24 h of exposure. Casualties who fail to respond to P2S should be given the second-line cholinesterase reactivator obidoxime (which is also indicated as a first-line drug for tabun [GA] exposure). In the UK, both drugs are available in multi-dose pods from the National Blood Service.

3 Benzodiazepines are used to control the CNS effects.

The exact treatment depends on the level of exposure and the type of poison. Organophosphates cause an almost irreversible phosphorylation of the active site of the cholinesterase enzymes; carbamates induce a much less stable carbamoylation of the binding sites which may be overcome by atropine alone. Patients with minimal symptoms and signs can be discharged after 4–6 h of observation. Those with respiratory distress will require intensive care.

Ricin and abrin

Ricin, the favourite poison of the old Soviet Secret Service, has recently been linked to terrorist activity. It is a toxalbumin that is extracted from the beans of the castor oil plant. Accidental poisoning has followed the ingestion of castor oil seeds; as few as eight seeds have killed an adult. Ricin is particularly toxic if injected, the fatal dose being only 1 mcg/kg. Although it is not volatile, it can be effectively spread and inhaled as an aerosol. Ricin inhibits protein synthesis, which rapidly leads to cell death and multiorgan failure. The onset of symptoms and signs may be delayed after absorption via any route, including:

- fever and widespread mucosal irritation
- abdominal pain, bloody diarrhoea and vomiting
- haematuria, proteinuria, raised creatinine and abnormal LFTs
- pulmonary oedema, pneumonia and acute respiratory distress syndrome (ARDS)
- fits and CNS depression.

Abrin is a similar toxin that is found in the Jequirity bean, the seed of the plant *Abrus precatorious*. The features of poisoning with abrin are almost identical to those with ricin but it is 75 times more potent. An ingested dose of just 3 mcg may be fatal.

Tx Patients should be removed from the source of an aerosol exposure (by personnel with full respiratory and body protection). Their clothing and personal effects should be removed and their skin decontaminated by washing with dilute detergent. Eyes should be irrigated. There is no antidote for ricin or abrin and so treatment is supportive. Patients who are still asymptomatic 8 h after ricin or abrin ingestion or 24 h after aerosol exposure may be safely discharged.

Biological agents

The Health Protection Agency (UK) considers a number of infectious diseases to have the potential for military or terrorist use. This is either because they are known to have been the subject of attempted weaponisation or because they have characteristics that make deliberate release a dangerous possibility. Such infectious organisms are invariably able to survive for long periods away from their natural host and can usually be distributed as an aerosol for subsequent inhalation by intended victims. Many of these unpleasant infections are zoonoses. The main diseases are as follows:

Anthrax → pp. 257 and 408.
Botulism → p. 234.
Brucellosis → p. 256.
Glanders and melioidosis → p. 256.
Plague → p. 256.
Q fever → p. 212.

Smallpox → p. 256.
Tularaemia → p. 408.
Viral haemorrhagic fevers → p. 254.

FURTHER CONSIDERATIONS IN POISONING

Mental state and psychiatric assessment

All patients who have deliberately poisoned themselves should be assessed for suicide risk (→ *p. 364*). This may entail immediate or delayed psychiatric referral. Most self-poisoned patients need help and so social and psychological follow-up should be offered (→ *p. 364*).

Child abuse

Poisoning in childhood is usually the result of accidental ingestion. Public safety measures have highlighted the need for care with the storage of noxious substances. However, there are three circumstances where isolated poisoning in a child may suggest the possibility of child abuse:

1 The ingestion has occurred in an environment of gross neglect. This may also be considered in some episodes of carbon monoxide poisoning after a house fire.
2 The child has been deliberately poisoned, usually as a case of Munchausen's syndrome by proxy → *p. 368*.
3 A crying child has been inappropriately sedated. This is increasingly recognised as the background to some cases of methadone poisoning in childhood. The parents do not intend to harm the child but a disturbed toddler, a bottle of methadone syrup and a rudimentary knowledge of pharmacology may prove to be a disastrous combination.

Suspected child abuse → p. 353.

Chronic poisoning

Heavy metals such as antimony, arsenic, bismuth, gold, mercury and lead are the most usual suspects in chronic poisoning. There have been cases of thallium poisoning in the 1990s among political refugees from unstable countries. Suspicion of chronic poisoning merits medical referral for detailed investigation. Antidotes for heavy metals include dimercaprol, penicillamine, sodium calcium edetate and dimercaptosuccinic acid (DMSA). There are usually local arrangements to measure the blood levels of heavy metals.

Mercury poisoning has been seen recently in the UK in women of Asian and African origin who have bought illegal skin-lightening creams over the internet. The active ingredients of these products are mercury (up to 3%), hydroquinone or corticosteroids. Blood concentrations of mercury can become elevated within 48 h of starting to use the cream and can remain detectable for 45 days after discontinuing it. Long-term usage causes dermatological disorders, hypertension, hypercorticism and mercurial nephropathy, including acute nephrotic syndrome.

Lead poisoning usually results from long-term occupational exposure (ingestion or inhalation) in professions such as plumbers, lead miners, shipbuilders, construction workers, pottery manufacturers and demolition workers. In addition, some hobbies (painting, soldering, target shooting and pottery), ingestion of lead weights, gunshot wounds and exposure to ethnic remedies and cosmetics may all be associated with lead poisoning. Elemental lead is less well absorbed than soluble lead salts, which are highly toxic. Lead poisoning causes a metallic taste, severe abdominal pain, diarrhoea with black stools, vomiting, hypotension, muscle weakness, cramps, fatigue, abnormal liver function tests, acute interstitial nephritis and encephalopathy in its acute form. Chronic features include anorexia, abdominal pain, constipation, headaches, irritability, fatigue, insomnia, depression, peripheral neuropathy, renal dysfunction and anaemia. There is little correlation between the blood lead level and total body lead content because the blood concentration reflects only recent exposure. Gastric lavage should be considered if acute ingestion of lead or lead salts has occurred within 1 h. A plain abdominal radiograph can be used to confirm effective decontamination.

Iron poisoning → p. 286.

Forensic aspects

If there is a suspicion of criminal poisoning, the police should be contacted. There are sometimes coexisting injuries or allegations of sexual interference. Specific urine and blood samples for toxicology may be required; the police will advise how these must be obtained. Criminal speculation is not part of your clinical assessment and must not form part of your recorded management.

ATYPICAL REACTIONS TO DRUGS AND OTHER SUBSTANCES

Allergic reactions

> Biphasic reactions, where a second wave of symptoms appears 4–8 h after the initial remission, are seen in a small proportion of patients with anaphylaxis. A single dose of oral prednisolone (1 mg/kg) may be given before discharge to ameliorate such an event, should it occur.

Drugs and foods, especially peanuts, are usually implicated in acute allergic reactions but a collapsed patient will give no history. In the UK, around 1 person in 200 (0.5% of the population) is allergic to peanuts. Even minute amounts of peanut allergen can cause very severe reactions.

The presentations of allergy can be divided up according to their immunological basis but for the emergency clinician it is the type and severity of the reaction that are of most significance. Any pattern is possible, combining elements of the following.

Airway (upper airway obstruction)

There is dyspnoea and stridor. This is usually the result of laryngeal oedema but swelling in the mouth or pharynx may also occur.

Tx
- Summon skilled anaesthetic and ENT help.
- Administer adrenaline parenterally (→ Box 15.11).
- Consider nebulised adrenaline (5 mg) in less acute cases.
- Give IV hydrocortisone (300 mg) and IV chlorphenamine (10 mg).

Breathing (bronchospasm)

The patient has dyspnoea and wheezing.

Tx
- Request anaesthetic help in severe cases.
- Administer a nebulised bronchodilator (e.g. salbutamol 5 mg).
- Give IV hydrocortisone (300 mg) and IV chlorphenamine (10 mg).

 Box 15.11 Adrenaline for anaphylaxis

- 1 in 1000 adrenaline contains 1 mg (1000 mcg)/mL; it is usually supplied as a 1-mL (i.e. 1-mg) ampoule
- 1 in 10000 adrenaline contains 0.1 mg (100 mcg)/mL; it is usually supplied as a 10-mL (i.e. 1-mg) ampoule

The intravenous dose of adrenaline is 1–3 mcg/kg given slowly under ECG control. For an adult this means giving 0.5-mL (50-mcg) aliquots of the 1 in 10000 solution. The IV (or intraosseous) route is only appropriate in situations that are immediately life threatening. In less acute situations, the IM route should be used. The IM dose of adrenaline is 5–10 mcg/kg (i.e. 500 mcg intramuscularly for an adult).

- Consider IV salbutamol or parenteral adrenaline (→ Box 15.11) in overwhelming reactions.

Circulation (shock)

The circulatory collapse is a result of vasodilatation and maldistribution of fluid. The presence of tachycardia may help to distinguish anaphylaxis from vasovagal syncope.

Tx
- Administer rapid IV fluids (20 mL/kg).
- Give IV hydrocortisone (300 mg) and IV chlorphenamine (10 mg).
- Consider parenteral adrenaline in severe cases (→ Box 15.11).
- Consider an infusion of IV ephedrine or even IV noradrenaline in prolonged shock.

> Cardiac arrest from acute anaphylaxis is treated in the same way as any other arrest. IV adrenaline will inevitably be given.

Patients who are taking β blockers appear to have an increased risk of anaphylaxis and may have severe reactions that are difficult to treat. Some effects – especially refractory hypotension – may be lessened by the use of IV glucagon.

Angio-oedema and rashes

Swelling of the face and hands is especially common. The lips and eyelids are often particularly badly affected. In these cases, consideration must be given to the airway. Rashes often occur as an isolated finding. The typical rash is that of urticaria or 'hives'. This is a blotchy, red 'nettle-rash' with raised whitish weals on it. It may persist or recur for several days or even weeks.

> Diffuse swelling of the face, hands and legs may be due to nephrotic syndrome, rather than allergy.

Tx
- IV or IM antihistamine (e.g. chlorphenamine 10 mg) should be given to all severely affected patients.
- IV or IM hydrocortisone (300 mg) should also be considered in patients with a very severe reaction.
- Supportive and symptomatic treatment should be given as indicated.
- Oral antihistamines are appropriate for continuing treatment or as the sole treatment in minor cases.
- Some patients will benefit from a short course of oral prednisolone.
- Follow-up must be that appropriate for the severity of the allergic reaction → *later*.

The allergen should be sought and removed as soon as possible. Some clinicians add an H_2-receptor antagonist (e.g. ranitidine) to the standard antihistamine therapy in severe cases.

Hereditary angio-oedema (C1 inhibitor deficiency): A congenital deficiency of C1 inhibitor causes episodes of soft-tissue swelling that may either arise spontaneously or be precipitated by factors such as trauma or illness. There may be swelling of the lips, tongue, mouth and pharynx as well as oedema of the face and abdominal symptoms. This hereditary angio-oedema (HAE) is resistant to standard therapy for allergic reactions.

Hereditary angio-oedema (HAE)/C1 (esterase) inhibitor deficiency → p. 263.

Aftercare of allergic reactions

1 Every patient must have a letter for the GP detailing the problem and the treatment.
2 The patient must understand the condition and be aware of the possibility of a further, more serious attack.

3 Patients with potentially serious reactions should be advised to avoid visiting areas where rapid medical help is unavailable – at least until specialist assessment of risk and standby medication has been obtained.

Acute dystonic reactions

Patients presenting with acute dystonic reactions are often misdiagnosed or labelled as hysterical. Young adults and children are most commonly affected. Symptoms vary from isolated problems with swallowing and talking, to generalised spasms of the face, neck and trunk (the oculogyric crisis). Usually, the dystonia is intermittent in severity. It is the reactions affecting only one cranial nerve area that are the most easily mistaken for hysteria. All patients will have recently taken antipsychotic or antiemetic drugs (dopamine-receptor antagonists). These may vary from regular depot major tranquillisers to one tablet of metoclopramide. Teenagers may occasionally have abused 'unknown' substances. Anticonvulsants and antidepressants have also been reported to cause extrapyramidal reactions.

Tx Symptoms are dramatically relieved by the intravenous injection of a centrally acting anticholinergic (e.g. procyclidine 5–10 mg or benzatropine 1–2 mg). The onset of these drugs, however, usually takes a few minutes and may take longer. Benzodiazepines (e.g. diazepam 10 mg) are also effective. It must be remembered that the antidote is unlikely to last as long as the offending substance. Patients therefore need admission or oral medication to take out.

Oculogyric crises may look very similar to the spasms of both tetanus and strychnine poisoning. *Tetanus and strychnine poisoning → p. 234.*

Neuroleptic malignant syndrome

This rare, idiosyncratic reaction is most commonly seen soon after starting phenothiazines and related neuroleptic drugs. The interrelationship of neuroleptic malignant syndrome, serotonin syndrome, severe dystonia and malignant hyperthermia (a life-threatening condition seen during general anaesthesia) is unclear. Typical features of neuroleptic malignant syndrome include:

- muscular rigidity
- hyperthermia
- dehydration
- autonomic instability – pallor, raised BP and tachycardia
- altered or fluctuating consciousness.

About 10% of patients with this syndrome die, usually as a result of:

- rhabdomyolysis (→ *p. 265*)
- acute renal failure (→ *p. 247*)
- pulmonary embolism (→ *pp. 190 and 214*).

Tx

- Give oxygen.
- Start vigorous rehydration.
- Begin cooling measures (→ *p. 271*).
- Send blood for electrolytes, glucose, blood gases and creatinine kinase assay.
- Give an antimuscarinic drug to reduce rigidity (e.g. IV procyclidine 5–10 mg).
- Sedate with a benzodiazepine if necessary.
- Consider correcting any acidosis with bicarbonate (→ *p. 252*).
- Consider arranging admission to a high dependency unit (HDU) or ICU.

Dopamine agonists such as bromocriptine and muscle relaxants such as dantrolene may also have a part to play (→ *p. 271*). Antipsychotic medication must be stopped.

Serotonin syndrome

Serotonin syndrome is a disorder that is seen infrequently in patients taking SSRIs. In most cases, it occurs when two or more drugs are taken that interfere with serotonin receptor systems (e.g. SSRI + monoamine oxidase inhibitor or SSRI + tricyclic antidepressant). Symptoms start insidiously within hours of commencing therapy with the second serotoninergic drug. The syndrome has also been reported after overdose of SSRIs. There are three main groups of symptoms:

1 *Mental changes* (seen in 40% of patients): agitation, confusion, hallucinations, drowsiness and coma
2 *Neuromuscular hyperactivity* (seen in 50% of patients): tremor, shivering and myoclonus
3 *Autonomic instability* (seen in 50% of patients): tachycardia, fever, hypertension or hypotension.

Flushing, diarrhoea and vomiting are also common. In severe cases, fits, hyperthermia, rhabdomyolysis, renal failure and coagulopathies may also develop.

Tx Most mild cases resolve spontaneously within 24 h. Serotoninergic drugs should be stopped and electrolytes and creatinine kinase monitored in all patients. Supportive therapy includes anticonvulsants, IV fluids and cooling measures. There are reported uses of both propranolol and cyproheptadine to control symptoms. Treatment of malignant hyperthermia with dantrolene (→ *p. 271*) may be required.

Poisoning with SSRIs → p. 279.

16

Abdominal pain

Pain in the abdomen is a common symptom that is managed by surgeons, physicians, gynaecologists, paediatricians and especially by GPs. Patients from all of these domains may present to an emergency department (ED); they may arrive critically ill and require resuscitation, they may have an acute illness that is best managed by admission or they may present with a problem that can be further investigated on an outpatient basis.

Abdominal injury → p. 83.
Children with abdominal pain → pp. 344 and 346.
Perineal problems → Chapter 17.

Immediate assessment and management

If the patient is distressed and in severe pain or otherwise clearly unwell:

- Give high-concentration oxygen
- Start an infusion of Hartmann's solution (or saline)
- Monitor pulse, BP, SaO_2 and temperature
- Consider 12-lead ECG
- Give intravenous (IV) analgesia with an antiemetic
- Pass a urinary catheter if there is a distended bladder or any suggestion of fluid depletion
- Consider inserting a nasogastric tube if there is abdominal distension
- Seek surgical advice.

Causes of collapse with abdominal pain → Box 16.1.

Further assessment

Ask about

- Site and speed of onset of the pain
- Character and duration of the pain
- Exacerbating and relieving factors
- Radiation of the pain
- Accompanying features such as nausea and vomiting
- General health, family and past history, drugs and allergies
- Travel abroad.

Think about the patient's anxieties. If there is a long history, why did the patient choose this moment to present to hospital?

Look for

- Abdominal tenderness and guarding
- Rebound tenderness
- Rigidity
- Bowel sounds
- Loin tenderness
- Hernias
- Perineal signs (→ Boxes 16.2 and 16.3)
- Chest disease.

A leaking abdominal aortic aneurysm is common but the symptoms and signs are often unremarkable. The diagnosis should always be considered in patients who either have collapsed or have trunk pain.

Sudden deterioration in a patient with abdominal symptoms is usually caused by acute blood loss, frequently from the upper GI tract or an aortic aneurysm. Rectal examination or the introduction of a nasogastric tube can be diagnostic.

Emergency Medicine Lecture Notes, Fourth Edition. Chris Moulton and David Yates.
© 2012 Blackwell Publishing Ltd. Published 2012 by Blackwell Publishing Ltd.

Box 16.1 Causes of collapse with abdominal pain

- Acute blood loss from the upper gastrointestinal tract (oesophageal varices and peptic ulceration)
- Perforation of a peptic ulcer, sigmoid diverticulum or the appendix
- Acute pancreatitis
- Leaking aortic aneurysm
- Mesenteric infarction
- Intra-abdominal sepsis with septic shock
- Ruptured ectopic pregnancy
- Hypovolaemia from any abdominal cause
- Diabetic ketoacidosis
- Cardiorespiratory pathology (e.g. myocardial infarction [MI] or pulmonary embolism [PE])

 Box 16.2 Rectal examination

This can provide information about:

- perianal pathology
- sphincter tone
- the rectal contents (empty, consistency of stool, presence of blood or melaena)
- the rectal wall (age >50 years, carcinoma is increasingly common)
- pelvic masses or tenderness, including the appendix
- the prostate gland

If the presenting symptoms and signs could not be expected to be associated with any of the abnormalities in this list, then there is no indication to undertake a rectal examination.

 Box 16.3 Vaginal examination

This is a very invasive procedure, particularly in young or nulliparous women. Do not consider undertaking any intimate examination unless you have:

- appropriate training
- an experienced chaperone
- privacy
- the confidence of the patient
- reason to believe that the findings of the examination will influence management

Before the examination
- Explain the need for the procedure and what it will entail (including any potential pain or discomfort)
- Give the patient an opportunity to ask questions
- Obtain the patient's permission
- Give the patient privacy to undress and later on to dress; use sheets to protect the patient's dignity

During the examination
- Do not make any irrelevant, personal or ambiguous comments
- Encourage questions and discussion
- Stop if the patient becomes distressed or requests that you terminate the examination

Oesophageal spasm is rare and should not be diagnosed in the ED. Myocardial pain is almost identical and is very common.

Investigations: Consider MI → *p. 177.* A normal ECG does not exclude an MI. A trial of antacids and observation may be helpful.

Tx Patients in whom MI cannot be excluded must be admitted for observation. However if:

- the history is indicative of oesophagitis
- the examination and ECG are normal
- the patient responds to antacid

then referral can be made to the GP for further care (weight reduction, small regular meals, stopping smoking, antacids and alginates). A course of a proton pump inhibitor (e.g. omeprazole 20 mg daily for 4 weeks) will give rapid relief of symptoms and promote healing.

PAIN AND BLEEDING IN THE OESOPHAGUS AND UPPER ABDOMEN

Oesophageal pain

Oesophagitis is caused by reflux of gastric contents. It is sometimes associated with a hiatus hernia. The patient is often overweight and experiences burning retrosternal pain on lying flat and bending down. The pain is relieved by antacids and sitting up. Severity of symptoms does not correlate well with endoscopic findings.

Oesophageal pain and bleeding after vomiting

Oesophageal injury may be caused by repeated vomiting, often after excessive alcohol consumption. A small tear of the mucosa may cause bleeding (Mallory–Weiss syndrome, which is usually seen in patients with chronic alcohol problems or after an alcohol 'binge'). Sometimes this is accompanied by diffuse, intense, retrosternal pain, suggestive of a transmural injury (Boerhaave's syndrome). Mediastinitis is then a common sequel and may be fatal.

Investigations: A plain chest radiograph (CXR) may reveal air in the mediastinum or a foreign body. Radiology after ingestion of contrast medium should be arranged. Oesophagoscopy is hazardous.

Tx Oral fluids are prohibited and an IV infusion should be commenced. Analgesia and systemic antibiotics are required and the patient should be admitted for observation.

Bleeding from oesophageal varices → p. 305.

Dyspepsia and gastritis

Epigastric pain and tenderness are often seen in young adults, especially after alcohol ingestion. Some cases will settle with minimal therapy, whereas others will subsequently prove to result from peptic ulceration. The non-endoscopic diagnosis of gastritis is dependent on the history and the magnitude and duration of the symptoms and signs.

Tx Most patients with a recent onset of dyspepsia will settle quickly with antacids. However, many GPs will treat undiagnosed dyspepsia in young adults (who have a low risk of gastric malignancy) with a short course of an oral H_2-receptor antagonist. Ranitidine (which can be bought 'over the counter' in the UK) is suitable; 150 mg twice daily for a maximum of 14 days should be prescribed. A similar course of a proton pump inhibitor (e.g. omeprazole 20 mg daily) is equally effective. Patients in severe pain will require analgesia and admission for investigation, including barium meal or gastroscopy. The eradication of *Helicobacter pylori* is now one of the main aims of long-term therapy.

Peptic ulceration

Dyspeptic pain and tenderness in the epigastrium are the cardinal features of peptic ulceration. Vomiting may also occur, especially with a gastric ulcer. Management depends on the severity and duration of the symptoms and signs. The differentiation between gastric and duodenal ulceration is of little clinical importance in the ED. Gastric carcinoma is associated with profound anorexia, weight loss and anaemia.

There are three other serious acute presentations of peptic ulceration, none of which necessarily follow episodes of dyspepsia:

1 *Gastrointestinal haemorrhage → below*
2 *Perforation and peritonitis → p. 307*
3 *Pyloric stenosis → p. 306*

Gastrointestinal haemorrhage

The patient with a GI bleed may present with any combination of:

- haematemesis
- melaena
- passage of bright-red blood per rectum
- hypotension, shock and collapse
- subacute symptoms (fatigue from anaemia, etc.).

Peptic ulceration is by far the most common cause of serious GI haemorrhage (more than half of all cases) but bleeding may also be seen in:

- gastritis and gastric erosions (e.g. after alcohol or non-steroidal anti-inflammatory drugs [NSAIDs])
- oesophagitis
- Mallory–Weiss syndrome (oesophageal tear after vomiting) → *above*
- oesophageal or gastric varices → *p. 305*
- diverticulitis (copious melaena or bright red blood)
- neoplastic and clotting disorders (variable presentations)
- minor conditions of the rectum (e.g. piles → *p. 326*).

Severe bleeding from the small intestine is rare.

> For patients admitted to hospital with upper GI bleeding, overall mortality is around 1 in 7; most deaths occur in older people. *High risk factors in patients with GI bleeding → Box 16.4.*

Tx
- Protect the airway and give oxygen.
- Start immediate volume replacement via two large-bore cannuli. Central venous access may be required. *Management of major haemorrhage → Figure 1.2 on p. 8.*
- Monitor vital functions.
- Discuss the patient with the admitting teams (usually both medical and surgical liaison is appropriate).

- Take blood for cross-matching (6 units), clotting screen, full blood count (FBC), glucose, urea and electrolytes (U&Es), and liver function tests (LFTs).
- Obtain a CXR and an ECG.
- Catheterise the bladder and monitor the urine output.
- Correct clotting abnormalities (vitamin K_1 or K_2, prothrombin complex concentrate [PCC] or fresh frozen plasma [FFP] → p. 258). Consider acquired haemophilia → p. 257.
- In suspected gastroduodenal bleeding, consider an IV infusion of omeprazole (40 mg diluted to 100 mL and given over 20–30 min), although this has not been shown to be effective.

Endoscopic assessment (which should be performed within 24 h of admission) usually precedes any decision to operate and may be life-saving in very severe bleeds.

Variceal haemorrhage

Haemorrhage from oesophageal (or gastric) varices is a devastating complication of portal hypertension that usually occurs in patients with chronic liver disease. The mortality rate is between 33 and 50%. Raised pressure in the portal vein usually develops as a consequence of increased intrahepatic vascular resistance and increased blood flow through the portal system. Venous collaterals enlarge, in an attempt to decompress the portal system. These varices occur mainly at the portosystemic anastomoses in the gastro-oesophageal junction and the rectum. Posthepatic causes of portal hypertension include the Budd–Chiari syndrome (hepatic venous obstruction) and constrictive pericarditis.

In diseases such as cirrhosis, collagen replaces the normal hepatic matrix and impedes intrahepatic blood flow. Thus 90% of patients with cirrhosis will develop gastro-oesophageal varices within 10 years.

The diagnosis should be suspected in patients with haematemesis or melaena who have signs of liver disease or a history of alcohol abuse. Unexplained thrombocytopenia may be due to portal hypertension.

Tx

The treatment is that detailed above for GI bleeding with special attention to the inevitable coagulopathy and thrombocytopenia. *Management of major haemorrhage → Figure 1.2 on p. 8.* Fluid repletion should be cautious, avoiding hypertension and transfusing to a haemoglobin of between 7 and 9 g/dL (over-transfusion increases portal venous pressure). There is no evidence that saline infusions are harmful in the presence of peripheral oedema or ascites. Prophylactic broad-spectrum antibiotics have been shown to reduce mortality (e.g. IV piperacillin with tazobactam or ciprofloxacin). Intensivists and GI specialists should be involved as soon as possible.

Vasoactive drug therapy controls bleeding by reducing portal venous pressure. This is achieved by vasoconstriction of the splanchnic bed, which reduces the blood flow into the portal circulation. Several drugs are used:

- Vasopressin (20 U IV over 15 min) induces vasoconstriction in almost all vascular beds. This causes inevitable side effects including myocardial and cerebral ischaemia. For this reason, nitrates are usually administered concurrently. However, the use of vasopressin has been largely superseded by terlipressin.
- Terlipressin (2 mg IV) is a synthetic analogue of vasopressin. It is a prodrug with a slower onset of action, a longer half-life and fewer side effects than the parent drug. It is still contraindicated in the presence of severe coronary heart disease, peripheral vascular disease or pregnancy.
- Somatostatin (250 mcg IV bolus followed by an infusion of 250 mcg/h) induces vasoconstriction in the splanchnic vascular bed. It is seldom used in the UK.
- Octreotide (50 mcg IV bolus followed by an infusion of 50 mcg/h) is an analogue of somatostatin. It is useful for patients who have contraindications to terlipressin.

Placement of a Sengstaken–Blakemore tube may be required as a temporising measure in continuing severe haemorrhage and is effective in up to 90% of patients. This device has two balloons and two aspiration ports (gastric and oesophageal in both cases). Inflation (with around 200 mL of air) and gentle traction on the gastric balloon alone is usually adequate to control bleeding. (The oesophageal balloon may cause damage, especially post-sclerotherapy.) However, if fresh blood continues to be aspirated from the oesophageal port, then the oesophageal balloon may be inflated to a pressure of 40 mmHg. Variceal tamponade with a Sengstaken–Blakemore tube is most appropriate and safest for patients under general anaesthesia with airway protection.

There are several ways of stopping variceal bleeding more definitively:

- Endoscopy (preferably under general anaesthetic [GA]) should take place within 12 h of the onset of bleeding or much sooner in severe cases. Variceal band ligation may be performed to achieve haemostasis. Injection sclerotherapy (with ethanolamine) is an alternative for oesophageal varices. Gastric varices (present in 20% of patients) are usually injected with cyanoacrylate glue or thrombin.
- An intrahepatic portosystemic shunt can be inserted via the transjugular route by an interventional radiologist. This decompresses the portal vein by creating an artificial shunt through the liver.
- Surgical interventions include oesophageal transection or creation of a splenorenal shunt.

Pyloric stenosis

In adults, pyloric stenosis is usually associated with a chronic ulcer history but there is often no recent pain. It presents with episodic projectile vomiting, unrelated to eating. Examination reveals undernourishment and a 'succussion splash' emanating from the full stomach. Hypochloraemia, hypocalcaemia and metabolic alkalosis are common. Initial management is directed at the correction of the dehydration and the electrolyte disturbance. The stomach should be emptied by a wide-bore oral tube before endoscopic assessment.

Hepatitis

Hepatitis is caused by the following:

- Viruses with an enteric mode of transmission (hepatitis A and E) → *below*
- Viruses with a parenteral mode of transmission (hepatitis B, C and D) (*immunisation against hepatitis B → p. 404*)
- Weil's disease (leptospirosis) → *below*
- Drugs.

Leptospirosis or Weil's disease: this occurs after mucosal contact with water that has been infected by rats' urine. It is sometimes fatal and should always be considered when a pyrexia and abdominal pain is found in:

- sewage workers
- farmers
- water board workers
- people who have been swimming in fresh water
- people who have been sleeping rough.

After an incubation period of about 10 days (range 4–21 days), there is a rapid onset of fever, headache, and limb and back pain. Jaundice occurs in 75% of cases with a purpuric rash and albuminuria.

Infectious hepatitis: hepatitis A is by far the most common cause of hepatitis. Transmission is by the faecal–oral route and the incubation period is 6 days to 6 weeks. Outbreaks may occur in primary schools and in other institutions.

Hepatitis causes a variable degree of:

- anorexia and malaise
- nausea and vomiting
- abdominal pain and right upper quadrant tenderness
- jaundice
- dark urine and pale stools
- pyrexia
- urticaria
- hepatomegaly and splenomegaly.

Investigations: There is bilirubin and urobilinogen in the urine.

Tx Admission is required for patients who:

- are significantly jaundiced
- are clearly very unwell
- have an uncertain diagnosis.

Those with hepatitis A (young, short duration of symptoms and limited signs) can be treated at home and followed up by the GP. Strict hygiene must be observed with a light diet and no alcohol.

Biliary disease

Biliary pain is usually associated with gallstones, is inevitably recurrent and may be precipitated by a fatty meal, often eaten some hours previously. The classic description of sufferers – female, forty, fat and fertile – is unflattering but, unfortunately, evidence based!

Biliary colic: this is caused by the passage of a gallstone through the bile ducts and presents as sudden, constant (not colicky), epigastric and right hypochrondrial pain radiating to the back. There is tenderness in the right upper quadrant; nausea and vomiting are common. Symptoms may be transitory or last for several hours, with the pain disappearing as suddenly as it started. Impaction of a stone in the common bile duct is unusual but associated with more prolonged symptoms and the gradual appearance of obstructive jaundice. Prolonged obstruction of the cystic duct leads to acute cholecystitis.

Acute cholecystitis: acute inflammation of the gallbladder with or without intermittent obstruction at its neck causes:

- constant right upper quadrant pain, referred to the back
- localised tenderness
- nausea and vomiting
- fever and malaise
- a palpable gallbladder with a positive Murphy's sign (sometimes).

The condition is differentiated from biliary colic by its less abrupt onset, longer duration, more profuse vomiting and the presence of a fever. (In more chronic cases, dyspepsia may be the presenting symptom. Pain is worse after a large, fat-laden meal, and heartburn and belching are common. If these are the only symptoms, then further investigation can be pursued on an outpatient basis.) Rarely, in elderly or diabetic patients, perforation of the gallbladder may occur with subsequent biliary peritonitis.

Cholangitis: infection of the biliary ducts is usually seen in elderly patients and is characterised by upper abdominal pain, fever and the development of obstructive jaundice (Charcot's triad). Hypotension and other signs of severe sepsis are common. Suppuration may lead to hepatic abscesses. *Escherichia coli* is the most common pathogen. The mortality rate is high (33%).

Investigations: Early ultrasound examination visualises the gallstones and the swollen gallbladder and/or bile ducts. Abdominal radiographs may show air in the biliary tree in cholangitis. Inflammatory markers (white cell count [WCC] and C-reactive protein [CRP]) may be raised in acute cholecystitis and cholangitis, although 50% of patients with infection of the biliary ducts have a normal or reduced WCC. The plasma amylase may be mildly raised.

Tx Analgesia, IV fluids and admission are required. In the presence of a fever, antibiotics (a cephalosporin, ciprofloxacin or gentamicin) should be prescribed. Patients with cholangitis may have severe sepsis ($\rightarrow$ *p. 260*) and IV piperacillin with tazobactam is appropriate antibacterial therapy.

Pancreatitis

The main predisposing factors are:

- chronic biliary disease (the most common cause in women)
- excess alcohol consumption (the usual cause in men).

The pain may begin suddenly but is then constant and very severe. It is accompanied by vomiting and may be relieved by sitting forward. The pain differs from that associated with perforation of a peptic ulcer in that it radiates to the back and extends from the epigastrium bilaterally. There is epigastric tenderness and guarding and decreased bowel sounds (due to ileus). Pyrexia is uncommon but tachycardia is usual. In severe cases the BP falls, cyanosis may be present and the patient is brought in as a 'collapse'.

Investigations:
- A serum amylase >1200 IU/mL is considered diagnostic. Lower levels may be caused by other abdominal conditions or by an MI.
- The sodium, potassium and calcium are usually low.
- The plasma WCC is invariably raised.
- The serum bilirubin may be raised.
- There may be hypoxia and an effusion on CXR.
- ECG may show non-specific abnormalities.

Tx Initial treatment is nil by mouth, nasogastric aspiration, IV fluids and antibiotics. Analgesia must be given. The patient may require intensive care and laparotomy for peritoneal toilet.

Pain and bleeding in the central and lower abdomen
Peritonitis

Generalised peritonitis usually occurs secondary to a perforated viscus following:

- peptic ulceration
- appendicitis
- diverticular disease
- neoplastic or inflammatory bowel disease
- trauma
- iatrogenic injury.

It causes:

- severe abdominal pain
- a rigid (board-like) abdomen
- hypotension and shock.

The pain of perforation begins suddenly. After a few minutes, its severity is reduced but the abdomen remains rigid, especially the epigastrium. The pulse is elevated and the patient is pale and anxious but not initially 'shocked'. Rigidity and pain may decrease after a few hours but bowel sounds remain absent. Symptoms increase again after around 6 h as bacterial peritonitis develops. Vomiting may occur. The patient is often elderly or has a recent history of NSAID ingestion.

Investigations: An erect CXR will show gas under the diaphragm in many (but certainly not all) cases. A CT scan of the abdomen is helpful, before laparotomy, to elucidate the cause of the peritonitis.

Tx Vigorous fluid resuscitation, analgesia and surgical referral are required. Antibiotics may be given: piperacillin with tazobactam (or a cephalosporin and metronidazole) are reasonable first-line choices.

Leaking abdominal aortic aneurysm

Leaking aortic aneurysm is most often seen in an older (>55 years) patient who has generalised vascular disease. Symptoms and signs are variable but include the following:

- Back pain (sometimes with a previous episode a few days before)
- Generalised abdominal pain with vague tenderness and fullness (pain may radiate to the groin)
- Hypotension
- Pallor and sweating
- Sudden collapse.

Classic features are often absent; an expansile, pulsatile mass may not be detected and the femoral pulses may be present and not delayed with respect to the radial ones. Pain may not be severe.

> Only about 50% of patients with a ruptured aortic aneurysm reach hospital alive. A further 10% are unsuitable for surgery. For the remainder, the surgical mortality rate is between 30 and 60%.

Investigations: Routine blood tests including clotting studies should be ordered. On admission, 60% of patients with a ruptured aortic aneurysm have coagulopathy, 40% have low platelets and 30% have impaired renal function.

The ECG usually shows ischaemic changes because 90% of this group of patients have coronary heart disease and the pre-existing coronary ischaemia is worsened by hypotension. (Atherosclerosis of other vascular beds is also common.)

There is no indication for a plain abdominal radiograph. However, if performed in cases where the diagnosis is not yet established, it may show the lumbar vertebrae notched by a chronically expanding aorta and an enlarged, calcified vessel wall.

If there is doubt about the diagnosis, then ultrasonography of the abdomen will show an aortic mass and free fluid if there is a leaking aneurysm. None of these investigations should delay surgical referral.

Tx
- Give oxygen.
- Start two infusions via large-bore cannuli. Volume replacement in the ED should be carefully controlled; the objective is to maintain adequate cerebral and coronary perfusion without increasing blood loss. Fluids should be given until large pulses are palpable, aiming to keep systolic BP around 70–90 mmHg but no higher.
- Monitor pulse, BP, SaO_2 and ECG.
- Call for surgical and anaesthetic help.
- Cross-match 8–10 units of packed red blood cells and order a similar number of units of both FFP and platelets (median transfusion requirements are 6–10 units). Excessive fluids may rupture a leaking aneurysm but anaemia will also be harmful in this low-output state. Therefore, transfusion with packed cells should begin as soon as possible (Hb should be kept around 10 g/dL and always >8 g/dL.)
- Send blood for FBC, clotting studies, U&Es and glucose.
- Obtain an ECG and a CXR.
- Give small increments of IV analgesia as required (but be careful because opiates will reduce vital sympathetic tone).
- Pass a urinary catheter and measure the urine output.

Management of major haemorrhage → Figure 1.2 on p. 8.

Other intra-abdominal bleeding

- Ruptured ectopic pregnancy → p. 320.
- The diseased and enlarged spleen may bleed dramatically after trivial injury or even spontaneously (e.g. during malaria or glandular fever).
- Patients with haemophilia and those on anticoagulant therapy may bleed spontaneously. Consider acquired haemophilia → p. 257.

Management of major haemorrhage → Figure 1.2 on p. 8.

Mesenteric vascular disease

Problems with the blood supply of the bowel are difficult to diagnose clinically and are often only found at laparotomy. These diagnoses should be thought of in older patients (usually >60 years) with other evidence of cardiovascular disease, who are disproportionately unwell and distressed for their clinical signs.

Mesenteric infarction: this usually involves the superior mesenteric vessels and is approximately equally split between cases of embolism and thrombosis. Symptoms are caused by infected, dying bowel in the abdominal cavity and are compounded by fluid loss into the bowel and perforation. Once the condition has developed, the patient is hypotensive and looks very ill. The pain is diffuse, severe and poorly localised. There is generalised abdominal tenderness and guarding with shifting dullness. Bowel sounds are decreased and there may be some abdominal distension. Vomiting is an early feature and bloody diarrhoea is passed per rectum. The mortality rate is very high (>50%).

Mesenteric angina: recurrent bouts of severe abdominal pain in elderly patients may be a result of ischaemia of the bowel. The pain may be followed by episodes of obstruction or bloody diarrhoea (ischaemic colitis).

Mesenteric venous thrombosis: venous occlusion gives rise to a similar clinical picture to infarction but is even more insidious in onset and in symptoms and signs.

Investigations: The haemoglobin and amylase are often raised, with a high WCC. An elevated D-dimer, although not very specific, is a very sensitive indicator of ischaemic bowel, so a normal D-dimer makes the presence of necrotic bowel extremely unlikely.

Plain radiographs are invariably unremarkable, although 'thumb printing' of the wall of the bowel is sometimes seen. ECG should be performed to rule out coexisting myocardial ischaemia and to look for a source of emboli. Mesenteric angiography may be used to confirm the diagnosis.

Tx Comprehensive resuscitation with early fluid replacement and analgesia is essential, together with prompt referral to the admitting surgical team.

Appendicitis

Appendicitis may occur at any age but is most common between the ages of 15 and 30 years and is uncommon under the age of 2 years. The usual features are:

- abdominal pain (initially periumbilical or epigastric, later radiating to the right iliac fossa)
- localised tenderness
- nausea and anorexia
- coated tongue and halitosis
- mild leukocytosis.

Pyrexia and tachycardia are unusual. The right iliac fossa is usually the most tender and guarded part of the abdomen but symptoms and signs may vary from the classic description:

- *Retrocaecal appendix*: pain may be elicited by right hip extension or be greatest in the right hypochrondrium.
- *Pelvic appendix*: rectal examination reveals tenderness high up on the right. There may be diarrhoea.
- *Gangrenous or perforated appendix*: signs of generalised peritonitis (→ p. 307).

Occasionally, an appendix mass will have developed. **Investigations:** The diagnosis is made on the basis of history and examination; special investigations are not indicated in the ED unless alternative diagnoses are being considered (→ Box 16.5).

Tx The patient should be referred for admission. If the appendix is thought to be leaking, then IV piperacillin with tazobactam (or a cephalosporin and metronidazole) should be commenced.

Diverticular disease

This usually occurs in patients age >50 years. There are three common acute presentations:

1 Inflammation (diverticulitis) causes periumbilical pain radiating to the left iliac fossa. There is

---

 Box 16.5 **The differential diagnosis of acute appendicitis**

- Urinary tract infection
- Mesenteric adenitis
- Ovulation pain (Mittelschmerz)
- Salpingitis
- Ovarian cyst torsion
- Constipation
- Pancreatitis
- Psoas haematoma (in patients with haemophilia)
- Perforated Meckel's diverticulum
- Non-specific abdominal pain
- GI upset in an athlete

localised tenderness and guarding in the left lower quadrant and a mass may be palpable. The patient may be pyrexial.

2 Perforation may occur without previous symptoms, producing acute peritonitis → *p. 307*.

3 Copious bleeding per rectum may cause profound shock → *p. 304*.

Tx Surgical referral is essential.

Inflammatory bowel disease

Ulcerative colitis: the patient with known ulcerative colitis may present to the ED with a fulminating attack. This is not usually associated with severe abdominal pain. Blood-stained mucousy diarrhoea is the most common feature with fever, tachycardia and hypotension.

Crohn's disease: this may rarely present as undiagnosed abdominal pain to the ED. There is usually a long history of recurrent diarrhoea and colic leading to anaemia and the development of an abdominal mass. The cicatrised small bowel may obstruct or perforate. If the patient presents with acute pain in the right iliac fossa, the previous history of diarrhoea should help to distinguish the condition from appendicitis.

Investigations: An abdominal radiograph may show a dilated colon in ulcerative colitis. Routine blood tests should be requested.

Tx Intravenous fluid replacement should be started and the admitting surgeons contacted.

Intestinal obstruction

The basic causes of intestinal obstruction are as follows:

- *Blocked lumen*: food, foreign body, faeces and very rarely a gallstone
- *Thickened wall*: carcinoma, Crohn's disease, tuberculosis
- *Altered geometry*: intussusception, volvulus
- *External compression*: herniae, inflammatory bands, adhesions
- *Absent peristalsis*: paralytic ileus, mesenteric infarction.

> The early features of intestinal obstruction can easily be mistaken for mild gastroenteritis. Small-bowel obstruction in the femoral hernia of an obese patient may be overlooked.

Paralytic ileus: this occurs after major abdominal surgery, but is most often seen in the ED in association with retroperitoneal haematomas, spinal and head injuries, and electrolyte disturbances.

Small bowel obstruction: this begins with periumbilical, intermittent, colicky pain. Vomiting is an early feature of jejunal obstruction but is delayed by a few hours in ileal obstruction. The patient usually presents at an early stage of the obstructive process; visible peristalsis may be seen and bowel sounds are increased. Later, the patient becomes dehydrated and oliguric. Central abdominal distension is occasionally evident. After the large bowel has been evacuated, there is 'absolute constipation' (no faeces or flatus per rectum).

Large bowel obstruction: this usually presents as an acute-on-chronic problem. Increasing constipation is the first symptom and abdominal distension is marked before the colicky pains become significant. The caecum becomes enlarged and tender unless the ileocaecal valve is incompetent. Vomiting is a late feature. Dehydration and major electrolyte abnormalities are often present by the time the patient is seen in the ED.

Strangulated bowel: when the blood supply to obstructed bowel is impaired, e.g. by the neck of a hernial sac, strangulation quickly ensues. Pain becomes more generalised and continuous and tachycardia increases. Rarely, these signs of impending necrosis and perforation are present without early evidence of obstruction if only part of the bowel wall is captured in a hernial sac (Richter's hernia).

Investigations: Clinical suspicion of bowel obstruction is one of the very few indications for an abdominal radiograph. Radiographs in patients with ileus, ischaemic bowel or pancreatitis are usually fairly normal but, in the presence of obstructed bowel, an abdominal radiograph may show dilated segments of intestine and fluid levels (although there are many causes of fluid levels). It is not always easy to differentiate between small and large bowel obstruction → *Figure 16.1*. A CT scan is no better at confirming obstruction than a plain radiograph although it may demonstrate the cause of the blockage. FBC, U&Es and glucose can be surprisingly normal or alternatively reveal gross dehydration and metabolic disturbance.

Tx
- Administer IV fluids. Fluid loss can be considerable, especially in small bowel obstruction.
- Give analgesia.
- Consider the need for a nasogastric tube.
- Measure urinary output (may need a catheter).

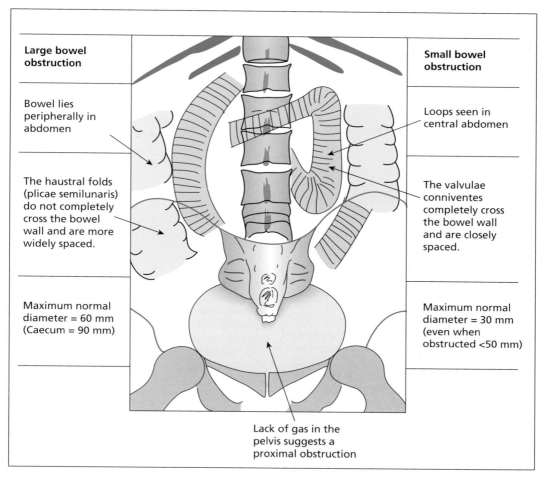

Large bowel obstruction		Small bowel obstruction
Bowel lies peripherally in abdomen		Loops seen in central abdomen
The haustral folds (plicae semilunaris) do not completely cross the bowel wall and are more widely spaced.		The valvulae conniventes completely cross the bowel wall and are closely spaced.
Maximum normal diameter = 60 mm (Caecum = 90 mm)		Maximum normal diameter = 30 mm (even when obstructed <50 mm)

Lack of gas in the pelvis suggests a proximal obstruction

Figure 16.1 Radiographs in bowel obstruction.

- Refer to the admitting surgical team. Small bowel obstruction often settles with conservative management whereas large bowel obstruction usually requires surgical intervention.

Intussusception in children → p. 349.

Gastroenteritis

Diarrhoea and vomiting in children → p. 348.

Gastroenteritis usually refers to a combination of diarrhoea with nausea or vomiting. Colicky central abdominal pain may also be present. The severity of the illness may vary from mild and inconvenient to severe and life threatening. In the developed world, 'D&V' is the most common reason for missing work, whereas, in developing countries, it remains a leading cause of death. Acute gastroenteritis is usually caused by infectious agents (or their toxins). Viruses are responsible for 50–70% of cases in the UK whilst a wide assortment of bacteria cause a further 15–20% and parasites are found in around 10%. These microbes produce GI upset by several different mechanisms: adherence to enterocytes, mucosal invasion, enterotoxin production and cytotoxin production (sometimes pre-formed before ingestion). All mechanisms result in increased fluid secretion and/or decreased absorption in the bowel. The increased luminal fluid content cannot be adequately reabsorbed, leading to dehydration and the loss of electrolytes and nutrients.

The history and examination are directed towards ensuring that the patient is not seriously ill and excluding other causes of GI upset such as:

- appendicis → p. 309
- pelvic abscess
- infective and travellers' diarrhoea → p. 254
- metabolic disturbance
- recent antibiotic therapy
- recent surgery
- athlete's diarrhoea (up to a third of athletes have a history of GI upset; the cause is usually not clearly defined, although gut ischaemia has been implicated).

Investigations: Further work-up is required only in patients who:

- appear seriously ill or dehydrated
- have a high fever, bloody stools, severe abdominal pain or persistent diarrhoea
- are immunocompromised
- are suspected of being part of a wider epidemic of gastroenteritis.

Tx Treatment in the ED is directed towards the following:

- Rehydration (oral or IV as required)
- Treatment of symptoms (especially fever and pain)
- Prevention of the spread of infection.

Oral rehydration is very successful, even for severe gastroenteritis. Small amounts of fluid can be given frequently, even while the patient is still vomiting. However, oral rehydration does not reduce the volume or the duration of the diarrhoea. A light diet should be reintroduced as soon as possible. Milk can be given safely. Despite the possibility of post-infective lactose intolerance, lactase deficiency is relatively uncommon, and most adults and children can tolerate non-human milk without any difficulty throughout a bout of acute gastroenteritis.

World Health Organization (WHO)-recommended oral rehydration solution → Box 16.6.

Antiemetics may be useful in the treatment of nausea and vomiting in adults with gastroenteritis but are not recommended for children. Antidiarrhoeals (antimotility agents) have traditionally been discouraged because of concerns about causing bacterae-

> **Box 16.6 WHO-recommended oral rehydration solution**
>
> Na^+ 90 mmol/L; K^+ 20 mmol/L; Cl^- 80 mmol/L; Glucose 20 g/L; Osmolarity = 310 mmol/L; $CHO:Na^+$ ratio = 1.2:1
>
> *The dose in severe diarrhoea is 250 mL (approximately 8 oz) every 15 min until fluid balance is clinically restored and then 1.5 L of oral fluid per litre of stool.*

mia. However, they may have a role in the symptomatic treatment of mild-to-moderate symptoms in adults. Patients who are clearly ill or significantly dehydrated will require admission

Norovirus is also known as Norwalk or winter vomiting virus and is the most common cause of gastroenteritis in the UK. The infection spreads rapidly in hospitals, other large institutions and cruise ships, with a short incubation period of between 12 and 48 h. Norovirus infection is usually diagnosed by the history. Some of the early symptoms include nausea, a sudden onset of vomiting, moderate diarrhoea, headache, fever, chills and myalgia. Uncontrollable vomiting is a classic sign and vomiting almost always predominates over diarrhoea. Spontaneous resolution occurs within 36–48 h. Strict hygiene is essential to prevent spread.

Rotavirus cause epidemics of gastroenteritis in children's schools and nurseries.

'Chinese restaurant syndrome' → p. 291.
Diarrhoea and vomiting in children → p. 348.
Scombroid fish poisoning → p. 291.
Travellers' diarrhoea and vomiting → p. 254.

Notifiable diseases: food poisoning, infectious bloody diarrhoea and suspected *Escherichia coli* O157 infection are all notifiable diseases. In around one in seven patients, haemolytic uraemic syndrome – also notifiable – follows verocytotoxin-producing *E. coli* infection (VTEC) (VTEC is also known as Shiga toxin-producing *E. coli* [STEC] and is usually type O157).

Acute bloody diarrhoea in children → p. 349.
Haemolytic uraemic syndrome and VTEC infection → p. 349.
Notifiable diseases → p. 388.

Non-specific abdominal pain

Some patients have abdominal pain for which no obvious diagnosis can be found. Non-specific abdominal pain should be diagnosed only in an adult aged <50 years, whose minimal symptoms and signs settle quickly. If discharged, the patient should be advised to visit his or her GP within a few days for follow-up.

Non-surgical causes of abdominal pain

Many conditions may present with abdominal pain as a feature. They include the following:

- *Cardiac pain*: myocardial ischaemia may present as acute upper abdominal pain. Right ventricular failure, leading to hepatic engorgement, may be associated with right hypochondrial pain → *p. 180*.
- *Diaphragmatic irritation*: pleurisy caused by a chest infection or pulmonary embolus may present with hypochondrial pain, worse on deep inspiration. There is usually referred shoulder-tip pain in addition → *p. 194*.
- *Pneumonia*: children with pneumonia may present with abdominal pain → *p. 339*.
- *Alcohol withdrawal*: This may cause surprisingly severe epigastric pain and tenderness → *p. 360*.
- *Poisoning* → *Chapter 15*.
- *Diabetes*: generalised abdominal pain associated with hyperglycaemia → *p. 242*.
- *Acute porphyria*: recurrent attacks of generalised or right-sided abdominal pain → *p. 264*.
- Hereditary angioedema (*HAE*): recurrent attacks of colicky abdominal pain, sometimes accompanied by diarrhoea and vomiting → *p. 300*.
- *Migraine* → *p. 226, epilepsy* → *p. 231, 343* and lead *poisoning* → *p. 298*. All may present with acute central abdominal pain.
- *Herpes zoster*: unilateral pain extending round either flank in the distribution of a cutaneous nerve. The herpetic eruption appears 24–48 h after the onset of pain → *p. 425*.
- *Collapsed vertebra*: usually the result of osteoporosis but may be caused by a secondary neoplastic lesion or tuberculosis. Pain may be generalised and not evidently arising from the spine.
- *Muscle injury*: rupture of part of the rectus abdominis or avulsion of the origin of the external oblique produces severe abdominal pain. It is exacerbated by attempting to sit up with the arms folded over the chest.
- *Sickle cell crisis* → *p. 257*.
- *Munchausen's syndrome* → *p. 368*.

> A patient who has presented with acute abdominal pain should not be discharged unless the diagnosis is confidently recognised as trivial or the patient has been discussed with and assessed by a senior colleague. Arrangements should be made for the patient to be followed up in a hospital clinic or by the GP.

PAIN FROM THE GENITOURINARY TRACT

Ureteric ('renal') colic

In the UK, renal calculi have a lifetime incidence of around 12% in men and 4% in women and these figures are doubled in those with a positive family history. The peak age for a first attack of ureteric colic is between age 35 and 45 years. It presents as severe and sudden bouts of pain radiating from the loin, around the flank, into the groin. Vomiting and sweating are usual and the patient may strain to pass small quantities of urine. The calculus is frequently held up proximal to the ureteric orifice in the base of the bladder at the trigone. The sensory nerve supply of the latter is identical to that of the external urethral meatus, because they share a common embryological origin. Hence trigonal pain is interpreted as arising from the tip of the external meatus. Renal and ureteric pain may also be caused by infections such as pyelonephritis and conditions such as renal carcinoma and renal infarction. It can be mistaken for the pain of a leaking aortic or iliac aneurysm and also that of biliary colic and peritonitis.

> Patients with Munchausen's syndrome commonly present with features of renal colic → *p. 368*.

Investigations: Around 85% of patients with ureteric colic have haematuria (usually microscopic). Urine should be tested for blood with reagent sticks and then sent for microscopy and culture. Blood tests should include serum calcium and uric acid levels as well as standard FBC and U&Es.

A plain abdominal radiograph may be requested to show the course of the ureters in the abdomen and pelvis (a 'KUB' or kidney–ureter–bladder radiograph). However, although nearly 90% of stones are radio-opaque, in reality, a plain film has a low sensitivity as a first diagnostic investigation. A non-contrast CT scan (CT-KUB) is both sensitive (96%) and specific (97%) for stones. As it has the added ability to rule out aneurysms and renal infarcts, it is the first investigation of choice for patients aged >60 years. Intravenous urography (IVU) has a similar sensitivity and specificity for calculi and also has the advantage of demonstrating renal function. An ultrasound scan can be used to rule out an aneurysm but will image only larger stones (>5 mm) in the proximal or distal (not mid) ureters.

> The absence of haematuria and/or lack of positive findings on a KUB radiograph does not rule out the possibility of pain due to renal calculi.

Tx Analgesia must be given as soon as possible. NSAIDs (e.g. intramuscular [IM] diclofenac 75 mg) are effective for lesser degrees of pain and should be added to IV opiates and antiemetics for more severe pain. Many patients will require admission for further analgesia and investigation, including those with the following:

- Pain that has not completely settled
- Fever or other signs of sepsis
- Recurrent attacks of ureteric colic
- A raised creatinine level
- Stones >6 mm in diameter (too large to pass).

Other patients can be followed up in a urology out-patient clinic.

Stones elsewhere in the urinary tract: bladder stones are rare in the UK. Stones in the renal pelvis are common but usually present to the outpatient clinic or are entirely asymptomatic. (They may cause chronic, dull pain and loin tenderness with intermittent infection or haematuria.)

Urinary tract infection

The symptoms of urinary tract infection (UTI) vary according to the site of infection and the age and sex of the patient. Pyelitis causes unilateral loin pain, tenderness and fever. Cystitis gives dysuria, frequency and urgency with or without haematuria. Both may cause some lower abdominal pain and tenderness. Some patients with UTI will be generally unwell, with evidence of systemic infection but few localising signs (especially infants and elderly people).

Investigation and treatment of UTI → p. 323.

Acute retention of urine

This causes severe abdominal pain, usually accompanied by a history of inability to pass urine. The enlarged bladder is easily palpable although it may be overlooked in the obese patient.

Causes and treatment → p. 325.

Pain from the testis and epididymis

Scrotal pain is usually referred to the lower abdomen. Always examine the perineum of a patient with abdominal pain.

Perineal problems → Chapter 17.

Pelvic inflammatory disease

Inflammation of the pelvic structures is usually caused by chlamydial or gonococcal infection and is therefore a manifestation of sexually transmitted infection in women of child-bearing age. Recurrent or chronic infections may cause ectopic pregnancy and infertility.

The presenting symptom is usually bilateral lower abdominal pain, although unilateral discomfort may be seen. The history may also reveal malaise, nausea, menstrual disturbance and vaginal discharge. Signs include fever, tenderness, guarding and cervical excitation (pain on moving the cervix). There may be tenderness of the uterus and in the fornices.

Investigations: FBC, erthrocyte sedimentation rate (ESR) and mid-stream specimen of urine (MSU) should be arranged, together with a pregnancy test. High vaginal, urethral and endocervical (chlamydial) swabs are also required but the acquisition of these is usually best left to a specialist. Laparoscopy may be needed to collect definitive specimens for culture.

Tx The condition is an inflammation and so injection of an NSAID (e.g. IM diclofenac 75 mg) can give considerable relief. Patients in severe pain or with hard signs should be admitted. Other patients can be followed up by the GP or in a gynaecology or genitourinary outpatient clinic. A short course of NSAIDs can be given to take out but antibiotics (usually doxy-cycline for 7 days or clarithromycin for 14 days) should be prescribed only after swabs have been taken. Ofloxacin and metronidazole are used for severe infections.

Other gynaecological causes of pain

Bleeding PV → p. 320.
Dysmenorrhoea → p. 323.
Ectopic pregnancy → p. 320.
Threatened and incomplete abortion → p. 320.

Rupture of an ovarian cyst causes sudden, lower abdominal pain with localised tenderness.

Torsion of an ovarian cyst causes lower abdominal pain and tenderness that may be recurrent. There may be a mass on abdominal or vaginal examination.

Endometriosis gives rise to recurrent abdominal pain, which is worse during menstrual bleeding. Other gynaecological symptoms are often present.

Obstetric, gynaecological and perineal problems → Chapter 17.

17

Obstetric, gynaecological, genitourinary and perineal problems

OBSTETRIC PROBLEMS

The abdomen in pregnancy → Figure 17.1.

Precipitant delivery

In the UK, most pregnant women have planned maternity care and so have made clear arrangements for the delivery of their baby. However, occasionally women arrive at the emergency department (ED) in the second stage of labour (i.e. after the cervix is fully dilated). Delivery of the baby may be imminent and

assistance must be given (→ *Boxes 17.1 and 17.2 and Figure 17.2*).

Further information about paediatric resuscitation → Chapter 11 on p. 151 and Chapter 18 on p. 329.

Antepartum haemorrhage

This is vaginal bleeding occurring after 24 weeks' gestation and is caused by placental abruption, placenta praevia or other less common lesions. The bleeding of placenta praevia is usually painless and starts around week 32 of gestation as the lower uterine segment is

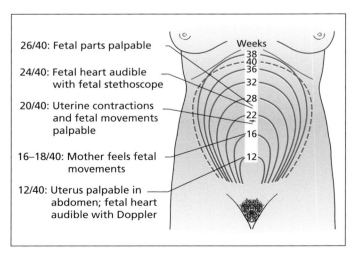

26/40: Fetal parts palpable

24/40: Fetal heart audible with fetal stethoscope

20/40: Uterine contractions and fetal movements palpable

16–18/40: Mother feels fetal movements

12/40: Uterus palpable in abdomen; fetal heart audible with Doppler

Weeks
38
40
36
32
28
22
16
12

Figure 17.1 Examination of the abdomen during pregnancy.

Box 17.1 **Precipitant delivery**

- Reassure the patient and take her to a private room
- Summon help (midwife and paediatrician)
- Keep a record of timing throughout
- Request a delivery pack, turn on the neonatal resuscitation trolley heater and get the Entonox apparatus
- Try to ascertain the gestational age of the baby and, briefly, the obstetric history of the mother
- Examine the abdomen to discover the position and number of babies
- Listen to the fetal heart with a Pinnard (or an electronic) fetal stethoscope. The rate should be >120 and if it slows with contractions it should recover quickly
- Allow the patient to adopt any position that she chooses
- Administer Entonox if required
- If liquor is draining, check the colour. Meconium staining indicates fetal distress
- Perform a vaginal examination to assess progress in labour, but NOT if there has been any bleeding (because of the risk of placenta praevia). If the cord is prolapsing, push it back into the cervix and hold it there until help arrives. Try to prevent cord compression by the head of the baby

- If the patient is 'pushing' (i.e. is late in the second stage) look to see if the fetal head, or other presenting part, is visible at the vulva. If it is, put on gown and gloves from the pack and place sterile towels around the delivery area. Cleanse the vulval area
- Control the descent of the head with the left hand while the right hand supports the perineum with a sterile pad
- As the head is delivered, encourage the mother to push more gently, while keeping the head flexed. If a breech appears, support the body gently without traction
- Check for the cord around the baby's neck and free it if necessary
- Allow the baby's head to turn laterally as the shoulders rotate. With the next contraction the body will be expelled. Deliver it by lifting the baby up and on to the mother's abdomen
- Tie or clamp the cord in two places at least 10 cm from the umbilicus and cut between the ties
- *For resuscitation of the baby → Box 17.2*
- Await spontaneous delivery of the afterbirth
- Keep the mother warm. If there is excessive bleeding, establish an IV infusion and give an ampoule of an oxytocic (e.g. Syntometrine 1 mL or ergometrine 0.5 mg IM)

beginning to form. With abruption, severe blood loss and shock may occur in the absence of significant external bleeding (concealed haemorrhage). There may be pain and a hard, 'wooden' uterus.

Tx The patient requires IV fluids, cross-match of blood and immediate referral to the obstetric service.

> Vaginal examination is contraindicated in antepartum haemorrhage.

Postpartum haemorrhage

Bleeding may occur soon after delivery or later on in the puerperium. It is the later bleeds (secondary

postpartum haemorrhage) that may present to the ED. The causes are retained products of conception and infection.

Tx IM Syntometrine (oxytocin 5 U and ergometrine 0.5 mg in 1 mL) may contract the uterus and control the bleeding. An IV infusion should be established and blood sent for cross-match before the patient is referred to the obstetrician.

Eclampsia

Eclampsia occurs in about 1 in 2000 deliveries in the UK and contributes to around 10% of maternal deaths. Women who are in late pregnancy or postpartum may occasionally present to an ED with eclamptic fits. The signs of pre-eclampsia (hypertension,

Box 17.2 Resuscitation of the newborn

Resuscitation Council (UK) algorithm for life support of the newborn infant → Figure 17.2.
Summon paediatric/anaesthetic help.
The assessment of the newborn infant depends primarily on three factors:
1 Colour
2 Respiratory effort
3 Heart rate

The Apgar score requires assessment of muscle tone and reflex irritability in addition to these three parameters.
A pink, crying baby needs no active resuscitation. The baby should be dried, wrapped up and given to the mother. Routine suctioning may cause reflex bradycardia and apnoea.
A blue baby who is gasping or apnoeic and has a heart rate >80 beats/min is in a state of primary apnoea. This will often respond to:

• warmth and peripheral stimulation
• gentle pharyngeal suctioning

• inflation of the lungs with oxygen using a bag and mask

A pale, apnoeic, floppy baby with a slow heart rate is in terminal apnoea. He or she needs:

• pharyngeal suctioning (meconium in the mouth indicates the need for inspection of the larynx and, if necessary, tracheal suctioning)
• ventilation with oxygen
• intubation if there is a skilled operator present (clumsy attempts may result in vagal bradycardia and laryngospasm) [endotracheal (ET) tube size = 3 mm after 28 weeks' gestation]
• cardiac compression if the heart rate is <60 beats/min (three compressions after each inflation with a compression rate of 120/min)
• adrenaline via the IV or intraosseus routes (the weight of a full-term neonate is usually about 3.5 kg and the dose of adrenaline = 10–30 mcg/kg)

oedema and proteinuria) may not be immediately apparent.

> In the UK, high-quality antenatal care has reduced the problems of pre-eclamptic toxaemia to such an extent that 75% of cases of eclampsia now occur in the postpartum period and a similar proportion occurs without pre-existing hypertension.

Tx
• Summon senior anaesthetic and obstetric help.
• Manage the airway and breathing.
• Establish venous access.
• Control the fitting with standard therapy (e.g. IV lorazepam) followed by IV magnesium sulphate (→ *below*).

Magnesium therapy: Magnesium sulphate is now the standard treatment for the control of recurrent eclamptic seizures. An IV injection of 4 g is given over 5–10 min, followed by an IV infusion of 1 g/h for at least 24 h. If fits recur then a further 2 g is given intravenously over 5 min; this dose is increased to 4 g if the

patient's weight is >70 kg. (Note that 1 g magnesium sulphate is equivalent to approximately 4 mmol ionised magnesium.)
Further information about magnesium → p. 158.

Major trauma in pregnancy

Management of major trauma in pregnancy → p. 31.

> When patients in late pregnancy are supine, the uterus may compress the inferior vena cava. This impairs the venous return to the heart and causes a profound fall in cardiac output. To avoid this problem, women in the last trimester of pregnancy should be tilted or wedged into a left semi-lateral position in the ED.

> Women who may have suffered abdominal trauma and who are rhesus D negative will require anti-D immunoglobulin.

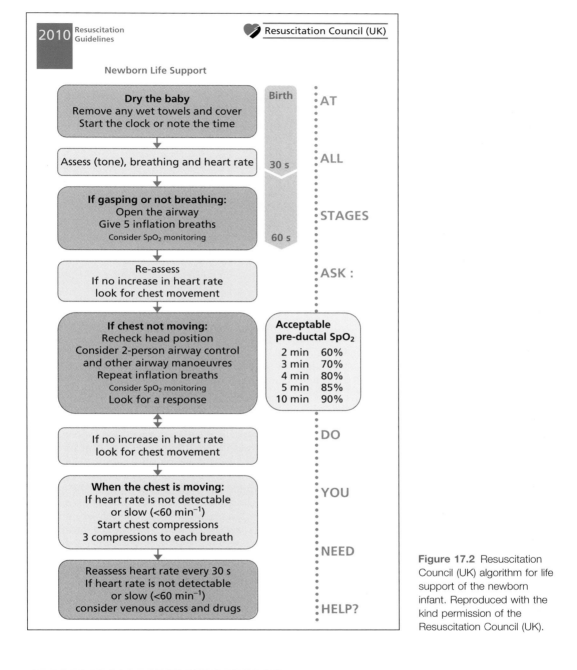

Figure 17.2 Resuscitation Council (UK) algorithm for life support of the newborn infant. Reproduced with the kind permission of the Resuscitation Council (UK).

GYNAECOLOGICAL PROBLEMS

Guidance about intimate examinations → p. 303.
Treatment of suspected rape or sexual abuse →
p. 373.

Hyperemesis gravidarum

Hyperemesis gravidarum is a severe form of morning sickness with intractable nausea and vomiting that prevents an adequate intake of food and drink. Around 75% of all pregnant women experience some degree of nausea and vomiting but hyperemesis occurs in only 0.5–2% of pregnancies and may affect the wellbeing of both the mother and the fetus. Weight loss, nutritional deficiencies and abnormalities in fluid and electrolyte and acid–base balance may occur. The peak incidence is at 8–12 weeks of pregnancy and symptoms usually resolve by week 20 in all but 10% of patients. Sufferers are more likely to be non-white and aged >30 years with a history of motion sickness, migraine or previous hyperemesis gravidarum. The condition is associated with multiple pregnancy, molar pregnancy and some fetal abnormalities; it may also have a genetic component. Strangely, cigarette smoking seems to be a protective factor! The cause of hyperemesis is unknown but is thought to be related to hormonal changes.

Investigations:

- Full blood count (FBC), C-reactive protein (CRP) and midstream specimen of urine (MSU) to exclude infection; routine blood chemistry
- Urine for ketones
- Ultrasound scan to assess fetal growth.

Tx Rehydration with IV fluids is usually required. Safe and effective antiemetics include IV metoclopramide, promethazine and ondansetron. Pyridoxine (vitamin B_6) has been found to be of help and avoidance of sensory triggers is important. Some women will require multiple admissions during their pregnancy.

Vaginal bleeding in pregnancy

Vaginal bleeding occurs in up to a fifth of all pregnant women but in over 50% of cases the pregnancy will continue successfully. After 24 weeks (and effectively after 20 weeks for the purposes of management in the ED) vaginal bleeding is classed as an antepartum haemorrhage ($\rightarrow$ p. 316). Before this time it may be:

- a threatened abortion
- an incomplete abortion
- a complete abortion
- other ($\rightarrow$ below).

Loss of the fetus is accompanied by:

- significant abdominal pain and tenderness
- heavy or continuing bleeding
- the passage of placental material in addition to blood clots
- an open cervical os
- the absence of a fetal heart on ultrasound examination.

Investigations: Portable Doppler ultrasound scanners are useful only at gestations of >12 weeks, although formal scanning may detect a heart beat at 7 weeks' gestation.

Tx Patients with the above features of imminent fetal loss require admission for observation. Severe bleeding necessitates IV fluids and, if fetal loss is assured, an oxytocic (e.g. Syntometrine 1 mL IM or oxytocin 5 U slowly IV). Pain must be relieved by appropriate analgesia, whatever the course of the pregnancy. Severe pain is sometimes caused by the passage of material through the cervix; great relief can be obtained by the removal of this tissue with sponge-holding forceps via a speculum.

> Loss of a fetus will be an important and sad event for most women; medical care must be accompanied by compassion.

Patients with threatened abortion without symptoms or signs of fetal loss may be referred back to the GP for bed rest at home, although requests for admission from patients must be given serious consideration. If possible, all such patients should be seen in a specialist pregnancy review clinic within 48 h. Early ultrasound scanning is essential.

The rhesus D antibody status of all patients with bleeding in pregnancy after 12 weeks' gestation must be ascertained. It may be recorded on the obstetric cooperation card in later pregnancy. If antibody status is unknown, then blood should be sent for urgent grouping. Patients who are RhD negative with a gestation of 12 weeks or more must be protected from developing anti-D antibodies to fetal RhD-positive cells, which may have leaked into the maternal circulation. This is achieved by the administration of anti-D immunoglobulin to destroy any RhD-positive cells before they can sensitise the mother. To be effective, the γ-globulin must be given within 72 h of the onset of vaginal bleeding. The dose is 250 IU by deep IM injection for patients with a gestation of <20 weeks and 500 IU for those with a gestation of ≥20 weeks.

Ectopic pregnancy

Sites for ectopic pregnancies $\rightarrow$ Figure 17.3.

There are 1.8 ectopic pregnancies per 1000 total pregnancies in the UK and it is still one of the most common causes of maternal death. The diagnosis must be considered in any woman of child-bearing age with abdominal or pelvic pain or unexplained collapse. There may be any of the following:

Figure 17.3 Sites for ectopic pregnancies: (1) Fallopian tube – isthmial; (2) Fallopian tube – ampullory; (3) cornual; (4) abdominal; (5) ovarian; (6) cervical.
- UK incidence, 1 in 200 pregnancies, almost all in the Fallopian tubes
- Pregnancy in isthmus of tube ruptures early (4–8 weeks' gestation) and causes sudden, acute lower abdominal pain and guarding with shock
- Pregnancy in ampulla of tube does not cause symptoms until 8–12 weeks' gestation. Blood leaking into the peritoneal cavity then causes intermittent pains over several days.

- A history of amenorrhoea (perhaps only for a couple of weeks and not by any means essential for the diagnosis)
- Vaginal bleeding (follows the pain but may be minimal and is absent in about 25% of cases of tubal pregnancy)
- Tenderness in the lower abdomen
- Tenderness in the fornices on vaginal examination
- Sudden onset of severe hypovolaemic shock.

Investigations: The absence of β human chorionic gonadotrophin (βHCG) in the urine makes the diagnosis of ectopic pregnancy very unlikely because its presence is a highly sensitive test for early pregnancy. Ultrasound scan (preferably a high-resolution transvaginal scan) or even laparoscopy may be needed to confirm the diagnosis.

Tx

- Establish an IV infusion.
- Cross-match blood.
- Refer the patient to a gynaecologist.

Patients with no abdominal tenderness who are haemodynamically stable may be a seen at an urgent clinic on the following day if local arrangements permit this course of action. In the presence of a low serum βHCG concentration (<1000 IU/L), nearly 70% of ectopic pregnancies will resolve without surgical treatment. Medical treatment with systemic meth-

otrexate raises this figure to around 80%. However, patients with tubal rupture, a mass >3.5 cm in diameter, free fluid >50 mL or a fetal heart beat on ultrasound scan still require conventional surgical treatment.

Other vaginal bleeding

Women with vaginal bleeding unrelated to pregnancy should be referred back to their GP for examination and cervical smear. Atypically severe menorrhagia may merit admission. Some reduction in the blood loss during a period can be achieved by taking a short course of oral NSAIDs at the time of the bleeding.

Emergency contraception

Some patients will present only on one occasion to one agency in their attempt to get the 'morning-after pill'. This 'window of opportunity' must be grasped by that agency in order to avoid the disaster of an unwanted pregnancy.

In England and Wales in 2010, more than 1 in every 100 young women between the ages of 13 and 16 years became pregnant. Pregnancy in the under-16s is not a planned event and half of these conceptions ended in therapeutic abortion.

Two main methods are currently used for emergency postcoital contraception:

1 Hormonal therapy → *below*
2 Immediate insertion of a copper-containing intra-uterine contraceptive device (IUCD) (this is more effective than emergency hormonal contraception and can be introduced up to 5 days after the earliest predicted ovulation).

Either of these therapies may be obtained by referral to the GP or a family planning clinic. For those women wishing to be treated in the ED, the hormonal method is the most suitable. It must be started within 72 h of unprotected sexual intercourse (preferably within 12 h) and consists of a single 1.5 mg tablet (or two 0.75 mg tablets) of the synthetic progestogen levonorgestrel to be taken immediately. This regimen can also be used between 72 and 120 h after unprotected intercourse but this is an unlicensed indication and its efficacy decreases with time. The dose of levonorgestrel should be doubled in women who are taking enzyme-inducing drugs. A second drug, ulipristal (a progesterone receptor modulator), is also licensed for emergency contraceptive use in the UK. It is as effective as levonorgestrel if taken (as a single 30 mg tablet) within 120 h of unprotected intercourse. Levonorgestrel for emergency contraception is available 'over the counter' in the UK but ulipristal is not. Emergency contraception with the Yuzpe regimen (combined oestrogen and progestogen tablets) is no longer recommended because the progestogen-only system is safer and three times more effective. There is no increased risk of ectopic pregnancy with emergency contraception using progestogens.

Before prescription, a medical and gynaecological history should be taken to discover the normal menstrual cycle and details of contraceptive usage. There are no absolute contraindications to the use of progestogen-only emergency contraception but caution should be exercised in women with porphyria or severe liver disease.

Women should be given verbal and written information on the following:

- The hormones work by making the lining of the uterus unsuitable for a pregnancy to develop, by delaying the release of an egg from the ovary or by preventing the egg from being fertilised by the sperm (i.e. by preventing ovulation, fertilisation and implantation).
- There is a failure rate of 1–3% with this method of emergency contraception. Expressed another way, levonorgestrel in the recommended dosage will prevent around 85% of expected pregnancies, if used within 72 h of unprotected intercourse. (The overall risk of pregnancy following one act of unprotected sexual intercourse at any time during the menstrual cycle is about 2–4%. However, around the time of ovulation [days 10–17] this figure climbs to 20–30%.)
- The next period may come earlier or later than usual and may be unusually light or heavy. A pregnancy test is required if proper menstruation has not occurred within 3 weeks.
- The main side effects of the tablets are nausea and occasionally vomiting. If vomiting occurs within 3 h of taking the pills, another dose must be taken as soon as possible.
- If the method fails and pregnancy ensues, there is no evidence that the hormones may harm the fetus.
- A barrier method of contraception should be used until the start of the next period.
- All women should attend the GP or family planning clinic as soon as possible to get definitive contraceptive advice.

Post-exposure prophylaxis after sexual exposure (to blood-borne viruses)

Post-exposure prophylaxis after sexual exposure (PEPSE) is the administration of antiviral therapy after possible sexual exposure to blood-borne viruses in the same way as with needlestick, splash or bite exposure (→ p. 402). In addition to consideration of hepatitis B immunisation (→ p. 404), there is 28 days of treatment with combination antiretrovirals which have considerable side effects and so, for this reason, it is crucial that the potential benefits of PEPSE outweigh the risks and that the affected individual is well informed.

Risk of HIV transmission
= Risk that the source is HIV positive
× Risk of exposure

Co-factors affecting the risk of transmission include coexisting sexually transmitted infections, high HIV viral load, breeches in mucosal membranes, bleeding, trauma and type of sexual activity. The use of PEPSE is recommended only when the individual presents within 72 h of sexual exposure and then the drugs should be administered as soon as possible. PEP is considered only after an isolated high-risk sexual exposure (ongoing regular exposure indicates the need for risk reduction advice rather than PEP). Such exposure includes the following:

- Condom accident in a discordant couple (one HIV positive, the other not)

- Rape, where the assailant is in a high-risk group ($\rightarrow$ *Box 21.7 on p. 403*). The probability of HIV transmission may be increased after aggravated sexual assault
- Unprotected penetrative sex with someone who then discloses HIV-positive status.

In these situations consider PEP when the source individual is known to be HIV positive and the following exposure has occurred:

- Receptive or insertive anal sex
- Receptive or insertive vaginal sex
- Ejaculation of semen into the mouth or splash of semen into the eyes.

Antiviral drugs to be given $\rightarrow$ Box 21.10 on p. 404 or consult local up-to-date (and frequently changing) guidelines.

Consider discussing all cases for possible PEPSE with a specialist genitourinary physician. All patients who have received PEPSE should be followed up at a specialist clinic.

Dysmenorrhoea

This complaint should be dealt with sympathetically even if definitive treatment cannot be offered. Other causes of abdominal pain must be excluded before the patient is referred back to their GP. NSAIDs may give great relief, both as drugs to take out and as a parenteral therapy in the ED.

Pelvic inflammatory disease

Pelvic inflammatory disease $\rightarrow$ p. 314.

Mid-cycle pain

Ovulation may sometimes be associated with pain and slight vaginal bleeding. This is called Mittelschmerz and can be followed up by the GP.

Vaginal discharge

A slight discharge is normal in women of reproductive age. It may be increased by the oral contraceptive pill. Candidiasis (thrush) causes an irritant creamy discharge.

Tx Suspected thrush may be treated by a short course of pessaries (e.g. miconazole). The partner will also need treatment to prevent reinfection.

Other patients should be referred to their GP for vaginal examination, swabs and cervical smear.

Vaginal foreign bodies

Women may present with retained vaginal foreign bodies, most commonly tampons or contraceptive sheaths. The posterior fornix is the site where such objects are often lodged.

Tx The foreign body should be visualised with the aid of a Cusco's speculum and removed with sponge-holding forceps. A digital examination must also be performed if the object is not found. It is worth noting that occasional cases of missed intravesical foreign body have been described.

Women who have had a retained vaginal foreign body for some days may be at risk of toxic shock syndrome ($\rightarrow$ p. 352). An unpleasant discharge may be treated with a short course of antiseptic pessaries (e.g. Betadine pessaries one twice daily for 5 days).

Labial abscess

An abscess may form in the Bartholin's gland, which is situated in the posterior third of the labia majora. The whole labia is swollen, inflamed and extremely tender. The patient must be referred to the gynaecologist on call for drainage and marsupialisation.

Breast abscesses and lumps

A combination of lactation and staphylococcal infection may lead to a breast abscess. The patient needs admission because the tender, red lump in the breast must be drained under general anaesthesia; anything less is inappropriate. Suppression of lactation may be required.

Breast lumps should be examined and the findings discussed with the patient. Referral should then be made to the GP who can arrange appropriate treatment, usually a surgical opinion and excision biopsy.

GENITOURINARY PROBLEMS

Urinary tract infection

Urinary tract infection (UTI) is more common in women than in men; when it occurs in men there is often an underlying anatomical or pathological abnormality. Recurrent episodes of infection, especially in children, are an indication for radiological investigation. Infection of the lower urinary tract is characterised by the classic symptoms of dysuria, frequency and urgency. Haematuria and proteinuria may be present but physical signs are usually minimal. Suprapubic pain and tenderness are sometimes seen. A patient with pyelitis or pyelonephritis is usually systemically unwell with pyrexia, loin pain, rigors and tenderness over the affected kidney.

> In children and elderly people, UTI may cause general malaise with non-specific features such as pyrexia, vomiting, abdominal pain and confusion.

Tx
- Test the urine for blood, protein, nitrites and glucose (to exclude diabetes).
- Send an MSU to the laboratory with the results forwarded to the GP.
- Commence antibiotic therapy in patients with positive findings → *below*.
- Advise the patient to drink an increased amount of fluids.
- Refer the patient to see the GP after 3 days for follow-up when the MSU result is available.

But note the following:

- Patients with features of pyelitis or pyelonephritis require admission under a general surgeon.
- Children with UTI should be followed up in the paediatric clinic. Investigations may reveal ureteric reflux or congenital abnormality.
- In men, UTI is often secondary to venereal infection and so genitourinary clinic follow-up should be arranged.

Antibiotics for UTI: the most common organism found in urinary tract infection is *Escherichia coli*. Other causative bacteria include Gram-negative bacilli of the *Proteus* and *Klebsiella* genera and enterococci. *Staphylococcus saprophyticus* is a common cause of UTI in sexually active young women. The sensitivity patterns of coliforms are changing – around half are resistant to ampicillin/amoxicillin and nearly a third are resistant to trimethoprim. Therefore, a 3- to 5-day course of cefalexin (cephalexin) or cefadroxil is a good first choice in uncomplicated cystitis; nitrofurantoin, nalidixic acid and trimethoprim are alternatives. Women aged >50 years and men are more difficult to treat and may require a longer course (7 days) of co-amoxiclav or a combination that includes ciprofloxacin (for *Pseudomonas aeruginosa*). Ascending infections of the urinary tract (pyelitis or pyelonephritis) should be treated with a quinolone or a broad-spectrum cephalosporin for 14 days.

Haematuria in the absence of signs of infection

Patients with mild haematuria may be referred back to their GP. Macroscopic, painless haematuria should be discussed with a member of the surgical team. Severe haematuria merits admission.

Prostatitis

Bacterial infection of the prostate gland can occur with *E. coli* and *Streptococcus faecalis*. The patient has the following:

1 The features of prostatism – frequency, hesitancy and poor stream – possibly leading to retention
2 Pyrexia, leukocytosis and a very tender prostate gland on rectal examination.

Tx The patient should be referred to the on-call surgical team. Acute prostatitis is treated with either ciprofloxacin or trimethoprim for 28 days.

Testicular swelling and pain

> A male patient aged <25 years with testicular pain must be assumed to have a torsion until proved otherwise.

Testicular torsion causes pain that is unilateral and usually, but not always, sudden in onset. It may radiate to the lower abdomen. There may have been previous episodes of the same pain. The testis is swollen and tender with a small hydrocele.

Epididymo-orchitis may be seen in older men after a UTI. The testis and cord are painful, tender and swollen and the patient is pyrexial. Orchitis may also occur as a feature of mumps → *p. 425*.

Investigations: An ultrasound scan of the scrotum can distinguish testicular swelling from paratesticular lesions and can demonstrate free fluid and tumours.

Tx Patients with testicular pain or swelling should be seen by the surgeon on call.

Sexually transmitted infections

Ulcers, warts or herpetic lesions of the genitalia may present to the ED. They should be assumed to be highly infectious. Referral should be made to the local genitourinary clinic.

Penile discharge is also invariably a symptom of sexually transmitted infection. It may be accompanied by dysuria. Referral should again be made to the genitourinary clinic.

HIV/AIDS → p. 261.

HIV post-exposure prophylaxis after sexual exposure (PEPSE) → p. 322.

Pelvic inflammatory disease (gonococcal or chlamydial infection) → p. 323.

Syphilis → p. 262.

Postcoital bleeding

Postcoital bleeding may occur in both sexes. Women with this symptom should be referred back to their GP for speculum examination and cervical smear. Men are usually found to have torn the frenulum of the foreskin. A small blood vessel may be bleeding profusely. It should be cauterised with silver nitrate.

Retention of urine

Acute retention of urine causes extreme distress. There is lower abdominal pain and an inability to micturate, although the patient may be unaware of the latter problem if obtunded. Usually, the enlarged bladder is obvious but it may be overlooked in the obese patient, especially if there is retention with overflow (i.e. a large volume remains in the bladder after voiding a small amount of urine).

In male patients, retention is most often caused by obstruction of the urethra by an enlarged prostate gland but a variety of other conditions may also cause it, including:

- urethral stricture (congenital or acquired)
- pain around the pelvis and perineum
- drugs (e.g. anticholinergics, antihypertensives and antihistamines)
- neurological problems.

Tx Treatment consists of careful, aseptic catheterisation and controlled drainage of urine. Most patients should then be admitted for investigation.

If transurethral catheterisation proves impossible or is contraindicated (e.g. in cases of traumatic injury to the lower urinary tract), then suprapubic catheterisation will be required. This requires considerable experience to avoid complications such as bladder perforation. High-risk cases should be performed in a controlled environment with a senior surgeon and anaesthetist present. Confirmation of bladder position by ultrasonography may be required. Suprapubic catheterisation is absolutely contraindicated in the absence of an easily palpable or ultrasonographically localised distended urinary bladder and it is relatively contraindicated in the following situations:

- Coagulopathy (until the abnormality is corrected)
- Prior abdominal or pelvic surgery (potential bowel adherence to the bladder or anterior abdominal wall; may recommend that a urologist perform an open cystostomy)
- Pelvic cancer with or without pelvic radiation (increased risk of adhesions).

After insertion of a suprapubic catheter, there should be a high index of suspicion for bowel perforation if the patient has abdominal pain, or is otherwise unwell and presents features of localised peritonitis.

In an emergency situation, with reduced senior support and limited access to equipment, it may be appropriate to consider bladder aspiration with a fine needle as an interim measure.

Catheter problems

Elderly male patients commonly present with blocked catheters. The catheter should be changed for a suitable long-term replacement and free drainage of urine confirmed. It is essential that arrangements are made with the district nursing team for follow-up and advice about future catheter care.

Balanitis

Infection of the prepuce and glans may occur, especially in boys with an unretractable foreskin.

Tx Severe infection or difficulty with micturition merits referral. Other patients require:

- a urine test for glucose to exclude diabetes
- a local swab to be sent to the laboratory
- a consideration of the possibility of infection with *Candida* or *Trichomonas* spp. – ask about symptoms in the partner
- cleaning of the infected area and advice on hygiene, especially in elderly people
- referral to the GP.

Some patients will go on to require circumcision.

Paraphimosis

Retraction of a tight foreskin can impair the venous return from the glans causing distal engorgement and extreme swelling.

Tx Reduction may be attempted in the ED. Analgesia and lubrication are obtained by the application of lidocaine gel. The thumb is placed on the prepuce and gentle but increasing pressure applied as the foreskin is drawn over it with the index and middle fingers. If this is unsuccessful, the patient should be referred to a general surgeon. Reduction under anaesthetic may be required and occasionally, in adults, a dorsal slit is needed.

'Fracture' of the penis

Trauma to the erect penis during intercourse may sometimes rupture one of the engorged corpora cavernosa. This is known as a 'fracture' of the penis. The patient presents with a history of increasing perineal discomfort and bruising after intercourse. The penis, scrotum and suprapubic area are found to be very swollen and bruised without any other external sign of injury. Patients with this condition should be referred immediately to a urologist for exploration of the damaged area. If left untreated, impotency can result.

Iatrogenic priapism

This problem is sometimes seen in patients who are under the care of a clinic that treats aspects of sexual dysfunction. Intracavernosal injections of papaverine (up to 120 mg) may be used by a patient as often as twice weekly to obtain an erection, which should subside spontaneously within 3 h. If this does not occur, the prolonged erection (priapism) becomes uncomfortable and distressing.

Tx Discuss the patient with a urologist or the doctor who prescribed the injections before contemplating treatment. If priapism is long standing, surgical evacuation of blood clots may be necessary. In cases of a shorter duration, decompression may be achieved by the following technique:

- Draw up 5 mg of the α agonist phenylephrine into a syringe, diluted with saline to 10 mL.
- Insert a 19 G butterfly needle into either corpus cavernosum.
- Withdraw 20–40 mL blood using a syringe. This will usually relieve the pain.
- Inject 1 mg of the phenylephrine solution (via the same needle) while monitoring the patient's BP. If there is no hypertension, inject a further 4 mg (to a total of 5 mg).
- Massage the penis gently. This may be painful.
- If there is little improvement, repeat the above procedure after 1 h.
- Observe the patient for an hour after the last treatment.
- Advise no further intracavernosal injections until the patient has consulted the doctor who prescribed the treatment.

PERINEAL PROBLEMS

Perianal abscess

Abscesses arising from the glands of the anal canal present as extremely painful swellings around the anus. Deeper infection in the ischiorectal fossa may cause a more diffuse swelling of the buttock. The patient should be referred to the surgical team for drainage under general anaesthesia. It is totally inappropriate to attempt incision under local anaesthesia in the ED.

Pilonidal abscess

This presents as a tender, red swelling in the upper part of the natal cleft. The underlying pilonidal sinus may not be visible. Inpatient care is necessary for this condition.

Gluteal abscesses may extend deep into the buttock and are also generally best treated in theatre.

Foreign bodies in the rectum

Rectal foreign bodies may be difficult to remove because of spasm of the sphincters. Removal under general anaesthesia is often needed.

Rectal bleeding

The loss of a significant amount of blood from the rectum should be treated in the same manner as any other bleeding, i.e. resuscitation, cross-match of blood and immediate specialist referral → *p. 304*.

Lesser amounts of bleeding, in an apparently well patient, can be referred back to the GP for investigation and referral as appropriate.

Haemorrhoids

Haemorrhoids or piles are enlarged cushions of anal mucosa accompanied by varicosities of the neighbouring (superior haemorrhoidal) veins. They may cause:

- bright-red blood with and after the motions
- pain on defecation and consequent constipation
- perianal irritation
- a prolapse of mucosal tissue (on straining – second-degree piles; or constant – third-degree piles).

Tx If the bleeding has stopped and abdominal and rectal examination is unremarkable, then further investigation can be undertaken by the GP. Extreme pain such as that caused by a strangulated pile or suppurative, ulcerated lesions should be referred to the duty surgeon.

Thrombosed external pile

This is a perianal haematoma caused by the rupture of a tributary of the inferior haemorrhoidal vein. There is pain and a dark-blue swelling at the anal margin. If it discharges or begins to resolve spontaneously then no further treatment is needed. If not, incision may be required either in the ED under local anaesthetic or in some cases by a surgeon in theatre.

Anal fissure

A tear at the anal margin may cause severe pain with defecation. It may be associated with a tag of anal epithelium known as a sentinel pile. Multiple fissures are a feature of Crohn's disease. Treatment is within the province of a general surgeon.

Perianal irritation

Pruritis ani is the predominant symptom of a perianal dermatitis. A build-up of moisture and small particles of faeces reduces the efficacy of the normal skin barrier in a manner similar to that which causes nappy rash. Scratching and secondary bacterial infection then compound the damage.

Tx
- The perianal skin must be kept clean and dry.
- Scratching and chemical irritants should be avoided.
- After every bowel action, the area must be cleaned by bathing or by using shower jets, a bidet or medicated wipes. Strong soap and abrasive methods of cleaning are not suitable.
- The area should be gently dried after cleaning with a soft towel or a hairdryer.
- Talcum powder, ointments and creams should not be used.

18

Children's problems in the emergency department

Patients aged <16 years account for about 25% of the attendances at a typical emergency department (ED) in the UK, with a disproportionate number of such children aged <5 years. Experiences of hospitals gained in childhood may influence patients throughout their lives.

In the UK in 2012

- Around 10% of children have a mental disorder
- Over 5% of children are disabled
- One in 400 children is on the child protection register (or equivalent)
- Over 80% of all illnesses in childhood are managed by the family
- Around 25% of calls to NHS Direct and 10% of walk-in centre attendances involve children
- Up to 50% of infants aged <12 months and 25% of older children will attend an ED
- One in 11 children will attend a hospital outpatient clinic each year and around 1 in 12 will be admitted

---

Assessment of the ill or injured child: the differences between adults and children

The principles of paediatric assessment are identical to those applicable to an adult. Problems arise because of the following.

The size of children

The variable age and hence size of children affects physiological measurements, drug doses and equipment sizes. An expected adult weight range might be 45–90 kg, i.e. a twofold difference. Children may easily vary from 3 kg to 60 kg: a 20-fold range. A factor of two is often disregarded – most adults are given a standard dose of drugs and assumed to have similar physiological parameters. A 20-fold difference is impossible to ignore; treatment must be tailored to the size of the child.

The age of a child is usually known but the weight is more difficult to ascertain. Because of this, it is important to be able to estimate a child's weight from a knowledge of his or her age.

Estimating a child's weight from his or her age → Box 18.1.

Emergency Medicine Lecture Notes, Fourth Edition. Chris Moulton and David Yates.
© 2012 Blackwell Publishing Ltd. Published 2012 by Blackwell Publishing Ltd.

Box 18.1 Estimating the weight of a child

- Average birthweight of a full-term infant = 3.5 kg
- Weight at age 5 months = double the birthweight
- Weight at age 12 months = triple the birthweight

Between the ages of 1 and 12 years the approximate weight of a child in kilograms can be calculated by the following formulae:

0–12 months: Weight in kg = (0.5 × Age in months) + 4
1–5 years: Weight in kg = (2 × Age in years) + 8
6–12 years: Weight in kg = (3 × Age in years) + 7

The causes of illness in children

The conditions with which children present are different. They do not generally suffer from the degenerative diseases of adult life but have more problems with infective conditions.

The causes of cardiac arrest in children

Children usually die from hypoxia, secondary to respiratory distress or depression, or from hypovolaemia (fluid loss or maldistribution). These lead to cardiac asystole, which has a very poor prognosis. Therefore, it is vital to recognise and reverse these conditions before terminal bradycardia supervenes. Coronary artery disease, and thus ventricular fibrillation, is very uncommon in children.

The anatomy and physiology of children

Children differ from adults in their body proportions. They also have a more elastic skeleton. This leads to a different pattern of injury and an airway that can be more difficult to manage. As a result of the elastic chest wall, children are far less likely to have rib fractures, although they may have severe underlying damage to the lung, liver or spleen (*also →* Chapter 6).

The fast metabolism and low reserves of children explain why they get ill, hypoxic, hypoglycaemic and hypothermic very quickly. However, their general health and high capacity for repair make for a speedy recovery.

The psychology of children

The interaction with the assessor is as variable as the age of the child. Only practice can teach the subtle parts of this relationship but those with children of their own have a distinct advantage.

IMMEDIATE ASSESSMENT AND MANAGEMENT

Cardiac arrest protocols for children → Chapter 11.
Principles of immediate assessment → Chapter 1.
Resuscitation of the newborn infant → p. 318.

> The skills required for the resuscitation of infants and children are best learned on an advanced paediatric life support course.

A – Airway

Checking for responsiveness

The presence of a response is usually immediately obvious. If it is not then gentle shaking may establish verbal communication with an older child. The young child will respond by eye movement, cry or body posture – the mother will know.

> Always consider the possibility of an inhaled foreign body in children who are unresponsive or dyspnoeic.

The child's airway

Children are particularly prone to airway obstruction because of the following:

- The airway has a small diameter. Its narrowest point is at the subglottis, rather than at the vocal folds as in an adult.
- The tongue and pharyngeal soft tissues are relatively bulky.

- The voice box (larynx) is more of a voice bag with a large, floppy epiglottis and pliable vocal folds. It lies more anteriorly than in an adult.
- In the submucosa of the airway there is a large amount of lymphoid tissue that can enlarge.
- The airway reflexes are particularly sensitive.
- Toddlers put things in their mouths.
- There is a high incidence of upper respiratory tract infection (URTI) in children, including several infections that target the airway.
- Children aged <6 months are compulsory nose breathers. Nasal obstruction is thus critical in this age group.

Choking protocols → p. 196.
Management of other laryngotracheal obstruction in children → p. 198.

Do not examine the throat with any instrument in children with stridor or suspected partial airway obstruction. Doing so may convert the problem to complete obstruction.

Maintenance and protection of the airway

The need for aids to maintain the airway is assessed on the same criteria in the child as in the adult. However, if a child's airway is maintainable by simple manoeuvres, an oropharyngeal (Guedel) airway is best avoided. This is because retching is easily induced in children and may be followed by laryngospasm or aspiration.

Artificial airway and endotracheal tube sizes → Box 18.2.

 Box 18.2 Artificial airway and endotracheal tube sizes

Oropharyngeal airway size = approximately the distance from the centre of the lips to the angle of the jaw.
Nasopharyngeal airway size = approximately the distance from the tip of the nose to the tragus of the ear.

Endotracheal tube size
Internal diameter (in mm) = (Age/4) + 4 [neonate 3 to 3.5 mm tube]
Oral tube length (in cm) = (Age/2) + 12
Nasal tube length (in cm) = (Age/2) + 15

Endotracheal intubation of infants

The large, floppy epiglottis of the infant prevents a standard intubation technique whereby the tip of the laryngoscope is positioned in the vallecula – the angle between the base of the tongue and the anterior surface of the epiglottis. Instead, the epiglottis must be lifted forward by a laryngoscope, which is placed posterior to it.

For this reason, paediatric laryngoscopes have relatively straight blades (e.g. Seward, Soper, Robertshaw, Miller or Wisconsin blades). The Robertshaw laryngoscope, which has characteristics of both typical adult and paediatric designs, is probably the easiest to use. After the age of about 18 months, a standard adult technique can be adopted, although many anaesthetists prefer to use a straight blade for children up to the age of 5 years.

The presence or absence of the gag reflex gives no useful information. Testing for it in children may easily induce retching or laryngospasm and create a certain airway problem.

B – Breathing

The oxygen saturation shown by the pulse oximeter should be close to 100% in a normal healthy child breathing air.

Normal respiratory rates in children → Table 18.1.

Very slow respiratory rates in children suggest imminent respiratory arrest or poisoning with narcotic drugs (e.g. methadone).

Table 18.1 Normal respiratory rates and pulse rates in children

Age (years)	Respiratory rate (breaths/min)	Heart rate (beats/min)
>1	30–40	110–160
1–5	25–30	95–140
5–12	20–25	80–120
>12	15–20	60–100

Note that the heart rate is roughly four times the respiratory rate at all ages.

Oxygen therapy

Almost all ill or injured children will benefit from high-concentration oxygen therapy. There is no need to assess risk as in adults with chronic lung disease. Only a small group of infants with duct-dependent congenital heart disease need controlled oxygen therapy.

> It is usually counterproductive to make an unwilling child wear an oxygen mask.

Therapy with brochodilators

All wheezy children should be given nebulised bronchodilators, whether or not they are known to be asthmatic. Ask the parents how much of this type of drug they have already had and look for agitation, tachycardia and tremor – the signs of overdosage. Remember, however, that these may also be signs of hypoxia.

Artificial ventilation

Ventilation is indicated as an emergency procedure for respiratory insufficiency in a child in the same way as in an adult.

Method of estimating appropriate ventilator settings → Box 18.3.

> **Box 18.3 Suggested ventilator settings**
>
> Tidal volume = 10 mL/kg
> Minute volume = 100 mL/kg

C – Circulation

Checking for a central pulse

The brachial or femoral pulses should be used in infants rather than the carotid pulse. The absence of a central pulse or a rate <60 beats/min in infants indicates the need to follow procedures for cardiorespiratory arrest (→ *p. 151*).

> In a child with ventricular fibrillation and no obvious precipitating factors, consider poisoning with tricyclic antidepressants.

Cardiac arrest and dysrhythmia protocols → Chapter 11 on p. 156.

Cardiovascular parameters

Normal heart rates in children → Table 18.1.

- Blood pressure varies with age. It can be difficult to measure in young, moving children. A useful formula is:

$$\text{Expected systolic BP (in mmHg)} = 80 + (\text{Age in years} \times 2)$$

- Blood volume is approximately 80 mL/kg.

The ECG is rarely as helpful in making a diagnosis in children as in adults. The exception is, of course, dysrhythmias. A cardiac monitor does, however, provide constant information about the heart rate.

Important signs of circulatory disturbance in children

- Purpura (meningococcal disease).
- Dehydration – a dry non-elastic skin or sunken eyes. In infants a floppy anterior fontanelle is a useful, if late, sign of severe fluid loss. Diarrhoea and vomiting can quickly dehydrate a small child.
- Wet nappies confirm urine output in young children. As usual, the mother will know their normal state.

Access to the circulation

The need for and site of this should be assessed carefully. There is nothing worse than looking for veins on a screaming child who is covered with bruises from previous attempts by someone else. Remember the possibility of intraosseous infusion and venous cutdown (→ *Box 18.4*).

Fluid replacement

- Bolus fluid therapy = 20 mL/kg, repeated as necessary after further assessment. (This is reduced to 10 mL/kg for children with trauma in hospital and 5 mL/kg for children with trauma in the prehospital setting.)
- Maintenance fluid therapy:
  - 4 mL/kg per h for the first 10 kg
  - 2 mL/kg per h for the next 10 kg
  - 1 mL/kg per h for subsequent weight.
  For example, a 25-kg child needs:

$$(4\text{ mL/kg} \times 10\text{ kg}) + (2\text{ mL/kg} \times 10\text{ kg}) + (1\text{ mL/kg} \times 5\text{ kg})$$
$$= (40) + (20) + (5)\text{ mL/h} = 65\text{ mL/h}.$$

Box 18.4 Intraosseous cannulation

This is recommended in children if intravenous (IV) access cannot be achieved rapidly. It is a safe technique and so every ED should have the equipment and expertise. The intraosseous (IO) route can be used for both volume resuscitation and drug therapy.

- Mark the anteromedial tibia 2–3 cm below the tibial tuberosity or the anterolateral femur about 3 cm above the lateral femoral condyle
- Prepare the skin and insert local anaesthetic in a conscious child
- Make a small cut in the skin
- Insert the special intraosseous needle with the trochar at 90° to skin. A gentle twisting motion results in penetration of the cortex. The needle should then be fixed in the bone. A special intraosseous drill makes this procedure easier
- Remove the trochar and use a 5-mL syringe to aspirate and confirm the cannula's position. Blood samples may be taken (although most hospital laboratories are reluctant to process them!)
- Connect an extension tube and three-way tap
- Fix the needle in position
- Give drugs or fluid in boluses from a syringe. A standard drip will not run adequately

Box 18.5 The Children's Coma Scale

Response elicited	Score
Best eye response	
Open spontaneously	4
Open to speech	3
Open to pain	2
No response	1
Best motor response	
Moves normally and spontaneously or obeys commands	6
Localises pain	5
Withdraws in response to pain	4
Flexes abnormally to pain (decorticate movements)	3
Extends abnormally to pain (decerebrate movements)	2
No response	1
Best verbal response	
Smiles, follows sounds and objects, interacts	5
Cries consolably or interacts inappropriately	4
Cries with inconsistent relief or moans	3
Cries inconsolably or is irritable	2
No response	1

As a routine maintenance and replacement fluid, children should be given 0.9% sodium chloride. This is because they can easily become hyponatraemic.

- The palm and adducted fingers of a child's hand are approximately equal to 1% of their body surface area and can be used to make a quick estimate of the fluid replacement required for a burn ($\rightarrow$ p. 137).

D – Disability

Always consider hypoglycaemia as a cause for a reduced level of consciousness in children.

Level of consciousness

AVPU scoring ($\rightarrow$ p. 7) is as useful for children as for adults. The standard, adult Glasgow Coma Scale (GCS) is suitable for children of school age but special variants of the GCS are more appropriate in children aged <4 years ($\rightarrow$ Box 18.5). Even sleepy children should be fairly easy to rouse.

Other signs

- Agitation or an odd cry or affect may be the first signs of cerebral irritation.
- Children may be flaccid or show abnormal posturing.
- Limb movements may be unequal – sometimes this is congenital but it is best never to assume so.

E – Exposure and environment

Comfort, warmth and the proximity of the mother or other carer are extremely important to children.

Attention to these details early on can radically change the wellbeing and demeanour (and hence ease of assessment) of a child. Clothing may have to be removed to facilitate assessment. However, it must be remembered that children easily become cold and embarrassed.

> In a child, cold limbs usually indicate a cold trunk and head.

F – Fits

Anticonvulsant therapy and cooling measures for children → p. 343.

In the apyrexic fitting child consider:

- hypoglycaemia
- meningitis
- poisoning
- cerebral oedema.

G – Glucose

Children are like fast-burning little engines and become short of oxygen and fuel very quickly. Their fuel is glucose and they have relatively low glycogen reserves.

All diabetic children will be on insulin; oral hypoglycaemic drugs are generally used only in adults. This does not mean, of course, that a child cannot take someone else's drugs and become hypoglycaemic.

Hypoglycaemia should be corrected with 2–5 mL/kg of 10% dextrose solution (0.2–0.5 g/kg of glucose) through a large vein. Intramuscular (IM) glucagon (20 mcg/kg) is an alternative if venous access is delayed.

H – History

The initial AMPLE history (→ p. 12) should be obtained from the child or from the carers.

Additional features of the history in children → later.

I – Immediate needs of the child

Some immediate needs will have been assessed as part of the 'environment'. These include the provision of warmth, the removal of wet clothing and the need to ensure psychological support from the mother or other carer. A position of comfort is also mandatory; it may be life saving in conditions such as epiglottitis.

As usual the relief of suffering is of paramount importance.

Assess

- *The need for analgesia*: exact localisation of pain is difficult in very young children but careful observation and discussion with the mother often help considerably. Analgesia can turn an unmanageable situation into a calm one. It also reassures the carers. It is far better to give analgesia freely to children who may be in pain than to withhold it on the spurious grounds that it alters conscious level or masks pupillary or abdominal signs.
- *The need for limb splintage*: simple limb support with troughs and pillows can be very helpful in children with limb injuries. Distal circulation should be assessed before and after positioning limbs in the same way in children as in adults.
- *The tolerance of cervical and other spinal splintage*: conscious children often do not tolerate this sort of restraint very well. If a collar is distressing a child significantly, it is better to remove it. The mother's hands and pillows can be more acceptable substitutes. A child who is struggling to remove a collar is actually moving his or her neck more than a child with no splint who is lying still. The indications for spinal immobilisation are the same in children as in adults, although young children are less accurate in localising the pain of spinal injury.

Ask yourself

Does this child need:

- drugs to relieve pain? (→ *Boxes 18.6 and 18.7*)
- splintage?
- freedom from splintage?

FURTHER ASSESSMENT OF THE CHILD

This will be greatly facilitated by a gentle approach and a child-friendly environment.

Additional features in a paediatric history

Maternal health and pregnancy

The health of the mother may affect the development of the fetus. Maternal infections (e.g. rubella) may lead to a damaged baby.

Box 18.6 Opiate analgesics for children

Children aged >12 months

Morphine injection	0.1–0.2 mg/kg
Fentanyl injection	increments of 0.5 mcg/kg
Pethidine injection	1–2 mg/kg
Diamorphine intranasal spray	0.1 mg/kg
Morphine elixir	0.2–0.4 mg/kg
Codeine elixir	1–1.5 mg/kg

Infants aged between 3 and 12 months
They should be given half the above doses of morphine

Infants aged <3 months
They are especially sensitive to opioids and so should be given a quarter of the usual paediatric dose

Codeine is best avoided in infants

 Box 18.7 Antipyretic analgesics for children

Paracetamol suspension
10–15 mg/kg every 4–6 h; paracetamol may also be given rectally as a suppository (loading dose = 15–20 mg/kg)

Ibuprofen suspension
5 mg/kg up to four times a day

Birth problems

A difficult birth (caesarean section or forceps delivery) may later manifest itself as developmental problems or fits. Was the child on the special care baby unit? If so, then the perinatal period was not as smooth as it might have been.

Siblings

The health of brothers and sisters may give useful information about a child's illness.

Development

The continuing rapid development of a child distinguishes him or her from the adult. Questions should be asked about relationships, behaviour, play, school, sports and activities.

Immunisations

Children in the UK benefit from the existence of a planned programme of immunisations (→ *Table 18.6 on p. 352*). The immunisations actually received should always be ascertained.

Communication with a child

Children vary widely in their ability to communicate. A neonate may make signals that are understood only by his or her mother whereas teenagers use the same system of communication as adults. The type and level of language used are also influenced by the child's intelligence and environment. Consequently, communicating with a child is a difficult art, which comes more naturally to some than to others.

Questions must be pitched at the right level and the responses of the child constantly reassessed. It is obviously a mistake to phrase a question in language that a small child cannot understand. However, it is equally inappropriate to patronise an older child.

A child's account of events can be extremely accurate. It should not be assumed that an adult's story of events is any more credible than an older child's.

Language problems

Children from ethnic communities may be multilingual and revert to their domestic tongue in a crisis. Gentle rephrasing of questions may reassure them and encourage dialogue but sometimes the help of a translator is required.

The needs of the parents

Children usually have someone in close proximity to look after them. Sometimes the worries of these carers predominate over the symptoms of the child. Requirements vary from simple reassurance to medical interventions. The satisfactory treatment of the child often depends on the support of those closest to him or her; the child's mental state may be inseparable from that of the mother. Parental anxiety or difficulty coping is a good reason for admitting a child to hospital.

Continuing assessment

Assessment must continue during initial treatment and transportation. Children may change their physiological status very rapidly. It is particularly important to assess the effect of any interventions.

Monitoring must be appropriate to the child's condition and should not replace careful observation. It needs to be considered in terms of: (1) usefulness of information obtained; and (2) acceptability to the child. In a conscious child, this probably means that:

- pulse oximetry is better than
- ECG monitoring, which is better than
- BP monitoring.

Consideration of other children in the vicinity

In many situations, such as severe infections, fires, poisoning and abuse, other children may have been exposed to the same agents as the patient. In such cases, it is appropriate to assess the risk to these children also.

RESPIRATORY PROBLEMS

Also → Chapter 13.

Respiratory disorders are responsible for around a third of all paediatric admissions to hospital in the UK.

Stridor

Angio-oedema → pp. 263 and 300.
Foreign body obstruction → p. 1.

Stridor is a harsh respiratory noise, which is loudest in inspiration and usually indicates obstruction of the extrathoracic airways. It can be caused by:

- epiglottitis (supraglottitis)
- laryngotracheobronchitis (croup)
- bacterial tracheitis
- foreign body obstruction
- angio-oedema
- thermal, chemical or other damage to the airways
- other rarer causes of obstruction (e.g. diphtheria, quinsy, glandular fever).

Accompanying features, including the degree of respiratory distress, depend on the cause of the stridor. They may include:

- hoarseness or inability to speak
- coughing
- drooling
- sternal and subcostal recession (this is a good indicator of the degree of obstruction whereas the intensity of the stridor is not)
- tachypnoea and tachycardia
- indicators of hypoxia such as cyanosis, agitation or drowsiness.

> Do not put anything, including a spatula or a thermometer, in the mouth of a child with stridor – it may precipitate complete respiratory obstruction.

Differences between epiglottitis and croup

Despite its name, the swelling of epiglottitis usually involves more than just the bright-red, cherry-like epiglottis. It is, in fact, a complete 'top of the larynx-itis'. This is different from the 'bottom of the larynx-itis' caused by croup. Spasmodic or recurrent croup is a variant form of the disease, which is more common in atopic children and is thought to have an allergic component.

Differences between the two most common infectious causes of stridor → Table 18.2.

Table 18.2 Differences between epiglottitis and croup

	Epiglottitis	Croup
Age of child	1–6 years	6 months–5 years
Onset of symptoms	Hours	Days
Runny nose	No	Yes
Cough	Slight	Characteristic barking
Speech	Difficult	Hoarse
Stridor	Soft	Harsh
Able to drink	No	Yes
Drooling	Yes	No
Pyrexia	>38.5°C	<38.5°C
Appearance	Pale and toxic	Variable
Respiratory distress	Severe	Variable
Site affected	Supraglottis	Lower larynx and trachea
Causative organism	*Haemophilus influenzae* b	Parainfluenza and other viruses
Decreased incidence (since Hib vaccine)	Yes – now rare in the UK	No – still common
Need for observation	Yes	Yes
Need for intubation	Yes	Sometimes (5%)
Need for antibiotics	Yes	No
Helped by steroids	No	Yes

XR There is no place for radiographs in the management of stridor.

Tx

- Leave the child in the position of comfort, usually sitting up and possibly on the mother's knee.
- Avoid interventions that may precipitate crying; oxygen may sometimes be tolerated but attempts at IV access will not.
- Ask for paediatric help.

If respiratory distress accompanies the stridor, then:

- summon skilled senior help immediately, including an anaesthetist and an ENT surgeon (a consultant anaesthetist is the most appropriate grade)
- notify theatre of the situation.

Gaseous induction of anaesthesia, with a volatile agent such as sevoflurane or halothane in oxygen, followed by gentle laryngoscopy is the only appropriate treatment in the distressed child who is still breathing. Intubation should, of course, be attempted if respiratory arrest occurs.

As a holding measure, 5 mg nebulised adrenaline may be life saving (5 mL of 1 in 1000 adrenaline nebulised in oxygen) with ECG monitoring. For young children, 0.4 mL/kg of a 1 in 1000 solution of adrenaline is appropriate (up to a maximum of 5 mL). The benefit of the adrenaline only lasts for 30 min and so, in suspected croup, it should be followed immediately by nebulised or oral steroids → *later*.

Croup

A croup score is used in some hospitals to describe the clinical severity of the illness. It is calculated by scoring five features:

1 Inspiratory stridor
2 Cough
3 Retractions
4 Dyspnoea
5 Colour.

Two alternative steroid treatments have been shown to lead to marked clinical improvement in croup. Either of the following should be administered as soon as the diagnosis is suspected:

- Nebulised budesonide 2 mg (4 mL) stat or 1 mg (2 mL) repeated after 30 min
- Oral dexamethasone (0.15 mg/kg).

Oral prednisolone (1 mg/kg) is also used by some units.

Bacterial tracheitis

Infection of the airway with staphylococci, streptococci or *Haemophilus influenzae* may cause bacterial tracheitis (pseudomembranous croup). The trachea contains copious purulent secretions with mucosal oedema and necrosis, features that can lead to severe airway obstruction. An affected child is unwell and toxic with a high pyrexia and stridulous breathing. Intensive care should be arranged immediately; three-quarters of such children require intubation. Antibiotic therapy should be a combination of cefotaxime and flucloxacillin.

Asthma in children

This section is mostly concerned with asthma in young children. Asthma in adults and older children → p. 201.

An acute attack of asthma is one of the most common reasons for admission to a paediatric ward in the UK, although admissions for asthma have been declining rapidly over the last 5 years. Throughout western Europe, around 13% of children and over 8% of adults have asthma. These figures confirm that childhood asthma often remits in adult life. Persistence into adulthood is more likely with the following:

1 Coexistent atopy
2 Female gender
3 Severe and frequent exacerbations of asthma in childhood
4 Smoking in adulthood.

The first severe episode of asthma usually occurs at around 18 months of age. Attacks are often precipitated by a viral infection; in older children exercise and emotional upset may be the triggers. Asthma is an allergic bronchitis and is not primarily an infectious condition. The inflammatory process causes smooth muscle irritability, oedema and sputum retention, resulting in obstruction of the intrathoracic airways. The clinical signs of this obstructive process are:

1 Increased work of breathing – wheezing, tachypnoea, recession and use of accessory muscles
2 Reduced efficacy of breathing – poor air entry and hyperexpansion
3 Failure of gas exchange – tachycardia, agitation and eventually drowsiness and cyanosis.

Clinical signs correlate poorly with the severity of airway obstruction; some very ill children do not appear to be distressed.

Severe attacks are characterised by the following:

- Child too breathless to talk or too breathless to feed (cannot complete sentences in one breath)
- Respiratory rate >50/min in children aged 2–5 years or >30/min in children aged >5 years (usually with marked recession and use of accessory muscles)
- Pulse rate >130/min in children aged 2–5 years or >120/min in children aged >5 years
- Arterial O_2 saturation (SaO_2) <92% on air, but any reduction in SaO_2 from the normal of ≥97% must be given serious consideration.

Life-threatening features include:

- fatigue or exhaustion
- agitation, drowsiness, confusion or a depressed level of consciousness
- cyanosis
- a silent chest
- poor respiratory efforts
- bradycardia or hypotension (bradycardia is often a preterminal sign)
- SaO_2 <85% on air.

It is very useful to know what has happened during previous attacks:

- Oral steroids? How many times? For how long?
- Admission? How many times? For how long?
- Intensive care unit (ICU) admission? How many times? For how long?

Investigations: Measurement of peak expiratory flow rate (PEFR) can usually be performed on children aged >5 years provided that they are not too breathless or too distressed to cooperate. *Predicted PEFRs in children → Figure 18.1*. Investigations, including chest radiograph (CXR), are not generally indicated in recurrent attacks of asthma, unless there is a possible history of foreign body inhalation or severe systemic upset. Close observation and pulse oximetry are more important. The aim should be to keep the SaO_2 >92%.

Tx

- *Nebulised salbutamol 5 mg or terbutaline 10 mg* in 100% oxygen (salbutamol 2.5 mg or terbutaline 5 mg if the child is aged <5 years). The oxygen flow rate should be around 5 L/min to produce small particles without excess loss of drug from around the facemask. In children with mild-to-moderate asthma and an SaO_2 >92% in air, there are some advantages in using a pressurised aerosol via a spacer device (± a facemask) to administer the β_2 agonist. Ten puffs are given, one at a time, and inhaled sequentially.

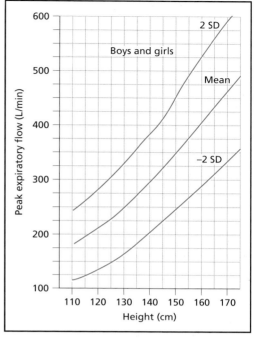

Figure 18.1 Predicted peak expiratory flow rates in children.

- *Soluble prednisolone 1 mg/kg* orally (up to a maximum of 40 mg). Children who are already receiving maintenance steroid tablets should be given prednisolone 2 mg/kg (up to a maximum of 60 mg). If the child is unable to swallow liquids or is vomiting, give IV hydrocortisone 4 mg/kg. This should be repeated every 6 h or followed by a continuous infusion of hydrocortisone 1 mg/kg per h.

With life-threatening features or in a deteriorating situation get senior help, including an anaesthetist or paediatric ICU (PICU) consultant, so that intubation and ventilation can be performed if the child does not improve. (Induction of anaesthesia may be performed with bronchodilating agents such as ketamine or halothane.) Children whose SaO_2 remains <92% on air after initial treatment should also be considered for PICU referral. Then consider adding:

- *Nebulised ipratropium bromide 250 mcg* (125 mcg if the child is aged <2 years). This may be repeated after every 20–30 min for children who are responding poorly to β_2 agonists.
- *Continuous nebulised β_2 agonists.*

- *IV salbutamol* 15 mcg/kg given over 10 min. This is an alternative to repeated salbutamol or terbutaline nebulisers for children aged >2 years. It is followed by a salbutamol infusion at a rate of 1–5 mcg/kg per min. ECG and electrolytes must be monitored to detect dysrhythmias and hypokalaemia.
- *Magnesium sulphate* 25–40 mg/kg given intravenously over 20 min (maximum dose 2 g; single dose only). *Further information on magnesium → p. 250.*
- *Aminophylline* 5 mg/kg given intravenously over 20 min under ECG control, followed by a maintenance infusion of 1 mg/kg per h in 5% dextrose. The infusion rate is reduced to 800 mcg/kg per h for children between the ages of 10 and 16 years and to 500–700 mcg/kg per h for adults. The initial loading dose should not be given to patients who are already receiving oral theophyllines.

Signs of clinical improvement include:

1 Improved activity levels or responsiveness: urge to eat, drink or play
2 Falling pulse rate
3 Rising peak flow rate.

Potential discharge

Even if a child responds very well to therapy, discharge from hospital needs careful consideration. No child should be discharged unless his or her SaO_2 is >94% on air and the PEFR is >75% of the predicted value. All children with features of severe asthma must be admitted. If the asthma attack was bad enough to come to an ED, then the child almost certainly requires the following:

- A period of observation (e.g. 4 h) in either a ward or a special area in an ED
- Oral (soluble) prednisolone for 3–5 days (1–2 mg/kg per day in either one morning or two divided doses up to a maximum of 40 mg/day)
- Follow-up in a paediatric clinic for reassessment and a review of his or her current therapy.

Further information about the discharge of a patient with asthma → p. 205.

Acute asthma in children aged <2 years

Attacks of wheezing in children aged <2 years are usually due to viral infection. The differential diagnosis includes bronchiolitis, pneumonia, aspiration pneumonitis, cystic fibrosis, tracheomalacia and other congenital conditions. Prematurity and low birthweight are risk factors for recurrent wheezing. A trial of bronchodilator therapy should be considered although children aged <18 months often respond poorly to β_2 agonists. Metered dose inhalers coupled to spacer devices fitted with facemasks may be more effective than nebulisers in this age group. Nebulised ipratropium bromide (125 mcg) may lead to some improvement in the clinical picture. Early use of steroid tablets in the ED has been shown to reduce both admission rates and the duration of hospitalisation. Soluble prednisolone 10 mg for 3 days is the recommended regimen. Many children with recurrent episodes of viral-induced wheezing in infancy do not go on to develop chronic atopic asthma, so they do not need regular prophylactic medication. The parents of these children should be advised about the relationship between exposure to cigarette smoke and the wheezy illnesses of childhood.

Bronchiolitis

Bronchiolitis is the most common serious respiratory infection of childhood, affecting 10% of all children at some time. It is a disease of infants; 90% of attacks occur in children aged <9 months and it is rare over the age of 2 years. Bronchiolitis is usually caused by respiratory syncytial virus and may occur in epidemics, invariably in the winter. Initial fever and upper respiratory tract symptoms progress to dry coughing and signs of dyspnoea:

- Poor feeding
- Tachypnoea (up to 100 breaths/min) with rib recession
- Hyperinflated lungs and thus easily palpable liver
- Fine inspiratory crepitations and expiratory wheezes
- Mild hypoxia on pulse oximetry
- Tachycardia.

Some infants with severe bronchiolitis (around 2%) will require ventilation, usually because of exhaustion. Signs of imminent deterioration include:

- pallor
- extreme tachypnoea (>60 breaths/min)
- exhaustion
- apnoeic spells
- significant hypoxia.

Some babies can be predicted to have a stormier course including those with a history of:

- heart disease
- failure to thrive
- prematurity.

XR CXR may show hyperinflated lungs and, in about a third of infants, areas of segmental collapse or consolidation.

Tx Many babies will require admission for observation, monitoring and therapy with humidified oxygen. The exceptions are those who are feeding adequately (>50% normal) with an SaO_2 >94% on air and appear to be otherwise stable. The disease usually settles over 10–14 days. Traditional bronchodilators and antibiotics are rarely helpful. Steroids, nebulised adrenaline and nebulised antiviral agents (ribavirin) are sometimes used but their role in bronchiolitis is still uncertain. However, the use of nebulised hypertonic (2.7%) saline looks very promising.

Pneumonia

Children with congenital abnormalities or chronic illnesses are at a high risk of pneumonia. Fever and cough may be accompanied by non-specific symptoms such as lethargy and abdominal pain.

XR CXR may show minimal changes, consolidation or widespread bronchopneumonia.

Tx Most children will require admission for assessment. A wide spectrum of pathogens may cause pneumonia in children and so the choice of antibiotic depends on the clinical features and the age of the child. IV cefotaxime or oral amoxicillin or oral clarithromycin are reasonable first prescriptions, depending on the severity of the illness (*Doses → Table 18.3*). Children with cystic fibrosis may present with complicated chest infections, which require specialist advice from the outset.

Pneumonia in older children and adults → p. 209.

OTHER MAJOR ILLNESSES IN CHILDHOOD

Meningitis

Bacterial meningitis occurs all year round although it usually peaks in winter months. Unfortunately, early diagnosis can be difficult and so the possibility of meningitis must always be considered in any patient with an unexplained illness or fever. Symptoms and signs in older children and adults include:

- severe headache
- nausea and vomiting
- fever
- back or joint pains
- drowsiness or confusion
- photophobia
- neck stiffness (often absent!).

Infants may have relatively non-specific signs such as:

- drowsiness and irritability
- poor feeding
- distress on handling
- vomiting or diarrhoea
- high-pitched or moaning cry
- tense or bulging fontanelle
- apnoeic or cyanotic attacks
- fever
- neck stiffness.

In meningococcal infection photophobia and neck stiffness are relatively uncommon features; the most common symptoms are fever, malaise and drowsiness (→ p. 341).

Table 18.3 Doses of common antibiotics for children			
	1–5 years	**<12 years**	**Adult**
Oral			
Amoxicillin (mg)	125 three times daily	125–250 three times daily	250–500 three times daily
Clarithromycin (mg)	125 twice daily	187.5–250 twice daily	250–500 twice daily
Trimethoprim (mg)	50 twice daily	100 twice daily	200 twice daily
Flucloxacillin (mg)	125 four times daily	125–250 four times daily	250–500 four times daily
Parenteral			
Cefotaxime	50–80 mg/kg three times daily	1–2 g three times daily	1–2 g three times daily
Benzylpenicillin (mg)	300 (0.5 MU) four times daily	600 (1 MU) four times daily	1200 (2 MU) four times daily

Prehospital treatment

In a patient with suspected bacterial meningitis, parenteral antibiotics (benzylpenicillin) should be administered before urgent transfer to hospital only if:

- The patient has a non-blanching rash or
- The patient does not have a rash but there may be significant delays in the patient getting to hospital, e.g. because of adverse weather conditions

It is no longer recommended that benzylpenicillin be given routinely to patients who do not have a rash before transfer to hospital.

Box 18.8 Contraindications to lumbar puncture

- GCS score <13
- Papilloedema
- Slow pulse, raised BP and irregular breathing (Cushing's triad)
- Impaired brain-stem reflexes
- Abnormal posturing
- Dilated pupils
- Prolonged or focal seizure
- Focal neurological signs
- Widespread purpuric rash
- Coagulopathy
- Shock
- Severe hypertension

Tx
- Give oxygen.
- Gain IV access. Shock must be treated but in its absence fluids should be given sparingly.
- Obtain routine blood specimens and blood cultures if possible.
- Control fits ($\rightarrow$ p. 343).
- Check for and treat hypoglycaemia ($\rightarrow$ p. 333).
- Start antibiotics. Ceftriaxone is used as a first-line monotherapy for meningitis in an IV dose of 80 mg/kg (maximum dose = 2 g). It is effective against meningococci, pneumococci and *Haemophilus influenzae*. Cefotaxime (in the same doses) is an alternative and is the first choice in infants aged <3 months with a history of prematurity or jaundice. About 10% of penicillin-sensitive patients will also be allergic to cephalosporins but, depending on the history, in this infection the risk may be worth taking. For those children (or adults) who have had a previous anaphylactic reaction to penicillin, chloramphenicol should be given intravenously in a dose of 12.5–25 mg/kg. To cover listerial infection, IV ampicillin (2 g four times daily) may be added for adults aged >55 years, pregnant women and immunosuppressed patients. The addition of ampicillin is also appropriate for infants aged <3 months (50 mg/kg four times daily). Consider the addition of aciclovir (10 mg/kg by IV infusion) if there is any suspicion of meningoencephalitis. Vancomycin should be given, as a supplement to the standard regimen, to patients who have recently been overseas. The possibility of tuberculous meningitis should also be considered.
- Give IV dexamethasone 0.15 mg/kg (to a maximum dose of 10 mg) four times daily for 4 days. This should be started with – or just before – the first

dose of antibiotics in adults, especially where pneumococcal meningitis is suspected (it may help to prevent deafness). In children, steroids can be delayed for up to 12 h, while awaiting a positive lumbar puncture. Dexamethasone should be discontinued if tuberculosis (TB) or a non-bacterial cause is identified.
- Refer the patient to in-patient physicians for further investigation and treatment. Consider the need for a CT scan of the brain to exclude other diagnoses. *Contraindications to lumbar puncture* $\rightarrow$ *Box 18.8.*

Viral meningitis

Many different viruses may cause a meningitis. The clinical picture is very similar to a bacterial infection although the severity of the illness is usually much less. Until the diagnosis is confirmed by lumbar puncture, the treatment is identical to that for bacterial meningitis.

Encephalitis

Coxsackieviruses, other enteroviruses, arboviruses and herpes simplex virus may all infect the brain. Drowsiness, lethargy and confusion are the most common symptoms, usually with very few hard signs. Lumbar puncture may be helpful; a CT scan is usually normal. The treatment is similar to that for suspected bacterial meningitis but with the addition of drugs directed against herpes simplex. Aciclovir 10 mg/kg is given by IV infusion every 8 h for 10 days (calculated on ideal body weight in obese patients).

Meningococcal disease

> Confusion, leg pain (!), photophobia, rash and neck pain/stiffness have been shown to be 'red flags' for the presence of meningococcal disease in children.

Meningococcal disease is the most common cause of death from infectious disease in the UK; the mortality rate in diagnosed cases is still 10%. The disease is on the increase and is most commonly seen in young children. However, in recent years, there has been a marked rise in incidence in young people aged 15–24 and the case fatality rate in this age group is twice as high as that in children aged <5. Meningococcal group B disease is responsible for >80% of cases with group C (since the introduction of the MenC vaccine) accounting for <10% of infections. There may occasionally be a history of travel to Saudi Arabia or sub-Saharan Africa or contact with Islamic pilgrims.

Endotoxin released by meningococci is responsible for many of the features of the infection. In the bloodstream, it triggers an intense inflammatory response, which causes vascular endothelium to become 'leaky'. Plasma then moves into interstitial spaces. Circulating endotoxin also activates the coagulation cascade and may cause disseminated intravascular coagulation (DIC). Together with cytokines, it depresses myocardial contractility. In the brain, endotoxin damages the blood–brain barrier leading to cerebral oedema. It causes microvascular thrombosis in the meninges and brain, with a consequent reduction in cerebral perfusion.

Meningococcal disease can present as either meningitis or septicaemia, or both, with a great variety of clinical features. A sudden onset of fever and malaise is characteristic. Alternatively, initially trivial symptoms may suddenly become more serious. In meningococcal meningitis, photophobia and neck stiffness are relatively unusual features; the most common symptoms are fever, malaise and drowsiness. Headache, vomiting and irritability are also often seen. Raised intracranial pressure (ICP) may lead to confusion, fits, abnormal posturing and florid neurological signs. Septicaemia can be very difficult to diagnose at first and patients can look relatively well and alert. Fever, malaise and weakness may be accompanied by myalgia, arthralgia and isolated limb pain. Rigors are common. Abdominal pain, diarrhoea and vomiting may occur; faecal incontinence has been described. As the infection takes hold, septicaemia manifests itself as shock with a vasculitic skin rash. A rapid increase in the distribution of the purpura is often associated with circulatory failure. Extensive purpura ('purpura fulminans') is indicative of coagulopathy.

> The characteristic purpuric skin rash can be found in >70% of cases of meningococcal septicaemia if a careful examination is made. However, the rash is macular and blanching in the early stages of the disease in 30% of cases.

Common mistakes in the diagnosis and treatment of meningococcal disease → Box 18.9.

Tx

- Call for senior help (including paediatrics and anaesthesia or PICU).
- Give oxygen (10–12 L/min by mask).
- Monitor and record continuously the heart rate, BP, temperature, respiratory rate, SaO_2, capillary refill time, GCS score, pupillary size/reactions and the spread of any rash.
- Start antibiotics – IV ceftriaxone 80 mg/kg or IV cefotaxime 80 mg/kg (maximum dose of either cephalosporin = 2 g). (For those children or adults who have had a previous anaphylactic reaction to penicillin, chloramphenicol should be given in an IV dose of 12.5–25.0 mg/kg.)
- Begin resuscitation with IV fluids (→ p. 331). Excess fluids should not be given if there is a possibility of raised ICP.
- Obtain routine blood specimens and blood cultures. If possible, also take blood for clotting studies, calcium, magnesium, phosphate, venous blood gases, meningococcal PCR (polymerase chain reaction) and blood grouping. (Low platelets, low WCC, raised urea and creatinine, coagulopathy and a base deficit > minus 5 mmol/L suggest a poor prognosis.)
- Check for and treat hypoglycaemia (→ p. 333).
- Control fits (→ p. 343).
- Give IV dexamethasone (0.15 mg/kg stat and then four times daily for 4 days) with the first dose of antibiotics to adults with clinical features of meningitis or raised ICP. In children with bacterial meningitis, steroids can be delayed for up to 12 h, until a positive lumbar puncture has been obtained.

All patients with raised ICP will require intubation and ventilation to control the $PaCO_2$ (at around 4–4.5 kPa). They should be nursed with a 30° head-up tilt and mannitol 0.25 g/kg and furosemide 1 mg/kg

---

 Box 18.9 Common mistakes in the diagnosis and treatment of meningococcal disease

1 *Expecting patients always to look very ill.* (They soon do!) In the early stages of meningococcal disease, patients may look relatively well and alert. Their mental state may remain unchanged until very late

2 *Expecting the signs of meningitis in all cases.* The bacterium would be better named the septococcus rather than the meningococcus! Symptoms of meningitis (neck stiffness and photophobia) are absent in pure septicaemia and in young children (especially those aged <2 years) with meningitis. Teenagers may be aggressive and combative rather than drowsy

3 *Expecting the rash to develop early and be purpuric and non-blanching in all patients.* It appears late and is blanching in 30% of cases of septicaemia – then early pinprick spots appear. The rash may be scanty, atypical or absent in pure meningitis. It is more difficult to see on darker skins – look at the soles, palms, palate and conjunctivae

4 *Failing to recognise the significance of common symptoms and signs.* Sudden onset of fever and malaise is typical. Rigors, weakness and muscle pains are common

5 *Failing to recognise the significance of uncommon symptoms and signs.* Isolated severe limb pain may occur in early septicaemia. In meningitis, ophthalmoplegia (new squint) is a sign of raised ICP caused by herniation of the brain through the tentorial opening

6 *Failing to recognise features that predict a poor prognosis (and the need for urgent action) at the time of presentation.* These features include depressed level of consciousness, absence of meningism, shock, rapidly progressive purpuric rash, coagulopathy, low white cell count (WCC) and thrombocytopenia

7 *Failing to anticipate and then treat pulmonary oedema promptly and effectively.* The oedema is caused by leakage from the adjacent capillaries and the treatment is intubation and ventilation with positive end-expiratory pressure (PEEP) to increase oxygenation – not diuretics

8 *Failing to treat impending shock aggressively.* Up to 60 mL/kg of fluid may be required in the first hour together with inotropic support of the circulation. The same problem that causes the shock – capillary leakage – may also cause pulmonary oedema. The fluid should be continued and the oedema treated as stated in the previous point. Most deaths result from shock and multiorgan failure; only a few are caused by raised ICP

9 *Failing to get PICU help early on.* PICU advice and invasive monitoring are essential as soon as possible

---

should be given intravenously to reduce the ICP. A urinary catheter will be required to monitor fluid balance. Lumbar puncture and insertion of internal jugular lines should be avoided. (*Contraindications to lumbar puncture → Box 18.8.*)

Septicaemic patients are very likely to require early intubation and ventilation with inotropic support. Boluses of colloid (10–20 mL/kg) should be given and a urinary catheter inserted. A urinary output of at least 1 mL/kg per h is the aim. Patients who do not respond to peripheral inotropes (dopamine or dobutamine at 10–20 mcg/kg per min) will require a central infusion of adrenaline (0.1 mcg/kg per min). There will be gross systemic and metabolic disturbance. Therefore, it is essential to anticipate, monitor and correct if required:

- *Worsening shock* (fluids and inotropes; → *previously*)
- *Pulmonary oedema* (ventilation with PEEP)
- *Raised ICP* (→ *before*)
- *Hypoglycaemia* (up to 5 mL/kg of 10% glucose)
- *Raised urea and creatinine* (secondary to inadequate renal perfusion – treat the shock and monitor the urinary output)
- *Acidosis* (1 mmol/kg of sodium bicarbonate if pH <7.2)
- *Hypokalaemia* (0.25 mmol/kg of potassium chloride over 30 min with ECG monitoring)
- *Hypomagnesaemia* (0.2 mL/kg of 50% magnesium sulphate over 30 min if serum magnesium <0.75 mmol/L)
- *Hypocalcaemia* (0.1 mL/kg of 10% calcium chloride over 30 min if ionised calcium <1.0 mmol/L)
- *Hypophosphataemia*
- *Anaemia, neutropenia and thrombocytopenia*
- *Coagulopathy* (fresh frozen plasma [FFP] 10 mL/kg or prothrombin complex concentrate → *Box 14.30 on p. 259*)

Prevention of transmission of the meningococcus

The meningococcus is carried in the nasopharynx of many healthy children and adults without causing any disease. Some people, however, may develop invasive disease within a few days of colonisation. Illness occurs in the first few days only after this colonisation and not during established carriage. The incubation period is generally 3–4 days with a range of 2–10 days.

Most cases of meningitis in this country are sporadic but, when a case occurs, the risk for other members of the immediate family is increased by up to 1000-fold. The risk factors for transmission are physical intimacy and prolonged close contact. The people most at risk are those who, within the 7 days before the onset of a patient's symptoms, have:

- slept under the same roof as the patient
- been 'kissing contacts' (friends and close relatives likely to have had mouth-to-mouth contact).

Childminders should be dealt with as part of the family unit but school contact or other community contact is not generally an indication for prophylaxis.

> Health-care staff require prophylaxis only when they have given a patient with meningococcal disease mouth-to-mouth resuscitation during the acute stage of the illness.

Chemoprophylaxis with antibiotics is given to eliminate nasopharyngeal carriage in order to reduce the likelihood of transmission in the community. It is a misconception that antibiotics are given primarily to protect the recipient of the drug. Ciprofloxacin is now the antibiotic of choice for close contacts of all ages, including during pregnancy. Rifampicin (or even ceftriaxone) is used when there is a hypersensitivity to ciprofloxacin. *Antibiotic dosages for prophylaxis against meningococci* → *Box 18.10*. The responsibility for tracing other contacts lies with the department of public health medicine.

Prevention of transmission of Haemophilus influenzae b

Invasive disease caused by this infection is most common in children aged <4 years and has a peak

> **Box 18.10 Antibiotic dosages for prophylaxis against meningococcal infection**
>
> **Ciprofloxacin by single oral dose:**
>   Adults and children aged >12 years = 500 mg
>   Children aged 5–12 years = 250 mg
>   Children aged 1 month to 4 years = 125 mg
>
> **Rifampicin by mouth:**
>   Adults and children aged >12
>   months = 10 mg/kg twice daily × 2 days
>   Children aged <12 months = 5 mg/kg twice
>   daily × 2 days (to a maximum dosage of
>   600 mg per dose or 1200 mg per day)
>
> **Ceftriaxone by single IM dose:**
>   Adults and children aged >12 years = 250 mg
>   Children aged <12 years = 125 mg

incidence between the ages of 3 and 12 months inclusive. The introduction of the Hib vaccine as part of the routine immunisations of childhood has resulted in a dramatic reduction in *Haemophilus influenzae* b infection. Prophylaxis with rifampicin (but at a higher dosage than in meningococcal disease) is indicated only for members of households where there is a child aged <4 years who is not immunised. Children in this category also require immediate Hib immunisation.

Fits

Around 7% of children have had a fit by the age of 3 years but only 0.5% of school-age children have epilepsy. In the neonatal period, birth injury, hypoglycaemia and hypocalcaemia are common causes of convulsions whereas intracranial infection, encephalopathy and poisoning occur at all ages. Children with congenital abnormalities often present with fits.

Febrile convulsions occur in about 3% of children between the ages of 5 months and 5 years. They are thought to be caused by a viraemia and are often recurrent. The child may present with prolonged fitting or there may have been a short period of clonic or tonic activity. Sometimes there is a story of an apparently well child suddenly becoming limp and falling to the floor. A history of stiffness, cyanosis, drooling or the eyes rolling upwards is extremely suggestive of a childhood fit. Children with known epilepsy are more likely to have a fit during a pyrexia.

Table 18.4 Rectal dose of diazepam

Age (years)	Dose (mg)
>1	5
>3	7.5
>5	10
>12	20
Adult	30

Investigations: The blood glucose should be checked in all cases at the bedside and the SaO_2 monitored. Children with atypical convulsions may need toxicological, septic and metabolic screening together with a CT scan of the brain.

Tx The fitting child must be protected from harm and IV access obtained. Anticonvulsant therapy should follow the following progression:

1 Lorazepam 0.1 mg/kg by slow IV injection (or by the intraosseus route). IV/IO diazepam emulsion 0.25 mg/kg is an alternative. This can be repeated after a few minutes if the fitting continues. Rectal diazepam (0.5 mg/kg) or buccal midazolam (0.5 mg/kg) can be given if IV access is delayed (→ Table 18.4). IV midazolam 0.1 mg/kg has a shorter duration of action than other IV benzodiazepines.
2 Paraldehyde 0.4 mL/kg per rectum (0.3 mL/kg for infants) diluted 50:50 with olive oil or saline (the diluted solution is thus given in a dose of 0.8 mL/kg). Paraldehyde must be given immediately if drawn up in a plastic syringe because it quickly degrades the plastic.
3 Phenytoin 18 mg/kg by IV (or IO) infusion over 30 min with ECG monitoring. This should not be given to any infants or children who are already on phenytoin. Instead, they should have IV (or IO) phenobarbital 15–20 mg/kg over 20 min (at a rate no faster than 1 mg/kg per min).
4 Thiopental (4 mg/kg given intravenously or intraosseously by an anaesthetist), usually with accompanying rapid sequence intubation and ventilation.

If cerebral oedema or intracerebral infection is suspected, then consider the need for the following:

- Intubation and ventilation to maintain a $PaCO_2$ of around 4.5 kPa
- Nursing with a 30° head-up tilt to facilitate cerebral venous drainage
- Dexamethasone 0.4–0.5 mg/kg IV (especially for oedema around a space-occupying lesion)

- Mannitol 0.25–0.5 mg/kg by IV infusion over 15 min, repeated as required to reduce cerebral swelling
- Cefotaxime and aciclovir intravenously for undiagnosed infection.

After the fitting has stopped, children with febrile convulsions should be cooled and given paracetamol or ibuprofen. Cooling measures will have only a transitory effect whereas antipyretic drugs 'reset' the hypothalamic temperature control mechanisms.

All children who have had prolonged or recurrent seizures should be admitted. Others may go home provided that:

- recovery is complete and sustained
- there is a definite diagnosis (known epilepsy or febrile illness in an appropriate age group)
- the parents agree to the discharge
- the home circumstances are satisfactory
- there are adequate arrangements for follow-up.

Some hospitals have a policy of admitting all children with a first febrile convulsion. In known patients with epilepsy, blood for anticonvulsant levels should be taken before discharge.

Diabetic ketoacidosis in children

Type 1 diabetes is on the increase in the UK, particularly in children aged <5 years. Almost 40% first present in diabetic ketoacidosis (DKA) with 20% having a pH of <7.1! This is the most common cause of death in children with diabetes with one death in every 300 episodes of DKA. Most deaths occur as a result of cerebral oedema (80%), hypokalaemia or aspiration pneumonia. There may be a history of increasing polyuria, polydipsia and weight loss, although more usually a concurrent infection precipitates the diabetic crisis. Abdominal pain and vomiting are common symptoms. The metabolic derangement may lead to coma, respiratory disturbance and ileus. Dehydration may be so profound as to cause shock.

Investigations: The clinical condition of the child is the best guide to severity. However, biochemical markers of severe DKA include:

- pH <7.2
- glucose >16 mmol/L
- ketones >2 mmol/L.

Tx A paediatric team should be involved as early as possible. To minimise the risk of cerebral oedema, metabolic abnormalities must be corrected slowly and rehydration should take place over 48 h.

- Protect the airway and give a high-concentration of oxygen.
- Monitor vital functions.
- Gain IV access and take blood samples (electrolytes, glucose, blood gases, full blood count and blood cultures; plasma chloride and phosphate levels should also be requested).
- If clinically shocked resuscitate with 10 mL/kg of 0.9% saline, repeated as necessary up to 30 mL/kg. Plasma is an alternative. Allow 30 min for each bolus of fluid.

> The administration of >40 mL/kg of resuscitation fluids is strongly associated with the development of cerebral oedema.

- Weigh the child and keep an exact record of fluid balance. Catheterisation may be required.
- Discuss the child with a paediatrician as soon as possible; intensive care should be arranged.
- Commence a 0.9% saline infusion with added potassium (20 mmol/L) → *Box 18.11*.
- One hour after starting the fluids for rehydration, start an infusion of soluble insulin at a rate of 0.1 U/kg per h. An initial bolus of insulin is now not recommended for children.
- Bicarbonate should be avoided unless the pH is <7.0. Acute gastric dilatation is common in DKA and so a nasogastric tube is often required, especially if the child is comatose or vomiting.

Once the blood sugar has fallen to <15 mmol/L, the IV infusion should be changed to 0.9% saline in 5% glucose with 40 mmol potassium in each 1000 mL. The insulin infusion can often then be reduced to 0.05 U/kg per h. If the blood sugar falls to <4 mmol/L, the insulin infusion should not be stopped because the insulin is needed to switch off ketone production. Instead, 10% glucose (2 mL/kg) should be given.

Note that children who are less than 5% dehydrated (dry mucous membranes and reduced skin turgor only) will often tolerate oral rehydration and subcutaneous insulin.

Recognition and treatment of cerebral oedema → *Box 18.12.*

> A third of children who develop cerebral oedema in DKA have permanent neurological sequelae.

 Box 18.12 Recognition and treatment of cerebral oedema

In DKA, cerebral oedema usually occurs in the first 24 h after starting rehydration. There are three major diagnostic criteria:

1 A reduced or fluctuating level of consciousness
2 Sustained episodes of bradycardia
3 Incontinence that is inappropriate for the age of the child

and five minor criteria: vomiting, headache, lethargy, hypertension and aged <5 years. *Two major or one major and two minor criteria strongly suggest the diagnosis.* Late signs such as papilloedema, convulsions and coma are associated with an extremely poor prognosis.

Treatment should be started immediately:

- Administer oxygen
- Exclude hypoglycaemia
- Nurse the patient with head elevated
- Give mannitol 1 g/kg over 20 min (5 mL/kg of 20% solution); hypertonic (2.7%) saline is an alternative (5 mL/kg given over 30 min)
- Restrict fluids to 50% of maintenance requirement only and replace the estimated deficit over 72 rather then 48h
- Discuss the need for intubation and hyperventilation (to reduce PCO_2) with an intensivist. It is a difficult decision
- Arrange a CT scan of the brain (to exclude other diagnoses)
- Repeat the dose of mannitol after 2h if no improvement

 Box 18.11 Fluids for a child with DKA

24-hour fluid requirement
= Maintenance fluids + Deficit

Fluid deficit in litres = Dehydration (%)
× Body weight in kg

Deficit should be calculated assuming a maximum of 8% dehydration and including the fluids given for resuscitation purposes. Remember that dehydration in DKA is often over-estimated!

Congenital abnormalities

Children with congenital abnormalities may present frequently with fits, chest infections and general illness. Their parents are under enormous strain, so admission should always be considered as an option. Background information from the GP may be useful.

COMMON COMPLAINTS IN CHILDHOOD

Herpes simplex stomatitis → p. 407.
Mumps → p. 425.

Upper respiratory tract infections and earache

Young children may have upper respiratory problems up to 10 times a year. Such infections may precipitate asthma attacks or lead to more serious chest infections. Symptoms of URTI include the following:

- *Cough and/or runny nose*: the most common signs of infection. The barking cough of croup is important to recognise because it may accompany stridor. Whooping cough is very distressing; severe coughing empties the lungs and is followed by an inspiratory 'whoop'. The problem may persist for weeks.
- *Sore throat*: this is caused by pharyngitis or enlarged lymph nodes in the neck.
- *Earache*: young children may pull at their ears if they have earache. Otitis media is a frequent accompaniment of URTI in children.
- *Abdominal pain*: this is caused by mesenteric adenitis and is common. There are usually no localising signs. Specific tenderness may be difficult to distinguish from appendicitis or urinary tract infection.
- *Non-specific symptoms*: pyrexia, poor feeding, malaise, crying and vomiting.

Tx Reassurance, fluids and paracetamol are the mainstays of treatment. The former is greatly enhanced if preceded by a thorough examination. Unilateral red eardrums are suggestive of bacterial infection and should be treated with antibiotics (amoxicillin or clarithromycin → *Table 18.3*). Some children with URTIs will need admission for a large variety of reasons.

The risk of sudden infant death syndrome

A high proportion of infants who die from sudden infant death syndrome (SIDS) will have had a minor infection in the previous few days. To minimise this risk the following advice should be given, without necessarily discussing the possibility of SIDS:

- The infant should be positioned on his or her back, or perhaps on the side if there are increased secretions or a risk of vomiting.
- The bedding should not be capable of causing restriction of movement or overheating.
- Infants should sleep within range of their parents' hearing.

Rashes

> The rash in meningococcal disease is classically purpuric but may be macular in the initial stages.

The common exanthemas (rashes) of childhood may baffle the staff of an ED. However, their recognition is important for prognosis, detection of severe illness and sometimes for credibility! The main types are the following:

- *Purpuric*: a non-blanching red or purple rash is caused by extravasation of blood. The septicaemia of meningococcal disease is the most serious cause (→ *p. 341*). It also occurs in vasculitis (Henoch–Schönlein purpura) and platelet deficiency (idiopathic thrombocytopenic purpura, leukaemia or drugs). All children with purpura must be seen by a paediatrician.
- *Urticarial*: blotchy, raised, itchy, red and hot. There is diffuse erythema and sometimes swelling of the face and hands. Areas may look like nettle-stings, which are also caused by histamine release (→ *p. 300*). Itchy scratch marks with either little else to see or some urticaria are usually caused by scabies infection (→ *p. 409*).
- *Vesicular*: small, itchy, fluid-filled vesicles that develop at different rates are typical of chickenpox. Later, they become pustular and, if badly infected, should be treated with flucloxacillin. (*Differences between chickenpox and smallpox → p. 256.*) Vesicles and blisters may also be seen in:

- herpes simplex (perioral and on the fingers) (→ *p. 407*)
- impetigo (→ *p. 406*)
- hand, foot and mouth disease: this is a Coxsackie viral infection that starts as painful red dots on the soles, palms and palate before small, clear, blisters develop
- staphylococcal scalded skin syndrome (Ritter's disease or fourth disease): this occurs mostly in infants. An epidermolytic toxin from a pathogenic strain of *Staphylococcus aureus* causes a widespread but superficial bullous eruption
- insect bites (most commonly found on the legs).

A single, dark, pus-filled vesicle is often found at the centre of a streptococcal cellulitis.

- *Morbilliform (or measles-like)*: the maculopapular rash of measles is diffuse, irregular and usually bright red. It is accompanied by an URTI, swollen watery eyes (conjunctivitis) and Koplick's spots (white dots on the buccal surface of the cheeks). The old name for this dreaded illness was 'first disease'. Allergy may sometimes cause a similar rash, which is unaccompanied by the high pyrexia of measles. *Measles → below.*
- *Pink, red, macular or papular*: scarlet fever is recognised by a diffuse, rough-feeling, red rash with circumoral pallor and a 'strawberry' tongue. These features are preceded by pharyngitis and pyrexia. The old name for scarlet fever was 'second disease' and a milder form of the illness is sometimes called 'scarlatina'. *Scarlet fever → p. 348.*

    A large variety of viral infections may cause a diffuse erythematous (and sometimes maculopapular) rash accompanied by pyrexia and upper respiratory symptoms including the following:

Rubella (German measles or third Disease): the erythematous rash is accompanied by characteristic postauricular and occipital lymphadenopathy.

Erythema infectiosum (slapped cheek syndrome or fifth disease): an infection with parvovirus B19, which begins with erythema of the cheeks and circumoral pallor. A 'lacy' rash then develops on the extremities, lasting for 7–10 days. This parvovirus can cause fetal loss in the second trimester of pregnancy and also affects the production of red blood cells.

Roseola infantum (exanthem subitum or sixth disease): there are discrete pink macules on the trunk.

    There are no 'seventh' and 'eighth' diseases!

Acute (guttate) psoriasis → p. 408.
Erythema nodosum → p. 408.
Lichen planus → p. 408.
Pityriasis rosea → p. 408.

> The diagnosis of Kawasaki's disease should be considered in any child with a febrile erythematous illness that persists for longer than 4 or 5 days (→ *p. 348*).

Measles

Measles is reappearing in the UK with a case fatality rate of around 1 in 5000. The patient has 2–3 days of severe cough, coryza and conjunctivitis, followed by a red maculopapular rash that starts on the hairline and behind the ears, before it spreads to the face, trunk and extremities. The temperature is usually >38.3°C and Koplick's spots may be seen on the buccal mucosa. In some areas of the body, the rash becomes confluent before starting to fade after 3–4 days. Around one in five patients with measles develops one or more complications including:

- pneumonia
- otitis media
- permanent loss of hearing
- diarrhoea (1 in 12).

Rarer complications include encephalitis and death. **Investigations:** Rapid diagnosis is required for both clinical and public health action but clinical diagnosis alone is unreliable. Therefore, one of the following specimens should be taken:

- Urine and/or throat swab (plain white swab not charcoal; ideally in virus transport medium [VTM] or a dry swab if VTM is unavailable) for PCR testing
- Blood (clotted) for measles IgM testing
- HPA (Health Protection Agency) salivary swab for both PCR and IgM testing.

Tx The treatment of uncomplicated measles is symptomatic – oral fluids and ibuprofen or paracetamol. Around 10% of cases require admission to hospital. The disease is notifiable in the UK and a list should be made of all the people who have been in the ED waiting room at the same time. The incubation period of measles is about 14 days from exposure to the appearance of the rash and it is infectious from 4 days before to 4 days after the onset of the rash.

> Measles is highly infectious. The virus can remain in the air for up to 2h after the patient has left the room. It is important that vulnerable (pregnant or immunocompromised) contacts of measles cases are identified as early as possible because they may require human normal immunoglobulin (HNIg).

Scarlet fever

Scarlet fever is caused by an exotoxin from *Streptococcus pyogenes* and is most common in children aged between 6 and 12 years. The illness starts with a sore throat, fever, cervical lymphadenopathy, headache, myalgia and general malaise. After 12–48 h, a fine, red, rough-textured rash appears on the chest, in the axillae and behind the ears. There is redness of the face with circumoral pallor. The 'sandpaper-like' rash then becomes more generalised but is worse in the skinfolds. It begins to fade after 3–4 days and a whitish coating on the tongue and throat peels away to leave a red 'strawberry' tongue. As the patient recovers, desquamation of the skin occurs, initially on the face and axillae, then on the palms, fingers and toes. Scarlet fever is treated with antibiotics (e.g. phenoxymethylpenicillin or clarithromycin). Septic complications such as pneumonia, sinusitis and local abscesses may occur. In rare cases, group A streptococci can also induce immune disorders such as rheumatic fever, glomerulonephritis and erythema nodosum. Scarlet fever is a notifiable disease in the UK (except in Scotland).

Kawasaki's disease

Kawasaki's disease is an acute febrile illness of unknown aetiology. Although uncommon, it is included in this section because of its non-specific features. Eighty per cent of cases occur in children aged <5 years, sometimes in small epidemics. There is an underlying vasculitis. The diagnosis is usually only confirmed if at least five of the following clinical features are present:

- Fever
- Reddening of the oropharyngeal mucosa including the tongue
- Dry, fissured lips
- Conjunctivitis
- Peeling fingers or toes
- Erythema of the hands and feet, which become swollen and indurated (oedema and pain in the extremities may be the predominant symptom)
- A morbilliform, maculopapular or urticarial rash on the trunk and limbs (within 5 days of the onset of the fever)
- Enlarged cervical lymph nodes (in over half of patients)
- Arthralgia
- Thrombocytosis.

During the illness, the coronary arteries can become dilated. This may result in the development of coronary aneurysms and delayed but sudden death.

Tx All patients in whom the diagnosis of Kawasaki's disease is a possibility must be referred to a paediatrician immediately. The administration of oral aspirin and IV human immunoglobulin can protect the coronary arteries from damage, but only if given within 10 days of the onset of the illness.

Urinary tract infection

Infections of the urinary tract in children are associated with vesicoureteric reflux and obstructive lesions. There may be an obvious urinary problem (dysuria, frequency, urgency, haematuria, enuresis or incontinence) or non-specific symptoms such as:

- pyrexia
- vomiting
- abdominal or renal pain.

Recurrent infections may lead to renal damage and chronic renal failure.

Tx A clean urine specimen for culture must be sent to the laboratory before antibiotic treatment is started (e.g. trimethoprim → *Table 18.3*). All children with urinary tract infections (UTIs) must be referred to a paediatrician via the GP for investigation of the urinary tract (micturating cystogram and renal imaging).

Diarrhoea and vomiting

> Children often vomit after minor injuries and during the course of many illnesses.

The main dangers of gastroenteritis are dehydration and electrolyte imbalance. Infants are particularly susceptible to dehydration because of their very high turnover of water relative to their size. An infant's normal daily fluid intake of 120–150 mL/kg represents up to 15% of his or her body weight. Gastoenteritis in an infant is thus similar in effect to cholera in an adult! *Signs of dehydration → Table 18.5.*

> Dehydration may be underestimated in hypernatraemia or in plump children.

In the UK, the most common infectious agents that are isolated from children with enteric infections are: rotavirus (56%), *Campylobacter* sp. (28%), *Salmonella* sp. (11%), norovirus (3%), *Shigella* sp. (1%)

Table 18.5 Signs of dehydration

Percentage of body weight lost	Signs
<5	Generally well: dry membranes, slight oliguria
5–10	Unwell: apathetic, sunken eyes and fontanelle, reduced skin elasticity, tachypnoea, oliguria
>10	Shocked: tachycardia and vasoconstriction
>15	Moribund

and verocytotoxin-producing *Escherichia coli* (1%). (Verocytotoxin-producing *E. coli* [VTEC] is also known as Shiga toxin-producing *E. coli* [STEC] or *E. coli* O157.) Bloody diarrhoea occurs in up to 30% of children infected with *Campylobacter jejuni* and in up to 90% of children with VTEC infection. *E. coli* infections should be suspected when there has been contact with ruminant farm animals (such as cattle, sheep and goats) or environments contaminated with their faeces or when an outbreak of VTEC is present locally. The incubation period for VTEC infection is usually 3–4 days but may be up to 14 days. VTEC infection leads to haemolytic uraemic syndrome in about 15% of cases (→ *p. 262*). This may occur up to 14 days after the onset of enteric symptoms.

Tx Most children can be managed at home with oral rehydration fluids (although clear liquids do not affect the frequency, amount or duration of loose stools). Vomiting may be reduced by giving fluids frequently and in small amounts. After 24 h (or even sooner), milk or a light diet can be reintroduced, although sometimes lactose intolerance will prolong diarrhoea.

Admission to hospital is required for children who are more than 5% dehydrated or whose parents are having difficulty in dealing with the problem. The type of fluid replacement will depend on the severity of the condition. In severe cases, the plasma electrolytes should be measured; hypoglycaemia may occur. **Acute bloody diarrhoea** in children is rare and is usually caused by intestinal infections, especially VTEC and *Campylobacter* sp. Around one in seven children infected with VTEC develops haemolytic uraemic syndrome. For this reason, all children with bloody diarrhoea should be admitted to hospital for specialist assessment. Antibiotics, non-steroidal anti-inflammatory drugs (NSAIDs), opiate analgesics and anti-motility drugs should not be given before referral.

Haemolytic uraemic syndrome and VTEC infection → *p. 262*.

Intussusception

Although not a common illness, this cause of intestinal obstruction is included in this section because of its often non-specific presentation. Intussusception usually affects children between the ages of 3 months and 3 years and is most common in the first year of life. It occurs when the terminal ileum and the ileocaecal valve invaginate into the caecum and ascending colon. The classic triad of intermittent colicky abdominal pain, vomiting and redcurrant jelly stools is seen in less than 10% of children with intussusception. Lethargy and malaise are the most common signs. There may be a palpable mass in the right hypochondrium.

Investigations: Redcurrant jelly stool is rare but the faeces usually test positive for blood. Ultrasound scan is the diagnostic study of choice; barium or air enema is a treatment.

Tx All children with suspected intussusception should be referred immediately to a surgeon. IV fluids are usually required.

Three months' colic

This is a condition that affects babies in the first few months of life. Spasms of severe crying and drawing up of the legs suggest a painful colic. Stools or flatus may be passed.

Tx No specific therapy has been shown to help. Paracetamol elixir and tummy rubbing are useful placebos. Admission should be considered for distressed parents, as discussed earlier.

Infants crying and parents not coping

Crying infants may be brought to the ED by their distraught parents. A thorough history and examination must be conducted, both to exclude serious illness or trauma and to reassure the parents. No tests are better than careful observation and taking the temperature.

> Occasionally, a hair or a thread that has spontaneously become wrapped around a digit is found to be the cause of the child's distress. *Treatment of a hair tourniquet* → *p. 402*.

Tx If no abnormality is discovered, then professional reassurance may be all that is needed. The GP should be notified. Some areas have the facility for late night visits by a health visitor.

Parents who feel that that they cannot cope with crying or minor illness must be taken seriously. The child should be admitted for care and assessment. A crying child causes enormous stress and may even in some cases provoke physical abuse.

Threadworms

Infestation with threadworms causes perianal irritation at night. This is the time when the mature female worm crawls out of the bowel to lay her eggs around the anus. Scratching transfers the eggs to the fingers, from where they find their way (via food, clothing and linen) back to the bowel. The small, white worms may easily be seen at the time of the symptoms.

Tx A single dose of 100 mg mebendazole will kill threadworms. All close contacts should be treated. The dosage may be repeated after 2–3 weeks to prevent reinfection. Mebendazole is not suitable for children aged <2 years or for pregnant or lactating women.

Hygienic precautions are necessary to prevent both reinfection and spread:

- Hand washing
- Daily bathing and washing around the bottom
- Wearing pyjamas in bed
- Having a personal towel
- Changing clothes and bedlinen frequently.

Injuries and accidents

Refer to the relevant sections in the appropriate chapters.

Burns → Chapter 10.
Fingertip injuries → p. 129.
Foreign bodies in the ears and nose → pp. 418 and 419.
Impetigo → p. 406.
Minor injuries → Chapter 21.
Poisoning → Chapter 15.
Swallowed foreign bodies → p. 420.
The child who is not moving an arm → p. 117.
The limping child → p. 92.

Poisoning

Detailed information about poisoning → Chapter 15.

Bizarre symptoms and signs and unexplained combinations of findings suggest poisoning. Younger children may ingest substances accidentally; older children may experiment with drugs. Either may have been given inappropriate medication by an adult. The most common non-specific signs are:

- confusion, agitation and drowsiness
- tachycardia
- dilated pupils
- evidence at the scene (which is of enormous help to hospital staff).

Gastric decontamination is rarely required in children. However, charcoal is now available in relatively palatable syrup suspensions. Milk is a simple treatment for many ingestions.

Osteochondritis

There are several conditions in which there is an abnormality of bone in an area of growth or at the site where a major tendon is developing its attachment to bone. Children with one of these diseases may present to the ED with pain and reduced movements, often exacerbated by a minor injury. There is often slight swelling around the affected area. These osteochondritides are most commonly seen in the lower limb:

- Head of the femur – Perthes' disease ($\rightarrow$ p. 92)
- Lower pole of the patella – Sindig–Laarson disease ($\rightarrow$ p. 99)
- Tibial tuberosity – Osgood–Schlatter disease ($\rightarrow$ p. 99)
- Posterior calcaneum – Sever's disease
- Navicular bone – Köhler's disease ($\rightarrow$ p. 107)
- Head of a metatarsal bone (usually the second metatarsus) – Freiberg's disease.

XR The affected area may be deformed or fragmented. It is thought that a deficiency in the blood supply of the growing bone leads to aseptic necrosis.

Tx Symptoms usually resolve with time. Rest from sports should be advised and an appointment at the orthopaedic clinic should be given.

Epiphyseal injuries

Injuries to the epiphyses are specific to childhood and adolescence. The epiphyseal plate is a weak area of the bone and so is often damaged. Bilateral or unilateral growth retardation may then occur. The Salter–Harris classification describes five types of epiphyseal injury, of which type II is the most common ($\rightarrow$ *Figure 18.2*).

Ankle injuries in children → p. 102.
Elbow injuries in children (and a description of the growing elbow) → p. 116.
Wrist injuries in children → p. 120.

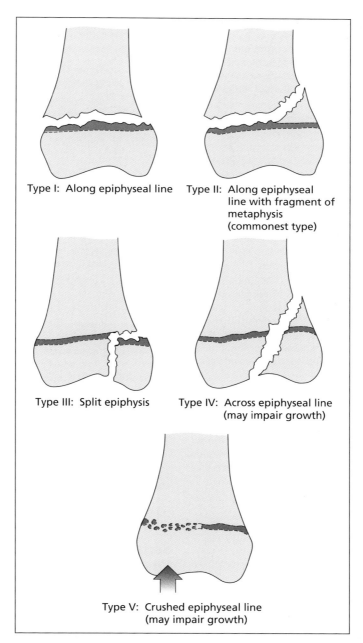

Figure 18.2 The Salter–Harris classification of epiphyseal injuries.

Immunisation in childhood

It is every child's right to be protected against infectious diseases. No child should be denied immunisation without serious thought as to the consequences, both for the individual child and for the community.

One in 10 children with meningococcal group C infection dies
One in 20 children with *Haemophilus influenzae* b meningitis dies
One in 500 infants with pertussis dies

For an ED, good practice in the area of immunisation is essential. No child should be given a single antitetanus vaccine. If protection against tetanus is needed, then this should be given together with the other vaccines indicated for that age group ($\rightarrow$ *Table 18.6*). Unimmunised children should be either immunised opportunistically or else referred to the GP and health visitor for follow-up.

Toxic shock syndrome

At any one time, around 3% of the population harbour a toxin-producing strain of *Staphylococcus aureus* on their skin. Infection of burns or other wounds with these pathogenic bacteria may lead to a life-threatening toxaemia. This toxic shock syndrome is characterised by:

- malaise, anorexia and lethargy
- dizziness or faintness
- pyrexia (usually >39°C)
- myalgia
- vomiting or diarrhoea
- a rash (often erythematous or maculopapular)
- peripheral shutdown and frank shock.

Burns information cards should advise parents of the possible dangers of these symptoms in their children. This syndrome may also be seen in women whose vaginal tampons have become infected.

Tx Resuscitation should be commenced immediately with oxygen and fluids. Anti-staphylococcal therapy must be instituted as soon as possible and purulent lesions should be drained. In severe cases, steroids have been used to limit the endogenous inflammatory response.

Table 18.6 UK immunisation schedule for children

Age	Target of immunisation	Name of vaccine
2, 3 and 4 months	Diphtheria, tetanus, pertussis, polio and *H. influenzae* type b	DTaP/IPV/Hib (5 in 1)
2 and 4 months	Pneumococcus	PCV
3 and 4 months	Meningococcus group C	MenC
Around 12 months	*H. influenzae* type b and meningococcus group C	Hib/MenC
Around 13 months	Measles, mumps and rubella	MMR
	Pneumococcus	PCV
3.5–5 years	Diphtheria, tetanus, pertussis and polio	DTaP/IPV or dTAP/IPV
	Measles, mumps and rubella	MMR
10–14 years	Tuberculosis	Tuberculin test then BCG if required
13–18 years	Tetanus, diphtheria and polio	Td/IPV

Td = tetanus vaccine combined with low-dose diphtheria vaccine. Low-dose (adult) diphtheria vaccine (d) should always be given after the age of 10 years rather than standard full-strength (paediatric) diphtheria vaccine (D). In older patients, use of the D vaccine results in a high number of both localised and generalised reactions.

Sedation and analgesia for children undergoing procedures in the emergency department

Midazolam elixir

This is an effective tranquilliser for minor procedures in children. The usual dose is 0.5 mg/kg. The onset of sedation occurs within about 20 min and the peak effect may be reached a few minutes later. Recovery is rapid – within <2 h – but, even so, the parents of all children who have been sedated should have written aftercare instructions to take home ($\rightarrow$ *p. 390*). Some children (around 10%) who have been given midazolam in the above dosage will become hyperexcited. As with all benzodiazepines, the effects of midazolam can be reversed with fluma-zenil ($\rightarrow p.\ 281$).

> Sedative drugs used in isolation do not provide analgesia.

Local anaesthetic agents

These must be used with care in children as the maximum safe dose is easily exceeded ($\rightarrow$ Box 18.13).

 Box 18.13 Maximum doses of local anaesthetic agents

Bupivacaine	2 mg/kg
Lidocaine	3 mg/kg
Prilocaine	4 mg/kg

Morphine elixir

This can be used to alleviate the pain of a procedure where local anaesthesia is not practicable, such as changing a dressing on a large burn. The dose is 0.2–0.4 mg/kg for a child aged >12 months. The elixir must be given at least 60 min before the procedure to give adequate time for it to work.

Parenteral doses of opiate analgesics

These can sometimes be useful in instances where a combination of sedation and analgesia is desirable and oral therapy is not suitable (*Dosages* $\rightarrow$ Box 18.6 on p. 334).

Gaseous analgesia and sedation

Analgesic gas from a premixed nitrous oxide/oxygen cylinder (e.g. Entonox) should be administered via a demand valve with a low opening pressure. An excellent sedative effect may be obtained with a continuous flow apparatus such as the Quantiflex machine ($\rightarrow p.\ 17$).

Ketamine

Ketamine given intramuscularly in a dose of 2.5 mg/kg creates a unique analgesic, dissociative and sedative effect. Although it is very safe, it should be used only by practitioners experienced in sedative techniques ($\rightarrow p.\ 17$).

Local anaesthetic creams

Topical local anaesthetic preparations are available. Mixtures such as 'EMLA' (lidocaine 2.5% and prilocaine 2.5% cream) and 'Ametop' (tetracaine 4% gel) are suitable for procedures on intact skin such as venepuncture and splinter removal. Cocaine and adrenaline cream may be used to provide analgesia for suturing of some small wounds.

Diversional therapies

These are a long-established psychological means of helping with difficult situations. Elaborate coloured pattern and bubble generators are now available as well as traditional diversions such as music and stories. Some departments employ a play specialist who can advise on this specific aspect of care.

Rewards such as balloons, badges and bravery certificates can help to soften the trauma of an unpleasant experience. Raisins and sweets – sugar free of course – are also used in some departments. As Mary Poppins said, in 1910, 'a spoonful of sugar helps the medicine go down'.

CHILD ABUSE

Five main types of child abuse are now recognised:

1 Emotional abuse
2 Neglect
3 Sexual abuse
4 Physical abuse (non-accidental injury or NAI)
5 Organised abuse.

The above list is in approximate order of prevalence, although the exact ranking is unknown.

Physical abuse

Child abuse occurs in every culture and is perpetrated by all social classes and by both sexes. Nevertheless, certain factors are associated with abuse and include:

- Parents abused as children (learned behaviour)
- Parents with alcohol or other drug problems (alcohol is a factor in most violence)
- Frequent address changes (without a permanent address a family has almost nothing)
- Undesirable and stressful living conditions or other poor social circumstances (of course).

The stress of looking after very young children also increases the risk and so:

- a third of NAI occurs under 6 months of age
- a third of NAI occurs between 6 months and 3 years of age
- a third of NAI occurs over 3 years of age.

A crying baby is an enormous strain and is the provocation for some cases of methadone poisoning.

> Diagnosis of abuse is a complex problem. False accusations may cause great distress. In suspicious circumstances, experienced advice should be obtained before a full examination is undertaken.

There are patterns of physical signs for some types of abuse but the history and the context in which the events occurred are the most important first indicators to alert the health worker. Some features of a history of injury that should raise a suspicion of abuse are the following:

- Inappropriate delay in seeking help and advice after a significant injury
- History of previous frequent accidents
- The history of the accident is not a likely mechanism for that injury
- Vague or absent history of an accident
- Different carers give different explanations for the same injury
- The history keeps changing
- The child gives a different history
- The child is supposed to have sustained the injury in a way that is inconsistent with his or her development (e.g. fell over before the child has started walking)
- The adults with the child are either unconcerned or hostile during questioning. Their attention is focused on their own needs throughout.

The following list of signs of child abuse is by no means comprehensive:

- Unexplained head, facial, chest or limb injuries, especially in children who are not able to walk and thus fall (few children walk under the age of 11 months)
- Multiple bruising
- Symmetrical bruising
- Linear bruising, especially to the buttocks or back
- Bruising around the eye, especially if bilateral
- Bruising around the ears, especially if bilateral

- Other facial bruising including in or around the mouth
- Facial petechiae/subconjunctival haemorrhages
- Tears of the frenulum of the upper lip
- Grasp marks or fingertip bruising especially to the face, arms or chest
- Unusual cuts and bruises; outline imprints of hands, sticks, cords, shoes, belts and teeth may be present
- Marks to the neck
- Marks to the genitalia
- A tender, red scalp (hair pulling)
- Unusual burns, e.g. those of a glove or stocking distribution or to the perineum or cigarette type
- Injuries of different ages
- Multiple old scars
- Any fractures in children aged <12 months
- Coexisting signs of neglect.

Non-accidental head injury in infants (previously called the 'shaken baby syndrome') → p. 41.

> All children in whom the diagnosis of abuse is suspected should be fully examined from top to toe by an experienced doctor. The investigation and management of a case of possible deliberate harm to a child must be approached in the same systematic and rigorous manner as the investigation and management of any other potentially fatal disease.

XR There are also typical radiological findings of abuse, which are more common in younger children:

- Old unsuspected fractures
- Fractures at different stages of healing
- Rib fractures (posterior rib fractures are particularly specific for abuse)
- Skull fractures in children who cannot walk (especially if multiple, depressed or in areas other than the parietal bones) (→ p. 41)
- Spiral fractures of long bones (twisting injuries)
- Injuries to the metaphyses of long bones (twisting injuries); these are very specific for abuse
- Periosteal injuries (twisting forces again).

A skeletal survey – to look for occult injuries – is usually indicated only in children aged <2 years. Dating of a fracture is a job for a radiologist (→ *Box 18.14*).

Box 18.14 Healing of fractures on radiographs

Periosteal new bone formation	10–14 days
Loss of fracture line definition	14–21 days
Soft callus formation	14–21 days
Hard callus visible	>21 days

Tx

> Look for a specific Child Protection Plan (or the child's name on the Child Protection Register) in the information held by the Local Safeguarding Children Board (or the Area Child Protection Committee) via the local social services portal (→ p. 384).

There will be a local protocol for the management of suspected abuse. The child should always be discussed with a senior member of the ED or paediatric staff. The duty social worker for child protection must also be notified of the concern as soon as possible. This should be followed up in writing within 48 h.

The child must be examined from head to toe and all findings measured and carefully documented (→ p. 370). Injuries should be treated and referred to other departments as appropriate. Specialised investigations in cases of abuse (e.g. clotting screen, platelets, liver function tests and calcium studies) are usually obtained by the paediatric staff at a later date.

The reasons for admission to hospital are the same as for non-abused children (unless admission is used as a method to prevent the child from leaving a place of safety). The Child Protection Unit now places most abused children in the care of the extended family or foster parents.

Legal aspects of child protection, including emergency powers, → p. 384.

Neglect and emotional abuse

Only gross forms of neglect can be recognised in an ED. Some of the characteristics are as follows:

- Short in stature and underweight for age
- Cold, mottled, discoloured extremities
- Poor skin condition (especially in the nappy area)
- Dry, sparse hair
- Wasting
- Diarrhoea
- Voracious appetite
- Flat affect and unresponsiveness
- Lack of energy and failure to play.

Emotional abuse is even more subtle than physical neglect.

Tx As for other forms of abuse, these children should be discussed with a social worker and a senior paediatrician.

Sexual abuse

> Before the age of 16, at least 1 in 10 girls and 1 in 15 boys will have been sexually assaulted. The peak incidence of first assault is at about 8 years of age.

Sexual abuse of children can occur in all socioeconomic, cultural and religious groups, and is associated with:

- acute perineal injury
- chronic perineal damage
- genitourinary infection
- sexually precocious behaviour
- sexualised drawings and play
- regressive patterns of behaviour
- eating and sleep disorders
- psychosomatic symptoms
- withdrawal and depression
- self-harm
- promiscuity
- running away from home.

> Profound anal dilatation can occur after failed cardiopulmonary resuscitation in children.

The most common victim is a girl of school age, the offender is usually male and disclosure to an adult is the most frequent way in which the abuse comes to light. A surprising number of patients who present with self-harm as teenagers or adults will later give a history of sexual abuse.

Tx All suspected cases should be referred for consideration of the need for child protection as described earlier. Examination of acute injuries should be left to a specialist police surgeon because forensic evidence must be collected.

Sudden infant death syndrome

One baby in every 1400 live births dies suddenly and unexpectedly for no obvious reason. This sudden infant death syndrome is the most common cause of death in the UK in infants aged >1 month. The diagnosis does not include all cot deaths because some infants die suddenly from well-understood causes.

- SIDS is more common among boys and with babies of low birthweight.
- It has a peak incidence at 2–5 months of age.
- It is more common in the winter months.
- Most deaths from SIDS seem to occur during sleep.
- Half of all babies who die from SIDS have had a recent URTI ($\rightarrow$ *p. 346*).

Tx Always bring an infant or young child into the resuscitation room and assess the situation properly, however cold or apparently dead. Children can withstand long periods of hypoxia and still recover. Parents often follow the ambulance not knowing the fate of their child. They need to know that the action taken was immediate and appropriate. Parents should have constant access to their child – even during resuscitation. A nurse should act as a communicator.

The principles of care of bereaved relatives are described on *p. 163*. After a child's death the following procedure should apply:

- A senior member of the medical staff should break the news. The baby's name should be used in conversation.

- The parents should be encouraged to sit with or hold their child in a quiet room – for as long as they want.
- They should be asked if they would like a photograph of the child or a lock of hair or a handprint.
- The parents should be given the Foundation for the Study of Infant Deaths (FSID) leaflet, *Information for parents following the unexpected death of their baby*, and also FSID local contact numbers.
- Contact should be made with other family members, the hospital chaplain and a translator if necessary.
- The coroner's officer must be informed. Postmortem examination is not always required by the coroner in cases of SIDS. The purpose of the coroner's procedures should be explained to the parents.
- The GP and the health visitor should be informed. They must ensure that the local health authority deletes the child's name from the immunisation register, etc. Suppression of lactation may be required for the child's mother.
- A senior paediatrician should be involved in the follow-up.
- Transport home should be offered to the relatives.
- The need for continued support should be recognised; a bereavement counsellor is invaluable in this respect.

> Infant death can be a very difficult situation for many doctors and nurses who may have children who are the same age as the deceased. Staff support should always be available.

The disturbed patient

Psychological disturbance can cause more upset to a patient, and his or her family and friends than a physical problem, and is just as valid a reason for seeking help in the emergency department (ED). The distress caused by mental illness should never be under-estimated.

> One person in seven has a diagnosable neurotic disorder, mainly depression and anxiety, and one person in 250 has a functional psychosis.

Behaviour is influenced by the interplay between the environment and the psyche, and is modified by drugs. A disturbed patient may have a psychiatric condition, an organic brain lesion, a personality disorder or an emotional upset → *Box 19.1 for common acute presentations of mental disturbance*. The task of the ED is to:

- identify those patients who need immediate therapy
- support the coping strategies of the patient
- liaise with the appropriate agency for further care.

Initial assessment and management of the disturbed patient

Ask about

- Presenting complaints as described by the patient and those accompanying him or her
- The history of the presenting complaints and any accompanying problems
- Current drug therapy and other management and support

- Previous psychiatric history: symptoms, duration, diagnoses, admissions and any treatment received
- Coincidental physical illnesses
- Social circumstances and support (e.g. one in four people with a mental health problem is also in debt).

Look for

- Abnormal appearance or behaviour
- Disorientation or altered conscious level
- Lack of attention or concentration
- Poor memory
- Unusual form or content of speech
- Depressed or elevated mood
- Disordered thought content
- Abnormal beliefs: delusions, misinterpretations and overvalued ideas
- Hallucinations (visual or auditory) and disorders of perception
- Obsessions and compulsions
- The level of insight that the patient has into his or her problems.

These are the main features of the mental state examination. Concise notes may be augmented by verbatim quotes of the patient's responses to questioning. A brief but comprehensive physical examination is also important to exclude organic causes of disturbance (→ *later*). This must include:

- temperature
- heart rate
- palpation of the scalp
- blood sugar
- gross neurological signs (walking and talking).

Therapeutic manoeuvres include the following:

- Correction of organic problems (e.g. hypoxia and hypoglycaemia)

Emergency Medicine Lecture Notes, Fourth Edition. Chris Moulton and David Yates.
© 2012 Blackwell Publishing Ltd. Published 2012 by Blackwell Publishing Ltd.

> **Box 19.1 The presentation of mental disorders to the emergency department**
>
> - Acute psychiatric disturbance (patient with little insight brought to ED by relatives, social workers or the police)
> - Psychological symptoms (patient usually self-referred with depression or anxiety)
> - Exacerbation of symptoms or loss of control in known psychiatric disease (patient usually has good insight and self-refers; may request admission)
> - Personality disorder (self-referred patient with no apparent insight; often manipulative)
> - Self-harm
> - Alcohol and drug abuse
> - Acute emotional upset

- Sedation: oral lorazepam (2 mg) should be tried initially; in extreme cases, intravenous (IV) benzodiazepines (lorazepam or midazolam) may be used. All normal precautions for sedation should be observed, as far as possible. If there is a confirmed history of previous significant antipsychotic exposure, and response, then the use of haloperidol in combination with lorazepam should be considered.
- Referral to a psychiatrist or other agency.

Distinction must be made between:

- responses to adverse life events that may appear logical to the patient, however bizarre to the doctor
- major psychiatric disease that may be distinguished by the history or examination
- other medical conditions that masquerade as psychiatric illness (e.g. head injury, hypoglycaemia, infection, drug disturbance, epilepsy and cerebrovascular disease).

Interaction with the disturbed patient

The image portrayed by staff is very important. The patient is extremely vulnerable and sees doctors and nurses as being in a position of power. Occasionally, this will provoke an aggressive response. It is important, therefore, not only that actions cannot be interpreted as threatening but also that staff are never put in a position of vulnerability themselves. Staff should avoid being judgemental and must be sensitive to a patient's affect. They need to be aware of the potential for manipulative behaviour but must not react to it in a critical manner.

> Promises should be made only if they can be visibly kept; unfulfilled promises increase distrust and the risk of further aggression.

The aim is to support the patient at a time of crisis and to identify appropriate agencies that can provide sustained care. The latter can include the patient's relatives and friends and the patient's own resources. Medication and admission – rarely against the patient's will – may be necessary but physical restraint can be justified only as a prelude to a specific therapy (e.g. holding down a patient while an injection of glucagon or IV glucose is administered).

The patient's behaviour must be responded to appropriately, e.g. if a patient is rude or abusive this must not be a cue for clever retaliation. Nor must it be ignored. The situation should be briefly summarised and an explanation that such behaviour is unacceptable given. Surprisingly, this sometimes works but, if it does not, lengthy interrogation must be avoided and an early decision made to seek further help from the duty psychiatrist.

Throughout care in the ED it is essential to reassure the patient constantly about the intended course of action and to keep the patient up to date with events.

CONFUSION AND PSYCHOTIC BEHAVIOUR

Acute confusional states

Delirium has four main features:

1 Disturbance of consciousness (reduced awareness of the environment and reduced ability to maintain attention)
2 Change in cognition (such as memory deficit, disorientation, language disturbance) or the development of a perceptual disturbance that is not accounted for by a pre-existing or evolving dementia
3 Rapid development over a short period of time (usually hours to days) with a tendency to fluctuate during the course of the day
4 Evidence from the history, physical examination, or laboratory findings that the disturbance is caused by the direct physiological consequences of a general medical condition, substance intoxication or substance withdrawal.

Delirium is under-recognised and associated with high rates of mortality and morbidity. Even after treatment of the underlying cause, delirium can persist for up to 6 months. Some patients will never regain full cognitive function.

Patients at risk include elderly people, and those with dementia, alcohol problems or impaired vision or hearing. A wide range of underlying conditions may be responsible for confusion and disorientation and so a full history and examination is required to establish the cause:

- Hypoxia may present as a toxic confusional state and a psychosis of rapid onset with disorientation, hallucination and delusions. There will be a clouding of consciousness and impairment of recent memory. These sudden alterations in cerebration are very frightening and sufficient to cause aggression in many patients.
- Hypoglycaemia may cause considerable violence and aggression.
- Infection, particularly of the central nervous system (CNS), can also cause an acute confusional state. Elderly patients with any infection (e.g. chest or urinary tract) can present in such a way that the underlying medical condition is completely masked.
- Drug intoxication ($\rightarrow$ *later and Chapter 15*).
- Gross metabolic disturbance, including that found with hepatic and renal failure.
- Organic brain lesions may occasionally present in this way.
- Post-ictal states: there may be aggression and agitation in a similar way to hypoglycaemia.
- Cerebrovascular accidents.
- Myocardial infarction (MI) may present with acute confusion in elderly people.

Dementia and depression may mimic delirium or may coexist.

Investigations:
- Full blood count (FBC), glucose, blood chemistry including calcium, liver function tests (LFTs), thyroid function tests (TFTs) and C-reactive protein (CRP)

- Consider the need for a troponin assay (12 h after the onset of symptoms) to detect an unsuspected MI ($\rightarrow$ *p. 185*)
- Consider the need for serum vitamin B_{12}, folate and ferritin levels
- Chest radiograph (CXR), ECG and mid-stream specimen of urine (MSU)
- Consider the need for a CT scan of the brain.

Tx A safe environment must be maintained and any possible improvement to communication ensured. Family and carers should be involved. Basic observations should be continued and oxygenation and hydration maintained. Retention of urine, constipation, pain and discomfort must be avoided and medications should be reviewed. If possible, catheterisation and sedation should also be avoided. However, it is often impossible to assess fully or manage an agitated patient. In addition, the patient may put him- or herself or others at risk of harm. Adequate sedation makes further therapy possible and may relieve the patent's distress. Small doses of IV lorazepam (or midazolam) are effective and have a rapid onset of action but careful observation and monitoring are necessary. Where there is a confirmed history of previous significant antipsychotic exposure (and response), haloperidol may be given. Hypoglycaemia is one of the few situations where rapid diagnosis and specific therapy obviate the need for sedation. The use of depressant drugs has been criticised in hypoxaemia because it may decrease respiratory effort. However, in situations of extreme restlessness, judicious sedation decreases oxygen requirements and makes possible the administration of high-concentration oxygen by mask.

Agitation can be greatly reduced if pain is relieved and so analgesia is often helpful. Splintage of injuries and drainage of a full bladder may have a similar effect.

Drug-induced psychiatric syndromes

Prescribed drugs

Mental disturbance caused by prescribed drugs is particularly common in elderly people but may occur with CNS-depressant drugs, β blockers, digoxin and cimetidine at all ages. Symptoms include fluctuating clouding of consciousness and restlessness with paranoid delusions and visual hallucinations in severe cases. Although usually a result of overdosage, these reactions may sometimes occur because of intolerance to the normal dose or after withdrawal of the drug.

Recreational drugs

Patients may retain full consciousness but experience paranoid delusions and visual hallucinations after ingestion of cocaine, amphetamines, lysergic acid diethylamide (LSD) and psychotropic fungi. Fear and restlessness lead to disruptive and aggressive behaviour. The condition can be distinguished from schizophrenia by the history and often by the extreme nature of the patient's behaviour.

Treatment of specific poisonings → Chapter 15.

Psychoses

A psychosis is defined as a significant mental illness that robs the patient of insight and distorts appreciation of the environment. It follows that a psychotic patient cannot be held responsible for his or her actions.

Schizophrenia is now no longer thought to be a single condition. The name embraces a heterogeneous group of clinical syndromes in which hallucinations, delusions and thought disorders are present. The intensity of these symptoms is constantly changing and they may be modified or abolished by drugs. Mood and behaviour are similarly fluctuant.

Patients with both schizophrenia and mania may present acutely to the ED with obvious psychotic behaviour. The distinction between the two conditions can be difficult at times but is not initially important because pharmacological control of symptoms is similar in both conditions.

More commonly, a patient with a known history of schizophrenia comes to the ED with an exacerbation of usually well-controlled symptoms. Loss of therapeutic control may be precipitated by:

- pressure of outside events
- moving area of residence away from long-term support
- omitting depot therapy
- absence of usual support (friends, relatives or care workers).

Tx Psychotic behaviour may necessitate the administration of neuroleptic drugs (e.g. IV or IM [intramuscular] haloperidol 5–10 mg), although oral lorazepam 2 mg and/or oral haloperidol 5 mg may be tried initially. These patients will subsequently require expert care from psychiatrists. In less acute cases, community psychiatric nurses can be a useful source of information and advice.

> It is important to distinguish patients with psychoses from those with neurotic conditions. Patients with neuroses are likely to be less disturbed and more amenable to therapy and advice from the non-specialist.

Medical conditions in psychiatric patients

Up to 50% of psychiatric patients have a medical condition and, in some cases, this may exacerbate psychiatric symptoms. In particular, patients with a diagnosis of schizophrenia have an increased incidence of:

- cardiovascular diseases
- endocrine diseases
- infections
- nutritional problems.

There is a corresponding increase in mortality from these conditions and thus medical symptoms in psychiatric patients should always be investigated appropriately.

ALCOHOL-RELATED PROBLEMS

Acute intoxication with alcohol

The patient who smells of alcohol may appear merely drunk and disorderly but never assume that this is the only pathology. A coexistent head injury or hypoglycaemia may look identical to the effects of alcohol. Diagnosis of alcohol intoxication must always be made by exclusion – never by neglect.

Alcohol absorption from the gastrointestinal tract will continue for some time after the last ingestion. In comatose patients, blood levels continue to rise for about 2 h after presentation. The patient may appear to be becoming quieter and more cooperative when he or she is in fact becoming more intoxicated. Respiratory depression and inhalation of vomitus can occur quite suddenly.

Signs of intoxication with alcohol and for the treatment of acute alcohol poisoning → p. 285.

Alcohol withdrawal states

Alcohol withdrawal is not synonymous with delirium tremens. There are in fact several possible presentations that can follow the cessation of drinking in patients who are physically dependent on ethanol.

Acute withdrawal syndrome

This occurs within 6–12 h of abstinence and presents as:

- agitation and restlessness (sometimes extreme)
- tremulousness
- sweating
- tachycardia
- anorexia, nausea and retching
- upper abdominal pain (but beware of pancreatitis or ulcer).

Tx Most of the symptoms respond well to IV diazepam. Enormous doses may be needed; the correct dose is apparent by the relief that it affords. Upper abdominal symptoms may be helped by antacids. The patient should be admitted for a reducing dose of oral chlordiazepoxide accompanied by IV fluids and parenteral high-potency vitamins B and C (e.g. Pabrinex two pairs of ampoules intravenously three times daily for 2–5 days). Oral vitamin therapy should be prescribed concurrently: vitamin B compound strong two tablets three times daily and thiamine 50 mg four times daily. The thiamine can be discontinued once the chlordiazepoxide detoxification regimen is complete but the high-dose oral vitamin B should be continued indefinitely.

Typical times of onset of alcohol withdrawal states →
Figure 19.1.

Generalised convulsions

Fits may be recurrent and require short-term treatment as well as a long-term management strategy.

Concurrent head injury must be excluded as a cause. Patients with withdrawal seizures should be prescribed carbamazepine 200 mg three times daily throughout the period of withdrawal. The drug can be reduced and stopped over 3–5 days when the detoxification is complete. If the patient is already taking an anticonvulsant drug such as phenytoin, there is no need to prescribe additional carbamazepine.

Acute alcohol hallucinosis

Around 10% of people withdrawing from alcohol will suffer from auditory and visual hallucinations while fully conscious and situationally aware. The onset is within 12–24 h of abstinence and resolution occurs within 24–48 h. The hallucinations are vivid and voices may be described such as those of family or friends, often threatening or degrading in manner. This is a distinct condition, separate from other withdrawal states, which should be discussed with a psychiatrist. Intravenous haloperidol (5–10 mg) may be helpful.

Delirium tremens

This occurs after 24–72 h of abstinence and is recognised by:

- agitation and restlessness
- tremulousness
- fever and tachycardia
- delirium (acute confusional psychosis with bizarre visual hallucinations often concerning animals or insects)
- fits.

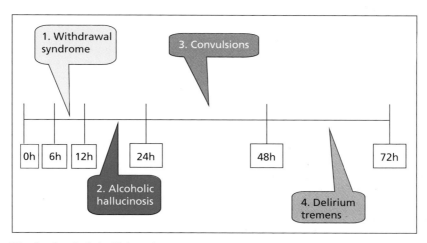

Figure 19.1 Timeline for alcohol withdrawal states.

Tx Delirium tremens has a high mortality rate (up to 5%), so intensive monitoring and observation are mandatory. The patient will need adequate sedation and supportive therapy.

Alcoholism

Alcoholism is a descriptive rather than a diagnostic term. The person with alcohol problems (alcoholic) continues to drink despite obvious harm to self and family. Addiction is a more specific description indicating tolerance, craving and withdrawal symptoms attributable to the drug. Every alcohol addict is an alcoholic but not every alcoholic is an addict. Many simply binge drink, wreak havoc with their lives for a brief period and then return to 'normality'. This, of course, is very disruptive to home and family. The following are the main features of true dependency on alcohol (addiction):

- Difficulty or failure to carry out daily life if there is an absence of alcohol
- Same daily pattern of drinking
- Increased tolerance to alcohol
- Compulsion for alcohol
- Priority in life is to maintain alcohol intake
- Symptoms of withdrawal ($\rightarrow$ p. 361).

Signs of chronic alcohol abuse include:

- poor nutritional status
- raised γ-glutamyl transpeptidase
- macrocytosis in the absence of folate or vitamin B_{12} deficiency
- multiple rib fractures at various stages of healing on CXR (pulmonary tuberculosis [TB] may also be present)
- atrial fibrillation.

A slow downward spiral often leads to the loss of driving licence, job and home, and then to residence in a hostel or on the streets.

Requests for detoxification are often made to ED staff. Unfortunately, there are very few acute facilities available for people requiring this sort of help and those that do exist require a completely sober individual. This is difficult to achieve because sobriety is usually accompanied by any one of the withdrawal states detailed above. The best policy is probably to advise the patient (ideally in the presence of carers) to continue drinking alcohol in sufficient quantities to hold off the worst of the withdrawal symptoms until attendance at a specialist clinic can be arranged. However, timely facilities for such help are in short supply in the UK.

Treatment of alcohol dependence is more effective if it is started early on in the downward spiral. Changes in funding for 'alcohol' services in the UK reflect a growing recognition that this help must be accessible by patients presenting to both primary and emergency care facilities.

Complications of chronic alcohol abuse

Many health problems accompany chronic alcohol abuse.

Wernicke–Korsakoff syndrome

In 80% of people with Wernicke–Korsakoff syndrome, the diagnosis is made only at *post mortem* examination.

The common causation of these two eponymous conditions (failure of cellular metabolism in the brain) has led to the description of one syndrome with two extreme forms:

1 Korsakoff's psychosis: severe loss of short-term memory causes the patient to invent his or her immediate past (confabulation). The patient may also be confused and disoriented.
2 Wernicke's encephalopathy: there is ophthalmoplegia, ataxia and peripheral neuropathy. In extreme cases hypothermia, hypotension and coma may also be seen.

The syndrome is often precipitated in alcohol-dependent patients by the stress of an intercurrent illness. It may be very difficult to diagnose and the classic triad of confusion, ataxia and ophthalmoplegia is rarely seen. Cerebellar degeneration (which is irreversible) may present a very similar clinical picture in intoxicated, alcoholic patients. If in doubt, it is better to treat as Wernicke–Korsakoff syndrome.

Tx There is an underlying imbalance between the brain's energy requirements and CNS B vitamin availability. Consequent failure of the citric acid cycle can lead to irreversible brain damage. Oral thiamine has little effect on its own in this situation. To restore CNS vitamin levels, high-dose parenteral vitamins B and C should be given two or three times a day (e.g. Pabrinex two or three pairs of ampoules intravenously three times daily for 2–5 days). Oral vitamin therapy should be prescribed concurrently: vitamin B compound strong two tablets three times daily and thiamine 50 mg four times daily. The patient should be admitted, rehydrated and observed. A CT scan of the brain should be performed.

Suicide and parasuicide

Suicide and parasuicide have an increased incidence in people with alcohol addiction. Therefore, possible ingestion of other drugs should always be considered.

Injury

People with an alcohol addiction are more prone to injury and very much more susceptible to assault than most people. A full physical examination is essential. Loss of reflex protective mechanisms when drunk contributes to the increased incidence of subdural haematoma as a complication of head injury in alcohol abusers ($\rightarrow$ p. 44).

Detection of alcohol abuse

Excessive alcohol intake is common throughout the world (also $\rightarrow$ p. 285). Its detection and control are a major global health problem. Patients may present to emergency services with a large variety of medical and traumatic complaints that are related to underlying alcohol abuse.

> The maximum recommended weekly intake of alcohol is 21 units for men and 14 units for women – with at least 1 or 2 alcohol-free days. (*Definition of a unit* $\rightarrow$ p. 375.)

The CAGE questions were designed as a quick and effective screen for use by health workers $\rightarrow$ *Box 19.2*. CAGE is an acronym made from the first letter of the key word in each question. More than one affirmative answer indicates problem drinking. However, for the purposes of an ED, the Paddington Alcohol Test is much more usable and informative.

DEPRESSED MOOD AND SELF-HARM

Depression

About one in seven people experiences some of the symptoms of depression in any one year and many

 Box 19.2 The CAGE questions

1 Do you feel that you should **C**ut down on your drinking?
2 Does anyone **A**nnoy you or get on your nerves by telling you to cut down your drinking?
3 Do you feel bad or **G**uilty about your drinking?
4 Do you have a drink first thing in the morning to steady your nerves or get rid of a hangover (**E**ye opener)?

If problems with alcohol intake are found to be the case, then the patient should be advised to reduce his or her consumption of alcohol and the relevant information communicated in writing to the patient's GP. Contrary to popular belief, confronting a patient with the evidence of an alcohol problem may limit further damaging behaviour.

more will experience an episode of a depressive disorder at some time during their lives. The problem is underdiagnosed and undertreated and so:

- enquire about depressed mood in anyone who seems 'low'
- enquire about suicidal thoughts in anyone who may be depressed.

> Questioning about suicidal intent will not encourage a patient to attempt self-harm.

Severe depression is usually accompanied by disturbance of eating, sleeping and working. Relationships are strained and retardation of all normal activities may be profound. The risk of suicide is paradoxically at its greatest during the early stages of recovery from depression.

Tx If suicidal thoughts are present or if there are profound somatic symptoms, psychiatric advice should be sought. Otherwise depression should be treated by the GP with antidepressants at full therapeutic dose. Supervision of a depressed person by a close relative or friend is essential for both his or her safety and mental wellbeing.

Suicide

Suicide has been called the ultimate act of the individual and, indeed, to attempt to take one's own life is to have lost all faith in the help offered by society and its members. The highest rates are in men aged 35–44 years and men aged >85 years. Some professions carry an abnormally high risk of suicide: doctors, pharmacists, vets, nurses and farmers. In the UK, the incidence of suicide is increasing in men aged <24 years and in young Asian women. Antiepileptic treatment is associated with a small increased risk of suicidal thoughts and behaviour. Most people who commit suicide have informed somebody of their intention before death.

Self-harm

Self-harm accounts for around 1.5% of all ED attendances in the UK and is one of the top five causes of acute medical admission. Patients may harm themselves by either poisoning or physical injury, the latter usually taking the form of cuts to the forearms or neck. In extreme cases it is obvious that there was a genuine attempt to commit suicide but often the intent of the patient is unclear. However, in the 12 months after attending an ED, about one in six patients will harm themselves again and almost 1% will die by suicide. It is therefore very important to distinguish between the different psychological states that underlie the self-harming behaviour:

- Depression and attempted suicide
- Psychosis and attempted suicide
- Emotional upset and impulsive self-harm (parasuicide)
- Psychopathic behaviour
- Sexual or other experimentation and unintentional self-harm.

> Around 40% of patients who poison themselves express a wish to die.

Tx The poisoning or injury must be treated appropriately and sensitively. Psychosocial assessment should take place in parallel to the physical treatment rather than waiting for its completion. In many hospitals, all patients who have harmed themselves are examined by a psychiatrist. This may follow admission for medical treatment or direct referral from the ED. If this is not the case, then the risk of suicide or further self-harm must be assessed before discharge (→ *Box 19.3*). The key psychological characteristics

 Box 19.3 Assessment of suicide risk

Certain features of the social and medical history coupled with aspects of the presentation suggest serious intention to commit suicide:

High-risk individuals
- Elderly (all self-harm in people >65 should be taken as evidence of suicidal intent)
- Male
- Widowed
- Recently bereaved
- Living alone with little support
- Unemployed

There are special risk factors in women:

- Three or more children under the age of 5 years
- Lack of either a close, caring relationship or a job

High-risk backgrounds
- Chronic disabling physical illness
- Previous psychiatric illness or suicide attempt
- Chronic pain
- History of alcohol or other drug abuse
- Family history of mental illness, suicide or alcoholism

Serious circumstances
- Overdose or injury performed in isolated circumstances
- Active precautions taken to avoid detection
- Self-harm timed to reduce likelihood of detection
- Did not confide in a potential helper
- Left a suicide note
- Modified a will or insurance, etc.

Suicidal thoughts
- Wanted, and still wants, to die (asking about this will not increase the risk of a repeat attempt)
- Has had these thoughts and planned suicide for at least 24 h
- Thought that the method used would succeed in killing him or her
- Is sorry that he or she has recovered
- Has intense feelings of hopelessness and worthlessness

associated with risk are depression, hopelessness and continuing suicidal intent. All discharged patients must be accompanied home and should be followed up by their GP.

Patients who harm themselves have a 100-fold increased risk of suicide in the following year.

Deliberate self-harm in young people aged <16 years

Self-harm is common in teenagers with as many as 1 in 10 affected. It is seven times more common in girls than in boys. There may be self-poisoning or various types of physical injury. The most common trigger is an argument with a parent or close friend. As in adults, self-harm in adolescents may reflect a variety of different underlying mental states and patients give many different reasons for hurting themselves. Unfortunately from a diagnostic perspective, the younger the child the less likely it is that the severity of the act that they perform reflects the actual seriousness of the urge to harm themselves. In all such cases, consideration needs to be given to the child's mental state, care and protection, and parental management. Thus it is the policy of the British Paediatric Association and the Royal College of Psychiatrists that all young people aged <16 years who harm themselves should receive a specialist assessment by an appropriately trained person, usually a child psychiatrist. This generally entails temporary admission to a paediatric ward.

> In the UK in 2005, 1 in 10 children had a recognised mental disorder, ranging from depression to autism. This prevalence of psychological disease doubles in children whose parents are both unemployed.

SPECIAL SITUATIONS

Compulsory admission and treatment → p. 379 and Box 20.5 on p. 380.

People with learning disabilities

Approximately 3% of the population has a learning disability (defined as an IQ <70). People with all levels of learning disability live in the community, in their family homes and in supported accommodation. Many lead independent lives in their own homes.

They develop similar physical and mental health problems to non-disabled people, although they have a higher prevalence of epilepsy, head injury, and difficulties with hearing and speech. Their presentations may be atypical because of difficulties in communication. This, coupled with apparent tolerance of quite severe symptoms, can make diagnosis challenging. Common presenting problems to the ED include physical injuries, medical illness, self-harm and alcohol misuse. Mental illness may manifest itself as a change in the person's usual pattern of behaviour. These patients should be treated as adults with a normal capacity for making decisions about their health, although simple language may need to be used. Family and carers may sometimes need to be involved but only with the patient's consent.

Personality disorders

People with a wide range of unusual or, in the statistical sense, abnormal personality types are seen in an ED. They may demonstrate features of histrionic, inadequate, sociopathic, psychopathic and other personalities.

> Brief assessment of a patient presenting with unreasonable behaviour tempts the busy doctor to attribute symptoms to long-term personality disorders and to make judgemental decisions. However, even patients who are known psychopaths can develop new treatable conditions.

Tx As with any patient, a careful assessment should be made at each attendance. The advice of a psychiatrist, even by telephone, can be very useful because many of these patients and their patterns of behaviour are well known to the mental health services. If it is concluded that the patient's presentation to the ED is exclusively caused by a personality disorder, then there is no therapy to be offered, although attempts should be made to ensure that community support is available and that appropriate agencies know of the patient's hospital attendance. Good records are essential to help at future presentations and to adjudicate in any dispute.

Neuroses

Patients with specific neuroses may present to an ED. They usually have some insight into their problems and so referral can be made to an appropriate agency, be it a psychiatrist, GP or psychologist.

Depressive states → p. 363.

Requests for drugs

Patients sometimes present to an ED with requests for psychotropic drugs. Generally speaking, it is inappropriate for such prescriptions to be dispensed by doctors who do not have ongoing care of a patient. However, there are no absolutes in medicine and every request should be listened to and dealt with according to the clinical situation.

> Never feel pressurised into prescribing.

It is helpful to remember that most patients who stop taking heroin do not experience major withdrawal symptoms. 'Cold turkey' is very unusual. According to many ex-users, the discomfort experienced during opiate withdrawal is no worse than a bad dose of flu and is certainly not akin to the life-threatening states caused by cessation of alcohol intake. However, staying away from recreational drugs in the long term is much more difficult than just stopping for a limited period.

Alcohol withdrawal states → p. 360.
Withdrawal from opiates → later.

Withdrawal from opioid drugs (narcotic analgesics)

> Why do people take heroin? Most users experience a pleasant, relaxing effect with a sensation of deep inner warmth and complete detachment from all of life's problems.

Patients with a physical dependence to opioids commonly present to an ED with psychiatric problems, drug overdose, alcohol intoxication, deep vein thrombosis (DVT) or infections secondary to drug injection. They may require admission to an observation area or ward. Symptoms and signs of withdrawal usually occur 6–12 h after the last dose of heroin or 18–48 h after a dose of methadone, as follows:

- Anxiety, restlessness, irritability, insomnia, cravings, dysphoria
- Lacrimation, rhinorrhoea, sneezing, yawning
- Muscle cramps, sweating, piloerection ('gooseflesh')

- Nausea, diarrhoea, vomiting
- Tachycardia, raised BP, dilated pupils.

The state of opioid withdrawal is unpleasant but not dangerous. However, failure to manage it effectively may limit the patient's compliance with other treatment or lead to self-discharge. Symptoms gradually decrease spontaneously over 5–10 days.

Tx The initial level of treatment depends on the clinical features but it is important to reassure the patient that any worsening of symptoms will trigger a review of the therapy. Oral methadone mixture (1 mg/mL) is usually prescribed. Buprenorphine is sometimes given as an alternative and, in an emergency, dihydrocodeine is reasonably effective. Benzodiazepines will also alleviate most of the symptoms of opiate withdrawal. The dose of methadone is 30 mg immediately followed by 10 mg every 4 h if signs of withdrawal recur (total daily dose up to 60–80 mg). Equivalent doses of methadone are:

> Oral methadone 2 mg = injectable methadone 2 mg = injectable diamorphine 1 mg (street heroin is not equivalent to medical diamorphine and so an empirical approach is necessary).

Lofexidine (an α-adrenergic agonist) is prescribed by specialists to control the symptoms of opiate withdrawal. The dose is 0.2–0.4 mg every 6 h. Naltrexone, a long-acting opioid antagonist, is used to prevent relapse in former addicts.

Patients who regularly abuse drugs should be referred to the community drug team. If already on a registered drug programme, their key worker should be contacted. It is important to consider the welfare of any children who may be in the care of people who abuse drugs.

Acute poisoning with opioids (narcotics) → p. 282.
Child protection issues → p. 384.

Withdrawal from other drugs

Patients with a physical addiction to sedatives and tranquillisers may display symptoms similar to alcohol withdrawal; these drugs should not be stopped abruptly. People who regularly use stimulant drugs such as amfetamines or cocaine will not usually suffer from a withdrawal state although they may become quite depressed.

Alcohol withdrawal states → p. 360.

Violent behaviour

Disturbed or violent behaviour may be provoked by environmental, organisational, situational or attitudinal factors. Some aspects of a person's past life are associated with an increased risk of violent behaviour:

- History of violent behaviour or of cruelty towards animals
- Relatives and carers reporting previous extreme anger or violence
- Previous expressions of intent to harm others
- Previous use of weapons
- Previous dangerous impulsive acts (including reckless driving)
- Denial of previous violent or dangerous actions
- Evidence of 'rootlessness' or social exclusion
- Evidence of recent stressful events
- History of misuse of drugs or alcohol
- Loss of a parent before the age of 8 years in association with any of the factors above
- History of bed-wetting in association with any of the factors above.

Certain behaviours indicate that a person's discontent may be escalating towards violence:

- Restlessness and pacing around the floor
- Increased volume of speech and erratic movements
- Refusal to communicate
- Prolonged eye contact
- Tense and angry facial expressions
- Delusions or hallucinations with a violent content
- Verbal threats or gestures.

Members of staff must realise that they are responsible for avoiding provocation in potentially violent situations. It is not reasonable to expect a person exhibiting angry behaviour to simply 'calm down'. ED staff must learn to monitor and control their own verbal and non-verbal behaviour such as body posture and eye contact. In addition, they must be able to defuse a difficult situation. De-escalation techniques include the following:

- Adopting a non-threatening but safe posture
- Allowing greater personal space than normal
- Relocating to a safer environment if at all possible
- Asking for weapons to be placed in a neutral location rather than just handed over
- Paying attention to non-verbal clues
- Attempting to establish a rapport and emphasising cooperation
- Offering and negotiating realistic options and avoiding threats
- Asking open questions and enquiring about the reasons for the person's anger
- Showing concern and attentiveness through both verbal and non-verbal responses

- Listening carefully and showing empathy
- Acknowledging any grievances, concerns or frustrations and not being patronising or minimising these concerns.

Protection of ED staff from violent people

It is the duty of all staff to ensure that they and their colleagues are not placed at unreasonable risk of injury during the course of their duties. For this reason, the police should be involved early on in any potentially violent situation. Many hospitals now have their own security personnel who can attend at short notice.

Most people who express aggression are completely responsible for their own actions. In the eyes of the law, intoxication with alcohol or drugs is no justification for unreasonable behaviour. The exceptions to this generalisation are functional psychoses and organic confusional states, which are not the direct result of the person's own actions. In schizophrenia, for example, auditory hallucinations and paranoid delusions may induce aggression as a defence mechanism. Thus, before an individual is removed from the ED, these conditions must be excluded. In a person who is not intoxicated this is usually fairly easy. However, it must be remembered that staff have a duty of care even to aggressive and 'unpleasant' patients.

Angry relatives

Dissatisfied or frankly aggressive relatives or friends of patients are not uncommon in an ED. There are several frequently met reasons for this:

- Inappropriate reaction to the stress of sudden illness or bereavement
- Guilt and redirection of blame
- Unrealistic expectations of a resource-limited system
- Misunderstanding of the situation (a failure of communication)
- Unexplained delays at any stage
- Understandable reaction to a failure of care.

The departmental staff must reply calmly, politely, clearly and firmly to all expressions of anger ($\rightarrow$ p. 366). If resolution cannot easily be achieved then the case must be referred to a senior member of staff. There is a clear procedure to be followed for all formal complaints, which will usually be directed through a central office of the hospital ($\rightarrow$ p. 387).

> Do not be frightened of saying that you are sorry. You can express regret that the patient is upset without implying that you are to blame.

Distressed relatives

Cot death → p. 356.
Sudden bereavement → p. 164.

In exceptional circumstances it may be appropriate to give distressed relatives a short course (3–5 days) of night sedation. If this is prescribed, the GP should be informed.

Munchausen's syndrome (factitious disorders)

Patients affected by this behavioural disorder display a recurrent need to adopt the sick role. Effectively, this means feigning illness to get attention, analgesia or admission to hospital. The underlying psychology of this behaviour is unclear but there is obviously a secondary gain to the patient. Presumably, Munchausen's syndrome is an acute form of the well-known disorder whereby an unrequited need for caring attention leads some healthy people to behave as chronic invalids. Vicarious forms of Munchausen's syndrome (Munchausen's syndrome by proxy) may be expressed as symptoms attributed to close relatives, especially children (→ *below*).

The diagnosis of Munchausen's syndrome should be made by exclusion (and in retrospect if necessary) by an experienced emergency physician. It must be distinguished from:

- psychopathic behaviour, including some self-harm
- hypochondriasis
- hysterical behaviour
- exaggeration of real symptoms
- genuine and unexaggerated illness.

Features associated with Munchausen's syndrome include the following:

- Apparently complex social background, no relatives
- Stranger to the district, 'passing through'
- Numerous previous hospital admissions elsewhere, usually undisclosed
- Classic textbook symptoms and signs, usually of painful conditions (e.g. renal colic)
- Scars from previous surgery

- Negative tests contrasting with positive history (beware of extraneous blood in urine specimens)
- Specific requests for opiate analgesia.

Tx If the diagnosis is strongly suspected, the case should be discussed with senior medical and nursing staff. Additional evidence may be obtainable. All departments should have a Munchausen's syndrome file in which letters about such patients from other hospitals are kept. The validity of distant addresses can be checked by the police.

The patient should be confronted; the response may clinch the diagnosis. The hospital management and/or department of public health should be sent details of the attendance together with a description of the patient and the presenting features; they will contact other hospitals. Wasting hospital time is illegal under UK law and the patient can be charged in court.

> It is better to give morphine misguidedly to a few patients with Munchausen's syndrome than to withhold it inappropriately from one patient with genuine pain. The doctor is not a detective; if there is a suspicion of genuine distress then analgesia should be given.

Munchausen's syndrome by proxy

This syndrome – which is more correctly called 'factitious illness by proxy' – occurs when a carer feigns illness in a child. The gain to the adults involved is presumably similar to that which would be obtained if they were the patients themselves. The factitious illness may be directly produced (induced illness), imitated with false signs or fabricated with misleading stories of colourful symptoms. This is an unusual form of child abuse and should be treated as such (→ *p. 353*).

Post-traumatic stress disorder

There are three main groups of people who may need psychosocial care after traumatic events:

1. Survivors/injured victims.
2. People who have participated in events as rescuers, emergency staff, etc.
3. The families of those who have died or been injured.

Adults, children and people from various ethnic groups may all have differing needs. Most people involved will have a normal emotional reaction with features of grief and distress; some may appear dazed and confused by events. The use of standardised individual or group 'debriefing' should be avoided because it is of no proven benefit and may do harm.

Some people will have features of acute stress soon after the traumatic event. Typical early symptoms include fear, anxiety, anger, guilt, sadness, feelings of helplessness, and distressing thoughts and dreams. Physical symptoms such as fatigue, muscle aches, tension headaches and dry mouth may also occur. Features may be accentuated by the presence of coexisting conditions such as depression or substance abuse, and anxiety, panic or phobic disorders. A few individuals may appear unaffected at first, only to experience problems hours or days later. For most people, symptoms subside without intervention. 'Psychological first aid' consists of the following:

- Information about possible symptoms that may be experienced
- Education for the individual and the family about the reasons for his or her altered attitude, mood and behaviour (including advice to avoid telling the sufferer to 'snap out of it')
- Advice to avoid using alcohol, tobacco or drugs to cope with anxiety
- Practical and social support as required.

The use of antidepressant drugs for adults in this early phase may be helpful if signs of depression are present.

All individuals with ongoing or worsening symptoms should be assessed if:

- symptoms have lasted longer than 1 month
- symptoms are complicated by other mental health problems

- the person has suicidal thoughts
- the person is unable to cope with normal activities
- there is marked hyperarousal.

Post-traumatic stress disorder (PTSD) is usually diagnosed only after a month of persistent symptoms. It is treated with cognitive–behavioural therapy by trained staff and this is associated with good long-term outcomes → *later*. Prolonged use of anxiolytic drugs should be avoided, although they may be helpful for adults in the first 2 weeks after a traumatic event to alleviate panic attacks or sleep disturbance. Antidepressant therapy may be required for many months in some patients.

Victim support → pp. 372 and 373.

Counselling

The constant recollection of distressing thoughts reinforces a negative perception of problems and further lowers mood. Counselling aims to break this cycle.

- Cognitive–behavioural counselling helps a patient to focus on positive rather than negative thoughts.
- Psychodynamic counselling takes a historical view of human mental processes and analyses the effect of past events on present thinking.
- Supportive counselling encourages the patient to focus on current daily problems rather than dwelling on traumatic events.

Bereavement counselling → p. 163.

20

Medicolegal aspects of emergency medicine

The information given in this chapter applies to the UK. In other parts of the world, the social and legal framework may lead to differences in some aspects of the practice and principles of medicine.

CLINICAL FORENSIC MEDICINE

Description of injuries

Many descriptions of injury are intended for lay people, the police or the legal profession. Medical terminology is unlikely to be familiar to them. It is therefore inappropriate to use the language of medicine in documents that are not medical records. A pair of erythematous haematomas on the pretibial area thus becomes two red lumps on the shin. Nevertheless, this simplification of terminology must not compromise accuracy. In both medical records and non-medical documents the description of a wound must include the following:

1 Site – described in everyday language
2 Side – left or right
3 Shape – circular, V shaped, etc.
4 Size – measured with a ruler
5 Structures that are also involved – such as nerves, tendon and bone, including radiological findings
6 Sutures – number inserted in the skin.

Drawings or photographs can be very helpful. Some idea of the age of a wound is also desirable, although with older injuries this can take a considerable amount of experience. Opinions as to causation should be expressed only if requested and then only if the doctor's experience makes this reasonable.

Types of wounds

According to the Offences Against the Person Act 1861, to wound is to destroy or damage, however superficially, a bodily surface, be it skin or mucous membrane. For the purposes of medicolegal description, there are five main types of wound:

1 *Bruises*: these are also known as contusions or ecchymoses. Blunt force applied to the body surface causes rupturing of small blood vessels and allows blood to escape into the surrounding tissues. This is dependent on the pressure in the vessels, so postmortem wounds are not associated with significant bruising. Petechial and subconjunctival haemorrhages are particular types of bruising that may be caused by direct trauma or by indirect force (e.g. strangulation). Bruises change in both colour and size with time. They are initially red–blue or purple–black and gradually become green–yellow over a few days. Older bruises have a blurred, fading edge. Tracking of blood along a tissue plane may result in bruising at a site well removed from the original injury.
2 *Abrasions*: an abrasion or graze involves only the outer layers of the skin. Unlike a bruise, it always indicates the exact point of impact. Direction may also be apparent, as may dirt from the source of trauma.
3 *Lacerations*: whenever blunt force splits the whole thickness of the skin, the wound is called a laceration. Such wounds may be inflicted with sticks or bottles or sustained in falls. The characteristic features are ragged, abraded, contused edges and irregular division of the tissue planes.

Emergency Medicine Lecture Notes, Fourth Edition. Chris Moulton and David Yates.
© 2012 Blackwell Publishing Ltd. Published 2012 by Blackwell Publishing Ltd.

4 *Incised wounds*: sharp cutting objects make even wounds with straight, unbruised edges. An incised wound is longer than its depth.

5 *Stab wounds*: a stab wound is different from an incision because its depth is greater than its length. The shape and edges of the wound depend on the object used. A puncture wound is a very small stab wound. The external dimensions of a stab wound are a very poor guide as to the size of the weapon (e.g. knife blade). This is because:

- the weapon may be tapered and not introduced to the full extent of its width
- the weapon may not have been used perpendicularly to the skin surface
- the skin contracts after the blade is withdrawn.

Areas of transient redness should also be noted. Erythema may be caused by pressure or a blow. There may be accompanying swelling or tenderness. Such injuries might include the red finger marks on a slapped face or the tender, red scalp that results from hair pulling. Fading occurs within a matter of hours.

Specific mechanisms of injury may give rise to a defined type of wound, such as a burn. Burns are distinct patterns of damage that result from thermal or chemical injury (*for types of burns → Chapter 10 for and child abuse → p. 353*). Gunshot injuries are usually self-evident, although the type of gun used can be more difficult to determine. Bite wounds also have characteristic patterns. Most wounds, however, can result from a variety of different mechanisms and so their causation is a matter of judgement.

> All clothing from a wounded patient should be preserved in a sealed, labelled bag for the attention of the investigating police officers.

Gunshot wounds

Airguns: these compressed air-driven weapons propel a small, blunt pellet that does not tend to penetrate very far, although it may severely damage the eyeball or even cause a pneumothorax.

Shotguns: there are several different sizes of shotgun; all fire a large number of lead pellets. The wound that they create depends on the distance from the gun, as a result of the fanning out of the shot. At up to 1 m the entry wound will appear as a single hole <3 cm in diameter. At such close range widespread tissue damage and skin burns will occur. Exit wounds are uncommon. At 2 m the shot is already beginning to disperse whereas at 6 m the shot will be spread over a diameter of about 15 cm. At 12 m the pellets are scattered over an area with a diameter of around 30 cm. These are only rough guides and should not be ventured as a definitive ballistics opinion in court.

Other firearms: differing types of firearm cause damage proportional to the amount of energy that their bullets transfer to the tissues. Handguns usually fire a large bullet at a relatively low velocity and so result in localised damage to the structures directly in the path of the missile. Military rifles have a high muzzle velocity and cause extensive damage. The high-energy transfer from the bullet to the surrounding tissues causes a large cavity to be formed along the track, which finishes in a large exit wound. Also the missile itself may roll and shatter in the tissues.

Taser injuries → p. 379.

Asphyxia

Attempted suffocation and strangulation may both cause a picture similar to traumatic asphyxia syndrome (*→ p. 78*). Signs of compression of the face or the neck may be present, as may the marks of a violent struggle. Hanging causes death through a mixture of asphyxia, cerebral ischaemia and spinal disruption. The asphyxia resulting from a bag over the head, seen in children and sexual asphyxia, usually causes death by hypoxia and subsequent bradycardia.

Drowning → p. 30.

Violent crime

Contrary to popular belief, most of the victims of violent crime who present to an ED are young men and not elderly women (*→ Box 20.1*). They are assaulted in a bar or a club or in the street and are often intoxicated, whereas 75% of the attacks on women occur in the home of either the victim or the assailant.

> **Box 20.1 Risk factors for violent crime**
>
> - Male sex
> - Age 16–29 years
> - Low income
> - Single
> - Member of ethnic minority group
> - Alcohol intoxication
>
> Only about half of all violent crimes are reported to the police, with men much less likely to report than women; 50% of victims suffer 80% of all recorded crimes and an unfortunate 4% suffer over half of these.

Injuries to the face, head and hands are the most common unless weapons are used in the assault. There may be long-term psychological and psychosomatic effects including:

- depression
- loss of confidence, fear and anxiety
- irritability, decreased concentration and mood changes
- lethargy, sleep and appetite disturbances
- headaches, nausea and muscle tension
- behavioural changes (e.g. withdrawal or increased alcohol consumption).

In some cases, the problems may be so severe and prolonged as to merit a diagnosis of post-traumatic stress disorder (PTSD) (→ *p. 369*). This diagnosis would not normally be made unless symptoms persisted for at least 1 month and caused impairment of normal life functions.

Domestic violence

More than 25% of all violent crime reported to the police is domestic violence of men against women, making it the second most common violent crime in the UK. It is thought to account for around 1% of all ED attendances. Up to one in four women will be physically assaulted by a partner during her lifetime and around one in ten will suffer an attack each year. It is estimated that a woman in an abusive relationship will suffer over 30 physical assaults before disclosing the abuse – usually when asked directly. Patterns of presentation with sufficient sensitivity to identify victims of domestic violence are few but facial bruising should always alert suspicion. Deliberate self-harm and pregnancy are associated with all types of abuse:

- Severe, repeated violence occurs in at least 5% of all long-term relationships in Britain. It affects women of all cultures, religions, ages and social groups.
- Over 45% of all murdered women are killed by their male partners; this amounts to one or two women per week in the UK. Women who leave their abusers are at a 75% greater risk of being killed than those who stay.
- Nearly half of all assaults against women are committed by a partner or former partner, compared with 4% of assaults against men.

Abuse may be:

- psychological – shouting, swearing, humiliation or enforced isolation from family and friends
- economic – withholding of money and transport

- sexual
- physical.

Physical injury is the most likely form of domestic violence to present to an ED. The following are possible signs of it:

- Delayed presentation of injuries
- Injuries that are inconsistent with the mechanism described in the history
- Multiple injuries, especially when symmetrically distributed or of differing ages
- Injuries such as bites, burns, scalds or bruises
- Injuries on areas of the body that are normally clothed
- Injuries to the face, neck, breasts, genitals or pregnant abdomen
- Perforated eardrums or detached retinas
- Evidence of rape or other sexual assault
- Pelvic pain
- Multiple somatic complaints
- Psychiatric illness
- Drug abuse.

> Domestic violence may occur in same-sex relationships and may be perpetrated by women against men.

Tx Injuries should be treated appropriately and social services contacted for advice and shelter if necessary. Specialist helplines to various organisations are now available. A friend or relative of the victim should be enlisted for support and enquiries made about the current safety of any children in the family. (The risks of violence to children growing up in an abusive household are substantial. Such children are much more likely than most to be listed on the Child Protection Register. Concerns about the welfare of children should lead to immediate contact with local child protection services.) The police can be involved only with the consent of the injured party.

> Reluctance by victims of domestic violence to involve outside help is common. This may frustrate staff who believe that immediate action is required. However, research has shown that information provided in EDs may be used at a later date when the patient finally feels that the time is right.

Rape and sexual assault

Around 17% of women and 3% of men in the UK state that they have been subjected to non-consensual sexual experiences as adults. About two-thirds of assaults of this type are committed by someone known to the victim. The experience of sexual violence can be life threatening and degrading. Not surprisingly, psychological upset and a specific form of PTSD (rape trauma syndrome) are common sequelae. Not all patients who have been sexually assaulted have visible genital (or oral) injuries, although around 50% have other physical injuries. Examination should be left to the police surgeon because forensic evidence will need to be collected in a way that does not contaminate it or render it invalid as evidence. Locard's principle states that 'every contact leaves a trace'. This includes ED staff!

Tx There should be early involvement of social services; there may be a dedicated rape crisis centre. Specialist police officers are allocated to this type of investigation.

> The police surgeon will also consider the need for emergency contraception (→ p. 321) and the exclusion or treatment of sexually transmitted infections.

Drug-assisted sexual assault

Alcohol (self-administered or in laced drinks) is by far the most common drug to be associated with sexual assault. However, gamma-hydroxybutyrate (GHB), ketamine, flunitrazepam and zopiclone have all been reported as being used to facilitate sexual assault. Patients drugged and assaulted in this way present a very difficult problem because they will have an impaired memory of events and may just feel that 'something wrong happened'.

Child abuse

Child protection procedures → p. 384.
Types of and signs of child abuse → p. 353.

Abuse of elderly people

Physical abuse of elderly people is surprisingly common; neglect and emotional abuse are even more common. The recent increase in the number of small, privately run nursing homes has done nothing to decrease the problem. Signs may be minimal or similar to those of other forms of domestic violence (→ p. 372). As soon as the diagnosis is suspected, advice should be sought from social workers and senior geriatricians.

Victim support and counselling

Details of local victim support schemes and the witness support service in the Crown Court can be found in the telephone directory, although the police will usually negotiate contact if asked. Victim Support (a registered UK charity) can help with:

- practical matters such as insurance and compensation
- personal and emotional support
- liaison with the police and other agencies
- explanation of the criminal justice system
- witness support.

People suffering from PTSD or depression should be referred to psychiatric services. Counselling is often advised (→ p. 369).

ALCOHOL AND OTHER DRUGS/ FITNESS TO DRIVE

Misuse of drugs

The Misuse of Drugs Act 1971 prohibits certain activities in relation to 'Controlled Drugs', in particular their manufacture, supply and possession. The penalties applicable to offences that contravene the Act are graded according to the harmfulness attributable to a drug when it is misused. For this purpose, the controlled drugs are divided into three classes called A, B and C (→ Box 20.2). The Misuse of Drugs Regulations 2001 define the classes of people who are authorised to supply and possess controlled drugs while acting in a professional capacity and lay down the conditions under which their activities may be carried out. In these regulations, drugs are divided into five schedules, each with its own specific legal requirements (→ Box 20.2).

The Misuse of Drugs (Supply to Addicts) Regulations 1997 instruct that only those medical practitioners who hold a special licence from the Home Office may prescribe, administer or supply diamorphine, dipipanone or cocaine in the treatment of drug addiction. This does not apply to the prescription of these drugs to known addicts for the relief of pain from organic disease or injury. Nor does it apply to methadone or dihydrocodeine.

Box 20.2 **The Misuse of Drugs Act 1971 and the Misuse of Drugs Regulations 2001**

The main offences under the Misuse of Drugs Act 1971 are as follows:

- Section 4 (2) Production of a controlled drug (i.e. Schedule 1, 2 and 3 drugs)
- Section 4 (3) Supplying or offering to supply a controlled drug
- Section 5 (2) Having possession of a controlled drug without a prescription or other authority
- Section 5 (3) Having possession of a controlled drug with intent to supply it to another person
- Section 6 (2) Cultivation of a cannabis plant
- Section 8 Being the occupier or manager of premises and knowingly permitting or suffering:
  - the production or attempted production of controlled drugs
  - the supply, attempt to supply or offer to supply a controlled drug to another person
  - the preparation of opium for smoking
  - the smoking of cannabis, cannabis resin or prepared opium

The penalties applicable to these offences are graded according to the harmfulness of a drug when it is misused. For this purpose, the controlled drugs are divided into three classes:

- Class A includes: cocaine, LSD (lysergic acid diethylamide), diamorphine, morphine, pethidine, methadone, opium, MDMA (3,4-methylenedioxymethamfetamine or ecstasy), methamfetamine, phencyclidine and class B substances when prepared for injection
- Class B includes: codeine, standard amfetamines and barbiturates
- Class C includes: buprenorphine, cannabis, cannabis resin, most benzodiazepines, zolpidem, anabolic steroids and some hormones

The Misuse of Drugs Regulations 2001 define the classes of person who are authorised to supply and possess controlled drugs in a professional capacity and lay down the conditions under which professional activities may be carried out. In these regulations, drugs are divided into five schedules, each with its own specific legal requirements:

- Schedule 1 includes: cannabis, LSD and other drugs that are not used medicinally
- Schedule 2 includes: diamorphine, morphine, pethidine, cocaine, amfetamine and secobarbital
- Schedule 3 includes: buprenorphine, most barbiturates and temazepam
- Schedule 4 includes: benzodiazepines (except temazepam), zolpidem, anabolic steroids and some hormones
- Schedule 5 includes: those preparations that (because of their strength) are exempt from virtually all controlled drug requirements

Requests for drugs in the ED and drug withdrawal → *p. 366.*

In England, health professionals are expected to report cases of drug misuse to their regional drug misuse centre as part of the National Drugs Treatment Monitoring System (NDTMS). Wales and Scotland have a similar national reporting system. All three countries require notification of misuse of all types of drugs including opiates, benzodiazepines and central nervous system (CNS) stimulants. In Northern Ireland, the Misuse of Drugs (Notification of and Supply to Addicts) (Northern Ireland) Regulations 1973 require doctors to send particulars of people whom they consider to be addicted to controlled drugs to the Department of Health and Social Services.

Misuse of Drugs Act 1971 and the Misuse of Drugs Regulations 2001 → Box 20.2 above.

Alcohol and trauma

Ethyl alcohol is probably the most dangerous substance in the world. It is freely available in many societies and, unlike other psychotropic drugs, it is dispensed by a barman rather than by a pharmacist. It is so frequently involved in the causation of accidents that no discussion of the work of an ED would be complete without it. In the UK, a tenth of all road accidents that result in injury are a result of the effects of excess alcohol in the blood and almost all other injuries have a significant association with alcohol usage (→ *Figure 20.1*).

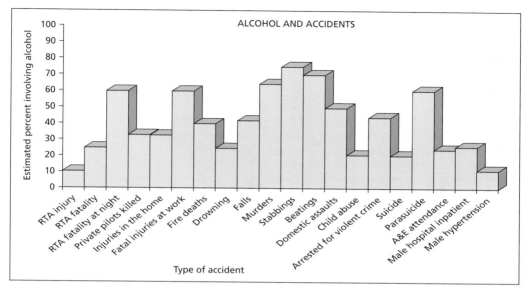

Figure 20.1 The involvement of alcohol in trauma. RTA, road traffic accident.

Detection and treatment of alcohol abuse → pp. 362–363.
Treatment of alcohol poisoning → p. 285.

Nearly a quarter of all ED attendances are alcohol related. Over a quarter of all male hospital inpatients have a current or previous alcohol problem.

 Box 20.3 Legal limits of alcohol for drivers in the UK

Blood 80 mg/dL of blood (= 800 mg/L)
Breath 35 mcg/dL of expired air
Urine 107 mg/dL of urine

Measurement of alcohol in the human body

Units of alcohol

A unit of alcohol has become the standard measure by which public health information on alcohol consumption is expressed. It is defined as 10 mL by volume (58 g by weight) of pure alcohol – roughly the alcohol content of a standard measure of 25 mL of many spirits. Half a pint of beer (3% strength) or a glass of wine (125 mL of 8% alcohol) is also roughly equivalent to 1 unit. Within the first hour, a unit of alcohol increases the blood level by approximately 15 mg/dL in an average man.

Elimination of alcohol

In a healthy person, about 90% of ingested alcohol is cleared from the blood by the liver. This occurs at a steady rate of about 15 mg/dL per h.

Laboratory units of alcohol

Several units of blood alcohol measurement are in use worldwide including milligrams/litre and millimoles/litre. The unit used in UK legal practice, although not necessarily in hospital laboratories, is milligrams/decilitre (i.e. mg/dL or mg% – 1 dL is 100 mL) (*legal limits for drivers → Box 20.3*).

Conventionally, breath alcohol levels are converted to equivalent blood alcohol levels by multiplying by a factor of 2300. The comparison is not strictly accurate because alcohol concentration in the breath rises faster and falls earlier than it does in venous blood.

Requests for specimens for analysis from patients in hospital

The Police Reform Act 2002 provided new powers concerning the taking of blood specimens from patients involved in road traffic accidents to test for levels of alcohol or drugs. As before, while a person is in hospital (as a patient!), he or she is not required to provide a specimen for breath or laboratory testing unless the medical practitioner in immediate charge of the case has consented. (It must be remembered, however, that there are very few medical circumstances that preclude sampling.) If there is no clinical objection, then a person from whom a police constable requires a blood sample and who (without reasonable excuse) refuses to consent commits an offence. Under the previous legislation, it was a statutory requirement to obtain consent for blood sampling from the person concerned. Therefore, when a patient lacked capacity to consent (usually because of a depressed level of consciousness), a specimen could not be obtained. This led to people escaping prosecution for very serious offences, such as causing death by careless driving while under the influence of alcohol.

The provisions of the Police Reform Act aimed to eliminate this inequity between those with capacity to consent and those without it. A police constable may now request that a blood sample be taken from a patient who, for medical reasons, is incapable of giving consent. This request would normally be made to a police surgeon but, in exceptional situations, may be made to another medical practitioner who is not directly involved in the clinical care of the patient. If the doctor considers it appropriate to take the specimen, then the police constable will provide a special kit to be used for this purpose. The location of all forensic specimens is required by law to be recorded at all times – 'the chain of custody'. As soon as possible, the police will inform the patient that a blood sample has been taken and obtain his (or her) consent for it to be analysed. In this case, failure to give permission for analysis may render the person liable to prosecution.

Driving and other drugs

Many drugs may impair the ability of a patient to drive or to operate machinery. Drowsiness and impaired psychomotor performance are the most common drug-related effects to interfere with driving, but postural hypotension, fatigue, hypoglycaemia and impaired vision may also occur. Drivers taking minor tranquillisers or tricyclic antidepressants are two to five times more likely to be involved in an accident than untreated control individuals. The early stages of treatment are associated with the highest risk and the effects of centrally acting drugs are often potentiated by alcohol.

As a result of these risks, patients must always be warned whenever their treatment could alter their ability to drive or perform other activities safely. A recommended list of advice is given in *Box 20.11 on p. 390*.

> Frequent users of cannabis are 10 times more likely to be injured or to cause injury to others in motor vehicle accidents than other road users.

Misuse of Drugs Act 1971 and the Misuse of Drugs Regulations 2001 → Box 20.2 on p. 374.

Driving and medical conditions

Medical conditions in drivers contribute to about 1% of the road accidents in the UK that result in injury or death (→ *Box 20.4*).

There are two sets of medical criteria for fitness to drive: one for an ordinary licence and another for a vocational licence (i.e. for a passenger-carrying vehicle [PCV] or for a large goods vehicle [LGV]). Licence holders have a statutory obligation to notify the licensing authority as soon as they become aware that they have any condition that might affect safe driving, unless the condition is not expected to last more than 3 months. Failure to notify is a legal offence.

> The General Medical Council advises that a doctor should notify the licensing authority when a patient is placing him- or herself or others in danger by continuing to drive. This does not constitute a breach of confidentiality.

The Road Traffic Act 1988, Section 92, lists prescribed disabilities that bar the sufferer from driving. They are:

A epilepsy
B severe learning disability

> **Box 20.4 Most common causes of collapse at the wheel**
>
> - Fits
> - Unspecified blackouts
> - Hypoglycaemia
> - Myocardial infarction
> - Strokes

C liability to sudden attacks of disabling giddiness or fainting (from any cause)

D disorder of the heart requiring a pacemaker

E inability to meet the eyesight requirements (the number-plate test).

In practice, a person with any of these conditions can drive once he or she has satisfied the licensing authority that he or she does not present any significant risk. The rules for vocational drivers are more stringent. Vocational licence holders are responsible for more than twice as many accidents that result in serious injury or death as ordinary car drivers, even when the statistics are corrected for mileage.

For the purposes of the ED, patients should be advised to (temporarily) refrain from driving whenever there is a possibility of a condition being diagnosed that could make driving or other complex tasks dangerous to themselves or others. Such problems may include:

- fits
- blackouts other than simple faints
- dizziness and vertigo
- head injury
- sudden cardiac dysrhythmias
- myocardial infarction
- CVAs (cerebrovascular accidents) and TIAs (transient ischaemic attacks)
- application of an eye pad in the ED (→ *p. 412*)
- decreased ability to use a limb (e.g. forearm in plaster)
- post-sedation or strong analgesia (→ *p. 15*).

Driving, or other prohibited activities, should only be recommenced when:

- the condition has resolved completely
- the diagnosis has been ruled out after specialist investigation
- the condition has been controlled and a symptom-free period has elapsed.

In the UK, the Medical Advisory Branch of the Driver and Vehicle Licensing Authority (DVLA) in Swansea supplies written and verbal advice for doctors on all aspects of fitness to drive.

Payment for emergency treatment of patients involved in road traffic accidents

The Road Traffic (NHS Charges) Act of 1999 allows hospitals to recover some of their costs for treating the victims of motor vehicle accidents from the insurers of the drivers involved. The value of this system to any particular hospital usually depends on the efficacy of local data collection systems.

LEGAL ISSUES

Consent

In the competent adult, treatment can be given only if the patient gives consent. Any physical contact or treatment without this consent may be construed as trespass or battery. These legal torts do not require harm to have resulted to the patient. Consent may be given verbally, in writing, by gestures or by actions. A signature on a consent form does not by itself prove that consent was valid. In addition, the following points should be noted:

- Valid consent or refusal is dependent on a patient's ability (capacity) to make decisions, namely to:
  1 understand and remember information
  2 believe this information
  3 evaluate this information.
- Capacity to give meaningful consent or make a valid refusal is a legal concept and not a medical one, and is governed by the following laws:
  England/Wales: Mental Capacity Act 2005
  Scotland: Adults with Incapacity Act 2000
  Northern Ireland: Common Law.

However, these laws presuppose that all registered medical practitioners are qualified to make an assessment of capacity. It also assumes that all adults have the capacity to consent or refuse unless proven otherwise.

> Conscious adults without serious mental dysfunction are always regarded by the law as capable of giving consent.

Children → p. 384.
Patients with mental illness → p. 357.

- Patients may be competent to make some health-care decisions, even if they are not competent to make others.
- Consent is valid only if the patient understood to what he or she was consenting (i.e. gave informed consent). However, a doctor must provide only that information about a procedure and its attendant risks that a reasonable group of doctors would disclose in the same circumstances. The concepts of the 'reasonable man' and 'the responsible body of medical opinion' pervade this type of law.

Compliance with the latter tenet forms the basis of the so-called Bolam test.

- The patient's right to self-determination takes precedence over the physician's duty to preserve life. A competent adult has the right to refuse any treatment or investigation even if it puts his or her life or health at risk. The patient has no obligation to justify this decision with valid and rational argument. The only exception to this rule is where treatment is for a mental disorder and the patient is detained under the Mental Health Act 1983 – and most such patients will lack the capacity to make decisions.
- A competent pregnant woman may refuse any treatment, even if this would be detrimental to the fetus.
- No one can give consent on behalf of an incompetent adult. However, such patients may still be treated provided that the proposed treatment is in their 'best interests' (England and Wales) or 'to the patient's benefit' (Scotland). 'Best interests' extend wider than best medical interests to include such factors as previous wishes and beliefs and general wellbeing. People close to the patient may be able to provide valuable information on some of these factors. Where a patient has never been competent, relatives, carers and friends may be best placed to advise on the patient's needs and preferences.
- An incompetent patient who has indicated in the past (while competent) that they would refuse treatment in certain circumstances ('an advance refusal') must not be treated should those circumstances arise.
- Consent obtained by deceit or with unreasonable pressure is invalid.
- Consent may be withdrawn at any time.

Treatment under common law

A patient who is incapable of giving consent (e.g. in cardiac arrest or coma) may be treated under common law. This means that, so long as staff perform only those procedures, which are reasonable to protect life and limb, then they are not liable to be sued for assault. Furthermore, to do less than this would be to neglect their duty of care. The law requires that all decisions must be made in accordance with the patient's best interests. Section 62 of the Mental Health Act 1983 codifies in statute this long-accepted practice.

Emergency treatment

The emergency treatment of physical and psychiatric problems in a fully conscious patient who cannot or will not give informed consent is an extremely difficult area. Treatment cannot be given without a patient's consent unless, by virtue of an abnormal mental state, he or she is incompetent to give or withhold consent. The difficulty is in deciding, in the acute situation, which patients are competent in the eyes of the law and which are not. In general, patients with frank psychotic symptoms can be detained and sedated under common law (→ *above*). Others are likely to be competent, even if depressed or agitated. The help of relatives and psychiatric specialists should be enlisted as soon as possible. Detailed records are essential.

Deprivation of liberty

In the past decade, people with learning difficulties, as well as some elderly and infirm people, have been the subject of rulings by the European Court of Human Rights that they have been unlawfully deprived of their liberty, contrary to Article 5[1] of the European Convention for the Protection of Human Rights and Fundamental Freedoms. This is a very difficult and grey area but factors that suggest deprivation of liberty may include the following:

- Restraint, including sedation, is used to admit a person to an institution where that person is resisting admission.
- Staff exercise complete and effective control over the care and movement of a person for a substantial period.
- Staff control assessments, treatment, contacts and residence.
- A decision has been taken by the institution that the person will not be released into the care of others, or permitted to live elsewhere, unless the staff in the institution consider it appropriate.
- A request by carers for a person to be discharged to their care is refused.
- The person is unable to maintain social contacts because of restrictions placed on his or her access to other people.
- The person loses autonomy because they are under continuous supervision and control.

The Mental Capacity Act (England and Wales) 2005 and the Adults with Incapacity Act (Scotland) 2000 provide strict rules about the capacity of adults to make their own decisions. There is also a judicial 'Court of Protection' that exists specifically to arbitrate about such matters.

Blood transfusion for Jehovah's witnesses

There are 140 000 Jehovah's Witnesses in the UK and Ireland; their faith does not allow them to accept the transfusion of blood or its primary components. Administration of blood in the face of a refusal by an informed and rational patient is obviously unlawful. Similarly, if written evidence in the form of a signed and witnessed advance directive exists, this should be acted upon. Such directive cards are commonly carried by Jehovah's Witnesses and usually state that the physician is released from liability if harm results from failure to transfuse. In the absence of verbal or written instructions from the patient, clinical judgement should take precedence over the opinion of relatives or friends.

Use of tranexamic acid and recombinant factor VIIa in severe bleeding → p. 26.

The children of Jehovah's Witnesses may be denied blood transfusion by their parents. If the wellbeing of a child is at risk, a court order (a specific issue order) may be applied for to provide legal sanction for an isolated treatment. However, in an emergency, blood should be given to a child as soon as it is needed to save life.

Compulsory detention for assessment or treatment

Part I of the Mental Health Act 1983 (England and Wales) and 1984 (Scotland) defines mental disorder as follows:

1 Mental illness
2 Mental impairment (learning disability)
3 Psychopathic disorder
4 Any other disorder or disability of mind.

In Part II, civil detention orders are specified (→ Box 20.5). The indication for these orders is that the patient is suffering from a mental disorder of a nature or degree that warrants detention of the patient in hospital in the interests of his or her own health or safety or with a view to the protection of others.

In the ED, the sequence of orders would usually be:

- Section 4 (Emergency Admission Order) or
- Section 136 (Police Admission Order) *(further information → later)* changed as soon as possible to:
- Section 2 (Assessment Order) converted later in hospital to:
- Section 3 (Treatment Order).

The patient in police custody

The fact that a patient is in police custody does not affect the duty of care that a doctor has towards him or her. Nor should reasonable constraints on his or her freedom prevent an adequate examination.

Handcuffs may cause a circumferential reddening of the wrists. Occasionally, abrasions and even anaesthesia in the distribution of the superficial radial nerve may be seen.

The decision of 'fitness to be detained' is one for a police surgeon to make, as is the similar examination for 'fitness to be interviewed'.

The police surgeon should also be involved as soon as possible in any case that looks as if it might have a complicated forensic element.

Taser injuries

'Tasers' are hand-held electrical devices that can be used to incapacitate dangerous offenders. They belong to a group of new non-lethal weapons designed as an alternative to firearms in critical situations. The taser fires two barbed probes into its target, which are attached to the 'gun' by a pair of thin wires. A high-voltage current is then immediately discharged down these wires, causing painful and overwhelming muscle contractions in the victim. The 'advanced tasers' used by most police forces rely on 'electromuscular disruption' technology, which uses higher energies than older 'stun guns'. A signal powered at 18–26W completely overrides the CNS to cause an uncontrollable spasm of skeletal muscle that even large and determined people cannot resist. Similar weapons have been used for over 20 years in the USA without significant harmful effects. However, they may be used against individuals suffering from drug intoxication, psychiatric illness or extreme agitation. Consequently, it is recommended that all recipients of a taser discharge should have a routine medical examination as soon as possible after the shock. Cardiovascular stability should be ascertained. The electrodes with their tiny barbs are easily removed by direct traction.

Patients detained under a Police Admission Order (Section 136 of the Mental Health Act 1983)

Police officers frequently bring disturbed people to an ED (if it is a designated place of safety) under Section 136 of the Mental Health Act 1983. This police admission order can be invoked by any police officer and has a maximum duration of 72h (→ Box 20.5). The stated purpose of the order is to allow police officers to remove a person who is apparently suffering from a mental disorder from a public place to a safe area where the person can be assessed by a registered medical practitioner and an approved social worker. The Code of Practice (which is not actually legally binding) says that the doctor examining the

Box 20.5 Orders (Sections) of the Mental Health Act (1983 England and Wales) with corresponding provisions for Scotland and Northern Ireland

Section 2
- Admission for assessment followed by treatment
- Duration up to 28 days
- Application by nearest relative or approved social worker
- Medical recommendation by two doctors (one Section 12 approved)

Section 3
- Admission for treatment
- Duration up to 6 months
- Application by nearest relative or approved social worker
- Medical recommendation by two doctors (one Section 12 approved)

Section 4
- Admission for assessment in cases of emergency
- Duration up to 72 h
- Application by nearest relative or approved social worker
- Medical recommendation by one doctor (preferably acquainted with patient) (must state that admission under Section 2 will involve undesirable delay)

Section 5 (2)
- Detention of patient already in hospital for any form of inpatient treatment
- Duration up to 72 h
- Invoked by doctor in charge of the case or one nominated deputy

Section 5 (4)
- Nurse's holding power applicable to any patient already receiving treatment for a mental disorder
- Duration up to 6 h while a doctor is found

- Invoked by nurses of a prescribed class (RMN and RMNH)

Section 136
- Police admission order that allows a police officer to remove a person apparently suffering from a mental disorder from a public place to a designated place of safety (usually a police station or a local hospital ED) for assessment by a doctor and a social worker
- Duration up to 72 h
- Invoked by any police officer

Section 135
- Under this order, and with a magistrate's warrant, a police officer, accompanied by a doctor and a social worker, may enter the residence of a person they believe to be suffering from a mental disorder to take him or her to a place of safety
- Duration up to 72 h
- A warrant must be obtained to use this order

Corresponding provisions of the relevant legislation in Scotland and Northern Ireland
The following information is given as guidance only:

Mental Health Act 1983 (England and Wales)	Mental Health Act 1984 (Scotland)	Mental Health Act (Northern Ireland) Order 1986
Section 2	Section 26	Article 4
Section 3	Section 18	Article 12
Section 4	Section 24	Article 6
Section 5(2)	Section 25	Articles 7 and 7A
Section 136	Section 118	Place of safety provisions

patient should, wherever possible, be approved under Section 12 of the Mental Health Act. Where the examination is conducted by a doctor who is not approved by Section 12, the reasons for this should be recorded. Social workers are understandably reluctant to see a patient whom the doctor does not recommend for detention. However, the Code of Practice states that the patient should not normally be discharged unless both professional assessments have been carried out. It then, rather confusingly, goes on to say: 'Where the doctor, having examined the individual, concludes that he or she is not mentally disordered within the meaning of the Act, then that individual can no longer be detained under the section and should be immediately discharged from detention.'

In our society, bizarre behaviour in a public place is not always a sign of mental illness. Many patients have 'calmed down' by the time they arrive at the ED. Such patients can be assessed and discharged by a responsible doctor after discussion with the accompanying police officers. Other patients will need to remain in the department while awaiting a detailed assessment by a psychiatrist (preferably Section 12 approved!). In extreme cases, the police officers must be asked to maintain their Section 136-empowered forcible detention until the psychiatrist has concluded his or her assessment and perhaps even arranged to detain the patient further under Section 2 of the Mental Health Act.

The violent and uncontrollable patient in police custody

Occasionally, a patient who is obviously dangerously disturbed and violent may be brought in by the police (usually without any Section 136 paperwork!). The most common causes are:

- drug intoxication (usually amfetamines or other stimulant drugs)
- hypoglycaemia
- post-ictal confusion
- head injury
- gross psychiatric disturbance.

There is a duty to protect the hospital staff, police and other patients in the ED. The patient is inevitably handcuffed and is best temporarily left so, while the above are excluded. Sedation is often necessary; the quickest and safest way of achieving this is with an intravenous benzodiazepine (e.g. lorazepam or midazolam). The usual rules regarding the administration of sedating drugs must be applied ($\rightarrow p. 15$). Once the patient is calmer, a more detailed assessment can be performed in relative safety.

Release of information to the police

> Police should be informed whenever a victim of an attack with a gun, knife or other dangerous weapon arrives at a hospital. This is to allow police officers to consider the risk of further harm to the patient, hospital staff or other members of the public. At this stage of initial contact, personal information should not normally be disclosed.

Most information requested by the police relates to injuries sustained by victims of assaults. It is provided on a standard form with the patient's written consent ('*Statements by professional witnesses*' $\rightarrow$ *p. 383*). However, police officers sometimes request information about patients who are suspects rather than

Table 20.1 Personal and sensitive information

Personal information	Sensitive information
Names or initials	Sexuality
Date of birth	Ethnicity
Gender	Physical or mental health conditions
Address or postcode	Religious or similar beliefs
Occupation	Political opinions or memberships
Identity number (e.g. NHS or National Insurance number)	Offences committed or court proceedings

Under the Data Protection Act 1998 and the NHS Caldicott guidance, there is a duty to keep personal and sensitive information on patients (and staff) confidential and secure.

victims (e.g. 'Did a young man attend with a hand injury last night?'). The vast majority of circumstances require the disclosure of personal rather than sensitive or clinical information ($\rightarrow$ *Table 20.1*). Clinical information should almost never be divulged without the informed written consent of the patient. The laws that control the release of information to the police in England and Wales and the situations in which they apply are described below.

Legal duty to disclose, even without consent

Terrorism: under the provisions of the Prevention of Terrorism Act 1989 and the Terrorism Act 2000, there is a statutory duty to immediately inform the police if any information is gained either personally or professionally about suspected terrorist activity.

Motor vehicle offences: Section 172 of the Road Traffic Act 1988 makes it a statutory duty to provide the police, on request, with the names and addresses of drivers who are allegedly guilty of offences under this act. Clinical information should not be given.

Court orders: where the courts have made an order, the required information must be disclosed unless the decision is challenged at a higher court.

Legal power to disclose, but must consider implications of gaining consent

Serious crimes: since the introduction of the Police and Criminal Evidence (PACE) Act 1984, the judicial system has accepted that Section 116 and Schedule 5

> **Box 20.6 Serious arrestable offences (PACE, Section 116)**
>
> An arrestable offence is 'serious' if its commission (or threatened commission) has led to or is intended or likely to lead to the consequences listed below:
>
> - Serious harm to the security of the state or to public order
> - Serious interference with the administration of justice or with the investigation of an offence
> - The death of any person (including by dangerous driving)
> - Serious injury to any person, which includes any disease or any impairment of a person's physical or mental state
> - Substantial financial gain to any person
> - Serious financial loss to any person. Loss is defined as 'serious' for the purposes of this section if, having regard to all the circumstances, it is serious for the person who suffers it

(parts I and II) of the Act, which describe offences that are always considered serious, can be used as suitable guidelines for the release of non-clinical information – without the need to obtain the consent of the patient. These crimes are known as serious arrestable offences and are defined by PACE, Section 116 (→ *Box 20.6*). If offences of this type have been committed, then the appropriate non-clinical information can be released by a consultant or his or her deputy at the request of a police officer of the rank of inspector or above. The request is usually made in writing on an agreed form of enquiry.

Aggregated data: the Crime and Disorder Act 1998 recognises that information may sometimes be required in the form of aggregated data (e.g. statistics) for the detection, prevention or reduction of crime. Such information may be required on an individual for the purposes of strategic cross-organisational planning to reduce crime or disorder in which that person is involved.

Child protection: under Section 47 of the Children Act 1989, a local authority must make all necessary enquiries (either directly or through the police) to safeguard or promote a child's welfare. In such a situation, information should be released without the consent of either parent or child (and without an obligation to inform them) unless 'to do so would be unreasonable in the circumstances of the case'. If you suspect that a child is being abused, then you have a legal power to disclose information to social services (under 'vital interest' conditions of the Data Protection Act) or to the police (under PACE Act).

Information where gaining consent may be prejudicial to an investigation: the police may also seek personal information under an exemption of the Data Protection Act 1998. A Section 29(3) Crime Exemption allows information to be provided by an organisation about an individual without consent. This is used when the police believe that the seeking of consent would prejudice their enquiries regarding either the prevention or detection of crime or the apprehension or prosecution of offenders. The police should produce a Section 29(3) form requesting the required information, signed by the police inspector who has decided to serve the exemption. This is now the most common legal power used by police to obtain information from an ED about suspects.

Information to protect vital interests: a similar clause of the Data Protection Act 1998, Schedule 2(4) and/or Schedule 3(3) (Vital Interests Disclosure) allows police officers to seek personal information without consent in order to 'protect the vital interests of the data subject or another person'. To release data under this Schedule, an appropriate form signed by a police officer of the rank of inspector or above must again be produced.

Injuries from firearms: gun-related crimes have a devastating impact on the communities where they occur. Current guidance from the UK General Medical Council (developed in conjunction with the Association of Chief Police Officers) requires that the staff of British EDs contact the police when a person attends with a gunshot wound. The patient's identity need not be disclosed, although his or her consent should be sought for both name and other information to be provided. Without this consent, information should be given to the police only where it is judged that disclosure is necessary to prevent serious harm occurring or to prevent, detect or prosecute a serious crime. This can be seen as a public health measure to protect staff, the police and the public, and to limit the likelihood of further injuries.

The Freedom of Information Act

The Freedom of Information Act 2000 gives everyone in the UK greater rights of access to the information held by public authorities such as NHS trusts. Requests can be made by anyone (e.g. members of the public, the media and pressure groups) to access information such as reports, policies, guidelines, correspondence, emails and minutes of meetings. The

Act applies to all public bodies and specifies that the request must be met within 20 working days. There are 23 exemptions from the Act, which may restrict the release of some types of information. Personal and sensitive information (→ *Table 20.1*) is still covered by the provisions of the Data Protection Act 1998.

Statements by professional witnesses

All doctors who work in British EDs will receive regular requests from the police for written statements about patients whom they have seen. These police statements should be carefully and legibly written using the case notes and should follow the format as shown in *Box 20.7* and use the correct description of injuries (→ *p. 370*).

The witness statement form must be signed and dated in the space provided at the top of the form and after the last handwritten word on the statement.

Going to court

Most doctors and nurse practitioners who work in an ED will have to go to court at some time to give evidence as a professional witness. This is different from appearing as an expert witness. The professional witness must give an accurate account of his or her findings and actions but is not expected to be the ultimate authority on the subject. He or she should be:

- punctual, smartly dressed and courteous
- well informed and willing to answer all questions without evasion
- in possession of copies of the relevant notes (however, these notes can be consulted in court only with the permission of the bench)
- honest about the limitations of his or her own knowledge of the subject
- able to describe the work of his or her profession in a way that everyone can understand.

> Attendance at court is not the same as going to an MRCP examination. The aim is to inform rather than to impress.

Rather more is expected of the expert witness. Both the defence and the prosecution may call their own expert but sometimes the judge will now request only one expert to give advice.

 Box 20.7 Statement by a professional witness

I am Dr [Name]. My qualifications are [Qualifications] and my GMC registration number is [Number]. I am employed as a [Grade of doctor] in the accident and emergency department of [Name of hospital]. On [Date of incident] I was on duty when I examined [Name of Patient, Date of Birth, Do Not Give Address (1)] who attended the hospital (or was brought to the hospital by ambulance) at [Time of registration using 24-h clock].

[Name of patient] alleged [Brief history and details of incident as reported to doctor (2)].

On examination there were [Clinical findings in layman's terms (3)].

These injuries were treated with [Details of treatment (4)].

He or she was referred to [Details of any referral or follow-up]. He or she was discharged from the hospital at [Time of departure using 24-h clock].

The relevant medical records can be produced to the court if required, labelled exhibit [Your initials with a number].

Notes on the above

(1) *No address*: to protect the victim from possible intimidation when the statement is made available to the defence.
(2) *Details of incident*: the history is part of the complete medical examination and so is more than hearsay evidence. A brief description such as 'said that he was hit on the head with a baseball bat' will suffice. Do not be tempted to expand this or other sections in relation to either causation or outcome. This statement is the evidence of a professional witness not the opinion of an expert witness.
(3) *Clinical findings* → *p. 370*.
(4) *Treatment*: including number of stitches, etc.

Different levels of court may be attended such as Magistrate's and Crown Courts in England and Sheriff's and High Courts in Scotland. The types of alleged crime that end up in each court again vary with the two legal systems.

RESPONSIBILITIES TO CHILDREN

Consent and confidentiality for patients aged <16 years

The Children Act 1989 changed the way that the law dealt with children by emphasising, for the first time, that the interests of the child must be paramount. For doctors, the biggest change was to the issues of consent and confidentiality as paraphrased below:

- Any competent young person, regardless of age, can independently seek medical advice and give valid consent to medical treatment.
- Competency is understood in terms of the patient's ability to understand the choices and their consequences, including the nature, purpose and possible risk of any treatment or non-treatment. Clearly, the more serious the procedure proposed, the more important it is that the doctor is sure that the child has a complete grasp of the situation.
- Parental consent to that treatment is not necessary, although it is obviously preferable for young people to have their parents' support for important and potentially life-changing decisions. It is the doctor's duty to discuss the value of this parental support with a young patient. However, if a competent child has consented to treatment, then a parent cannot override that consent.
- Legally, a parent (or legal guardian) can give consent for treatment even if a competent child refuses – a situation that is best avoided. A refusal can also be overridden by a decision of the High Court.
- The duty of confidentiality owed to a person aged <16 years is as great as that owed to any other person. Regardless of whether or not the requested treatment is given, the confidentiality of the consultation should still be respected, unless there are convincing reasons to the contrary.
- When young people consult a doctor other than their usual GP, they are unlikely to refuse a request for details to be passed on to their GP, provided that the chain of confidentiality is maintained.

The legal framework for the above was established in the 1985 House of Lords' ruling in the Gillick case. This was particularly concerned with contraceptive advice but in general allowed for a person aged <16 years to submit to examination and treatment without a parent being informed, provided that this was the wish of the child.

These guidelines are obviously applicable to teenagers but, for younger children, consent for examination and treatment should still be obtained from a person with parental responsibility. It should also be obtained from the child if he or she is of sufficient understanding to make an informed decision. Lawyers generally believe that in a normal child this would be at 10 years of age or more.

Blood transfusion in the children of Jehovah's Witnesses → p. 379.

Child protection procedures

The Local Safeguarding Children Board (Area Child Protection Committee)

Under the legislation of the Children Act 2004, every local authority in England and Wales has to maintain a Local Safeguarding Children Board (LSCB). This is known as the Area Child Protection Committee (ACPC) in Northern Ireland and the Child Protection Committee (CPC) in Scotland. The Board (or Committee) is a forum that has representation from many different agencies and takes an overview of child protection issues in the area in which it has jurisdiction (governed by the LSCB Regulations 2006). It is staffed and administered by the local social services department; there is usually a specialist child protection unit. A Child Protection Conference (CPC) will be convened in the case of all children where there is reason to believe that there may be a need to formulate a Child Protection Plan (CPP) for their welfare. The Board (or Committee) also has a responsibility to conduct Serious Case Reviews (SCRs) for all children aged <18 years who are significantly harmed or who die in its area of jurisdiction.

Safeguarding information: the Child Protection Plan or Register

The compilation and maintenance of information about children's welfare and safeguarding issues is the responsibility of the LSCB or the (Area) CPCs in Scotland and Northern Ireland. Computerised access to this important information from departments of emergency medicine is becoming much more common (and simple). The Child Protection Register (CPR; often colloquially called the 'at-risk' register) has now been replaced by specific CPPs in England and Wales, but is still maintained in other parts of the UK.

Before a child is subject to a plan, the CPC must decide that there has been, or is a likelihood of, significant harm leading to the need for this measure.

The cause of the harm must be established as far as possible. If the risk can be applied to other children living in the same household, then it may justify their having a CPC also. The plan may be reconsidered at review conferences, which are usually held at least every 6 months. Reasons for disenactment of the plan include the following:

- The original factors that led to the plan no longer apply
- The child and family have moved permanently to another area and the child's plan has been transferred to the new LSCB or ACPC
- The child has reached 18 years of age or has married.

The Emergency Protection Order

The Emergency Protection Order (EPO) (Children Act 1989, Sections 44 and 45) replaced the Place of Safety Order. It may be made for a maximum of 8 days and extended for up to a further 7 days. Any person may apply for this order but applications are usually made by employees of either a social services department or the NSPCC (National Society for the Prevention of Cruelty to Children). The court will make the order only if there is reasonable cause to believe that the child is likely to suffer significant harm if:

- he or she is not removed to another place
- his or her removal from a safe place (e.g. a hospital) is not prevented
- enquiries being made are frustrated by access to the child being unreasonably refused.

EPOs exist in all four countries of the UK; in Scotland, the equivalent is the Child Protection Order (CPO).

The Police Protection Order

The Police Protection Order (PPO) (Children Act 1989, Section 46) gives a police officer the power to take a child 'into police protection' for up to 72 h if he or she believes that the child is at risk. This useful order can be used to prevent the removal of a child from the ED – at much shorter notice than the EPO.

Discharge of children from the ED

Section 11 of the Children Act 2004 places a duty on all NHS trusts and other NHS organisations to make arrangements to ensure that, in discharging their functions, they give regard to the need to safeguard and promote the welfare of children. This applies to all children and young people who are aged <18 years and so will also impact on some hospital adult services.

The National Institute for Health Clinical Excellence (NICE) provides a specific *Discharge advice sheet for carers of children younger than 5 years old who have a fever*, because this group is known to have special problems with safe discharge from urgent care services.

DEATH

Reporting of death and the role of the coroner

About three-quarters of all the deaths in England and Wales each year are certified by a doctor and the remainder by a coroner. The local coroner must be informed if death is associated with any of the following:

- suspicion of homicide
- suspicion of suicide
- recent violence or other trauma
- any accident (road traffic, domestic or industrial)
- drugs, poisons or alcohol
- abortion
- infancy
- self-neglect or neglect by others
- death in police custody or in prison
- recent surgical procedure
- allegation of medical negligence
- industrial or occupational disease.

In such cases, a death certificate should not be issued without the coroner's permission. The coroner, or more usually a police officer acting on his or her behalf, must also be informed of any sudden death or in cases where the cause of death is uncertain. This includes most patients who are brought to hospital dead or who arrive in cardiac arrest and are not able to be resuscitated. A death from AIDS or of an HIV-positive individual does not need referral to the coroner unless there are other grounds for concern as detailed above.

> If in doubt, discuss the patient with the coroner or his deputy.

The role of the coroner is set out in the Coroner's Act 1998 and coroners are also subject to the Coroner's Rules (1984). A coroner is obliged to hold an inquest if there is reasonable cause to suspect that the deceased has died:

- a sudden death of which the cause is unknown
- a violent or otherwise unnatural death

- in prison or in such a place or in such circumstances as to require an inquest under any other Act.

In Scotland, the procurator fiscal fulfils the office of the coroner, the main difference (for doctors) being that he or she is less likely to request a postmortem examination than his or her English counterpart.

Clinical diagnosis of death

For most purposes, death is signalled by the irreversible failure of respiration, circulation and innervation. Diagnosis of death in an apparently lifeless patient should thus depend on the following:

- Absence of respiratory movements or breath sounds
- Absence of central pulses or heart sounds
- Absence of the protective reflexes of the eye (e.g. the corneal reflex)
- Absence of the pupillary response to light.

The Academy of Medical Royal College's Code of Practice for the diagnosis and confirmation of death recommends that the patient should be observed by the person responsible for confirming death for a minimum of 5 min to establish that irreversible cardiorespiratory arrest has occurred. Digital palpation of a central pulse is not sufficiently reliable to confirm absence of the circulation; terminal changes on ECG are also required.

A state of near-death simulated by hypothermia, cold-water drowning or sedative poisoning must be excluded. Rigor mortis is usually fully established 12 h after death, lasts about 12 h and then wears off over the next 12 h.

Brain-stem death

Sometimes a patient may be brought to an ED with a functioning circulation but no other apparent signs of life. The criteria necessary for the diagnosis of brain-stem death were laid down in a statement issued by the Conference of Medical Royal Colleges and their Faculties in the UK on 11 October 1976.

Loss of brain-stem function is diagnosed by:

1 coma
2 no spontaneous respiration
3 no abnormal postures or epileptic jerking
4 no brain-stem reflexes.

Essential preconditions to testing

Before a diagnosis of brain-stem death can be considered all of the following must coexist:

1 The patient is deeply comatose.
2 The patient is maintained on a ventilator because spontaneous respiration had previously become inadequate or had ceased.
3 There is no doubt that the patient's condition is caused by irremediable, structural brain damage.

Necessary exclusions

Before proceeding to testing, the following must be ruled out:

1 Coma secondary to drugs, hypothermia or metabolic disorder
2 Respiratory failure and unresponsiveness secondary to neuromuscular blocking agents. Spinal reflexes should still be present.

Testing for absent brain-stem function

Seizures and abnormal posturing (decorticate or decerebrate) imply that there is a passage of nervous impulses through the brain stem, which therefore has live neurons in it.

The oculocephalic reflex ('doll's eye phenomenon') is a brain-stem reflex not mentioned in the UK code. If positive, the brain stem is still alive. There is often confusion about what is a positive reflex. Any deviation of the eyes with head movements is positive. In a dead patient, the eyes (obviously) always move in a fixed way with the head.

The brain-stem findings used to confirm death in the UK code are as follows:

- No pupillary response to light
- No corneal reflex
- No vestibulo-ocular reflexes
- No motor responses within the distribution of the cranial nerves in response to adequate stimulation of any somatic area
- No gag reflex or reflex response to bronchial stimulation by a suction catheter passed down the trachea
- Apnoea over a 10-min period during which the patient is oxygenated by diffusion and attains a $PaCO_2$ level of at least 50 mmHg (6.7 kPa); failure of the respiratory centre is the ultimate sign of loss of brain-stem function.

Tests should be carried out by an experienced clinician, usually in the presence of another doctor. Re-testing is performed after an interval of 2–3 h for the purposes of ensuring that:

- there is no observer error
- there is no change in signs.

The decision to remove life support is a difficult one to make in an ED unless gross cerebral disruption is visible. A patient maintained on a ventilator whose brain stem is dead will inevitably develop asystole within a matter of hours.

Organ and tissue donation

There are two main types of organ donation:

1 Donation after brain death (DBD): heart-beating donation; death certified on neurological criteria
2 Donation after cardiac death (DCD): non-heart-beating donation; death certified on cardiorespiratory criteria.

DCD may be 'controlled' (withdrawal of life-sustaining treatment) or 'uncontrolled' (failed cardiopulmonary resuscitation or CPR)

Patients initially assessed in EDs in whom organ donation is a possibility should be admitted wherever possible to an intensive care unit (ICU) in order that their clinical and broader interests (including the potential for donation) can be fully assessed. Potential donors should be cared for by staff with the appropriate competencies, particularly with regard to end-of-life care. The decision to withdraw life-sustaining treatment on the grounds of 'futility' should be made transparently and consistently, regardless of the potential for organ donation. There are absolute contraindications to all types of organ donation ($\rightarrow$ *Box 20.8*).

The law requires that treatment be given only if it is 'in the patient's best interests' (England and Wales) or 'to the patient's benefit' (Scotland). However, if an

individual expressed a wish to be an organ donor, treatments that facilitate that wish and do not cause the person harm or distress are regarded as in their best interests. Guidance to this effect was published in England and Wales in 2009 and in Scotland in 2010. No treatment specifically aimed at organ donation should be instituted before the decision to withdraw treatment has been made and no intervention that can potentially restore cerebral circulation and function is allowed under any circumstances. Tracheal re-intubation, to facilitate lung donation, may be performed after the declaration of death and before the start of abdominal organ retrieval.

OTHER ED ISSUES

Complaints

Any effective organisation that serves the public must have a well-structured system for dealing with complaints. Problems that are dealt with in a rapid, efficient and courteous manner will often resolve satisfactorily. The current NHS complaints system aims to achieve this by using several levels of response.

Local resolution

Verbal discussion of the problem usually follows a direct approach to a member of the clinical or reception staff at the time of treatment. A senior member of the medical or nursing staff should be involved from the outset.

Written complaints, which should be made within 6 months of the problem revealing itself, are forwarded to the hospital complaints manager who then gathers information from the relevant clinical staff. The chief executive subsequently replies in writing and a meeting with the patient or the relatives may be convened.

Investigation by the Health Service Commissioner

The next level of the system is a complaint to the Health Service Commissioner or Ombudsman. The Ombudsman is independent of the NHS and acts as a final arbiter of both complaints and complaints procedures.

The most common areas of complaint to a department of emergency medicine are:

- waiting times
- attitude of staff
- communication and information given

Box 20.8 Patients who are not suitable for organ donation

Patients with one or more of the following conditions should not be referred as potential donors:

- Active invasive cancer in the last 3 years (excluding non-melanoma skin cancer and primary brain tumour)
- Haematological malignancy (myeloma, lymphoma or leukaemia)
- Untreated systemic infection
- Variant Creutzfeldt–Jakob disease (CJD)
- HIV disease (but not HIV infection)

- aspects of clinical care, such as failure to obtain a radiograph.

Staff dealing with a complaining patient or relative should consider the following guidelines in an attempt to defuse the situation:

- Do not be confrontational or defensive.
- Listen attentively and sympathetically.
- Do not be afraid of saying that you are sorry. You can empathise with a patient's distress without admitting liability or error (e.g. 'I am sorry that you are not happy with your treatment').
- Ask questions and obtain the full facts about the perceived problems.
- Do not attempt to justify; explain if appropriate.
- Agree a course of action and ensure that it is carried out quickly and efficiently, and moreover that it is seen to be carried out.
- Provide written information about the NHS complaints system if the complainant wishes to take the matter further.

The content and conclusion of the discussion should be recorded in the patient's case notes.

Notifiable diseases (and other notification duties of registered medical practitioners)

In the UK, registered medical practitioners attending a patient are required to notify the proper officer of the local authority in which the patient resides when they have 'reasonable grounds for suspecting' that the patient:

- has a notifiable disease as listed in the Notification Regulations (→ Box 20.9)
- has an infection not included in the Notification Regulations which, in the view of the doctor, could present significant harm to human health (e.g. emerging or new infections)
- is contaminated (such as with chemicals or radiation) in a manner that, in the view of the doctor, could present significant harm to human health
- has died with, but not necessarily because of, a notifiable disease, or other infectious disease or contamination that could present harm to human health.

Notifications of cases of infection not included in the Notification Regulations and of contamination are expected to be exceptional occurrences. Doctors should not wait for laboratory confirmation or results of other investigations in order to notify a case. This ensures prompt transfer of information so that health protection interventions and control measures can be initiated as soon as possible. Legal action may be taken by an infected person if the index case has not been notified. Notification requires the completion of the appropriate form but urgent cases should be notified by telephone as well (within 24 h of any suspicions at the latest). Books of notification certificates are available and there is also a template notification document on the Health Protection Agency website. In Scotland, written notification should be undertaken electronically via the Scottish Care Information (SCI) Gateway. Throughout the UK, there is no longer a fee payable for notification.

In England and Wales, the notifiable circumstances are designated by the Public Health (Control of Disease) Act 1984, as amended by the Health and Social Care Act 2008 and the Health Protection (Notification) Regulations 2010. There are some differences in Scotland and Northern Ireland where the notifiable diseases are listed by the Public Health (Notification of Infectious Diseases) (Scotland) Act 2008 and the Public Health (Notifiable Diseases) (Northern Ireland) Order 1990 respectively. (*Notifiable diseases in the UK* → Box 20.9). HIV infection/AIDS is not a statutorily notifiable disease in the UK. There is, however, a voluntary confidential reporting scheme (with a special form) to the Public Health Laboratory Service Communicable Disease Surveillance Centre.

Sick notes

> Work is good for health. It is an essential part of individual identity and social status. It promotes recovery and rehabilitation and leads to better health outcomes. Long-term unemployment is associated with a two- to threefold increase in poor general and mental health and a 20% excess mortality rate.

Most patients who attend an ED will need only a few days away from work. Self-certification allows for 7 days' absence before a doctor's note is required. The relevant forms are the following:

- Form SC1 for people who are self-employed or unemployed. It is usually available in the ED.
- Form SC2 for people who work for an employer. It is obtained from the place of work. Medical

Box 20.9 **Notifiable diseases in the UK**

[Schedule 1 of the Health Protection (Notification) Regulations 2010 with additions for Scotland and Northern Ireland]

Acute encephalitis (not Scotland)
Acute viral meningitis (not Scotland)
Acute bacterial meningitis***
Acute poliomyelitis***
Acute infectious hepatitis*** (not Scotland)
Anthrax***
Botulism***
Brucellosis***
Chickenpox (Northern Ireland only)
Cholera***
Diphtheria***
Enteric fever (typhoid or paratyphoid fever)***
Food poisoning*** (not Scotland)
Gastroenteritis in children aged <2 years
    (Northern Ireland only)
Haemolytic uraemic syndrome (HUS)***
Haemophilus influenzae type b (Scotland only)
Infectious bloody diarrhoea*** (not Scotland
    unless *Escherichia coli* O157)
Invasive group A streptococcal disease***
Legionnaires' disease*** (not Scotland)
Leprosy (not Scotland or Northern Ireland)
Malaria (not Scotland)
Measles***
Meningococcal septicaemia***
Mumps
Necrotising fasciitis (Scotland only)
Plague***
Rabies
Rubella
Severe acute respiratory syndrome (SARS)***
Scarlet fever (not Scotland)

Smallpox***
Tetanus***
Tuberculosis
Tularemia (Scotland only)
Typhus
Viral haemorrhagic fever (VHF)***
West Nile Fever (Scotland only)
Whooping cough***
Yellow fever

***URGENT = notify immediately by telephone and then send paper/electronic version within 3 days.
It is no longer a requirement to notify cases of dysentery, ophthalmia neonatorum, leptospirosis and relapsing fever.

Special circumstances
Some normally non-notifiable diseases may need notification if there are circumstances that put others at significant risk, e.g. chickenpox in a health-care worker who is in contact with immunosuppressed individuals or a patient with parvovirus B19 infection who is in contact with pregnant women. Another example would be suspected cases of carbon monoxide poisoning. It is also considered good professional practice to report any suspected clusters of cases of normally non-notifiable diseases. There are separate ways of notifying cases of:

- Healthcare-associated infections
- HIV/AIDS and other sexually transmitted infections (via genitourinary medicine clinics)
- Creutzfeldt–Jakob disease (National CJD Surveillance Unit)

certificates (doctor's statements) should be issued to patients who will clearly be away from work for a longer period without seeing another doctor.
- Form Med 3 is the usual doctor's statement. It should be issued by the doctor who, at the time, has clinical responsibility for the patient. The rules governing its use are described in *Box 20.10*.
- Form Med 5 is the doctor's special statement. It should be used when Form Med 3 is not appropriate:

    – The patient requires a statement for a past period during which he or she saw the doctor but no statement was issued.
    – The doctor wishes to advise a patient whom he or she has not examined to refrain from work for up to 1 month on the basis of a written report that is not more than a month old from another doctor.
- Form Med 4 is used for illnesses lasting longer than 28 weeks.

Box 20.10 Form Med 3

Closed statements – has return to work date
The note is for less than 2 weeks from the day of examination. It should indicate the earliest day on which the patient is likely to be fit for work.

Open statements – no return to work date
If a doctor is unable to issue a closed statement as above, then an open statement may be issued by entering a period during which the absence from work is likely to continue. This period may not be for more than 6 months from the date of issue unless the patient has been certified as unfit to work for the previous 6 months. When a patient who has been given an open statement recovers, he or she must be given a closed statement as above to terminate the spell of incapacity and allow a return to work:

- The statement must be based on an examination of the patient and issued no later than the day after this examination
- The 'remarks' space of the statement can be used for any additional background information that may be relevant
- Only one statement can be issued for one period of absence. If this is lost, it can be replaced by another marked 'duplicate'

Conditions for safe discharge

To send a patient home you must be sure of the following:

- The patient does not have a life-threatening condition.
- The symptoms can be adequately controlled in the environment in which the patient lives.
- Any further investigation or treatment that the patient may need can be reasonably carried out at or arranged from home.
- The patient has access to further help, and carers, should it be necessary.
- You have communicated your plan for present and future management to both the patient and any others necessary for this care (e.g. relatives, GP, health visitor, district nurse, social worker).

Box 20.11 Instructions about the care of a patient who has received sedative medicines in the ED

Your relative/child/friend has received sedative medicines or injections in the ED. These drugs may cause:

- drowsiness
- unsteadiness and loss of balance
- poor coordination and clumsiness

Some of these effects may last for up to 24 h. as a result of this, a person who has received sedatives should:

- be accompanied home
- be escorted when going upstairs
- take care when using the toilet or bathroom

They must NOT:

- be left alone in the house until fully recovered (e.g. overnight)
- drive or go cycling
- go out walking alone
- use machinery or go into situations where poor balance or coordination could be dangerous
- drink alcohol
- sign any legally binding documents

However, they can:

- eat and drink light meals
- sit around the house
- take painkillers and regular medicines

If you have any worries or problems with this patient, then telephone the ED helpline.

Patients who have received sedative or opioid drugs in the ED

Many patients receive drugs likely to cause sedation as part of their treatment in the ED. For both practical and medicolegal reasons, these patients need to be given verbal and written warnings about the possible residual effects of these drugs. *Box 20.11* summarises this information as it should appear on a card for the patient to take home.

Small wounds and localised infections

SMALL WOUNDS

Small does not mean trivial. The wound may be:

- the only visible manifestation of a significant deep injury
- simple yet serious if not treated promptly or properly
- capable of leaving a considerable amount of disfigurement or loss of function
- of no consequence in the doctor's eyes but worrying to the patient.

> Inadequately treated small wounds cause much distress for patients, a lot of worry for doctors and a considerable amount of work for lawyers.

Assessment of wounds

Certain features of a wound are associated with a high risk of complications. The following must always be considered:

- *Mechanism of injury*: excessive force, high speed, retained glass, dangerous weapon
- *Site of injury*: trunk, perineum, neck, near a joint, over a neurovascular bundle
- *Time of injury*: wounds more than 6 h old are more likely to get infected
- *Place of injury*: field or garden injuries carry a greater risk of contamination with tetanus and gas-forming organisms.

> A butcher's knife may be contaminated with many organisms from animal carcasses. When boning a carcass and holding the knife with both hands, it is possible to receive a deep, penetrating and highly contaminated wound.

Also ask about

- Allergies to drugs including antibiotics
- Previous injuries: if the patient is a child, always consider child abuse (→ *p. 353*)
- Current medication, because some drugs may affect local treatment (e.g. anticoagulants)

Look for

- Site, extent and character of the wound
- Evidence of contamination, non-viable tissue or foreign bodies
- Involvement of deep structures. Assess distal neurovascular and tendon function and record the findings.

Bleeding is exacerbated by alcohol, anticoagulants, partial (rather than complete) tears of vessels and continued interference with wounds. If there is a potential for significant bleeding, intravenous (IV) access should be established.

Pain may be extreme with some small injuries. Less painful and more serious injuries may have been inflicted in the same incident and can easily be missed. Local anaesthetic may be needed before further investigation; sensory loss must be recorded first.

Emergency Medicine Lecture Notes, Fourth Edition. Chris Moulton and David Yates.
© 2012 Blackwell Publishing Ltd. Published 2012 by Blackwell Publishing Ltd.

Anaesthesia for wounds

All wounds must be explored and cleaned before closure is contemplated. This usually requires anaesthesia, as does the subsequent closure. A general anaesthetic will be required when the areas involved are multiple or large, or belong to children or anxious adults (→ *Boxes 21.1 and 21.2*).

Cleaning and exploration of wounds

Wound cleaning must be extensive and thorough. Particulate matter and contamination must be me-chanically removed. This can be achieved by high-pressure irrigation or by scrubbing with a sterile nailbrush or toothbrush and an antiseptic solution. Hydrogen peroxide is not recommended nowadays. Dirt left in a wound may cause infection or be taken up by inflammatory cells to produce a permanent tattoo effect.

Exploration of a wound is essential to identify:

- the depth and extent of damage
- structures exposed or damaged
- foreign bodies.

An appreciation of the direction and force of the injuring agent will facilitate exploration.

 Box 21.1 Local infiltration

Maximum doses of local anaesthetics →
  p. 353.
Treatment of severe local anaesthetic toxicity
  → Box 21.3.

- Use lidocaine, always without adrenaline:
  - 2% is suitable for nerve blocks; in a digital ring block this reduces the volume required and hence the risk of vascular compression
  - 1% is appropriate for general use
  - 0.5% should be used when large areas of tissue are involved and more than 10 mL anaesthetic are required
- Clean the wound edge with an antiseptic solution. If local anaesthetic is injected before the antiseptic has dried then the patient will be given a painful subcutaneous injection of both
- Always trim hair for at least 2 cm around the wound, before injecting local anaesthetic. The aim is to expose the wound fully and to prevent hair from interfering with the sutures. Scissors are usually adequate. A razor is sometimes necessary. Never shave the eyebrows
- Using a short 23 G needle, inject a small amount of lidocaine under the wound edge, either through the wound edge if the wound is fresh and socially clean, or through the skin if the wound is grossly contaminated or contused (safer but more painful)
- Once this small area is anaesthetised inject through it to raise a weal a little further on. Wait and then repeat. In this way, the patient feels only the first injection

---

 Box 21.2 Ring block

This is effective for procedures involving distal wounds of the finger. There is a risk of damage to, or spasm of, the digital arteries and it must not be used if there is a history of upper limb circulatory problems.

- Use only plain lidocaine (2% for an adult). Adrenaline added to the lidocaine may produce irreversible spasm of the digital arteries and loss of the finger
- Clean the base of the finger with antiseptic solution
- Insert a 23 G needle into the dorsolateral border of the base of the finger. The tip of the needle should end up near the bone on the palmar side of the finger. Aspirate and if blood is seen withdraw the needle and start again
- Inject no more than 2 mL of solution and much less in a child. The more fluid that is introduced the greater the risk of vascular damage. Repeat on the opposite side of the finger
- Wait for at least 5 min for full anaesthesia of the finger
- If digital artery spasm occurs stop the procedure. Massage the base of the finger where the anaesthetic has been injected and instruct the patient to move the finger vigorously. These manoeuvres should dissipate the fluid and release the spasm

The risk of digital artery spasm is increased if digital tourniquets are used. Most procedures on fingers in the ED do not require them.

Box 21.3 The treatment of severe local anaesthetic (LA) agent toxicity

Signs of severe LA toxicity include sudden loss of consciousness, convulsions, cardiovascular collapse, cardiac conduction disturbances, tachydysrhythmias, asystole and ventricular fibrillation (VF).

- Institute cardiopulmonary resuscitation (CPR) if required
- Attend to the ABCs
- Control convulsions with standard drugs
- Control cardiac dysrhythmias with standard therapy
- Treat cardiac arrest with lipid emulsion, continuing CPR throughout for up to an hour. (This is a relatively new approach. Intralipid 20% has been shown to reverse LA-induced cardiac arrest in animal models and in some human case reports. It has also been used successfully in life-threatening LA toxicity without cardiac arrest.) An intravenous bolus of 20% Intralipid 1.5 mL/kg is given over 1 min followed by an infusion of 0.25 mL/kg per min. The bolus injection can be repeated twice at 5-min intervals if an adequate circulation has not been restored and the rate of the infusion can be doubled.

Resection of tissue:
- Use a scalpel to remove dead tissue and trim the edges of old wounds.
- Be very cautious in the face, scalp, foot and hand. Skin is at a premium here. Always ask for help with complex wounds in these areas.

Radiographs for foreign bodies

Foreign bodies are often surprisingly difficult to locate. The radiograph request card must indicate that a foreign body is being sought so that the radiographer can adjust the exposure accordingly. Glass is usually radio-opaque. Some thin metals (e.g. razor blades) can be surprisingly difficult to visualise on the film. Conversely, small fragments, obvious on a radiograph, can be very difficult to find and remove. Occasionally, less damage is done by leaving them *in situ*. This decision must be made after consultation with a senior colleague.

All wounds involving glass must have radiographs to exclude retained fragments.

Closure of wounds

- *Primary*: for most recent incised wounds
- *Delayed primary*: after 3–10 days, for crush injuries
- *Secondary* (i.e. by natural processes): when surgical closure is impossible and granulation and epithelialisation are encouraged.

Monofilament synthetic sutures are more difficult to handle than silk but are resistant to infection tracking up the thread and will give a better cosmetic result. Polyglycolic acid and catgut sutures evoke a pronounced tissue response as a necessary part of their autodestruction and are unsuitable for skin closure in an emergency department (ED). For most wounds 4/0 G sutures are used, with finer gauges for cosmetically sensitive areas. Absorbable sutures should be used to close subcutaneous spaces.

- Plan sutures strategically – do not just start at one end.
- Use interrupted sutures – not continuous or subcuticular because these cause increased risk of infection tracking along the suture.

Suturing skills cannot be learned from a book.

Tissue glue, adhesive strips and skin staples are alternative methods of closure with several advantages:

- Less traumatic for children
- Sometimes less scarring but only if good apposition is achieved
- Sometimes cheaper
- Sometimes quicker to apply.

However, wounds closed with these methods still require thorough cleaning, possibly under local anaesthesia.

Tissue glue is applied to the carefully opposed skin surfaces and not to the open wound.

Skin loss: When closing defects in the skin, excessive tension should be avoided at all costs. If there is extensive skin loss or any loss on the face or hand, seek advice. Small skin defects elsewhere may be closed by undermining. This is achieved using a scalpel about 3 mm below the skin in the horizontal plane. A tissue plane may then be opened up using blunt scissors.

Aftercare of wounds

Dressings may not be required (e.g. on the face) or may be of simple non-adherent type. Splintage should be minimal but may be necessary if a wound is over the extensor aspect of a joint.

Removal time for sutures varies with the site: 3–4 days on the face, up to 14 days in lower limbs or over joints, but usually about 7 days for most other parts of the body. Earlier replacement with adhesive strips may avoid permanent puncture-mark scars. Sutures may be removed in the GP clinic provided that adequate documentation accompanies the patient.

Postoperative analgesia depends on the patient's needs. Efficacy, suitability of formulation and cost should all be considered.

Resuturing wounds

Patients returning with wounds that have broken down should have a senior opinion. Such wounds must be cleaned and dressed until ready for resuture. Anything more than local infection requires oral antibiotics. Facial wounds need a specialised opinion and wounds in children may need reclosure under general anaesthetic. The possibility of a retained foreign body should always be considered.

Skin grafts

These can be full thickness (Wolfe) or partial thickness (Thiersch); only the latter is generally used in EDs. The objective is to transplant the tops of the dermal papillae from the donor site, leaving the bases and skin appendages as a partial-thickness defect. This will heal by secondary intention. The donor skin must be applied directly to a clean, granulating wound. It will be nourished initially by direct tissue perfusion and then later by new capillary buds. The technique may not be suitable for patients on steroids with very thin, friable skin → Box 21.4.

Reimplantation of body parts

Successful reimplantation of amputated body parts is possible using microsurgical techniques. Clean injuries without contamination or contusion have the best chances of success. Suitable structures for reimplantation include:

- the whole or part of a finger (with amputations proximal to the distal interphalangeal joint only)
- the penis
- ears
- large pieces of scalp
- hands, feet and more extensive parts of a limb.

Patients with these injuries should be discussed as soon as possible with the nearest plastic surgery unit. The amputated part should be wrapped in saline-soaked gauze and then put in a plastic bag in a container full of crushed ice. The body tissue must not come into direct contact with the ice as tissue necrosis may occur.

Prevention of wound infection

This is achieved in most cases by:

- cleaning the wound
- excising necrotic tissue
- closing the wound as appropriate
- dressing the wound carefully
- using antibiotics when indicated (→ Box 21.5)
- anticipating the presence of spore-forming organisms (→ later).

Patient compliance in aftercare is essential.

The most common wound contaminants are bacteria from the skin, so flucloxacillin or clarithromycin is adequate cover. In bites, however, a wider spectrum of organisms is involved and so co-amoxiclav or clarithromycin should be prescribed.

Spore-forming organisms are more likely to contaminate wounds incurred on sports fields or in gardens, and also injuries of the lower limb. They will flourish in areas of hypoxia, e.g. deep, penetrating and contused wounds. Primary prevention involves scrubbing all wounds under effective anaesthesia and surgically removing all necrotic tissue. Contused wounds should not be closed. All foreign material must be removed.

Gas gangrene can be prevented if wounds are managed as outlined above. Long-acting penicillins are no substitute for adequate wound toilet.

Prevention of tetanus

Diagnosis and treatment of tetanus → p. 233.
Routine UK immunisation schedule for children →
    Table 18.6 on p. 252.
Summary of tetanus prophylaxis → Table 21.1.

Box 21.4 **Skin grafting**

A clean theatre with a good light is essential. Aseptic theatre technique must be followed, with the operator using gown and gloves. Infection is the most common cause of graft failure. Antibiotics should not be used routinely.

Anaesthesia: this may be general or local. The latter is often preferable. Lidocaine 0.5% or 1% is infiltrated subcutaneously around donor and graft sites.

Donor site: the donor site should be discussed with the patient. Upper arm and inner thigh are usually appropriate.

Graft site: the graft site should be clean and granulating. Avascular eschar should be removed. Clinical evidence of infection precludes surgery. Any doubt should be resolved by prior bacteriological investigation.

Technique of removing graft: a small graft knife designed to take a razor blade is appropriate for most cases (a Silva knife). The thickness of the graft is determined by the distance between the blade and the underlying roller. The donor site is dressed with paraffin gauze, a non-adherent dressing and crepe.

Application of graft: the graft is reversed on to paraffin gauze which is then trimmed to the graft size to provide support. Postage stamp-sized grafts are ideal, the defect being covered by a number of grafts with minimal overlapping. Any subsequent haematoma formation then lifts and devitalises only one small area and most of the graft survives. Apposition of graft and granulating bed is maintained by suturing the edges and tying in antiseptic-impregnated cotton wool (→ Figure 21.1).

Follow-up: the outer dressing of the grafted area is removed after 2–3 days to check for infection. Smell and exudate warrant further investigation. In the absence of either, the top dressing is replaced and neither this nor the wound is disturbed for 10–14 days. Fiddling with the dressings greatly increases pain at the donor site and the risk of failure of the graft.

When the dressings and sutures are removed the graft should not be cleaned vigorously but merely examined and then covered with a non-adherent dressing. Small defects usually close quickly by secondary intention. The graft will take months to stabilize. Initially, it will need constant protection by a dressing. Later, a hand cream should be applied. The split skin will not sweat or produce grease and tends to dry out and break down easily. The patient should be advised to protect it while sunbathing for at least a year.

Box 21.5 **Indications for antibiotics in wound care**

Antibiotics are indicated for wounds that:

- are already showing signs of infection when seen
- are more than 12h old and in need of primary closure
- have a definite history of contamination with problem organisms (e.g. human and cat bites)
- are possibly contaminated with deep areas that are not amenable to cleaning (e.g. some puncture wounds)
- have exposed or damaged deep structures (e.g. bone in compound fractures, tendon or nerve)

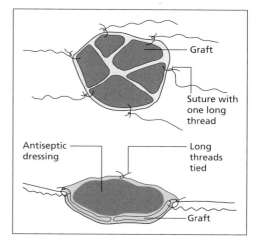

Figure 21.1 Application of a split-skin graft.

Table 21.1 Tetanus prophylaxis

Patient immunisation status	Tetanus-prone wound	Other wound
Has had five or more doses of vaccine during lifetime	Nothing required (HTIg if very high risk of contamination)	Nothing required
Has had complete course of three doses or booster dose within the last 10 years	Nothing required (HTIg if very high risk of contamination)	Nothing required
Has had three-dose course of vaccine or single booster >10 years ago	Booster dose + consider HTIg if wound contaminated	Booster dose
Has never had complete course of vaccine or immune status unknown	Complete course of vaccine + HTIg if wound contaminated	Complete course of vaccine

HTIg, human tetanus immunoglobulin.

 Box 21.6 Tetanus-prone wounds

Wounds that are particularly tetanus-prone include those that:

- are >6h old at presentation
- are deeper than they are long (stab or puncture wounds)
- contain devitalised tissue
- are possibly contaminated with soil or manure
- show clinical evidence of sepsis

There are still several cases of tetanus in the UK every year, although prophylaxis against tetanus is cheap and safe. Infection is caused by contamination of a wound with the spores of the bacillus *Clostridium tetani*. Days or even weeks after infection, local multiplication of the organism occurs with release of its neurotoxin → *p. 233*. Until recently, most cases of tetanus in the UK were in people aged >65 years who had not been previously immunised. In the last few years, tetanus has also been seen in young adults who abuse IV drugs. Even the most trivial of wounds can introduce tetanus into the body but some wounds carry a particularly high risk. *For factors that identify tetanus-prone wounds → Box 21.6.*

With diphtheria on the increase in eastern Europe, single antigen tetanus vaccine (T) has been replaced by the combined tetanus and low-dose diphtheria vaccine for adults and adolescents (Td) for all routine uses. Td replaced single tetanus as the standard booster for UK school leavers in 1994. For both diphtheria and tetanus, a total of five doses of vaccine are considered to give life-long immunity. These may have been given either as the primary three-dose course in childhood followed by school entry and school-leaving doses, or as a primary course at any time followed by a booster dose 10 years later and a second booster 10 years after that. Polio vaccine is usually also included in the booster doses.

Unscheduled booster doses are therefore indicated only for the following indications:

1 After a tetanus-prone wound (→ *Box 21.6*) where the patient has not received a full five-dose course and is due a further dose
2 After a tetanus-prone wound (→ *Box 21.6*) where the patient's immunisation status is unknown (e.g. elderly patients and immigrants to the UK)
3 For travellers to areas where medical attention may not be accessible, should a tetanus-prone injury occur, and whose last dose was more than 10 years previously.

Tetanus toxoid vaccine confers active immunity. It stimulates the production of antibodies, which may take several weeks to reach a peak. Therefore, in the case of contaminated wounds, patients receiving Td vaccine in the first two categories above should also be given passive immunisation with human tetanus immunoglobulin (HTIg) → *later*. The two injections should be given into separate areas. Patients with impaired immunity may not respond to active immunisation and may therefore also need HTIg.

Active immunisation against tetanus was introduced into some areas of the UK as part of the primary immunisation of infants from the mid-1950s and was adopted nationally from 1961. It was provided by the British armed forces (mostly to men!) from 1938 onwards. Knowledge of these dates and the age of the patient will help to determine the likelihood of previous immunisation.

Patients with doubtful or unknown immune status to tetanus and diphtheria require a full primary course of Td vaccine (three doses at 1-month intervals). Notification should be sent to the patient's GP to this effect. Two further booster doses at 10-year intervals will also be required to confer life-long immunity.

Td vaccine is given by deep subcutaneous or intramuscular (IM) injection. Local reactions such as pain, redness and swelling around the injection site may occur and persist for several days. Acute allergic reactions (anaphylaxis or urticaria) are uncommon; peripheral neuropathy is a rare but recognised side effect. Vague post-immunisation symptoms such as headache, pyrexia, lethargy, malaise and myalgia may also occur occasionally. Persistent nodules at the injection site may arise after shallow injections.

The contraindications to Td vaccine are as follows:

1 Coincidental acute febrile illness – unless there is a tetanus-prone wound. Minor infections without fever or systemic upset should not postpone immunisation.
2 Severe reactions (e.g. anaphylaxis or peripheral neuropathy) after a previous dose.

HIV-positive status is not a contraindication to immunisation.

Human tetanus immunoglobulin

Human tetanus immunoglobulin (HTIg) gives passive immunity. It is a preparation of human antibodies, which is not associated with significant side effects or allergy, unlike the previously used horse serum. The dose is 250 IU by deep IM injection. This may be increased to 500 IU if more than 24 h have elapsed or if there is a risk of heavy contamination or after large burns.

Tetanus and diphtheria immunisation for children

The administration of an unscheduled tetanus and diphtheria immunisation to a child may cause great difficulty with the correct timing of other immunisations. For this reason, concurrent administration of the other recommended immunisations for that age group or referral to the child's health visitor is usually the better practice.

*Routine UK immunisation schedule for children →
Table 18.6 on p. 352.*

Wound botulism

This related clostridial infection has recently re-emerged in the UK.

*Diagnosis and treatment of wound botulism → p. 234.
Treatment of clostridial and other necrotising soft-tissue infections → p. 266.*

SPECIFIC TYPES OF WOUNDS

*Abdominal wounds → p. 81.
Burns → p. 136.
Chest wounds → p. 72.
Facial wounds → p. 64.
Forensic aspects of wounds → p. 370.
Neck wounds → p. 62.
Scalp wounds → p. 37.
Serious hand injuries → p. 128.
Wrist wounds → p. 119.*

Abrasions

Motorcyclists and children may present with dirty abrasions.

Tx The basic care is as for any wound. However, the ingrained dirt must be removed to prevent infection and to avoid the development of a permanent 'tattoo'. Scrubbing with a swab or a small brush may be necessary. Analgesia for this purpose can be obtained by:

• application of local anaesthetic gel
• infiltration of local anaesthetic
• general anaesthesia.

Crush wounds

Where there is an element of crush or bursting in the mechanism of injury there is widespread damage to tissues. Extracellular fluid accumulates and the tissues continue to swell for 24–48 h.

Tx The wound should be cleaned, explored and then dressed.

If crush wounds are closed immediately, interstitial pressure will rise, resulting in tissue necrosis and infection.

The patient must be reviewed on the following day. Severe crush injuries require admission for elevation and observation. Decompression may sometimes be needed, especially if the crush has damaged deep tissues without tearing the skin or if there is a deep, closed compartment.

Compartment syndrome → p. 110.

Degloving injuries

When skin is traumatically removed from limbs in this way it is tempting to simply replace and suture it. However, the injured skin is always contused and often dead. The risks of necrosis and sloughing are very great. A patient with a degloving injury must be referred for inpatient surgical management.

Roller injuries

These have features of both degloving and crush injuries. The injury may seem trivial at first but widespread tissue necrosis can occur. Admission, elevation and careful observation are essential. Vascular compromise is suggested by:

- failure to blanch on pressure
- failure of capillary refill
- paraesthesia.

Flap wounds

Flaps are caused by initial contact at the apex of the wound and then a tearing of the skin towards the base. Contusion of the skin flap is inevitable. Narrow, distally based flaps have a poor blood supply.

Tx If the flap has a wide base or is thick with obviously viable tissues, it may be sutured in the normal way. If not, consider defatting the flap and replacing it as a skin graft with a pressure dressing. The skin of children is very elastic and a V-shaped cut may appear to have lost tissue or have a narrow base as a result of contraction. The skin flap should be stretched back to its normal position without undue tension before viability and skin loss are assessed.

Stab wounds

Stab wounds are defined as wounds that are deeper than they are long. As such they have an invisible deep part. The risk of severe damage relates to the anatomical site of the injury, but particular areas of concern are:

- the chest – back or front (→ *pp. 62, 73, 78*)
- the neck (→ *p. 62*)

- the abdomen (→ *p. 82*)
- near joints
- near large limb vessels.

> The presence of distal pulses does not exclude vascular damage. Swelling is always worrying.

Xr Radiographs are used to show air shadows:

- Pneumothorax and surgical emphysema on chest X-ray (CXR) with chest wounds
- Air under the diaphragm on CXR after an abdominal injury
- Surgical emphysema on the lateral soft-tissue view of the neck after a neck wound
- Air in a joint showing synovial penetration after a wound to a limb.

Tx Stab wounds must be assessed by an experienced doctor. Uncomplicated injuries are best treated by cleaning and simple dressing; immediate closure tends to trap any haematoma that forms. All patients with this type of injury should be either admitted for observation or reviewed on the following day.

Legal aspects of stab wounds → Chapter 20.

Gunshot wounds

Gunshot wounds have a twofold potential for damage:

1 Direct injury to structures along the track
2 Damage to neighbouring structures from dissipated kinetic energy. This depends on the type of weapon involved. High-velocity weapons fire bullets that transfer a large amount of energy to the surrounding tissues. Damage is greatest to solid organs in closed spaces. Bone splinters may cause secondary damage. Vascular injury can be overt and extensive or confined to the endothelium (with intact pulses); delayed thrombosis may result.

Xr As for stab wounds above.

Tx All patients with gunshot wounds require:

- resuscitation
- assessment
- admission and observation.

Most need surgical exploration of the bullet track to remove necrotic tissue and clothing fragments.

Legal aspects of gunshot wounds → Chapter 20.

Animal bites in the British Isles

Bite wounds account for up to 2% of all attendances at an ED. Dog bites are the most common and bites from humans and other primates are usually the worst.

Tx Teeth produce dirty, contused wounds, which must be cleaned thoroughly; this can be difficult with deep puncture wounds. Once cleaned and irrigated, bites are often considered for delayed closure. However, gaping wounds should always be approximated with adhesive strips or loose sutures (not tissue glue). On the face, the excellent blood supply usually prevents infection and this rule can be ignored – especially as the cosmetic results of delayed closure are poor.

Shallow dog bites do not need antibiotics at first presentation. Patients with cat bites, human bites or deep puncture wounds should be given a short course of co-amoxiclav (or clarithromycin or doxycycline and metronidazole if allergic to penicillins) to protect against anaerobic infections. All patients must be covered against tetanus infection (→ *p. 394*). Cat bites may be followed by a painful, fulminating cellulitis that is due to deep inoculation with *Pasteurella multicida*. In penicillin-allergic patients, a combination of clindamycin and ciprofloxacin may be used to treat this infection.

> Human bites may carry a risk of hepatitis B transmission. *For prophylaxis against blood-borne viruses* → *p. 404*.

Envenoming (especially adder bites) → *p. 292*.
Rabies → *p. 253*.

Insect and spider bites in the British Isles

The horsefly *(Haematopota pluvialis)* is also known as the cleg fly and has a very painful bite for a small creature. The female flies use their sharp mandibles to rip a triangular hole in the skin of humans and other mammals and then suck up the blood that oozes out of the wound. These insects easily spread bacteria from host to host and so a bite of this type may often become cellulitic → *p. 406*.

The Blandford fly *(Simulium posticatum)* is a species of black fly. It is small and dark and is usually found near water, mostly in the south of England. Unlike other biting flies, Blandford flies will crawl through clothing and often bite in the middle of the day rather than the evening. The females use their jagged mouths to bite through skin and then feed on blood, just before mating. Allergic reactions can occur and, if the bites are contaminated with bacteria, then local infection is possible.

The false black widow spider *(Steatoda nobilis)* is the most venomous of the 12 biting spiders found in the British Isles. It arrived in Britain 200 years ago and is closely related to the true black widow spider. It is mostly found in the south of England and only the female spiders bite. Enough poison is delivered by a single envenoming to cause severe pain and inflammation. Victims describe a burning sensation that spreads out from the bite and also flu-like symptoms lasting for up to 3 days. This is thought to be a mild form of neurotoxic araneism (spider poisoning). Antihistamines provide some relief of symptoms.

Stings in the British Isles

Wasp and bee stings: the stings from almost all arthropods of the *Hymenoptera* cause local pain, redness and swelling but rarely result in severe problems. Exceptions are anaphylactic reactions and intraoral swellings, both of which need appropriate treatment (→ *pp. 299 and 424*). (It is said that up to 0.5% of the population is hypersensitive to either bee or wasp venom.) Unlike wasps, bees leave their stings imbedded in the skin and these should be removed with splinter forceps. The acid bee venom may then be neutralised by the application of bicarbonate, while vinegar may help to soothe the caustic wasp sting. The inflammation from all stings can be treated with local applications of calamine lotion, antihistamine cream or hydrocortisone 1% cream.

Caterpillar stings: the brown tail moth *(Euproctis chrysorrhoea)* is common throughout central and southern Europe, including the south of England, and is found in all types of habitat. The hairs of its caterpillars may cause an extremely painful rash if touched. (This ordinary-looking caterpillar is brownish grey with red spots along its back and is not particularly hairy.) Hydrocortisone cream may ease the pain. The oak processionary moth *(Thaumetopoea processionea)* has a similar distribution to the brown tail moth but the toxin on its insignificant-looking brown caterpillars is irritant to the skin, eyes and bronchi of humans and animals. These moths are considered to be a significant human health problem when populations reach outbreak proportions, such as those in The Netherlands and Belgium in recent years.

Weever fish stings: the lesser weever fish *(Trachinus vipera)* is found in shallow sandy water around the shores of the British Isles; the greater weever fish *(Trachinus draco)* is caught by anglers in deeper water. The dorsal and gill cover spines of both fish may give a very painful sting. The venom can be denatured by immersing the injured part in very hot (but not >45°C) water.

Jellyfish stings: the Portuguese man-of-war jellyfish *(Physalia physalis)* has friable and venomous tentacles, as do several other jellyfish found in British waters. Adherent tentacles should be removed with forceps and then a strong solution of sodium bicarbonate applied to the injured area. The stings from other British species of jellyfish, e.g. the lion's mane jellyfish *(Cyanea capillata)*, are also treated with alkaline solutions unlike tropical species (such as the box jellyfish [*Chironex fleckeri*] of Australasia) for which vinegar is an essential first-aid remedy.

Bites and stings from exotic creatures

Exotic pets may inflict exotic bites and stings on their keepers. In addition, world travellers may encounter poisonous insects, spiders, snakes, fish, corals, hydroids, anemones, jellyfish and octopi.

Tx All such wounds must be cleaned thoroughly and then dressed. Tetanus prophylaxis must be ensured. It may occasionally be necessary to give antivenom and it is important that each ED knows where the nearest supply is kept (the *British National Formulary* contains up-to-date telephone numbers of regional depots). In the UK 24-hour help and advice can be obtained from the following centres:

1 The Liverpool School of Tropical Medicine
2 The Hospital for Tropical Diseases in London.

In the case of travellers, expert local advice is essential for both diagnosis and treatment.

Envenoming (especially adder bites) → *p. 291.*
Non-venomous injuries from the spines of sea urchins and other marine creatures → *p. 402.*
Rabies → *p. 253.*

Cutaneous myiasis

Travellers (and military personnel) from tropical regions may present with large red boils with a central aperture through which a living creature is visible. The inhabitant of the cutaneous swelling is a fly larva that has developed from an egg laid (or deposited by a carrier mosquito) in the clothing or bedding of the host. The back and the buttocks are most commonly affected and there may be surrounding inflammation or even cellulitis. (This suggests that the larva is dead because it is unable to survive and develop in inflamed or infected tissue.) The torsalo or human bot fly *(Dermatobia hominis)* is found in Latin America and the tumbu fly *(Cordylobia anthropophaga)* is resident in Africa, Arabia and southern Europe. Tumbu maggots may be partially asphyxiated by the application of petroleum jelly and then squeezed out of their home. Bot fly larvae are more resistant but will usually crawl out of the central punctum of the burrow if 2% lidocaine is injected around and into the swelling (the lidocaine seems to reduce the maggots' ability to grip the sides of their burrows → *Figure 21.2*). No other treatment is required unless there is significant surrounding infection.

Pretibial lacerations

Pretibial lacerations are common in elderly women and often follow comparatively minor trauma. The area has a poor blood supply and little deep tissue to support the skin. Despite this, most pretibial wounds heal well, albeit slowly. More problems can be anticipated with:

- distally based flaps
- very contused flaps
- very elderly patients
- patients with very thin skin or those on steroids.

Tx Most pretibial lacerations should not be sutured – the stitches tear the thin skin. Adhesive strips are ideal but must not be applied until the wound has been adequately cleaned, usually under local anaesthesia. Tension should be avoided when laying back the skin. Blood clots must be removed and the flap laid closely on to a clean bed. A secure non-adherent pressure dressing can then be applied.

The patient should be encouraged to continue ankle movements but to elevate the foot when at rest. Initial follow-up should be arranged for a couple of days post-injury and then as appropriate. Admission for bed rest may be required for frail patients with extensive wounds. In extreme cases, plastic surgical advice may be needed.

Pretibial haematomas

After injury, patients occasionally present with a large tender, pretibial haematoma.

Tx Waiting for this swelling to resolve taxes the patience of both the doctor and the patient. A better

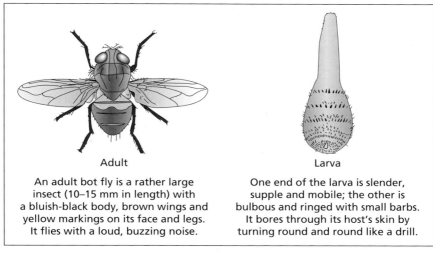

Adult	Larva
An adult bot fly is a rather large insect (10–15 mm in length) with a bluish-black body, brown wings and yellow markings on its face and legs. It flies with a loud, buzzing noise.	One end of the larva is slender, supple and mobile; the other is bulbous and ringed with small barbs. It bores through its host's skin by turning round and round like a drill.

Figure 21.2 The human bot fly and its larva.

outcome may be achieved by draining the blood clot through a surgical incision. Needle aspiration is unlikely to succeed. The mode of anaesthesia for the procedure depends on the patient and the size of the haematoma. Observation in clinic over a few days will help to determine the best form of treatment.

Puncture wounds of the feet

Puncture wounds of the feet are common and often caused by nails, needles and glass. There is usually a tender but unremarkable wound on the sole.

XR Radiographs are indicated for any suspicion of foreign body and with all glass wounds. A retained fragment is common with wounds from a needle and with glass but not when a nail is involved. A skin marker, applied to the skin at the site of entry, will greatly help with localisation on a radiograph.

> Retained foreign bodies can be very difficult to locate, even if they appear superficial on a radiograph.

Tx The wound must be cleaned, an antiseptic dressing applied and antitetanus prophylaxis given if indicated. The patient should be instructed to return if there are any signs of infection.

Foreign bodies must be removed in a suitable environment – usually an operating theatre – by an experienced doctor working in good conditions (fine instruments, a bloodless field and adequate anaesthesia).

Patients returning with obvious infection must be seen by a senior member of staff. Antibiotics, further consideration of the possibility of foreign bodies and follow-up are indicated. Infections in puncture wounds can be very difficult to treat. Exploration of the track and IV antibiotics may be required in some cases.

> *Pseudomonas* sp. likes to live in the damp environment of training shoes and similar footwear.

Nails through hands or feet

It is quite common for a patient to present with a nail protruding from a finger or a foot. The patient should be asked if the nail is from a nail-gun. The nail fired from this tool has two copper barbs on it, which impede withdrawal. Sensation must be assessed before local anaesthesia is administered and then movements assessed after the nail is removed.

XR Initial radiographs can be helpful if there is difficulty removing the nail. Otherwise they should be obtained after removal to look for bony damage.

Tx The nail should be removed under local anaesthesia and the wound protected with an antiseptic dressing. If there is bony damage, antibiotic cover is indicated (flucloxacillin or clarithromycin).

Foreign bodies in the feet or hands

The removal of a foreign body from the palm of the hand or the sole of the foot can be particularly difficult despite often appearing to be easy. It may require:

- a bloodless field and hence a tourniquet
- good anaesthesia, usually general
- skill and experience
- adequate equipment – a metal detector may be helpful.

Management should be discussed with a senior colleague; inpatient care may be required.

Some foreign bodies can be removed in the ED. These will be:

- superficial
- easily palpable
- recently implanted
- discussed with a senior member of staff.

Other foreign bodies

Other foreign bodies (e.g. airgun pellets) need localisation and then a similar consideration given to the mode of removal.

Sea urchin spines

Patients may present with sea urchin spines imbedded in their hands or feet, usually acquired while swimming in the Mediterranean Sea. The dark-brown spines are very friable and so are difficult to remove intact. Softening the skin with either acetone or salicylic acid 2% ointment, applied overnight, may facilitate the process. Analgesia can be achieved with local anaesthetic cream before attempting to remove the larger pieces with a hypodermic needle. Smaller pieces may be scrubbed out with a toothbrush but most of the remaining debris usually ends up being left *in situ*. Fortunately, with appropriate dressings and analgesia, the injury settles down very quickly.

Other spine-bearing marine creatures including stingrays, scorpion fish, stonefish, weever fish, catfish and crown-of-thorns starfish may inflict painful puncture wounds on the unwary. The pain is usually very marked in the case of venomous species. Expert local advice is essential for both diagnosis and treatment.

Envenoming → p. 291.
Stings from weever fish spines → p. 400.

Fish hooks

Fish hooks can be removed under local anaesthesia (ring block or infiltration of lidocaine). The barbed end of the hook should be pushed forwards through the anaesthetised skin and the hook cut in two with K-wire cutters. It can then be withdrawn easily.

Splinters under the nail

Splinters under the nail should be removed under ring block. Attempts may be made with splinter forceps initially but it is often necessary to trim back or remove the nail. Thorns can cause serious infection including tetanus and must be removed.

Subungual collections

Subungual haematomas can be drained by trephining (→ p. 134). This procedure does not introduce infection and thus antibiotics are not required for an associated fracture. Collections of pus under the nail are usually treated by removing the nail under a ring block.

Hair tourniquets around the digits

An infant is sometimes found to have a tight ring of hairs (usually an adult's long thick hairs) wrapped around the base of a finger or toe (this can be the reason for a crying or otherwise distressed child). The hair tourniquet has often eroded deeply into the skin but distal ischaemia is rare. The constricting band of hair must be removed carefully with a stitch cutter, ensuring that no residual hair rings remain buried in the circumferential wound.

Injection injuries to the digits

EpiPen adrenaline injection injuries → p. 129.
High-pressure hose injection injuries → p. 129.
Oil-based veterinary vaccine injection injuries → p. 129.

Blood and body fluid exposure incidents ('needlestick injuries')

Post-exposure prophylaxis after sexual exposure (to blood-borne viruses) (PEPSE) → p. 322.

Both hospital staff and members of the public may present after a needlestick injury or other body fluid exposure incident. Hepatitis B, hepatitis C and HIV are the major blood-borne viruses (BBVs) but several other pathogens may also be transmitted by this route. Exposure incidents include the following:

- Piercing of the skin by any contaminated sharp objects
- Splashes into the eyes with body fluids
- Contamination of broken skin by body fluids
- Significant human bites
- Ingestion by mouth of body fluids.

An assessment of risk must be made. People at a high risk of having (and thus transmitting) BBVs are listed in *Box 21.7*. However, all patients in an ED should be regarded as potential sources of BBVs because some apparently benign groups contain a high number of hepatitis B carriers (e.g. elderly ex-servicemen). Around a third of IV drug abusers in the UK carry hepatitis C but HIV prevalence in this group is still less than 1%. The features of an injury or other incident that increase the risk of transmission of BBVs are listed in *Box 21.8*. The estimated risks of seroconversion are shown in *Table 21.2*. The HIV risk with an unknown source is generally minimal and so patients can be reassured. Hepatitis B is the major problem because transmission can occur with much smaller quantities of blood and with older blood.

Tx Skin punctures should be encouraged to bleed freely. If the eyes are involved, they should be irrigated with water. Wounds must be cleaned and dressed and prophylaxis against tetanus ensured. The patient should be informed of the general risks from BBVs, the risk from this particular incident and the benefits of the proposed treatment. Counselling can be arranged in special situations. In all cases, the patient's GP and occupational health department must be notified of the type and date of the injury, the action taken and any further action or follow-up required.

Unknown source of needle: Send 10 mL unclotted blood from the patient to the Public Health Laboratory Service for storage and possible later testing. (In the unlikely event of seroconversion, this sample can be used to prove that the disease was occupationally acquired.) Ensure protection against hepatitis B → *later and Box 21.9* – but assume the source of the needle to be low risk for this and other BBVs.

Known source of blood or body fluid: Take 10 mL unclotted blood from the patient and the same from

Box 21.7 High-risk sources for transmission of BBVs

- Known carriers of BBVs
- Close family contacts or sexual partners of known carriers of BBVs
- Children of mothers who are known carriers of BBVs
- Homosexual or bisexual people (especially men)
- Intravenous drug abusers
- Workers in the sex industry
- Recent residents of sub-Saharan Africa (and Egypt for hepatitis C virus or HCV)
- People who have had sexual contact or a blood transfusion in sub-Saharan Africa
- Inmates (or past inmates) of custodial institutions
- Residents of enclosed units for people with learning disabilities, including staff
- Health-care workers and trainees (especially from developing countries)
- Morticians, embalmers and tattooists
- Patients on long-term renal dialysis
- Patients with chronic liver infection
- People with haemophilia or others receiving regular blood products, and any relatives responsible for the administration of these products
- Patients with jaundice under investigation

Almost all body fluids should be regarded as high risk. Exceptions (where exposure to the fluid would not justify the risk of post-exposure prophylaxis [PEP]) are: vomitus, saliva, tears, urine and faeces (unless any of these fluids are visibly blood stained).

the person who was the source of the blood or body fluid. Send both samples together to the Public Health Laboratory Service for storage and possible later testing. (In the unlikely event of seroconversion, these samples can be used to prove that the disease was occupationally acquired.) Ensure protection against hepatitis B → *later and Box 21.9*. All cases that involve a known HIV-positive source must be discussed with a consultant virologist who may recommend prophylaxis with zidovudine and other antiretroviral drugs → *Box 21.10*. Treatment with these drugs – ideally started within 2 h of exposure – reduces the transmission rate of HIV by over 70%.

Box 21.8 High-risk exposure incidents for transmission of BBVs

- Percutaneous rather than mucocutaneous exposure (puncture wound rather than splash)
- Exposure to blood rather than blood-stained fluid or any other body fluid
- Injury from hollow-bore rather than solid needle (wider gauge = worse)
- Injury from hollow-bore needle that has directly entered a blood vessel
- Visible blood on the injuring device
- Deep wound rather than shallow abrasion
- No protective equipment used
- Immediate washing and/or bleeding not performed
- Highly infected source (HBV e-antigen [HBeAg] detectable, HCV RNA detectable, HIV high viral load)
- Source terminally ill
- Source infected with more than one blood-borne virus
- Exposed person not immunised

 Box 21.9 Post-exposure prophylaxis against hepatitis B infection

- If immunised within the last 5 years with a known level of antibodies (≥100 U) no further action need be taken
- If more than 5 years have elapsed since immunisation or if the antibody level is low (between 10 and 100 U) give a booster dose of hepatitis B vaccine
- If the antibody status is unknown after a previous course of vaccine, then give a booster dose of hepatitis B vaccine. Assess the risk of the source and the exposure (→ Boxes 21.7 and 21.8) and if high, give hepatitis B immunoglobulin (HBIg) in addition
- If the patient has not been immunised against hepatitis B, then start an accelerated course of hepatitis B vaccine. Assess the risk of the source and the exposure (→ Boxes 21.7 and 21.8) and, if high, give HBIg in addition

Table 21.2 Estimated risks of seroconversion after blood exposure

Infection	Route	Risk (%)
HIV	Mucocutaneous	<0.1
HIV	Percutaneous	0.3
HCV (detectable RNA)	Percutaneous	0.5–1.8
HBV (HBeAg +ve)	Percutaneous	30 (for non-immune individual)

Hepatitis B immunisation

The usual course is three doses of 1 mL (20 mg), the second 1 month and the third 6 months after the first dose. For children (birth up to 12 years) this is reduced to three doses of 0.5 mL (10 mg). The deltoid muscle is the preferred site of injection in adults whereas the anterolateral thigh is used in children. The buttock must not be used because vaccine efficacy may be reduced. An accelerated course of hepatitis B vaccine

 Box 21.10 Post-exposure prophylaxis against HIV infection

The risk of HIV transmission through occupational exposure in health-care workers is approximately 0.3% from a percutaneous injury and <0.1% after mucous membrane exposure. Prophylaxis with drugs reduces the risk of infection by >70%. Triple or quadruple therapy with antiretroviral agents is usually offered to health-care workers after high-risk exposure to body fluids from a HIV-positive source. Drugs include:

1 Zidovudine (AZT) 250 mg twice daily or 200 mg three times daily
2 Lamivudine 150 mg twice daily
3 Nelfinavir 1250 mg twice daily
4 Indinavir 800 mg three times daily

These drugs are continued for 28 days and are not without side effects. Zidovudine and lamivudine are nucleoside reverse transcriptase inhibitors ('nucleoside analogues'). Nelfinavir and indinavir are protease inhibitors.

is the preferred schedule for emergency usage; one dose is given immediately and then two more doses with an interval of 1 month between each injection.

Indications for hepatitis B immunisation in an individual patient → Box 21.9.

Hepatitis B immunoglobulin

Hepatitis B immunoglobulin (HBIg) is usually obtained from the nearest Public Health Laboratory. It must be given as soon as possible after the incident for maximum effect and certainly within 48 h. The dose of HBIg varies with age:

- Age 0–4 years: 200 IU (2 mL)
- Age 5–9 years: 300 IU (3 mL)
- Adults and children aged ≥10: 500 IU (5 mL).

The large volume of HBIg should be given by deep IM injection into the upper outer quadrant of the buttock. Concurrent hepatitis B vaccine should be given into a separate site (e.g. the deltoid area of the upper arm). *Indications for HBIg in an individual patient → Box 21.9.*

> Hepatitis B immunisation should be considered for all IV drug injectors who attend an ED.

LOCALISED INFECTIONS AND INFLAMMATIONS

Hot red joints

Patients may present to an ED with a single acutely inflamed joint. This may be caused by:

- septic arthritis including gonococcal arthritis
- crystal arthropathy (e.g. gout or pseudogout → *below*)
- a bursitis in the area of the joint (→ *pp. 99 and 119 and also bunions → below*)
- a connective tissue disorder (rarely).

Septic arthritis

This is most likely to occur following:

- trauma, often minor
- soft-tissue infection
- osteomyelitis
- a non-septic joint inflammation.

The most common joints to become infected are the interphalangeal joints and the knee. The joint is held in flexion and all movements are restricted by intense pain.

XR Loss of joint space may be seen in septic arthritis. It is apparent early on in small joints. However, a normal radiograph does not exclude infection.

Tx If there is doubt then the patient should be assumed to have a septic arthritis until proved otherwise. Diagnostic joint aspiration is not recommended in the ED. Admission must be arranged under the care of either the orthopaedic or the rheumatology department, as seems most appropriate from the likely underlying pathology.

Acute gout

The first metatarsophalangeal joint is the most common site for acute gout although the knee may sometimes be primarily affected. The patient presents with severe local pain and a red, swollen joint. There is extreme tenderness such that even the weight of the bedclothes can be unbearable. A pyrexia often accompanies the inflammation. Other causes of a painful joint must be excluded.

Tx A wool and crepe bandage is required to protect the joint, together with non-weight-bearing crutches. The inflamed area must be rested and elevated. A makeshift 'cage' to protect a painful foot at night can be made by cutting a hole out of a large cardboard box. Initial analgesia and anti-inflammatory activity is provided by non-steroidal anti-inflammatory drugs (NSAIDs). A first parenteral dose can be very beneficial. In severe cases, an additional short course of oral steroids (prednisolone 30–40 mg a day) gives fast and effective relief.

The patient should be referred back to the GP in order that he or she can:

- assess progress
- measure serum urate
- exclude precipitating causes (full blood count and erythrocyte sedimentation rate [ESR] indicated)
- consider allopurinol therapy.

Bunions

Hallux valgus with varus deformity of the first metatarsal bone causes prominence and osteoarthrosis of the first (big toe) metatarsophalangeal joint. An enlarged bursa develops on its medial aspect – this is termed a 'bunion'. The patient may present to the ED with an acute exacerbation of this chronic condition.

Tx An infected bunion should be treated with oral antibiotics (e.g. flucloxacillin) and the patient advised to consult the GP about an orthopaedic referral.

Osteomyelitis

This diagnosis should always be considered when there is spontaneous or unresolving bony pain. The distal phalanges of the hands and the feet are the most common sites of osteomyelitis in ED patients. There is usually a history of a minor injury, but then pain, swelling and redness persist beyond the expected time of resolution. An accompanying septic arthritis is common. The inflammatory process can be relatively acute or more chronic. The major risk factor for developing osteomyelitis is an immunosuppressive state (such as diabetes mellitus, chronic steroid use, AIDS or alcoholism) and the most commonly isolated pathogen is *Staphylococcus aureus*.

> Bone tumours may masquerade as bone or joint infection.

XR Plain radiographs are the best initial mode of imaging to detect osteomyelitis. After 10–14 days, radiographs show absorption of the underlying bone, giving a characteristic moth-eaten appearance. However, almost 50% of the bone structure must be destroyed before there is detectable radiological lucency. Elevation of the overlying periosteum may also be seen. The neighbouring joint space may be lost if infection has spread to the joint.

Tx All patients with suspected osteomyelitis must be referred to the orthopaedic department immediately. Treatment consists of IV antibiotics and surgical debridement.

Cellulitis

Infection of the skin may arise around a wound or without any obvious port of entry. The patient is usually tired and anorexic with a raised temperature; slight nausea is common. The skin is red, swollen and hot but the degree of pain is variable. A cause should be sought but is usually not found.

Tx Antipyretic analgesics and antibiotics should be prescribed. The infection may be streptococcal or staphylococcal and so a combination of flucloxa-cillin and phenoxymethylpenicillin is appropriate (phenoxymethylpenicillin is probably unnecessary because flucloxacillin has good activity against streptococci). Clarithromycin can be given to patients who are allergic to penicillins. Admission for observation and IV therapy may be required for extensive or progressing infections. Lesser cases can be treated with oral antibiotics at home but should be reviewed within 24–48 h. The limits of the infection should be marked on the skin with a pen so that changes are obvious at review.

Athlete's foot: is a fungal infection, which gives rise to an itchy whitish area between the toes, usually in the space between the middle and the ring toes. It may be the cause of an ascending cellulitis and should always be excluded whenever there is cellulitic infection of the lower leg. Athlete's foot is treated with a topical antifungal cream such as clotrimazole.

Erysipelas

Erysipelas is a type of skin infection that is caused by group A β-haemolytic streptococci *(Streptococcus pyogenes)*. It was formerly known as St Anthony's fire. It differs from cellulitis in several ways:

- The affected skin is fiery-red, swollen, hot, tender and indurated.
- The affected area has raised edges and a sharply demarcated border. Vesicles, bullae and petechiae may occasionally occur.
- There is regional lymphadenopathy and, sometimes, lymphangitis.
- Fever and systemic upset are common (rigors, headaches, nausea and muscle pains). These symptoms may be prodromal.
- It involves the dermis rather than deeper subcutaneous tissues.
- It is caused by streptococci rather than by staphylococci.

Erysipelas targets the face (20%) and the legs (70%), usually in older adults. Immunodeficiency or general ill health predisposes an individual to the condition. Erysipelas is treated with phenoxymethylpenicillin, clarithromycin or clindamycin. The infection recurs in around 25% of patients.

Impetigo

A localised staphylococcal infection of the skin may cause an area of weeping inflammation with a yellow crust. This is impetigo and is a highly infectious condition. It is most commonly seen in children in the area around the mouth but may spread to other parts of the patient or to relatives and medical staff.

Tx All patients should be advised of measures to contain the spread by:

- frequent and appropriate hand washing
- avoidance of contact with the infected area
- using own towel and cutlery, etc.

An anti-staphylococcal cream should be prescribed (e.g. mupirocin or fusidic acid). Severe cases or those with systemic upset will need oral flucloxacillin.

Herpes simplex infections

Herpes simplex may cause painful yellow blisters with surrounding inflammation on the fingers or face. There is often accompanying malaise, pyrexia and enlargement of related lymph nodes. Treatment is symptomatic – hygiene, dressings, analgesia and flucloxacillin for superadded infection. However, extensive gingivostomatitis in distressed children may necessitate admission.

Large abscesses

A great variety of large abscesses is inevitably seen in patients presenting to an ED. Among the most common types are found in the following areas:

- Axillary – often loculated and may be recurrent
- Breast → p. 323
- Perianal → p. 326
- Pilonidal → p. 326
- Gluteal → p. 326
- Labial → p. 323.

These painful and distressing conditions should be treated under general anaesthesia in the privacy of an operating theatre. Recurrent abscesses of the groin, perineum and axilla may be a result of hidradenitis suppurativa – a condition of unknown aetiology that leads to blockage and infection of apocrine sweat glands. There may be local fistulae and skin tags. The problem is treated by excision of all the surrounding hair-bearing skin and its related apocrine glands.

Boils (furuncles)

A boil is an abscess arising from a hair follicle. The problem may be multiple or recurrent.

Tx Small abscesses in appropriate sites in adults may be drained in the ED under local anaesthesia. Others need inpatient care.

Most abscesses should be drained with an incision along the lines of cleavage of the skin. In the limbs, a longitudinal incision is more appropriate to avoid damage to nerves, vessels and tendons. A surprising amount of lidocaine may be needed to achieve adequate anaesthesia for this procedure. The cavity should then be cleaned out and a ribbon coated with antiseptic inserted. This stops any bleeding and allows free drainage (the cavity should not be packed too tightly because this impairs both drainage and healing). A dressing should be applied over the whole area.

The patient will require oral analgesics to take out. The wound should be reviewed on the following day and the dressing changed.

Infected sebaceous cysts

Sebaceous cysts may become infected and painful. The resulting tender, red lump may be distinguished from a boil by:

- the history of a pre-existing swelling
- the site (cysts are common in certain areas such as the back and the neck)
- the presence of a central punctum (only sometimes visible)
- the contents of the swelling (white, cheesy material).

Tx In the early stages of infection, the inflamed cyst may respond to antibiotics (e.g. co-fluampicil). However, incision and drainage are often necessary and management is then identical to that detailed above for a boil. Sometimes an infected sebaceous cyst will disappear after discharging its contents but often the wall will need surgical removal at a later date.

Carbuncles

A carbuncle is a deep multiloculated infection of the skin, which involves a group of hair follicles. It has several openings, each of which discharges pus. The patient is often a middle-aged man and the most common site is the back of the neck. The infection is painful and slow to settle; it may become chronic or recurrent.

Tx The area should be cleaned and then pus gently extruded. Debridement or deroofing under local anaesthesia may be required. The patient will need oral antibiotics (e.g. flucloxacillin) and analgesia to take out. The carbuncle must be reviewed and frequent dressing changes arranged; this may be undertaken at the local health centre.

Skin lesions acquired from animals (zoonoses)

Orf begins as painless vesicles, which progress to red nodules with sunken centres containing pus. The lesions then gradually discolour, crust and heal. No specific treatment is required. The causative virus is acquired from sheep and goats.

Cutaneous anthrax starts as a small vesicle, which becomes purulent. A painless skin lesion then develops at the site with a black eschar and a considerable amount of surrounding oedema and induration. Anthrax can be an occupational disease of people who work with large herbivorous mammals or their hide products, but has also been spread by terrorist action. If inhaled, the spores of *Bacillus anthracis* cause a haemorrhagic pneumonia and septicaemia. Anthrax is a notifiable disease.

Systemic anthrax → p. 257.

Anthrax should be considered as a possibility in IV drug users with severe soft-tissue infections or other sepsis including meningitis.

Tularaemia presents as pyrexia and indurated skin ulcers with lymphadenopathy. It is transmitted to humans by close contact with rabbits. Tularaemia is not endemic in the UK, but occurs in Scandinavia, eastern Europe and the USA. If inhaled, *Francisella tularensis* may cause a plague-like pneumonia.

Other skin lesions

Patients with an enormous variety of other skin lesions present to an ED over the years. Their detailed description is beyond the scope of this book. However, four lesions cause confusion more often than most:

1 **Erythema nodosum:** the characteristic fiery-red, infiltrated lesions of erythema nodosum are seen on the knees, shins and forearms. They are very tender with an ill-defined border. Bruising may occur. Erythema nodosum is sometimes mistaken for an allergic reaction; larger patches may look like cellulitis. The condition is a reactive vasculitis to systemic diseases, infections and drugs. A recent streptococcal illness is by far the most common precipitant.

2 **Acute guttate psoriasis:** this is most common in children and adolescents. A shower of small, round, erythematous papules appears 1–3 weeks after an infection (usually streptococcal in nature). It is thought that streptococcal superantigens may resemble an antigen on keratinocytes. Crops of papules appear over about 2 weeks and soon develop characteristic psoriatic scaling. The lesions are most prominent on the trunk but may also affect the scalp, face and limbs. The rash settles slowly over several weeks and is often mistaken for a reaction to antibiotics.

3 **Pityriasis rosea:** this self-limiting benign illness occurs in clusters in spring and autumn and is most common in women aged 15–40 years. A primary plaque (the 'herald' patch) first appears, usually under the costal margin. It is oval shaped, 1–2 cm in diameter and salmon coloured with a dark-red periphery. The two areas are separated by a fine, scaly ring. This primary lesion is sometimes accompanied by vague prodromal symptoms and is followed after 3–21 days by a distinctive rash that appears in crops following the lines of cleavage of the skin. The secondary lesions are smaller than the herald patch but similar in appearance. They are distributed symmetrically on the truck, neck and proximal limbs, and last for between 2 and 6 weeks. There is a variable amount of pruritis. Despite the clustering of contacts, no causative agent has ever been identified. No treatment is required other than reassurance.

4 **Lichen planus:** this dermatosis of uncertain aetiology is encountered far more frequently in MRCP examinations than in reality. Shiny pink papules appear on the wrists, shins and lumbosacral area, often with involvement of the mucous membranes. Itching is a variable feature. The rash can look non-specific with an atypical distribution and so often gives rise to confusion. Treatment is aimed at controlling the itching with steroid creams and calamine lotion.

Common rashes of childhood → p. 346.

Paronychial infections

Infections around the nailfolds of the fingers are a common cause of presentation to an ED.

Tx Occasionally, the infection can be treated with antibiotics (e.g. flucloxacillin). More usually an abscess has formed, which requires drainage rather than antibiotics. The finger should be ring blocked and a longitudinal incision made into the abscess such that the cut extends across the nailfold (→ *Figure 21.3*). An antiseptic dressing is then applied and changed on the following day.

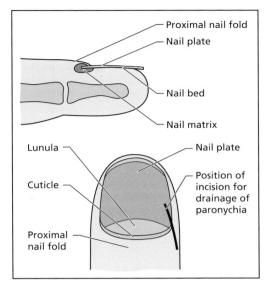

Figure 21.3 Direction of incision for paronychia. Divide the nailfold (but not the nail!).

Ingrowing toenails

This paronychial infection of the big toe commonly presents to an ED. The area alongside the distal toenail is red and tender. There may be a yellow exudate and, in chronic cases, tissue granulation.

Tx Local policy varies according to the availability of chiropody services. A chiropodist will usually perform a wedge resection of the side of the nail and give advice on foot care. Recurrent cases should have the germinal matrix of the nail destroyed with phenol.

In the absence of a chiropodist, severe infection is best treated by removal of the entire nail under ring block. The patient then requires an antiseptic dressing, crutches and analgesia. He or she must be told to rest and elevate the foot. The dressing should be changed on the following day.

Frostbite

Cold injury is most likely to affect peripheral exposed parts such as fingers and toes and is not only seen in extreme climates. The frostbitten area is initially pale and extremely painful but, if exposure continues, the pain subsides. On re-warming, there is erythema, oedema and blistering and eventually a line of demarcation will appear at the junction with the undamaged tissue.

Tx Analgesia should be given (together with IV fluids if more than fingers or toes are involved). Rapid rewarming of acute cases is achieved by total immersion of the affected part in warm water. The degree of permanent damage cannot be assessed when first seen and so admission for observation may be indicated.

Trench foot

This is a similar condition where tissue damage and maceration result from prolonged contact with cold, wet, muddy footwear. Treatment follows the same principles.

Wanderer's foot

No discussion of foot problems in a textbook of emergency medicine would be complete without a mention of this condition. The patient presents with macerated soles of the feet that are causing pain while walking. The shoes and socks are usually in poor condition and extremely smelly. There may be a history of homelessness and prolonged walking.

Tx The feet should be washed and then soaked in antiseptic for an hour. Blisters should be slit open and any obvious infection treated. Crutches may be needed. Definitive treatment necessitates a place to stay so as to rest and bathe. New footwear may be required.

Homelessness → p. 14.

Scabies

Infestation by the scabies mite causes intense itching, which is worse at night. Other close contacts may be affected.

If it itches, think of scabies.

At first, the mites affect only the areas where they burrow – between the fingers, wrists, genitalia, buttocks, axillae, waistline and the soles of the feet in children. Small linear tracks of papules may be the only evidence. Later, a sensitivity reaction to the mite causes a widespread papular eruption.

Tx Malathion 0.5% aqueous lotion is applied to all areas of the body including the head and the face. It is left to dry naturally and then washed off after 24 h. Only one application is necessary provided that all areas are covered (e.g. the web spaces and under the fingernails). This will eradicate scabies in around 75% of cases. For those with persistent symptoms, a second application after 1 week is recommended. Permethrin 5% cream is a more expensive – and possibly more effective – alternative. It is applied to the whole body, washed off after 8–12 h and then reapplied after a week. The whole family and any close contacts must be treated, whether or not they have a rash; the GP should be asked to coordinate this. An oral sedative antihistamine may be required at night to control the itching.

Ophthalmic, ENT and facial conditions

THE EYES

Ophthalmic problems account for over 5% of all emergency department (ED) attendances.

Assessment of the eye

- Obtain an accurate history.
- Ask about vision.
- Test the visual acuity ($\rightarrow$ *Box 22.1*).
- Examine the eye with a pen torch looking for redness, discharge and other gross abnormalities. Look also for asymmetry and irregularity of the pupils.
- Note the pupillary response to direct light. Switch on the light after it has been placed in front of the eye. This is more likely to detect a small pupillary response than the more usual method of moving a light across the front of the eye.
- Test the cross-pupil reflex. When the damaged eye is illuminated, absence of pupil constriction in the opposite eye indicates interruption of the visual pathway.
- Assess ocular movements, noting any diplopia, visual fields and eyelid movements.

In the presence of blepharospasm (inability to open the eyes), further examination may require the application of local anaesthetic eyedrops, e.g. tetracaine (amethocaine) 1% or oxybuprocaine 0.4%.

- Evert the eyelids to allow examination of the fornices.

- Instil orange-coloured fluorescein drops to highlight any corneal damage – the injured epithelium appears green. A blue light makes a shallow pool of fluorescein much more easily visible.
- Examine the eye systematically from front to back using a slit-lamp and an ophthalmoscope. This may sometimes necessitate the administration of a short-acting mydriatic (a drug that dilates the pupil) such as tropicamide.

The anterior chamber may contain blood, which collects inferiorly in the erect patient to produce a fluid level. This haemorrhage is called a hyphaema ($\rightarrow$ *Figure 22.1*). Damage to the lens or pupillary muscle will result in irregularities in the shape of the iris and disorganised or absent constriction to light. A laceration through the cornea will allow aqueous humour, muscle and even part of the lens to herniate anteriorly. Vitreous humour may be opacified by bleeding and the fundus thereby totally obscured.

> Whenever local anaesthetic has been applied to the conjunctival sac in the ED, it is advisable to pad the eye for protection for a few hours.

Corneal abrasions

Corneal abrasions may result from a scratch or other injury to the eye. Sometimes they follow prolonged rubbing of an irritating eye:

Emergency Medicine Lecture Notes, Fourth Edition. Chris Moulton and David Yates.
© 2012 Blackwell Publishing Ltd. Published 2012 by Blackwell Publishing Ltd.

Box 22.1 How to test visual acuity

Test each eye separately with patient wearing normal spectacles.

Acuity equation = Distance from eye to print in metres/Number adjacent to smallest line of print readable on chart

- Snellen letter chart is 6 m in front of patient (or equivalent distance using a mirror)
- Largest print on top line is usually 60
- Smallest print on bottom line is usually 5
- A patient with normal acuity can read down to line 6 and has '6/6' vision
- With excellent acuity this may be '6/5' vision
- A patient who cannot read the top line has vision 'worse than 6/60'
- If the test is repeated at 3 m and the top line can now be read, vision is '3/60'
- The bigger the fraction, the better the vision

Additional information can be obtained by asking the patient to look at the chart through a pinhole. This improves vision in patients with a refractive or corneal abnormality but worsens vision in those with macular problems.

 Box 22.2 Padding an eye

- A single pad will not keep an eye closed
- To apply a double pad, fold one pad in half and place it over the closed eyelids. Place a second, flat pad over the first and secure it in place with three pieces of tape
- The patient must be advised not to drive. Monocular vision impairs judgement of speed and distance. Patients who intend to drive (without a pad) must be instructed on how to apply the pads at home
- If both eyes require pads, leave this until the patient is at home
- All patients require spare pads and tape to take away

Never give a patient local anaesthetic drops for outpatient use. They impede epithelial healing and invite additional injury. Similarly, non-steroidal anti-inflammatory drug (NSAID) drops or ointment is very effective at relieving pain but has the same effect on the corneal epithelium as oral NSAIDs have on the gastric mucosa.

- The eye is red, injected, painful and watering.
- There is often pronounced blepharospasm (spasm of the eyelids).
- There may be a sensation of a foreign body.

Tx A foreign body must be excluded, especially a subtarsal one (→ *below*). The patient then requires the following:

- Dilatation of the pupil of the affected eye with a medium-duration mydriatic (e.g. cyclopentolate)
- Antibiotic ointment or viscous drops (e.g. fusidic acid) – three times a day for 3 days is sufficient and also easy to remember. The first dose should be instilled in the ED
- A firm eyepad overnight (→ *Box 22.2*)
- Instructions not to drive or operate machinery
- Either a review appointment or instructions to return if there is not a marked improvement within 24 h.

Most abrasions heal spontaneously within 2 days. Remember to check tetanus immunisation status.

Contact lens abrasions

Contact lens wearers may present with bilateral, large, shallow abrasions. There is often a history of prolonged use of hard lenses in a hot, dry, smoky atmosphere such as a nightclub.

Tx This is similar to the treatment for any other abrasion but is complicated by the fact that the lesions affect both eyes. Bilateral pads leave the patient without vision and can be deferred until safely home. Glasses should be used instead of contact lenses for at least a week. The patient should be advised to get a supply of artificial teardrops to lubricate the eyes whenever they are in similar circumstances to those in which the problem occurred.

Subtarsal foreign body

Foreign material may lodge in the conjunctival sac. There is an anatomical trap under the upper eyelid. The signs are those of corneal damage:

- The eye is red, injected and watering.
- There is pain and blepharospasm.

- There is a marked foreign body sensation.
- There is increased discomfort on blinking (but small children may keep their eyes tightly shut for relief).
- Linear scratches to the superior cornea are extremely suggestive of a subtarsal foreign body.

Tx Evert the eyelid, remove any foreign material, swab the tarsal conjunctiva and then treat as for a corneal abrasion. Local anaesthesia should be avoided if possible because the pain and foreign body sensation are dramatically relieved by the removal of the offending particles – a useful confirmation of the diagnosis.

Superficial foreign bodies imbedded in the eye

Fragments may fly into the eye while working (e.g. grinding) or may be blown in by the wind:

- The patient complains of a red, painful, watering eye.
- There is marked blepharospasm (it may be necessary to instil local anaesthetic drops before the eyelids can even be opened satisfactorily).
- The eye is injected and vision may be slightly blurred.

Always consider the possibility of deeper damage with higher-velocity injuries (→ *below*).

Tx Superficial fragments may be removed from the anaesthetised cornea using a cotton bud or a hypodermic needle. The resulting corneal ulcer should then be treated in the same way as a corneal abrasion.
Rust rings: metallic, ferrous, foreign bodies produce rust rings if left in the cornea for more than a few hours. If the rust is not removed completely, the patient should be reviewed at the eye clinic after 48h when the softened area of damage will easily 'shell out'.

'Arc' eye

This occurs in a welder, skier or ultraviolet sunbather with inadequate eye protection. The condition is caused by corneal absorption of ultraviolet light. Problems usually start several hours after exposure:

- Both eyes may be affected.
- The eyes are painful, weeping and red.
- There is usually blepharospasm and a sensation of a foreign body.
- Fluorescein may reveal multiple tiny corneal erosions.

Tx Symptoms can be relieved by the instillation of local anaesthetic and dilatation of the pupil. The patient is then given topical antibiotics and an eye pad. The condition should settle within 48h.

Chemical splashes

Chemicals may cause inflammation of the conjunctiva or even a corneal burn. Patients present with an irritant or painful, watery, red eye. Alkalis may cause a penetrating eye injury.

Tx Irrigate the eye with copious amounts of saline. This is best achieved by emptying a 500-mL bag into the conjunctival sac through a standard giving set or by using a purpose-built irrigator. Ensure that both fornices are thoroughly washed and remove any lime or other fragments. Fluorescein drops will help reveal the extent of the damage. Antibiotic ointment should then be prescribed. Serious injuries must be referred to an ophthalmologist immediately.

Penetrating injuries to the eye

Deep, foreign bodies are difficult to identify, produce greater morbidity and yet, initially, may not be as painful as superficial lesions. A good history is essential. There is a high risk of intraocular damage in patients with eye pain who have worked with:

- a hammer and chisel
- glass
- machinery that emits high-speed fragments
- high-pressure water jets.

Fragments from grinding wheels rarely cause eye perforation.

The presence of hyphaema or prolapse of intraocular contents indicates severe injury, as does distortion of the pupil. Retained ferrous fragments will cause blindness because they are neurotoxic.

> The degree of pain that follows ocular trauma is not a reliable indicator of the severity of the injury.

XR Fluorescein-aided corneal examination is followed by radiology of the eye. Lateral views with the eye looking up and down (so that the foreign body appears to move) are particularly helpful in distinguishing foreign bodies from the normal bone pattern and from specks on the film.

Tx Immediate specialist referral is essential but acuity should be assessed first and an eye pad applied. Pressure on the eyeball and coughing and straining by the patient must be avoided for fear of dislodging intraocular structures.

Severe blunt trauma to the eye

Damage to the globe of the eye most commonly results from sports injuries and assaults. Squash balls are particularly dangerous in this respect because they are small enough to enter the eye socket. Urgent ophthalmic referral is required in all cases. Pressure on the eyeball and coughing and straining by the patient must be avoided for fear of dislodging intraocular structures.

Hyphaema: blood in the anterior chamber is caused by rupture of internal blood vessels (→ *Figure 22.1*). The patient is at risk of acute (secondary) glaucoma and requires bed rest and observation. A hyphaema may occasionally be accompanied by iridodialysis – rupture of the insertion of the iris.

Traumatic mydriasis: fixed dilatation of the pupil is a relatively common observation after blunt injury. The pupil may be distorted. Mydriasis is sometimes permanent. Traumatic miosis (constriction of the pupil) may also occur.

Dislocation of the lens: this is uncommon, although trauma is the most common cause. Cataract may also occur.

Posterior segment injuries: the best sign of this type of trauma is a sudden reduction in visual acuity. Injuries include vitreous haemorrhage and retinal damage such as tears, haemorrhage and detachment.

Choroidal rupture and even globe rupture are occasionally seen.

Tx The presence of any of the above conditions is an indication for an urgent ophthalmic opinion.

Blow-out fractures of the floor of the orbit → p. 71.

Subconjunctival haemorrhage

Post-traumatic subconjunctival haemorrhage is common and usually trivial. Fluorescein may be used to reveal any conjunctival lacerations. Failure to visualise the posterior border of the haemorrhage may suggest orbital or retro-orbital trauma.

Spontaneous subconjunctival haemorrhage may follow coughing or straining. It is alarming to the patient but is usually of no consequence. Hypertension should be excluded.

Tx No specific treatment is required but the patient should be warned that the discoloration may take several weeks to resolve.

- Topical anaesthetics inhibit epithelial healing and protective ocular reflexes
- Topical steroids may exacerbate herpes infections or precipitate glaucoma

---

Assessment of the red eye

In the absence of a history of trauma, the cause of a red eye can be difficult to determine. Key observations are shown in *Box 22.3*. Minor trauma is the most common cause of a red eye in the ED.

** Box 22.3 Assessment of the acute red eye: key observations to help in diagnosis**

- Is the problem bilateral?
- Is there any associated visual loss?
- Is there a sensation of a foreign body?
- Is the eye uncomfortable and irritating or is it painful?
- Are the eyelids puffy or the conjunctiva oedematous?
- Is there any photophobia?
- Is the pupil irregular, dilated or unreactive?

Fluid level

Figure 22.1 Hyphaema – blood in the anterior chamber of the eye.

Infective conjunctivitis

This may be caused by several different agents:

- It is often bilateral.
- The eye is red, injected and uncomfortable with a gritty feeling.

Bacteria cause the classic, sticky eye, which is worse on waking.

Viral conjunctivitis results in itchy, watery eyes. There may be a concurrent upper respiratory tract infection (URTI). Injected follicular swelling in the lower fornix and a preauricular lymph node are characteristic findings

Adenovirus causes a painful, puffy, watery red eye. The condition is slow to resolve and very infectious.

Tx As it may be difficult to differentiate between the types of infectious conjunctivitis, it is usual practice to treat them all with a topical antibiotic (e.g. chloramphenicol ointment or gentamicin eyedrops).

> Ocular conditions that have not significantly improved after 24 h merit a specialist opinion.

Allergic conjunctivitis

This is caused by exposure to eyedrops, plants or other allergens, and is associated with atopy. Chloramphenicol, neomycin and atropine are the most common drug offenders:

- It is the most common cause of a puffy, red eye.
- There is lid swelling and conjunctival oedema (chemosis).
- It is irritating but not painful.

Tx Remove the offending substance. Eyedrops containing a vasoconstrictor and an antihistamine (e.g. Otrivine–Antistin drops) may be helpful.

Acute conjunctival oedema

Acute conjunctival oedema is sometimes seen without other signs of allergy, especially in children. The conjunctiva may balloon out of the lower fornix in a very alarming way.

Tx Local application of vasoconstrictor drops may be dramatically effective (→ *before*).

Episcleritis

This condition is idiopathic and self-limiting:

- It is uncomfortable and may be painful.
- A discrete area of conjunctiva is injected and swollen.

Tx Ophthalmological referral is required. NSAIDs can be helpful.

Orbital cellulitis

This is most common in young children and arises from an infection of an adjacent sinus or eyelid. There may be a history of a URTI:

- The eye is red and the eyelids are puffy.
- Swelling may be painless at first but within hours there is pain, fever and distress.

Tx Admission and treatment with intravenous (IV) antibiotics is required. Referral may be made to an ENT (ear, nose and throat) surgeon, ophthalmologist or paediatrician, as suggested by the most likely origin of the infection and local policy.

Corneal ulcers (keratitis)

Dendritic ulcers: these are caused by herpes simplex infection of the cornea:

- The eye is red and photophobic.
- There may be a foreign body sensation.
- There is a branching ulcer that stains with fluorescein.

Referral and therapy with aciclovir is required. Inappropriate steroid therapy can lead to corneal destruction and the need for a graft.

Bacterial corneal ulcers: these may occur in patients with chronic corneal disease or corneal exposure as a result of lid disorders:

- The eye is red and painful.
- There is an intracorneal opacity.

The patient should be referred without antibiotic prescription.

Uveitis (iritis)

This is an idiopathic inflammation of the anterior intraocular structures. It is often recurrent and in young adults may be associated with ankylosing spondylitis. There is:

- a red and painful eye with circumcorneal injection

- tenderness of the eye
- photophobia
- adhesions between the pupillary margin and the lens (synechiae), which may cause irregular dilatation of the pupil
- a haze over the cornea, especially the lower half.

Tx Local anaesthesia does not relieve symptoms; mydriasis may help. Urgent referral to an ophthalmologist is required.

Glaucoma

Acute angle-closure glaucoma is a disease of the over-40s and especially elderly people. It is associated with severe long-sightedness. Impaired outflow of aqueous humour from the anterior chamber of the eye causes raised intraocular pressure. Clinical features include the following:

- A red, painful eye, which is injected and tender and feels hard on palpation through the lid
- Visual loss, with the appearance of haloes around lights
- A semi-dilated, ovoid pupil, which does not react to direct or consensual light stimuli
- Corneal haze caused by oedema
- Malaise, nausea and vomiting.

Tx Immediate ophthalmic referral is essential. Discuss initial treatment that may include the following:

- Parenteral analgesics and antiemetics
- Pilocarpine eyedrops every 5 min for up to an hour
- Acetazolamide 500 mg orally or by slow IV injection
- Mannitol 20% (up to 500 mL) by slow IV infusion.

Recurrent corneal erosion

There is usually a history of a previous minor corneal injury. The patient describes a sharp discomfort on waking that settles after a few hours and then worsens over a few days. The signs are those of corneal damage.

Tx Referral and lubricating eye ointment at night for several months.

Marginal keratitis

This is a recurrent condition. There is:

- a red, injected eye
- photophobia

- a sensation of a foreign body within the eye
- small, white patches within the cornea, close to the limbus, which do not stain well with fluorescein. These are sterile inflammatory infiltrates.

Tx Referral to the next eye clinic.

The eyelids

Injuries → p. 71.

Blepharospasm

Spasm of the muscles that close the eye should immediately suggest an underlying problem, such as a corneal abrasion. The application of local anaesthetic drops through the narrow palpebral fissure will usually result in relaxation after a few minutes. The eye can then be examined properly.

Blepharitis

Inflammation of the eyelids should be treated with a topical antibiotic and advice on bathing the eyelids.

Lumps on the eyelids

Small cystic swellings of the eyelid glands are common (meibomian cysts or chalazia). They may become inflamed. The patient should be given a topical antibiotic ointment and referred to the ophthalmology outpatient clinic.

Sudden loss of vision

Sudden visual loss is distressing for the patient as he or she fears that it will herald permanent blindness.

Retinal detachment

- Visual loss often described as 'like a curtain'
- Sensation of flashing lights
- Detached retina appears dark through an ophthalmoscope
- Associated with severe short-sightedness.

Retinal venous occlusion

- Sudden visual loss of varying degrees
- Congested, haemorrhagic retina
- May only involve one tributary of the retinal vein and hence one quadrant of the retina
- Increasing incidence with age
- More common than arterial occlusion.

Retinal arterial occlusion

- Acute, unilateral, visual loss
- Pale, ischaemic retina with a 'cherry-red spot' at the macula and a swollen optic disc
- May be associated with temporal arteritis (need for urgent erythrocyte sedimentation rate [ESR]) → p. 225
- Pressure on the globe may dislodge the obstruction, which can be thrombus or embolus
- After about an hour, optic nerve atrophy will result in permanent blindness.

Amaurosis fugax

- Visual loss with the same mechanism and associations as a transient ischaemic attack of other regions of the brain → p. 229
- Often wrongly diagnosed in place of the previously cited conditions.

Vitreous haemorrhage

- Occurs in people with diabetes who have new vessel formation
- Absent red reflex/retina cannot be visualised.

Macular disease

- Sudden visual reduction with distortion
- May be related to diabetes or other ocular pathology
- May need urgent laser photocoagulation.

Cortical blindness

This worrying condition may follow a head injury and may persist for several hours → p. 45.

Migraine

This may cause visual distortion or field defects → p. 226.

Tx All patients with acute visual loss require an immediate ophthalmological opinion. Thrombolysis (with streptokinase) may be recommended for central retinal venous or arterial thrombosis.

THE EARS

Barotrauma → p. 236.
Haemotympanum and bleeding from the ear canal → p. 43.
Injuries to the pinna → p. 71.
URTI in children → p. 346.

Earache

Pain in the ear is distressing for both adults and children. Examination of the canal and drum will usually differentiate between otitis media and otitis externa, although the presence of a discharge may make the distinction more difficult. Pain following pressure on the tragus or gentle otoscopy strongly suggests that the canal is inflamed. Pus in the meatus usually comes from the middle ear via a ruptured tympanum, although a boil in the canal may also leak pus.

Tx Otitis media should be treated with analgesic antipyretics and amoxicillin (or clarithromycin). Some patients will require stronger analgesia (e.g. an injectable NSAID). Tympanic rupture should be reviewed after 2 weeks (GP or ENT follow-up). Otitis externa is treated with drops containing both an antibiotic and an anti-inflammatory steroid (e.g. gentamicin and hydrocortisone). Oral flucloxacillin should also be prescribed. The inflamed ear must be kept clean and dry. Patients with debris in the canal should be referred for aural toilet.

Rupture of the tympanum

Rupture of the tympanic membrane can occur in a wide variety of conditions, some with pain and bleeding and some without:

- *Infection*: otitis media, mostly in children → *above*
- *Direct trauma*: in adults and children who have been poking something in their auditory canal
- *Indirect trauma*: usually a slap to the pinna that sends a pressure wave down the auditory canal; this may occur in domestic violence → p. 372
- *Barotrauma*: diving or air travel in susceptible individuals → p. 236
- *Blast injury*: a primary injury from blast overpressure (shock) waves → p. 30
- *Lightning strike or other high-voltage shock*: often bilateral rupture → p. 144
- *Fracture of the base of the skull*: more commonly a haemotympanum occurs → p. 43.

Tx Management of the underlying cause is essential. Some degree of hearing loss is inevitable after damage to the eardrum and ENT follow-up is usually advisable.

Problems with earrings

Earlobe piercing may introduce infection, including serum hepatitis, but more often it causes problems because of inadequate hygiene in the postoperative period. Not uncommonly, a patient complains of a lost 'butterfly' – the rolled clip used to secure the stud or 'sleeper'. The missing metal can be felt embedded in the inflamed earlobe.

Tx The earlobe should be anaesthetised by slowly injecting it with 1–2 mL lidocaine 2% without adrenaline.

> Do not inject local anaesthetic solutions containing adrenaline into the ear or nose.

The foreign body can then be easily and painlessly removed from behind using splinter forceps. The area should be treated with a local antiseptic.

Foreign bodies in the ear

Patients may present acutely with a missing foreign body or chronically with a discharging ear. In an adult, the lost object is usually the tip of a cotton bud; in a child, more variety can be expected!

Tx The ear should be examined gently but no attempt made to remove anything but the most superficial objects in a struggling child. Loops can be used as can Hartmann's 'crocodile' forceps and wax hooks. Syringing is another option (→ *Box 22.4*). The method used depends on personal experience, although attempts to remove foreign bodies lying close to the eardrum should be limited to syringing only. If removal is unsuccessful, referral should be arranged to the next ENT clinic. A slight delay before removal is not important but inexpert manipulation, with inadequate instruments, a poor light and a struggling child can produce major injuries to the tympanic membrane. The chronically discharging ear should also be seen in the ENT clinic.

Insects can crawl or fly into the auditory canal where their movements cause great distress. Before removal, they can be killed by pouring olive oil into the canal or paralysed by instilling 2% lidocaine.

Sudden hearing loss

Sudden hearing loss is commonly caused by the movement of accumulated wax in the external auditory canal. This causes an obstructive type of deafness. Wax can be removed by syringing, a procedure usually performed at the local health centre. The removal can be eased, and the patient helped, by

Box 22.4 How to syringe an ear (→ *Figure 22.2*)

- Ask about past history (e.g. known perforation). A strong jet of water may perforate a scarred drum
- Warm some 0.9% sodium chloride solution to 38°C. Temperature deviation of any significance from core temperature may cause profound vertigo
- Examine the canal with an auroscope
- Drape the patient with towels and position the ear tank or similar receptacle. An assistant is usually necessary
- Straighten the canal by pulling the pinna upwards and backwards
- A manual or, preferably, a pulsed electric ear syringe should be used. Direct the water jet upwards and backwards along the roof of the canal, aiming for the patient's occiput not the eardrum
- Stop immediately if the patient complains of pain or vertigo or if there is any bleeding
- During the procedure, re-examine the canal periodically
- Mop away excess fluid afterwards

Figure 22.2 Direction of fluid stream to wash out an aural foreign body.

recommending the purchase of drops to loosen the wax (e.g. Exterol).

Sudden hearing loss of the sensorineural type is an indication for urgent ENT referral. Occasionally, it may be caused by a cerebrovascular accident.

THE NOSE

Nasal foreign bodies

These usually accompany small children and anxious patients. If superficial they can be removed in the ED but often they are deep and surrounded by crusty exudate, having been in place for some days. There may be a purulent discharge.

> Unilateral nasal discharge in a small child is usually caused by a retained foreign body, even if this history is denied.

Tx Try occluding the unblocked nostril with gentle alar pressure and getting the child to blow with his or her mouth closed. This is often successful. An alternative is to suck the object out with a Yankauer sucker with the side holes taped up. If these measures fail, early specialist referral is recommended. Inexpert probing with forceps or artery clips may push the object further back and cause airway obstruction. Any forceps used for even proximal removal should be of the Tilley type with a parallel blade, which will not apply a force in a backward direction.

Epistaxis

Epistaxis is common and affects most people at some time in their lives. Arterial bleeding from Little's area on the anterior wall of the nasal septum is responsible for around 90% of epistaxis in adults. However, in children, nasal bleeding usually comes from the retrocolumellar vein and follows infection or trauma (with a finger). Only 10% of nosebleeds are posterior but they can be very severe and appear to be bilateral. Clotting disorders including drug therapy and telangiectasia must be considered in all patients. Epistaxis can be associated with regular excessive consumption of alcohol and hypertension. The blood pressure should be measured.

> Pressure to stop a nosebleed should be applied by firmly squeezing the soft part of the nose between the fingers. The most common reasons for failure are misplaced compression over the nasal bones and lack of constant pressure.

Tx
- Attempt to arrest haemorrhage with alar pressure. A swimmer's nose clip can be used for this purpose.
- Resuscitate if necessary (IV fluids).
- Consider the need for cross-match, full blood count (FBC) and clotting studies. FBC and cross-match are required only with prolonged bleeding and where admission is anticipated. Clotting studies are indicated only when there is a history of a bleeding disorder or liver disease, when the patient is taking anticoagulants or with very prolonged bleeding.
- Cauterisation with silver nitrate can be useful for small anterior bleeds.
- Anterior bleeding may also be limited by a wet nasal tampon or a pack (→ *Figure 22.3*). A hydrocolloid gel balloon tampon (e.g. the 'Rapid Rhino') is ideal. It is comfortable for the patient and excellent at achieving haemostasis by both platelet aggregation and direct tamponade.
- Bleeding from a more posterior site can be controlled by the careful insertion and inflation of a balloon catheter (→ *Figure 22.4*). However, long (7-cm) hydrocolloid gel balloon tampons are now available that are both effective and comfortable for the patient.
- Antiseptic cream (e.g. Naseptin) should be prescribed to prevent recurrent bleeding, especially in children.

Urgent ENT referral is required for severe nasal bleeding of any causation. Recurrent epistaxis merits follow-up in the ENT clinic. Patients who have been seen earlier in the ED and who then return with a further episode of epistaxis are also best discussed with an ENT surgeon.

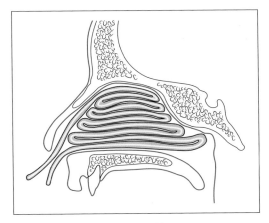

Figure 22.3 Anterior nasal packing.

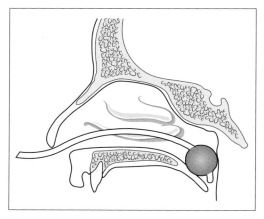

Figure 22.4 Foley catheter in the nasopharynx.

THE MOUTH AND THE THROAT

Management of choking → p. 196.
Other airway obstruction, including foreign bodies →
* p. 201.*

Small foreign bodies stuck in the throat

Patients commonly complain of a foreign body stuck in the throat, usually after eating fish. Ask about the ability to swallow solids, fluids and saliva; this is usually unaffected. *For oesophageal obstruction →* *below.*

Examination requires a good light and a cooperative patient. An instrument tray for ENT use should be available. Dentures are removed and examined for completeness. The mouth is inspected; the area around the fauces is a common site to find a fish bone. Foreign bodies often lodge in the piriform fossae and are usually radiolucent. A mucosal tear may produce identical symptoms to an impacted foreign body.

XR A lateral radiograph of the soft tissues of the neck will occasionally show a radio-opaque foreign body such as a chicken bone. Calcified laryngeal cartilages are a source of confusion.

Tx Any obvious foreign body should be removed; a topical anaesthetic spray may help. Patients with a foreign-body sensation in whom no cause is found should be discussed with an ENT surgeon; they can usually be reviewed in the next clinic. Difficulty swallowing suggests bolus obstruction of the oesophagus → *below.*

Oesophageal food bolus impaction

A patient may have sudden onset of dysphagia during a meal – often after an attempt to swallow a lump of meat. The blockage is usually reported to be in the 'upper chest'. In the most severe cases, the obstruction extends to fluids (including saliva) as well as to solids. In such cases, a drink of water causes regurgitation within a few seconds. Patients with disorders of oesophageal motility are particularly prone to this problem. Dental plates and other devices that reduce palatal sensation also predispose to it. The problem may be recurrent.

XR An oblique radiograph of the chest is the best projection for the detection of radio-opaque material in the oesophagus. Neck films may show an oesophageal fluid level. Surgical emphysema may also be seen.

Tx Some cases resolve spontaneously. Effervescent agents (e.g. fizzy drinks or a mixture of citric acid and sodium bicarbonate) are often advocated but there is little hard evidence for their efficacy. IV metoclopramide 10 mg or IV hyoscine butylbromide 20 mg is also sometimes recommended. Most patients should be referred for surgical assessment and oesophagoscopy in theatre. Oesophageal tears may produce mediastinitis, which is often fatal.

Swallowed foreign bodies

This is generally a problem of children and some patients with psychiatric conditions. Rounded objects such as coins are the most frequently swallowed. There may be initial coughing but thereafter the patient is usually symptomless. An oesophageal foreign body sometimes – but not always – causes dysphagia and retrosternal discomfort. Examination should include the fauces, upper airways and lung fields.

The narrowest sites for obstruction are at the cricopharyngeal sphincter, the upper third of the oesophagus at the level of the aortic arch and the cardia. Objects that pass into the stomach will usually traverse the entire gastrointestinal tract within 2–6 days, but may not uncommonly take 2–4 weeks. The two exceptions are:

1 Irregularly shaped articles such as open safety pins, which may impact, especially on the pylorus

2 Very long, straight objects, which may not be able to negotiate the duodenal loop.

> Most foreign bodies that cause a problem are lodged in, or have damaged, the oesophagus.

XR In the case of radio-opaque objects (the majority), radiographs should be obtained of the chest, abdomen and neck (in that order) until the foreign body is located. For a small child this takes only one film. In an anteroposterior view of the neck, a coin in the larynx appears side on as a bar, whereas a coin in the oesophagus appears as a round disc.

> Thin aluminium objects (e.g. can ring-pulls) and some dental prostheses are not radio-opaque.

Tx
Airway → p. 219.

Pharynx or oesophagus: refer to an ENT surgeon immediately for removal at oesophagoscopy.
Stomach or bowel: usually pass uneventfully, although this may take several weeks. If in a child, parents should bring the child back if abdominal symptoms develop.
Sharp objects: require observation and either removal or tracking with frequent radiographs.
Glass: sometimes swallowed by patients with psychiatric problems or personality disorders. Glass may be seen on a radiograph; it is usually harmless.

Ingestion of 'button' batteries

Small 'button cell' batteries are sometimes swallowed by children. They may stick and damage the bowel electrically or disintegrate and release toxic contents.

> One in 20 children who have ingested button batteries will have swallowed more than one cell.

There are four main types of button cell:

1 Mercury (1.5V)
2 Silver (1.5V, usually non-toxic)

3 Alkaline manganese (1.5V)
4 Lithium (3V, but more resistant to corrosion; not usually swallowed because it is used inside watches and replaced by a jeweller).

Used cells are less likely to leak or cause tissue injury than new ones. New mercury batteries are the most dangerous. When discharged, the mercuric oxide has been mainly converted to elemental mercury, which is not absorbed. Late signs of ingestion include:

• fever
• abdominal pain
• vomiting
• blood in the stools.

XR Obtain radiographs of the chest, neck and abdomen until the exact position of the battery is established. Children with button cells in the stomach need daily abdominal films to show transit and to detect disintegration. Batteries in the bowel should be tracked every 3 or 4 days.

Tx
Foreign bodies in the airway → pp. 1, 201.

> Chemical burns in the mouth suggest that the battery was leaking before ingestion.

• Identify the type of battery involved from the packaging or a matching or similar battery and determine whether it is new or old. Not all button cells are marked with numbers.
• Get more information about the battery contents from:
– a poisons information service by phone or via the internet
– the national battery ingestion guidelines, which are produced by the British Battery Manufacturers' Association and distributed to all EDs in the UK.
• Oral antacids or milk may help to reduce battery corrosion. Emesis is contraindicated.
• Button batteries in the stomach usually pass from the bowel without problems but all children who have swallowed button cells should be followed up after 24 h with a repeat radiograph.

Button batteries that are localised above the stomach or are not passing through the gut satisfactorily or are leaking may require removal. *Indications for referral for the removal of button cells → Box 22.5.* Endoscopic or magnetic removal is often possible.

Box 22.5 Indications for referral for removal of button cells

- Any button cell in the airway
- Any button cell in the oesophagus
- Any button cell remaining in the stomach for more than 48h, especially new, undischarged ones
- Any button cell static in the gut for a prolonged period, especially new, undischarged ones
- Any button cell where the ingestion is accompanied by signs of peritonitis
- Mercury cell in the stomach for more than 24h
- Mercury cell that appears (on radiograph) to be disintegrating in the stomach (it is advisable to measure mercury concentrations in the blood and urine when leakage is thought to have occurred)

All children who have swallowed button-cell batteries must be admitted or followed up in clinic.

Sore throat

Pharyngitis, laryngitis and tonsillitis are common and usually result from a viral infection. Some patients will have a bacterial infection but clinical differentiation is almost impossible.

Tx Symptomatic relief with paracetamol is usually sufficient. Pragmatic treatment is to give antibiotics to patients who are systemically unwell or have severe local symptoms and signs. Phenoxymethylpenicillin, an oral cephalosporin or clarithromycin is appropriate.

Amoxicillin or ampicillin may cause a florid rash in patients with glandular fever.

Infectious mononucleosis, cytomegalovirus infection and toxoplasmosis may cause a prolonged sore throat with systemic symptoms.

Diphtheria

Diphtheria is still a major cause of death in the world; it has re-emerged in eastern Europe because of falling levels of immunisation.

Diphtheria is caused by infection with the bacterium *Corynebacterium diphtheriae*, which is droplet spread with an incubation period of 1–5 days. Following the introduction of immunisation against diphtheria on a national scale in the UK in 1940, there was a dramatic fall in the number of notified cases of the disease. From 1986 to 2002, 103 cases of diphtheria were identified and 2 deaths were reported. The first symptom of diphtheria is usually a mild pharyngitis causing pain with swallowing. The following are other typical features:

- Low-grade fever (<38.5°C)
- Headache, nausea and vomiting
- Inflammation of the larynx and nasal passages
- Pharyngeal exudate forming a thick greyish 'pseudomembrane'
- Swollen lymph nodes ('bull-neck' appearance)
- Pallor and tachycardia.

Complications include:

- respiratory obstruction
- pneumonia
- otitis media and sinusitis
- myocarditis, peripheral neuritis and nephritis
- shock and organ failure.

Tx Patients with suspected diphtheria should be admitted and discussed with a specialist in infectious diseases. Impending respiratory obstruction may require intubation or even tracheostomy. Diphtheria is treated with benzylpenicillin and sometimes with a specific antitoxin. It is a notifiable disease →p. 388.

Epiglottitis

This condition appears to be on the increase in adults. *Haemophilus influenzae* B, β-haemolytic streptococci or even staphylococci may be responsible. It should be suspected when the degree of hoarseness and dysphagia appears to be disproportionate to the other signs.

Tx This is the same as in children → p. 335:

- Reassure the patient and work calmly. Do not examine the throat.

- Summon skilled anaesthetic and ENT help immediately.
- Position the patient for maximum comfort.
- Administer high-concentration oxygen by mask.
- Consider using nebulised adrenaline (5 mg) by mask until help arrives.

IV cefotaxime or chloramphenicol is used to treat *Haemophilus influenzae* epiglottitis.

Stridor in children → p. 335.

Retropharyngeal abscess

This condition usually occurs in infants and young children, typically aged between 2 and 6 years. Infection of the upper respiratory tract leads to a pyogenic adenitis of the retropharyngeal lymph nodes. The resulting abscess is limited to one side of the midline by a median raphe → *Figure 22.5*. The child is obviously unwell and has:

- a high pyrexia
- a sore throat with dysphagia or odynophagia (including for saliva)
- hoarseness, noisy breathing or stridor (but not always!)
- restricted neck movements (the head may be held flexed to one side)
- cervical lymphadenopathy (a smooth unilateral swelling of the posterior pharyngeal wall may sometimes be seen).

XR A lateral soft-tissue view of the neck may show marked soft-tissue expansion in the retropharyngeal space which, in severe cases, can push the trachea forwards. (The pre-vertebral soft tissue, anterior to C1–4, should normally be no wider than a third of the adjacent vertebral bodies.) A CT scan may be performed to provide more information about the swelling.

Tx ENT referral is required for IV antibiotics and, possibly, surgical drainage. Sepsis (including mediastinitis) may occur. Airway compromise is rare.

Dentoalveolar abscess

A dentoalveolar abscess is an acute lesion characterised by localisation of pus in the structures that surround the teeth. Odontogenic infections are polymicrobial, with an average of five different causative bacteria. In most cases, residential bacteria cause infection when the host's defences are breached. The dominant isolates are strictly anaerobic Gram-negative bacilli and Gram-positive cocci, in addition to facultative and microaerophilic streptococci. They include genera such as *Bacteroides*, *Fusobacterium*, *Peptococcus* and *Peptostreptococcus*, and also *Streptococcus viridans*. Anaerobic bacteria outnumber aerobes by a factor of two or more and the strictly anaerobic Gram-negative rods are more pathogenic than the Gram-positive cocci. Three types of infection are seen:

1 A periodontal abscess involves the supporting structures of the teeth (the periodontal ligaments and the alveolar bone). It is the most common dental abscess in adults but may occur in children with impaction of a foreign body in the gingiva.
2 A periapical abscess originates in the dental pulp and is usually secondary to dental caries. It is the most common dental abscess in children. Dental caries erodes the protective layers of the tooth (enamel and dentine) and allows bacteria to invade the pulp, producing a pulpitis. This can progress to necrosis, with bacterial invasion of the alveolar bone, causing an abscess. Dental abscess is rare in infants because abscesses do not form until teeth erupt.
3 Pericoronitis is infection of the gum that overlies a partially erupted third molar (a 'wisdom tooth').

The tooth that is most frequently involved is the lower third molar, followed by other lower posterior teeth. Upper posterior teeth are involved much less frequently and anterior teeth are only rarely involved. There is localised pain, tenderness and swelling, extending towards the buccal side of the gum and into the gingival–buccal reflection. Severe facial swelling, pyrexia, trismus and dysphagia may also occur.

XR Panoramic radiography (an orthopantomogram) is the most useful investigation in emergency

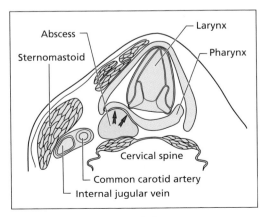

Figure 22.5 Retropharyngeal abscess.

situations because it provides the most information about all the teeth and their supporting structures.

Tx Most patients should be treated with analgesia, antibiotics and referral to a dentist or maxillofacial surgeon. Clarithromycin or co-amoxiclav is probably the best first-line antibiotic; metronidazole, phenoxymethylpenicillin or clindamycin is an alternative.

Other swellings in the mouth

Swollen salivary glands

Salivary glands may swell because of obstruction, tumour or infection. Obstruction by a stone may cause increased symptoms when the production of saliva is increased (i.e. eating). Mumps must be remembered as a common parotid infection → *p. 425*. Bacterial parotitis may occur in debilitated patients.

Quinsy

Peritonsillar abscess presents as a large, unilateral swelling in an unwell patient with a history of tonsillitis. The oedematous uvula is displaced to the opposite side. Dysphagia, halitosis and trismus are inevitable. The throat pain is often accompanied by earache and the cervical nodes are enlarged and tender. Sometimes the head is flexed to one side.

Intraoral soft-tissue infections

Cellulitis of the floor of the mouth may cause dangerous swelling (Ludwig's angina). It is most common in young children. There may be associated dental sepsis. Vincent's angina may affect the pharyngeal and tonsillar area.

Diphtheria → p. 422.

Tx Acute intraoral swellings with pain or pyrexia are indications for immediate referral to the appropriate specialist. Surgical drainage may be required in addition to IV antibiotics. Conditions compromising the airway should be treated in exactly the same way as epiglottitis → *p. 422*.

Other throat and neck symptoms

Several conditions can be associated with unusual symptoms in the throat. In particular:
Dystonia: bizarre intermittent problems with speech and swallowing may be the only signs of an acute dystonic reaction → *p. 300*.
Tetanus: tetanus ('lock-jaw') may start with jaw stiffness and trismus → *p. 233*.

Pneumomediastinum: the most common symptoms caused by air in the mediastinum are neck pain and dysphagia → *p. 194*.

Bleeding after tonsillectomy

Patients (usually children) may be brought to an ED with post-tonsillectomy bleeding. This may occur a few hours after the procedure or, if secondary to infection, after a few days. Bleeding may occasionally be severe enough to threaten the airway. The patient should be placed in the recovery position (unless unhappy with this posture in which case a position of least resistance should be sort) and oxygen administered. Gentle suctioning may help to clear the airway. FBC and blood grouping should be requested and IV access obtained. Immediate ENT referral is appropriate; an anaesthetic opinion may also be required.

Acquired haemophilia and anticoagulation problems → pp. 257, 259.

Bleeding after dental extraction

Bleeding is usually from a tooth socket; it must be localised with the aid of a good light and suction. The patient should be:

- sat upright
- reassured
- asked to bite on a gauze pad for 5 min.

If this does not stop the bleeding, an adrenaline pack or a piece of gel foam may be tried. Rarely, the socket may require oversewing. Post-extraction bleeding is more likely to occur in the presence of infection and will itself increase the risk of infection. Antibiotics should be prescribed. Contributory factors such as haemophilia and anticoagulant therapy must be considered → *p. 259*.

> The Dentists Act 1984 used to allow registered medical practitioners to practise dentistry but the Dentists Act (Amendment) Order 2005 restricted dental practice to registered dental professionals only. However, doctors still have an ethical and contractual obligation to offer appropriate treatment (e.g. antibiotics, analgesia and arrest of haemorrhage) in a dental emergency.

Toothache

This condition is usually seen in an ED 'out of hours'. The patient is distressed and in pain. The teeth may be generally carous and in need of dental care or show little sign of any problem. The cause of the pain is usually local inflammation – pulpitis or pericoronitis – and gentle tapping of the tooth or gum may exacerbate the pain. Sometimes, a periapical or periodontal abscess may be forming.

Tx Considerable relief may follow the injection of an NSAID (e.g. IM diclofenac 75 mg). Antibiotics (amoxicillin, clarithromycin or metronidazole) and strong analgesia should also be supplied. The patient must see his or her own dentist as soon as possible.

Dental injuries → p. 70.
Dentoalveolar abscess → p. 423.
Numbering system used to describe teeth → p. 70
(Box 5.2).

THE FACE

Facial pain

Sinusitis

This can occur in any of the four groups of sinuses. There may be facial pain and tenderness in the affected area together with headache and pyrexia. The pain may be periodic. Chemosis, proptosis and other eye signs may be seen. The urgency of referral should depend on the signs. First-line antibiotics for sinusitis are amoxicillin, clarithromycin and doxycycline.

Shingles

Herpes zoster infection may cause acute facial pain. Oral aciclovir therapy is effective in limiting prolonged symptoms but is expensive. Shingles of the ophthalmic division of the trigeminal nerve (Va) may damage the cornea and thus requires ophthalmic advice. The usual treatment is with topical aciclovir.

Trigeminal autonomic cephalgias

This is a comparatively rare group of conditions that are characterised by severe unilateral pain in a trigeminal distribution associated with ipsilateral cranial autonomic features → p. 227.

Facial palsy

Bell's palsy is an idiopathic condition causing a unilateral lower motor neuron paralysis of the face. It is associated with discomfort in the vicinity of the

mastoid and develops over 48 h. It must be differentiated from a stroke affecting the face. The classic sign used for this purpose is the failure to wrinkle the forehead on the affected side in Bell's palsy. In an upper motor neuron condition this movement is likely to be unaffected because the upper part of the face has bilateral cortical representation.

> Look in the ears of patients with facial palsy. A herpetic infection of the meatus and tympanic membrane may be identified (the Ramsay Hunt syndrome). Severe earache and malaise precedes the development of the palsy by 24–48 h. Vertigo, deafness, loss of taste and vesicles in the fauces may also occur.

Tx Bell's palsy resolves spontaneously over a few weeks in 90% of patients. To prevent residual problems in the remainder, early prophylactic treatment with steroids has been advocated. Although there is little evidence to support this therapy, many doctors prescribe a short course of high-dose oral prednisolone (40 mg for adults or 1 mg/kg for children daily for 5 days). Patients who have difficulty in closing one eye also need a supply of eye pads to protect the cornea at night.

Suspicion of cerebrovascular disease should prompt medical referral. Patients with facial palsy accompanied by a discharging ear, a cholesteatoma or vesicles should be referred to an ENT specialist.

Mumps

Infection with the mumps virus has a long incubation period (≥18–21 days) and seems to be on the increase. Mumps parotitis causes pyrexia, malaise and progressive tender facial swelling around the angle of the jaw. In 80% of cases, both parotid glands are affected. There may also be cervical adenitis, intraoral swelling of the orifice of the parotid ducts and occasionally presternal oedema. The illness usually resolves spontaneously within 7–10 days. Complications include meningoencephalitis, pancreatitis and inflammation of almost any other glandular tissue. Orchitis is seen in about a quarter of postpubertal males with mumps. It is usually unilateral and may lead to testicular atrophy.

Diphtheria → p. 422.
Facial swellings originating from the mouth → p. 423.

Index

Emergency Medicine Lecture Notes, Fourth Edition. Chris Moulton and David Yates.
© 2012 Blackwell Publishing Ltd. Published 2012 by Blackwell Publishing Ltd.